THE DENTAL ASSISTANT

SIXTH EDITION

PAULINE C. ANDERSON, C.D.A., M.A.
Professor Emerita, and formerly Chairperson
Department of Allied Health, Pasadena City College
Pasadena, California

Life Member, American Dental Assistants Association

MARTHA R. BURKARD, C.D.A., R.D.A., M.A.
Professor (Retired), Dental Assisting Program
Department of Allied Health, Pasadena City College
Pasadena, California

Life Member, American Dental Assistants Association

Cynthia Wittman, C.D.A., B.S., M.Ed.
Contributor (Chapters 28 and 29)
Forbes Road East Area Vocational-Technical School
Monroeville, Pennsylvania

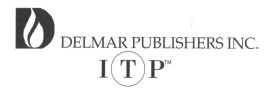
DELMAR PUBLISHERS INC.
I(T)P™

NOTICE TO THE READER

Delmar staff:
Publisher: David C. Gordon
Acquisitions Editor: Adrianne C. Williams
Project Editor: Melissa A. Conan
Production Coordinator: Barbara A. Bullock
Art and Design Coordinator: Timothy J. Conners
Editorial Assistant: Jill Rembetski

For information, address
Delmar Publishers Inc.
3 Columbia Circle, Box 15015
Albany, NY 12203-5015

COPYRIGHT ©1995 BY DELMAR PUBLISHERS INC.
The trademark ITP is used under license.

Certain portions of this work
© 1987, 1982, 1974, 1970, and 1965.

Printed in the United States of America
Published simultaneously in Canada
by Nelson Canada,
a division of the Thomson Corporation

1 2 3 4 5 6 7 8 9 10 XXX 01 00 99 98 97 96 95

Library of Congress Cataloging-in-Publication Data
Anderson, Pauline Carter.
    The dental assistant / Pauline C. Anderson, Martha R. Burkard. —
6th ed.
      p.   cm.
    Includes bibliographical references and index.
    ISBN 0-8273-5281-6
    1. Dental assistants. 2. Dentistry—Outlines, syllabi, etc.
  I. Burkard, Martha R. II. Title.
  RK60.5.A5   1995
  617.6—dc20   93-40765
                                                                       CIP

THE DENTAL ASSISTANT

Contents

SECTION 11   DENTAL SPECIALTIES

SECTION 12   DENTAL RADIOGRAPHY

Preface

In this sixth edition of THE DENTAL ASSISTANT, the philosophy and objectives of the material presented remain the same, while the format and content have been updated.

As with previous editions, our first priority is to present a combination text and workbook, while providing the student with sufficient knowledge and the skills needed to qualify as an entry-level dental assistant. Emphasis continues to be placed on the *what*, *why*, and *how* in the development of manipulative skills, based on the selection and application of theoretical knowledge.

Our second priority is to present the material in understandable terms as they apply to the practice of dentistry. The reader is introduced to terminology in sequence, as the subject matter is presented. The text material is kept within the knowledge required in a basic, yet scientific, approach to dentistry. The student is encouraged to use additional sources of information, and to seek continuing education in the quest for professional growth.

The facts, techniques, and methods, as they apply to clinical or laboratory procedures, are provided for the student. Review exercises and suggested activities are included. Since all education now stresses literacy for the entire populace, regardless of age or gender, review questions in this book continue to require a written response. The completed statements tend to reinforce learning, provide a basis for quick review, and eliminate the possibility of an incorrect answer as so often occurs with true-false and multiple-choice questions.

Several new chapters added to this edition include dental management, human cell structure and function, dental/medical emergencies, preventive dentistry, nutrition, infectious diseases in the dental environment, OSHA regulations, and an introduction to the dental specialties. Coverage of dental instruments has been updated and expanded with new illustrations, included is the chapter on surgical instruments.

The authors believe the text is one that can be effectively used for the dental assistant who is trained on-the-job, whether in a private dental office or clinic setting. For those dental assistants who wish to upgrade their skills and increase knowledge, the information is current.

The reader will observe that he/she and his/her have been used interchangeably in the text. No intention to favor gender, whether with reference to a patient or member of the dental health team, has been made.

Acknowledgments

Many people contributed their talents and gave invaluable assistance in preparing this text. They all took unexpected time and effort to ensure that each chapter fit the format, theme, and objectives of the book. It is our pleasure to express thanks and appreciation to:

Alice E. Pendleton, C.D.A., R.D.A., R.D.A.E.F., M.A., Linda C. Teilhet, C.D.A., R.D.A., R.D.A.E.F., and the students of the Registered Dental Assisting program, Pasadena City College, Pasadena, CA.

Joan E. Brandlin, B.A., R.D.H., and the students of the Registered Dental Hygiene Program, Pasadena City College, Pasadena, CA.

Christopher V. Chapman, Pasadena College of Design, for his artistic renderings in the book.

Oscar Chavez, official photographer and audio-visual technician, Pasadena City College, for his specialized advice and artistic contributions.

James Harrah, Professional Publishers, dental charts/forms.

Paul Thompson, Rinn Corporation, radiography illustrations/diagrams.

The staff at Delmar Publishers: Adrianne Williams, Melissa Conan, Barbara Bullock, and Timothy Conners.

Chapter 1: The Dental Auxiliaries

OBJECTIVES:

After studying this chapter, the student will be able to:
- Identify the members of the dental health team.
- Discuss the basic qualifications and requirements for all members of the dental health team.
- State the shared goal of the dental health team.
- State the responsibilities of the chairside assistant.
- State the responsibilities of the secretarial assistant/receptionist.
- Discuss the eligibility pathways for dental assistant certification.
- State the one common requirement for all the eligibility pathways and dental assistant certification.
- Discuss the requirements for the registration and licensure of the dental hygienist.
- Determine the educational requirements for the dental technician.
- Define the concept of ethics
- Discuss the role of the State Dental Practice Act and its relationship to the Board of Dental Examiners.

INTRODUCTION

Given the ever-increasing demand for dental care, the modern dental office is designed with a dental team approach for the delivery of dental care. Although this chapter covers in detail the dental auxiliaries, their requirements, and functions, it seems appropriate first to introduce the dental health team.

THE DENTAL HEALTH TEAM

Members of the Team

The dental team is composed of dentist(s), dental assistant(s), dental hygienist(s), and dental technician(s). Although the composition of the team may vary from office to office, it is the dentist who always supervises the delivery of services to the patient.

Basic Qualifications and Requirements

The first requirement for any member of a dental health team is that person's good physical and mental health. A dental practice cannot afford to have an employee who is not physically well, has less-than-average ability to reason, or is unable to adjust to the dental environment. Failure to care for his or her own person cannot be tolerated.

Second, each team member must know, and practice, the rules of professional **ethics** and con-

1

duct. Each team member must exhibit social and professional self-assurance. Such proper behavior invites the confidence of the patient, and that confidence and trust must be treated with sincerity. A friendly approach is highly desirable and is shown by a smile and a pleasant, calm, and patient attitude. Friendliness, rather than familiarity, indicates to the dental patient that the team members are courteous representatives of dentistry. Courtesy is capable of attracting many persons to a dental practice. Patients tend to come back to a dental office for help, empathy (feelings, thoughts, and motives that can be understood by another), and assurance. In contrast, patients will not permit a disinterested or egotistical dental team. Patients need to know they have a team that is honest and interested in their welfare.

All members of the dental team have specific duties and responsibilities. As a team they are working together with the shared goal of providing the best possible dental care. The success of such a team depends on the attitudes and cooperation of all team members. The efficiency of the team depends on the ability of each member to contribute those particular talents and capabilities required in providing quality dentistry to patients.

THE DENTAL AUXILIARIES

The Dental Assistant

With the modernization of dental equipment and improved operating techniques, such as sit-down, four-handed dentistry, qualified assistants are required.

Whether the office is a private (solo) or group practice, more than one assistant is needed. The delegation of responsibilities can be divided into separate areas.

Chairside Assistant. An assistant who works directly with the dentist in the operatory (treat-ment room) is the chairside assistant. The chairside assistant is also responsible for infection control and sterilization, preparation of restorative materials, exposing, processing, and mounting dental radiographs, care and maintenance of dental equipment, and other delegated tasks permitted under the State Dental Practice Act of the state in which he or she practices, figure 1–1.

Secretarial Assistant/Receptionist. A secretarial assistant or receptionist handles all business procedures and is responsible for the smooth operation of the office. The duties include office management, answering the telephone, control of the appointment book (scheduling all appointments), financial arrangements for patient fees, banking, bookkeeping, office correspondence, and dental insurance billing, figure 1–2. Some offices may employ a third assistant. This person may have specific duties or assist wherever needed, at chairside or front office.

Certification

For those dental assistants who meet the eligibility and examination requirements, certification may be earned in one or more areas. In order to earn any of the available certifications, a

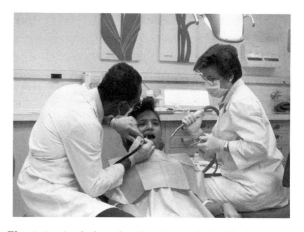

Fig. 1–1. Assisting the dentist at chairside (Courtesy Registered Dental Assisting Program, Pasadena City College, Pasadena, CA)

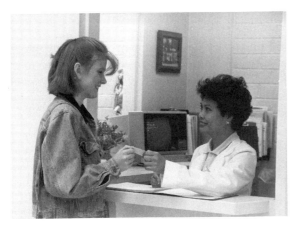

Fig. 1–2. The secretarial dental assistant handles dental office business procedures. (Courtesy Registered Dental Assisting Program, Pasadena City College, Pasadena, CA)

dental assistant must (1) meet one of the eligibility pathways for the certification being sought; and (2) pass the certification examination directly related to the area of certification. Documentation for each of the requirements in the eligibility pathway sought must be submitted to the Dental Assisting National Board.

The Certified Dental Assistant (CDA) credentials will include certification in chairside duties plus radiation health and safety. All pathways require verification of current cardiopulmonary resuscitation (CPR) certification from the American Heart Association or the American Red Cross.

Eligibility Pathways for Certification.

Certified Dental Assistant (CDA)

Pathway I:

Graduation from a dental assisting or dental hygiene program accredited by the ADA Commission on Dental Accreditation

Current CPR certification

Pathway II:

High school graduation or equivalent

Two years of full-time work experience (3,500 hours) as a dental assistant, along with recommendations from the dentist employer

Current CPR certification

Certified Oral and Maxillofacial Surgery Assisting (COMSA)

Pathway I:

High school graduation or equivalent

Successful completion of 500 hours of postsecondary education in oral and maxillofacial surgery assisting, plus six months of full-time work experience (875 hours) in an oral and maxillofacial surgery office, or the equivalent over the past three years

Current CPR certification

Pathway II:

High school graduation or equivalent

Work experience in an oral and maxillofacial surgery office, plus one of the credentials of CDA, LPN, RN, RDH, or RDA

Current CPR certification

Pathway III:

High school graduation or equivalent

Two years of full-time work experience (3,500 hours) in an oral and maxillofacial surgery office, or the equivalent

Current CPR certification

Certified Dental Practice Management Assisting (CDPMA)

Work experience in a dental office

Current CPR certification

Certified Orthodontic Assisting (COA)

Pathway I:

High School graduation or equivalent

Work experience in an orthodontic office, plus a CDA, RDH, or RDA credential

Current CPR certification

Pathway II:

High school graduation or equivalent

Two years of full-time work experience (3,500 hours) in an orthodontic office or the equivalent

Current CPR certification

Certification is in no sense a degree, nor does it hold any legal status. However, it does carry with it knowledge in the dental field and the ability to apply it.

Some states require the dental assistant to pass a written and/or clinical examination to become registered or licensed. Rather than requiring a second exam, some states will accept the Dental Assistant National Board (DANB) examination and grant registration to those assistants. Having met the requirements, the assistant is known as a registered dental assistant (RDA).

Many states require registration or licensure for all dental personnel who expose dental radiographs. Most registration or licensure requires periodic renewal.

Areas of Service

Dental assistants currently serve the profession in dental offices, in federal agencies, or in facilities of the armed services. The majority of assistants are employed by dentists in private (solo) practice. These offices are maintained by both general practitioners and specialists in the dental profession.

Other assistants are employed by the rapidly growing group-practice system. In the group-practice setting, several general practice dentists or specialists join and share one receptionist, one business office, and one dental laboratory. Federal agencies, including clinics and hospitals of the Veterans Administration and the U.S. Public Health Service, also employ dental assistants.

The Dental Hygienist

The dental auxiliary member employed specifically to perform oral hygiene care is the dental hygienist. The hygienist is trained to record health histories, scale and polish the teeth, apply fluoride treatments, and expose, process, and mount dental radiographs, figure 1–3. In addition, the hygienist provides health education to patients on plaque control, oral hygiene instruction, and diet and nutrition counseling, figure 1–4.

Another important responsibility of the hygienist is to maintain an active recall system. Such a system is used to inform patients, either by postcard or telephone, of their next **prophylaxis** (teeth cleaning) appointment. The recall system is most vital in that it affords the patient an opportunity to be involved in his or her own preventive dentistry program.

Although the dental hygienist is licensed and sees patients on an independent basis within the

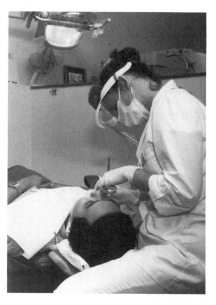

Fig. 1–3. The dental hygienist performs prophylaxis. (Courtesy Registered Dental Hygiene Program, Pasadena City College, Pasadena, CA)

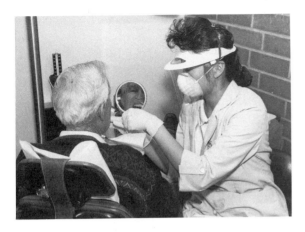

Fig. 1–4. The dental hygienist provides oral health instruction. (Courtesy Registered Dental Hygiene Program, Pasadena City College, Pasadena, CA)

dental office, clinic, or hospital, the responsibilities remain under the supervision of the dentist. Hygienists must comply with the regulations within the State Dental Practice Act. In certain states the hygienist is permitted to perform various other tasks and may assume some chairside duties when necessary.

Requirements for Sitting for the National Board in Dental Hygiene (NBDH) Written Examination

Graduation from a dental hygiene program accredited by the ADA Commission on Dental Accreditation

Current CPR certification

Successful completion of the state licensure examination in dental hygiene (a practical examination)

(*Note*: some states may have a written component to the licensure exam, i.e., exposing, processing, and mounting dental radiographs, and other clinical procedures.)

or completion of a state regional practical board examination (for participating states): applicant, for a fee, may be licensed in more than one state; applicant may complete a state regional board examination in more than one state.

Results of the examination will be sent to member state boards in which the person holds state licensure.

A hygienist uses the title of registered dental hygienist (RDH) and is licensed and governed by the State Dental Practice Act of the state in which he or she practices.

The Dental Laboratory Technician

Unlike other auxiliary members of the dental team (assistants and hygienists), dental technicians do not perform work directly on the patient, but in a laboratory.

A dental technician is trained to perform the mechanical and technical tasks necessary to prepare dental restorations and appliances, such as fabrication of gold and porcelain restorations, partials, or full dentures. However, the dental technician is under the guidance and supervision of the dentist and must have a written prescription from the dentist to complete the required laboratory procedures. Generally, the technician is not a member of the dentist's immediate staff but is either self-employed or works in a commercial laboratory, figure 1–5.

Dental laboratory technicians may complete programs approved by the ADA Commission on Dental Accreditation. Programs approved by the ADA last two years and are usually conducted in a two- or four-year college or post-high school institution. Upon successful completion of an ADA-approved program, the technician receives the Certified Dental Technician (CDT) certificate.

Dental technicians may also receive their training through apprenticeship (by agreement, the learner agrees to work for a specific amount of time for instruction in the area of concern). Apprenticeship is offered by commercial dental laboratories, leading to employment.

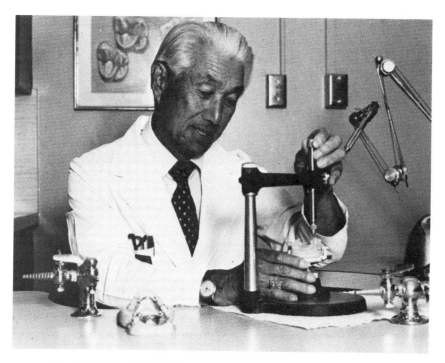

Fig. 1–5. A dental technician surveys a case for a partial appliance.

ETHICS

Ethics may be defined as that part of philosophy (love of learning) that deals with moral conduct (knowing right from wrong), judgment (the mental capacity to make reasonable decisions), and being able to apply these capacities. As a result, one is able to feel a sense of duty (moral obligation).

A *code of ethics* is the standard of moral principles and practices that a profession closely follows. Although they are voluntary controls, rather than laws, they serve as a method of self-policing within a profession.

Principles of Ethics

Highlights of the Principles of Ethics, Adopted in 1980 by the American Dental Assistants Association (ADAA):

Each individual involved in the practice of dentistry assumes the obligation of maintaining and enriching the profession. Each individual may choose to meet his or her obligations according to the dictate of personal conscience, based on the needs of the human beings the profession is committed to serve. (The spirit of the Golden Rule is the basic guiding principle of this concept.)

Each individual must strive at all times to maintain confidentiality and to exhibit respect for the dentist and coworkers. Each individual shall refrain from performing any professional service that is prohibited by state law and has the obligation to prove competence before providing services to any patient. Each individual shall constantly strive to upgrade and expand technical skills for the benefit of dentistry and the consumer public.

Each individual should seek to sustain and improve her or his local, state, and national professional organizations by active participation and personal commitment.

THE STATE DENTAL PRACTICE ACT

The State Dental Practice Act contains the legal restrictions and controls on the dentist, the dental auxiliaries, and the practice of dentistry. It is specific regarding the requirements for, and restrictions placed on, the practice of dentistry within that particular state.

The State Board of Dental Examiners, created by the act and designated as an administrative board, usually interprets and provides a definite procedure to ensure that regulations are fulfilled.

THE STATE BOARD OF DENTAL EXAMINERS

The **State Board of Dental Examiners** is the body responsible for the administration of examinations for licensure, for enforcement of statutes (laws), rules, and regulations, and for the establishment of the standards for quality continuing education for license renewal.

The board adopts rules and regulations that define, interpret, and provide a plan that follows the intent of the dental practice act. The State Board of Dental Examiners supervises and regulates the practice of dentistry within the state.

REVIEW

1. List the members of the dental health team.

    a. _____

    b. _____

    c. _____

    d. _____

2. List at least three basic qualifications/requirements for all dental health team members.

    a. _____

    b. _____

    c. _____

3. The shared goal of the whole dental health team is to _____

_____.

4. The success of the dental team depends on the _____

_____.

5. The efficiency of the team depends on the ability of each member to _____

_____.

6. The chairside assistant is responsible for

a. _____

b. _____

c. _____

d. _____

7. The duties of the secretarial assistant/receptionist are

a. _____

b. _____

c. _____

d. _____

e. _____

f. _____

g. _____

8. Certification for dental assistants may be earned in one or more areas. What are they?

a. _____

b. _____

c. _____

d. _____

9. All eligibility pathways for dental assistant certification require_____

_____.

10. Educational requirements for the dental hygienist include _____

_____

_____

11. Hygienists must successfully complete the _____

_____before qualifying

for the written examination of the NBDH.

12. The dental technician may receive education by

a. _____

_____

or

b. _____

13. Ethics may be defined as _____

_____

_____.

14. A "code of ethics" is the standard of_____

    _____.

15. The basic guiding principle of the concept of ethics is_____

    _____.

16. The state dental practice act contains legal restrictions and controls on _____

    _____

    _____.

17. The state board of dental examiners is the body responsible for

    a. _____

    b. _____

    c. _____

18. The board of dental examiners supervises and regulates the _____

    _____.

Chapter 2: The Dental Office Routine

OBJECTIVES:

After studying this chapter, the student will be able to:
- Define *rapport*.
- Discuss the acceptable personal appearance of a well-groomed dental assistant.
- Describe the manner in which a visitor/colleague of the dentist should be received.
- Discuss the housekeeping procedures for maintaining an attractive dental office.
- Describe the daily function of handling the mail.
- Discuss the various indexing and filing procedures.
- Discuss the methods used for maintaining dental supplies.

INTRODUCTION

The first individual a prospective patient meets in the dental office may be the dental assistant. Many people base their first impression of the dental practice on the dental assistant's personal appearance. It is at this first meeting that the dental assistant has the opportunity to build patient confidence and a pleasing atmosphere. Both are necessary for proper patient and practice rapport. *Rapport* can be defined as having a relationship of mutual trust and confidence between persons.

PERSONAL APPEARANCE

A neat, well-groomed dental assistant is an asset to any dental practice. In many offices the assistant wears a uniform that must be kept immaculate. Dental uniforms vary from the traditional dress-type to pants and a top and may be in white or a color. The hair should be attractively styled and easy to control. Comfortable duty shoes of standard design must be kept clean and polished. Nails must be clean, short, and with smooth cuticles. Nail polish is discouraged; colored nails have proven offensive and nonprofessional in the eyes of patients and doctors.

Using a chamois buffer to give a sheen to the nails is recommended. If the dental assistant is female and uses cosmetics, any makeup should be in good taste and not readily noticeable.

Good grooming and personal cleanliness are vital to the success of a dental assistant. Spending a few minutes each day will ensure that the dental assistant's appearance is orderly.

THE RECEPTION ROOM

When greeting a dental patient, a dental assistant should always check the appointment book to know the correct name of the patient. The patient should be greeted by name, promptly, upon arrival. The dental assistant should enter the reception room to greet each patient rather than just peeking around the door. A business-like dignified, courteous manner should be kept at all times.

Conversation in the reception room between patients and the dental assistant should be kept to a minimum. Personal comments are in order only when the patient and dental assistant are well acquainted. Lengthy conversations are time-consuming and do not contribute to the atmosphere of the office. The fears of apprehensive patients cannot be reduced by idle chatter.

11

An efficient assistant is considerate and concerned about the patient's welfare but does not talk too much. The assistant makes certain the patient is as comfortable as possible and offers special help when necessary. In dismissing the patient, the chairside assistant will accompany the patient to the secretarial assistant for any necessary appointments, then thank the patient for coming in. The assistant should also have a special good-bye for children, praise them for being good patients, and, if it is the dentist's routine, reward them with a small token.

Should an individual enter the reception room and introduce herself or himself as a doctor (colleague) or personal friend of the dentist, the assistant should offer a seat in the reception room. The dentist should be notified as soon as it is convenient to do so. Professional colleagues of the dentist who are not members of the office staff should not be allowed into the dental operatory unless the patient and dentist have given permission.

Reception Room Reading Material

A variety of magazines with different subject matter should be provided for patients in the reception room. It is suggested that several areas of interest be included in the magazine selection:

- sports
- homemaking
- business
- pictorials
- children's books
- children's coloring books (with colored pencils or crayons)

Reading material must be updated and kept orderly at all times. The dental assistant should sort the magazines and discard all except the last two editions of each periodical. Current issues, if damaged, should be repaired or discarded.

HOUSEKEEPING

The dental office should be completely and periodically cleaned. Woodwork, tables, and table lamps must be checked daily for finger marks and kept clean. Furniture should be free of dust and soil. When the reception room is carpeted, the carpeting should be inspected daily for tread marks left by foot traffic and soil. Routine vacuuming and spot cleaning should keep maintenance at a minimum.

Proper lighting and ventilation in the dental office, with a mid-morning and a mid-afternoon temperature check will ensure comfort for the patients and staff.

Secretarial Assistant's Desk

Because the secretarial dental assistant's desk is usually in view of the patients in the reception room, it is essential that the desk be kept free of clutter. Everything should have its place—and be kept in its place. Personal belongings must be kept out of sight. Papers, patient records, dental radiographs, and like items must not be allowed to pile up on the assistant's desk. Tiered desk trays will help greatly in keeping order, figure 2–1.

Doctor's Office and Treatment Rooms

Good housekeeping in the inner office provides the dental staff with the proper environment for conducting dental treatment. As each patient is dismissed, the assistant should quickly clean the room before the next patient is seated. Any evidence of the preceding patient must be removed.

ADMINISTRATIVE DUTIES

Handling Mail

An important function of the dental staff is the handling of mail. The mail includes display

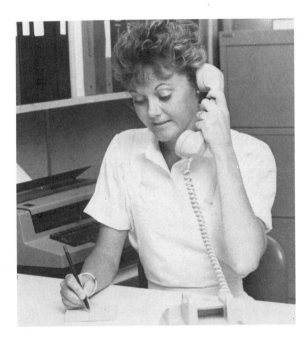

Fig. 2–1. The secretarial dental assistant controls the appointment book.

advertisements, personal letters, bills, checks, professional announcements, magazines, laboratory reports, samples from drug houses, and so forth. Most often, it is the dental assistant who opens this mail.

As a general rule, every doctor has a preference for the way the office mail is handled. For instance, the dentist may prefer to open certain mail and delegate the rest of the responsibility to the dental assistant. There are certain classes of mail separated according to their importance:

- telegrams
- special-delivery letters
- payment envelopes
- personal letters
- advertising material
- magazines and newspapers
- other routine mail

Once the routine has been established, the dental assistant can direct telegrams, special-

delivery letters, and personal mail to the doctor's office without opening them. Occasionally, there is some doubt in the assistant's mind regarding a particular piece of mail. A good rule to follow in such cases is this: if you are uncertain about opening a letter or parcel, *don't*. Discretion in handling the mail is very important, and it is essential that communications containing personal items for the doctor be routed unopened to the doctor's desk.

The dental assistant will then group the mail into the mentioned categories and handle as necessary. Magazines, for example, should be placed in the reception room in exchange for dated magazines. Payment envelopes from patients can be separated and recorded immediately in the day's receipts. Other items may need to be filed, shown to the doctor, or thrown away. The more accomplished the dental assistant becomes with this routine, the more time the dentist can devote to professional duties.

There are fewer problems involved in handling outgoing mail than there are with incoming mail. Letters, for example, that are sent from the doctor's office should *always* be checked for correct spelling and punctuation. Care must be taken that the correct letter goes into the right envelope. A copy of all outgoing correspondence is maintained and filed in the office. However, copies of letters should not be filed until the doctor has signed the original letter. Should a particular letter be one the doctor prefers not to sign (because of an inaccuracy), both letter and copy can be destroyed without having to remove the copy from the file.

When mailing letters, local mail should be separated from out-of-town and foreign mail that may require special postage. Such letters or parcels should be taken directly to the post office for mailing. Group the mail together, and schedule a time each day to send it on its way.

In the event that the doctor is not at the office and cannot be contacted when important mail arrives, the dental assistant should try to get in touch with the sender immediately, explain the reasons for the delay, and ask for the sender's cooperation. It is wise when forwarding mail to the doctor to inform the sender that the mail has been forwarded and that there will be some delay. In some cases, the doctor will respond directly to the sender. In other cases, the doctor will dictate a message to you for forwarding to the sender. Other mail not requiring special handling that arrives during the doctor's absence can be placed in a folder and held until the doctor returns.

Supplies

To keep the supply area well stocked, it is necessary to have a record, or inventory, of supplies on hand and supplies to be ordered. Accurate records, systematically kept, will enable the dentist and office staff to devote more time to patient care.

Recent surveys of various manufacturers of dental products indicate that the dental assistant is in charge of ordering and maintaining supplies.

Ordering Supplies. It is important to set up a method of inventory and to maintain a well-balanced stock. A spiral notebook may be used as an inventory logbook, with additional information retained on file cards.

The inventory log should include the following:

- date order is placed
- name of supplier
- reference or ID number for each order
- name and quantity of product
- projected cost of each item
- items on back order, and approximate shipping date
- name of the supply house and individual taking the order
- check-off column for items received

A complete inventory should be conducted on a monthly basis.

When ordering by mail or phone, the name, address, and telephone number of the doctor's office should be included with the ordering information. These orders should also be indicated in the log.

Keeping a separate index of file cards on which product name, price of item, supplier name, address, and telephone number are recorded provides easy reference when ordering.

A complete inventory once a month (in addition to the daily routine checking of supplies) before an order is placed is highly recommended.

Storing Supplies. After the supplies have been ordered and received, it is necessary to have a storage plan. A neat, well-arranged supply cupboard will aid in better and more efficient dental assisting. As a rule, supplies should be stored according to accessibility, temperature, light, and effects of moisture on each item. When an article is removed from its place, care should be taken that it is returned to the same place. Expiration dates of chemicals and other supplies that deteriorate during storage must be checked periodically and replaced as a routine part of ordering.

REVIEW

1. Define *rapport*. _____

   _____

2. What is considered an acceptable appearance for a dental assistant? _____

   _____

   _____

   _____

3. What procedures should be followed when greeting a patient in the reception room?

   a. _____

   b. _____

   c. _____

   _____

   d. _____

   _____

4. To ensure comfort for patients and office staff, what factor(s) are of greatest importance? _____

   _____

5. The test of a good file clerk is the ability to _____

   _____.

6. The person in charge of ordering and maintaining supplies is _____

   _____.

7. An inventory log for dental supplies should include

   a. _____

   b. _____

   c. _____

   d. _____

   e. _____

   f. _____

   g. _____

   h. _____

8. How often should a complete inventory of supplies be taken? _____

   _____

9. Supplies should be stored according to

   a. _____

   b. _____

   c. _____

   d. _____

10. An important daily function of the dental assistant is_____

    _____.

11. Certain classes of mail are separated according to their importance

    a. _____

    b. _____

  c. _____

  d. _____

  e. _____

  f. _____

  g. _____

12. Mail that should be directed to the doctor's office includes

  a. _____

  b. _____

  c. _____

After studying this chapter, the student will be able to:
- Define *communication*.
- Discuss human relationships as they apply to the practice of dentistry.
- Determine the skills necessary to establish a sound professional relationship.
- Discuss the need for dental patient questions.
- Determine the role of dental staff when verbally communicating with a patient.
- Discuss time management.
- Define the term *patient's advocate*.
- Determine the influence of office environment on the patient.
- Discuss the method used for emergency coverage of dental patients.
- Determine the meaning of *division of responsibilities* as it applies to dental patients.
- Define proper distance from patients.
- Discuss making appointments.
- Evaluate the need for keeping good dental records.
- Understand the necessity of sound financial management.
- Discuss how a dentist/patient relationship is terminated.

Dentistry is both a technical- and person-oriented profession. The success of a dental practice and the satisfaction enjoyed by the dentist, the staff, and the patients largely depend on how well needs and expectations can be shared and adjusted. Patients find dentistry more rewarding when they understand the importance of sound personal oral hygiene, and appreciate the value of the technical work performed. When the dental staff shares a common system of values and goals, only then can the needs of the patient be met. These goals are all more likely to be achieved when there is good communication.

COMMUNICATION

What is communication? *Communication* is an exchange of information, ideas, views, meanings, and understanding, be it *verbal* (spoken, written) or *nonverbal* (actions, attitudes, gestures).

Patients look for competence, commitment, and caring. Dental professionals must be able to communicate through words and actions that the dentist knows what he or she is doing, that the team is committed to the patient's health and care about him or her as a person, as well as about his or her overall health. Communicating these values to the patient will improve patient satisfaction.

Communication can also be seen as a way to involve others in the problems faced in the practice of dentistry. Good interpersonal (between people) communication skills are essential for getting better control of what goes on in the dental office. *Control* involves the capacity to predict and influence the present environment adequately enough to get one's work done. Control implies less hassle, fewer surprises, and a greater sense of accomplishment. Consequently, control benefits all concerned. The dental professional who is at ease, effective, and predictable, because he or she communicates well, helps the dentist, patients, and coworkers gain control.

HUMAN RELATIONSHIPS

Rather than stressing the technical aspects of dentistry when speaking with patients, the focus should be on human relationships. Dental health professionals can find great satisfaction in their work when they make a conscious and continuous effort to study human behavior—both their own and that of other people. _Behavior_ is the manner in which a person conducts him- or herself under specified circumstances.

With some patients, it will be easy to establish a pleasant relationship, one in which the patient believes that he or she is understood and that everyone in the dental office is concerned. This relationship is termed _rapport_.

Good rapport may be more difficult to establish with other patients. Perhaps, the patient's behavior arouses unfavorable feelings in the staff. Perhaps, the patient is not found to be "interesting" to staff. It is easy to project blame or label the patient "difficult."

The patient who has been labeled "difficult" is probably most in need of special attention from the dental team. The behavior that causes the patient to appear difficult may actually be signals that the patient's needs are not being met. On the other hand, the pleasant, agreeable patient may be covering up true feelings and may have just as much need for concern and understanding. In other words, providers of dental care will need to apply interpersonal skills to establish rapport with each patient as an individual. Some patients will present more of a challenge than others, but all need to be shown understanding and a sincere interest in making a positive contribution to their health care.

During the first visit, the patient and dentist establish a rapport that will assist them in their future professional relationship. As a result, all dental staff will want to make this initial visit as successful as possible. The following are suggested ways in which dentist and staff can let patients know that they will be taken care of, that their questions will be answered, and that their concerns will be addressed.

Listening Skills

Three things that dentists and staff can do to make patient relationships stronger are: (1) listen; (2) listen; and (3) listen. Listening takes work and it takes time. It may be that changes in the office scheduling procedures may need to be made to allow time for adequate listening.

Eye Contact. When listening, maintain good eye contact with the patient. Good eye contact is recognized by the public as representing honesty, cooperativeness, regard for others, and self-confidence. These are characteristics that the dentistry team wants to have associated with it. When dentist and staff have developed a comfortable and effective eye contact with the patient, the doctor/patient/staff relationship will increase in value.

Avoid Distractors. When patients are talking, make every effort to avoid shuffling papers, viewing radiographs, or doing anything that would indicate to patients that they do not have the full individual attention of the listener.

Sitting with the Patient. Another technique that helps the patient feel that he or she has been given ample time for discussion is the simple act of sitting down in the patient's presence. It is customary for this to occur during a prophylactic appointment with the hygienist, but less likely when the dentist enters the operatory to check the patient's chart and mouth after the prophylactic exam is completed.

Allowing the patient to sit upright and at a level where the dentist and patient have good eye contact will help the communication process. The patient who receives information of extreme importance regarding dental care, while staring at the acoustical tiles of the ceiling or the nose of the dentist, will not gain much from this kind of communication and may, in fact, resent such inconsiderate behavior.

Body Posture. Keeping a body posture that is open and relaxed is also important when listening to a patient. Slouched or closed posture habits, such as sitting or standing with only one side facing the patient rather than full-face, could suggest a disinterest in patient's problems and concerns.

Patient Questions

Dental professionals should avoid becoming defensive about questions asked by the patient. Questions are opportunities for better patient satisfaction and should be encouraged. Often, the patient is looking for a way to better understand, to remove doubt, or for various reasons to feel comfortable with treatment recommendations. Patient questions are often opportunities for the dental personnel to help rid the patient of perceived notions about dental care.

Patients who leave the dental office with unanswered questions may not be happy with the recommendations, which can lead to discontent with completed treatment. How can the patient be encouraged to ask questions? Simply ask for them.

Careful listening to patient questions and concerns can often help the dentist and staff recognize a problem or realize that the patient is unhappy at a very early stage of treatment. Before the patient leaves the office, every effort should be made to determine any questions the patient might have and to mutually agree on the appropriate solutions.

SPEAKING SKILLS

Language and Terminology

Adjusting language and terminology to the level that the patient understands will assist both the dentist and the staff in communicating with the patient. While some patients understand technical terminology, others will need "lay terms" for complete comprehension. Patients should be asked if they are following the explanation being offered. Answering questions or clearing up information will help patients recognize that they have a part to play in their health care. Patients need to understand their role in the treatment process.

Staff Communication

The dentist will set the tone for the communication style of the office and direct the interaction with the patients. However, all dental personnel are responsible for good communications with the patients. Staff should check on the patient on a regular basis to make certain the patient is not left alone for long periods of time. They can also help to reassure the patient even when the doctor is present. Often, the patient is more willing to seek support from a staff member rather than from the dentist. Thus, the staff member becomes the *patient's advocate*, one who will speak in the patient's behalf.

TIME MANAGEMENT

Time management is another technique for making the patient feel comfortable. Patients should not have to wait for lengthy periods of time in the reception room nor be kept waiting in a treatment or consultation room or at the front desk to make future appointments or pay their accounts.

When an emergency alters an orderly schedule, demonstrate concern for the scheduled patient by letting her or him know immediately by offering the opportunity to reschedule. Tardiness reflects an uncaring attitude, and such timely explanations will go far in soothing ruffled feelings.

NONVERBAL COMMUNICATION

Office Design and Decorative Style

The office environment will often influence how the patient feels about the treatment offered by a particular dental practice. Is the office kept clean? Has it been decorated in a manner that is suitable to the clientele? Are the furnishings updated or decades old?

Since patients do not have the technical expertise to judge the clinical competence of the dentist, they will use other unspoken clues to assess his or her abilities. If the dental office has the appearance of being a bit untidy or dirty, patients may suspect that sterilization techniques are not thorough.

Matching the office decor to patients' taste will assist in reducing the pressure or strain felt by many patients. The mere fact that they have a dental appointment produces stress-related disturbances. If the office is decorated like one in Beverly Hills, when the practice is predominantly suburban and where patients come directly to the office from varied types of employment, these patients may feel uncomfortable in such surroundings. On the other hand, if the furnishings are not up to the acceptable standards of modern dentistry, the patients might think the dental practice is not keeping up with current trends and techniques in dentistry.

Personal Hygiene

All dental personnel must have a commitment to personal hygiene. Patients will be offended by poor hygiene habits of health care providers. If they think that the dental professional does not take health care recommendations seriously, they may not accept any treatment recommendations. Consider the example of working with the patient on improving daily oral health care, while the dentist or staff member explaining these procedures has bad breath!

The message is clear: many factors contribute to the way patients think about the dental office, the dentist personally, and the staff. These thoughts affect the patients' attitude about treatment success, coupled with how comfortable the patient feels within the environment.

Written Communications

Written communication to the patient will emphasize the dentist's concern for the patient's health. Follow-up letters after a treatment consultation summarizing the discussion and agreements made during the appointment, serve to assure the patient that his or her needs are being met. The secretarial dental assistant will play an important role in all correspondence to the patient.

Phone Communications

A phone call at the end of the day to check on patients after a long or difficult procedure or treatment will communicate the concern about total patient care, not just a mouth or some teeth.

Emergency Coverage

In the event the doctor is unavailable to the patient (such as during vacation or illness), arrangements should be made by the office for another dentist to see emergency patients. When patients realize their dentist is arranging for their health care in his or her absence, they will feel reassured.

PATIENT EDUCATION

The patient must understand the division of responsibilities of care. The dentist's responsibility is to make a diagnosis, establish an acceptable treatment plan, and provide adequate dental care. The patient's responsibilities include making and keeping timely appointments, caring for his or her oral health before, during, and after care, and for the financial obligations associated with the treatment. Patients should also know that they must promptly report to the dentist any problems they might experience.

INTERPERSONAL DISTANCE

There are distances that are appropriate for certain relations between people and for certain activities. Any departure from these socially expected distances may cause tension and contribute to misunderstanding, table 3–1.

Intimate Distance

A distance of 0 to 18 inches is usually reserved for close friends and family members. The individuals are well known to each other and express warmth and concern; they share private feelings and secrets.

Much of dentistry is performed within this intimate distance. Since no personal or emotional intimacy is intended, it is important that dentists, hygienists, and assistants be always

TABLE 3–1
INTERPERSONAL DISTANCE

Type	Distance	Relationship
Intimate	1 to 18 inches	Close friends, family
Personal	18 inches to 4 feet	Friends, equals
Social	4 to 12 feet	Acquaintances
Public	12 feet or more	Strangers

conscious of their professional conduct. The dental team can calm the patient's fears by responding with the blend of confidence, caring, and warmth that is expected of all professionals.

Personal Distance

A distance of 18 inches to 4 feet is the range at which dental professionals often talk to patients, usually pushing the stool back from the dental chair to present diagnostic findings or give instructions.

Every individual carries a personal space, usually 2 to 4 feet. Because dental personnel must constantly break into that space to perform dental treatment, they should be careful to observe the professional precautions of courtesy and formality when doing so.

Personal distance is suitable when greeting patients, scheduling appointments, or collecting fees. More than likely, there will be office furnishings between the assistant and the patient.

When the dentist presents a treatment plan, make every effort to have it presented in a consultation room. The room should have comfortable chairs, positioned facing each other, and be barrier-free (no desk or table) between doctor and patient. Keep a distance of 3 to 4 feet between the two.

When scheduling a consultation, keep a comfortable distance of 3 to 4 feet between the two people, as well. Regardless of the place for the consultation, distractions such as phone calls or staff interruptions should never interfere with the meeting. The patient must understand that the dentist will provide undivided attention during the discussion. The dentist must establish and maintain direct communication with the patient.

Personality and mood can alter the requirements for personal space. Stress and anxiety increase the required distance as an interpersonal buffer. Some individuals will not tolerate closeness or being touched when they are angry, frightened, or tired. Professionals who are sensitive to the needs of patients and coworkers who are under pressure can effectively improve their communication by adding 1 or 2 feet of distance.

Social Distance

Most patients would prefer 4 to 7 feet between them and the dentist when speaking. This is the distance the dentist would normally stand from the receptionist or other office staff when they are discussing the day's activities. Social distance is used less frequently in performing dental treatment. The dental assistant may come within the intimate distance to place a radiographic film into the patient's mouth but will then leave the room or stand behind a lead barrier when exposing the film.

Public Distance

Distances over 12 feet express formality and influence. Public distance is used when speaking to a group or to strangers. Public distance is not usually applied in the practice of dentistry.

TOUCHING

Touching is an important part of dental care. Positioning the patient's head, assisting the patient in and out of the chair, and unexpected contact at the front desk are examples.

Professional Touching

The contact with patients and coworkers that cannot be avoided during dental care is called *professional touching*. Retracting cheeks, positioning radiographic film, and registering bites are all professional touching. The contact pattern never changes and is predictable. The dental professional devotes full attention to the task, often explains the procedure, and avoids eye contact with the patient.

Social Touching

Social touching, as with the handshake, shows trust and mutual respect. This type of touching occurs when giving advice or information. In a dental office it happens when greeting patients and when advising patients on home care or postoperative instruction. The backs of hands and arms, shoulders, top of the head, and the back are places where social touching is most likely to occur and least likely to be misunderstood.

Emotional Touching

On occasion, patients or coworkers are so choked with emotion that normal communication is impossible. Such display of emotion may be triggered by grief, a feeling of hopelessness and defeat, or frustration. Emotional touching is used by some professionals to signal that social rules may be momentarily suspended. Emotional touching includes hugging, holding another person's hand in yours, or grasping the arm of another. This touching carries with it an obligation for intimate listening, offering support, and a willingness to accept without criticism any emotional message.

MAKING APPOINTMENTS

Service to dental patients is at its best when there is complete mutual understanding and cooperation. When a series of treatments is provided to the patient, the secretarial dental assistant can expect complete cooperation in making and keeping appointments. Generally, there is a customary sequence of procedures that is followed in making appointments for new patients, recall patients, emergency cases, and special cases. To keep a dental practice running smoothly, appointments and the handling of the appointment book are usually assigned to the secretarial dental assistant. If appointments are made systematically and efficiently, there will be more productive time available. The dentist will be able to handle emergencies, which results in more new patients. There will also be sufficient time allowed for each operation. A more evenly spaced day for both the dentist and the chairside dental assistant is the outcome.

When scheduling an initial appointment for the new patient, allow for a complete dental and medical history to be obtained. Adequate time should be allotted so that the dentist can make a thorough examination of the patient's mouth and teeth. Diagnostic radiographs and study models are usually reviewed on a subsequent appointment. It is preferable to allow an additional fifteen minutes to fill out the patient history card, which includes health information. The dental assistant should also determine who referred the patient to the office and the reason for the appointment.

The dental hygienist may first see the patient for **prophylaxis** and radiographs. Many offices will routinely take impressions for study models prior to a second diagnostic appointment. Findings from radiographs, diagnostic models, and clinical findings obtained during the first appointment are studied and diagnosed prior to the second appointment. The conditions present and the recommended proper treatment are discussed with the patient at the time of the diagnostic appointment. If more than one method of treatment warrants consideration, the alternatives are thoroughly discussed, and the patient is informed of what can be expected from each type of service. The exact fee for the services is discussed at that time. When the method of treatment has been decided, additional time is then set aside for the most efficient and the earliest possible completion of the case. In addition, a definite arrangement for the payment of fees is made by the patient. The secretarial dental assistant is usually given the responsibility for this agreement.

Emergency appointments are frequently made by patients who are suffering from some dental discomfort or pain. It is the duty of the dental assistant to determine the extent of the dental problem and to do the utmost to arrange for an appointment. If certain hours of each day are allotted for emergency appointments, the emergency patient should be scheduled at that time. It is recommended that one-half hour of each day be scheduled for such emergencies. In nonindustrial areas, 11:30–12:00 A.M. or 1:00–1:30 P.M. may be set aside. If the day is fully appointed, the patient should be so advised. The patient should also be told that there is a scheduled emergency time when the doctor will be available. As with all cases, the assistant should never indicate to the patient that the office staff and the dentist are in a hurry because of a full schedule.

Generally, it is a good idea to notify all patients twenty-four hours in advance of an appointment. However, if a patient has a tendency to break appointments, the following suggestions may help in keeping such broken appointments to a minimum: (1) *always* notify the unreliable patient twenty-four hours in advance of each appointment; (2) impress such a patient with the fact that a broken appointment results in considerable inconvenience to the dental routine; (3) remind the patient that the doctor works on a schedule; (4) if the doctor has such a policy, inform the patient that there will be a charge for broken appointments; and (5) if the patient habitually breaks appointments, suggest that no more appointments be made until the patient feels that the appointments can be kept.

Should a patient cancel an appointment, the dental assistant should remain courteous. The patient should be thanked for calling, and another appointment should be scheduled. In the event the patient does not wish to make another appointment at the time of cancellation, the dental assistant should ask if it is all right to call the patient in a week or two to reschedule the appointment. If the patient desires this service, the dental assistant should note this and be certain to call the patient at that time to reschedule the appointment.

KEEPING PATIENT RECORDS

It is essential to keep accurate patient records. Several items are necessary to have these records complete.

1. Correct name, address, home telephone number
2. Place of employment and telephone number
3. Dental insurance carrier (if applicable)
4. Birthdate (month, day, and year)
5. Dental and health histories
6. Mold and shade of teeth used in denture and bridgework; shade of synthetics and plastics

Such records should be posted on the patient's record and kept up-to-date.

Current trends in record keeping involve use of the computer, thus enabling rapid retrieval of patient records, figure 3–1.

Indexing and Filing

Accurate indexing and filing in a dental office are both a convenience and a necessity and are the bulk of most dental office filing procedures. All dental offices, whether large or small, should

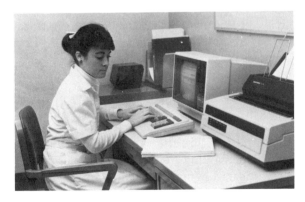

Fig. 3–1. Using a computer to store dental records

keep all letters received and make copies of all letters that are sent out. In addition to correspondence, much other important information is carefully kept, such as receipts, canceled checks, purchase orders, duplicate sales slips, invoices, statements, and catalogs. There is always a chance that such items will be needed for quick reference. They must be properly indexed and filed if they are to be located quickly.

Many offices keep separate folders or sections in file drawers for correspondence, auditor information (income tax returns, bank statements, and social security information), invoices, paid statements, unpaid statements, and catalogs. These papers should be filed properly and promptly to ensure that they can be located quickly when they are needed.

FINANCIAL MANAGEMENT

Successful financial management is the key to a successful dental practice. Such management is based on establishing a practical arrangement with each patient and includes diagnosis, case presentation, and an estimate of work to be done. A definite understanding of what is expected of both doctor and patient is essential to financial management. Even though the patient has selected a dental program and the method of payment, certain unforeseen situations may arise, causing the account to become delinquent. The secretarial dental assistant, in many instances, has the responsibility of collecting the delinquent accounts.

Delinquent accounts are usually caused by one or more factors:

- dissatisfaction with service
- misunderstanding of fees and work to be done
- poor money management by the patient
- poverty
- dishonesty

Delinquent accounts may be collected by phone or mail solicitations. Generally, contact is made each month following the last payment of the overdue account. The method should be persuasive, and the communication should be simple. The purpose is to have the patient willing to pay the account.

Collection Problems

Collection problems can be minimized by satisfying the patient. If the estimate is correct and the payment schedule is realistic, patients are appreciative and more apt to pay their accounts promptly. The paying habits of new patients should be investigated to determine their occupations, earning power, and credit histories. If a doctor is a member of a credit union, this information is readily available.

The Case Presentation

The case presentation is the responsibility of the dentist. The staff should prepare and gather all the materials needed for the meeting. These include patient charts, radiographs, study models (if any), visual aids, booklets, brochures applicable to the case, schedule of fees, and "consent" form for the patient's acceptance of the treatment plan.

A treatment plan will include proposed treatment with options to that plan, if options exist. The fees associated with each treatment option should be presented during the treatment discussion.

Once the plan has been agreed upon and accepted by the patient, the payment schedule of fees will be discussed by doctor and patient. Long-term patient benefits rather than the financial aspects of the treatment should be stressed.

RECORDING DOCUMENTARY

Good record keeping is important, to support not only the clinical aspect of the treatment but also the dentist/patient/staff relationship. The doctor's notations on the patient chart should include patient questions, how a mutually agreed-upon solution was achieved or determined, and any satisfactory comments made by the patient. Such entries in the chart must be made accurately and without personal prejudice.

Staff entries can be beneficial to the patient's entire record. Staff can note on the chart additional information or comments made by the patient directly to them. Any questions concerning appointments, follow-up visits, and other nontreatment concerns the patient expressed should be noted. Entries should be signed by the person making them. Staff notations should be reviewed by the dentist, signed, and dated. Once an entry is made in the patient record, it becomes documented evidence of what has transpired.

ENDING THE RELATIONSHIP

Sometimes the dentist/patient relationship must be terminated. Termination of the relationship involves three considerations: (1) the health of the patient must not be jeopardized by the termination of care; (2) there must be written notification to the patient that treatment is to be discontinued; and (3) the patient must be given ample time to secure the services of another dentist.

It is recommended that this written notification be sent by registered mail, with a return receipt to be permanently filed in the patient's chart.

Ways to find another dentist should be offered to the patient. The local dental society may maintain a referral service or have a list of dentists' names within the same geographic area. The patient should be notified that copies of dental records, radiographs, and other materials that would be helpful and beneficial to future care will be forwarded to the new dental practice.

REVIEW

1. Define communication.

   _____

   _____

   _____

2. Good interpersonal communications are essential to gaining _____ in the dental office.

3. A key to building positive doctor/staff patient relationships is_____

   _____.

4. Providers of dental care will need to apply interpersonal skills to _____ with each patient as an individual.

5. Listening is a skill that takes _____ and _____.

6. Good eye contact when listening is recognized by the public as representing

   _____.

7. When listening, body posture should be _____ and _____ rather than _____ and _____.

8. Often, when a patient asks questions, he or she is looking for a way to

   a. _____

   b. _____

   c. _____

9. Language and terminology should be adjusted to the level that the patient

   _____.

10. The staff member that becomes the patient's advocate will speak _____

_____.

11. How can the dental environment influence a patient? _____

_____

_____

_____

12. Updated furnishings are an indication that the dental practice is _____

_____.

13. All dental personnel should have a commitment to personal _____

_____.

14. Written communication to dental patients is the responsibility of the
    _____ and _____.

15. List the four types of interpersonal distance.

    a. _____

    b. _____

    c. _____

    d. _____

16. Much of dentistry is performed within the _____ distance.

17. The contact with patients and coworkers that cannot be avoided during
    dental care is called_____.

18. Touching that is most likely to occur, and least likely to be misunderstood, is
    _____ touching.

19. The case presentation is the responsibility of the_____.

20. The division of responsibility for the dentist includes

   a. _____

   b. _____

   c. _____

21. The division of responsibility for the dental patient includes

   a. _____

   b. _____

   c. _____

22. The doctor's notations on the patient chart should include

   a. _____

   b. _____

   c. _____

23. Staff entries made on the patient record should include

   a. _____

   b. _____

   c. _____

   d. _____

24. All entries made on the patient record should be

   a. _____

   b. _____

25. When a dentist/patient relationship is terminated, the understanding should be that

    a. _____

    b. _____

    c. _____

    d. _____

Chapter 4: Human Cell Structure and Function

OBJECTIVES:

After studying this chapter, the student will be able to:
- Discuss the role of genes in the development of body cells.
- Describe the sequence of cell division (mitosis).
- Describe the basic structure of human body cells.
- Discuss the role of proteins in cell development and maintenance.
- Describe the four basic tissues of the body.
- State the single most important substance of the body and its function.
- Discuss the development and life span of the red blood cells (erythrocytes).
- Discuss the development and life span of the white blood cells (leukocytes).
- Describe the human circulatory system.
- Compare the human lymphatic system with the circulatory system.
- Discuss antigen-antibody reactions as they pertain to immunity.
- Discuss blood clotting.
- State the difference between active immunity and passive immunity.

INTRODUCTION

The understanding of cell structure and function does not consist of learning a vast number of scientific names but in comprehending the process that is taking place in the body. We have meant this chapter to be functional rather than anatomical. It is intended for those who have had no previous contact with **anatomy** (study of structures and parts of the body) and **physiology** (study of the functions of the body systems) and provides only a review by those who have. Microscopic descriptions have received little emphasis, as they are apt to be meaningless to one who has not himself or herself studied changes under the microscope.

The human body has been likened to a machine. The machinelike nature of the body was recognized some four centuries ago by René Descartes (1596–1650), a French philosopher. In his *Treatise of Man*, Descartes compared the body to the mechanical devices of his age.

Any study of human body systems must have a logical place to start. Having established that fact, the logical place to start is at the beginning, with the cell, the basis of life. The *cell* is a unit of structure, of development, and of function, both normal and abnormal.

CELLS

Each human adult body, "that miracle of mechanical perfection," is composed of minute units of life, or cells, too numerous to measure. Together these cells give the body its appearance, shape, and form. Each human cell, except for mature red blood cells that lose their nucleus soon after their cell division is completed, has a potential capability of forming a complete human being.

The cells are controlled by *genes* (units of heredity), and every cell in an individual has the same set of genes. There are many thousands of genes within each cell, just how many is uncertain.

The genes are biologic blueprints that form and shape the body on a production line making identical cellular models, millions of them every day. In the internal world of the body, there are no new cellular models; each new cell is a replica of an old one.

Cell Division and Differentiation

All the cells of the body originate from a solitary cell created by the union of a sperm from the father and an *ovum* (fertilized egg) from the mother. This cell divides to create more cells, and then they divide and subdivide. The process of cell division is called *mitosis*.

The first cells formed by the fertilized ovum are identical. Then a complicated, almost endless, process called differentiation occurs. *Differentiation* is a series of changes whereby the cells acquire completely different individual characteristics. Thus, cells of different shape, size, and texture are created, each with a specific task. All the cells of the body become specialized in form and function, with the exception of the sex cells that are set aside at a very early stage of development for the purpose of reproduction of the race.

Cell Structure

Although cells may be highly specialized in their function, they all have the same basic structure. That is to say, they have an outer covering

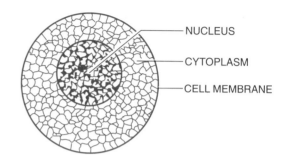

Fig. 4–1. Structural plan of the cell

called the *cell membrane*, a main substance called the *cytoplasm*, and a *nucleus*, figure 4–1.

The *cell membrane* is a very fine layer of tissue that regulates entry of raw materials into and discharge of waste material from the cells. *Tissue* comes from the French word *tissu*, which means fine gauze or weave. The cell membrane possesses membrane gateways or minute perforations through which substances such as oxygen pass into the cell and waste products such as carbon dioxide pass out. Cell membranes are capable of selection in the passage of substances into and out of the cell. This mechanism is termed *diffusion*.

Beneath the cell membrane is the *cytoplasm* (cyt-, cell; plasm-, basic material of the cell), or cellular fluid. Cytoplasm is a watery gelatinlike substance that gives the cell its bulk and provides the medium in which chemical changes occur.

The *nucleus* is the control center of the cell and influences growth, repair, and reproduction of the cell. The nucleus is where the blueprints of life are stored in a "library" composed of 46 chromosomes arranged in 23 pairs of different shapes and sizes. A *chromosome*, a large collection of genes, may be thought of as one volume in this library, and the genes as the pages that provide building instructions.

The cytoplasm and the substance of the nucleus are collectively termed *protoplasm*.

Protoplasm is composed of water (75 percent) and protein (25 percent), along with various minerals. *Proteins* are any group of organic compounds (combined natural elements) containing carbon, hydrogen, oxygen, nitrogen, and usually sulfur and phosphorus. Proteins exist in the cell in the form of *molecules*, the smallest units of a compound.

Proteins, named from the Greek word meaning "first importance" are the chemical basis of life on earth. They account for about 12 percent of body weight and shape the characteristics of individual cells. Proteins also control the multitude of chemical changes taking place simultaneously within cells. None of the body cells can survive without an adequate supply of proteins.

Products such as hormones and enzymes are formed from proteins. **Hormones** are chemical messengers produced by cells of the body and transported by the bloodstream. Hormones regulate growth, the biologic clock, and basic drives and emotions. *Enzymes* are catalysts that stimulate biochemical reactions (chemistry of vital processes), without taking any direct part in them. Every cell contains several thousand kinds of enzyme molecules, all of which are essential for building up the cell, maintaining it, and helping it carry out its specific duties.

Proteins are formed by linking together hundreds of amino acid molecules. Twenty-three different sorts of *amino acids* (building blocks) are found inside the body, and all but ten can be manufactured by cells. During digestion, the proteins consumed are broken down into simpler compounds (amino acids) the body can use; this is the *catabolic phase* (cata-, down; bol-, food), or the chemical change that food undergoes. This change is also referred to as **catabolism**. The *anabolic phase* (ana-, upward) converts the simpler compounds obtained from the nutrients into living, organized substances the body can use. This chemical change is also referred to as **anabolism**. These two phases combine as the process of body metabolism. **Metabolism** (meta-, changed, involving change) is the total of the complex physical and chemical processses involved in the maintenance of life.

HINDS OF CELLS AND TISSUES

The various types of cells that make up the tissues of the body possess the general features common to all cells; but each kind has, in addition, certain characteristics and specialized functions, figure 4–2.

Epithelium [Covering Tissue]

Epithelium is made up of cells that may be thin and flat, or tall, in the shape of columns, or varied shapes between the two. Epithelium may be a single layer in thickness, or it may be composed of several layers of cells. It covers the exposed surfaces of the body—the skin, the eyes, the lips; it also lines the cavities, the ducts (passageways) of glands, tracts, vessels and makes up linings in the interior of the body. It lines the digestive tract, the blood vessels, the abdominal and chest cavities, as well as the secretory cells of glands. Epithelial tissues serve to protect, absorb, and secrete (to generate and separate out a substance from cells of body fluids). For secretion, there are groups of cells that have grown down from the surface epithelium to form glands. A *gland* is composed of a specialized group of cells that draws specific substances from the blood and alters them for later release. The characteristic thing about epithelial tissue is that one of its surfaces is usually "free," exposed either to the exterior of the body or to the cavity of a hollow structure.

Muscle [Contracting Tissue]

There are three varieties of muscle tissue: the *striped* muscles, which move the skeletal parts; the *smooth* muscles of the internal organs and blood vessels; and the *muscle of the heart*.

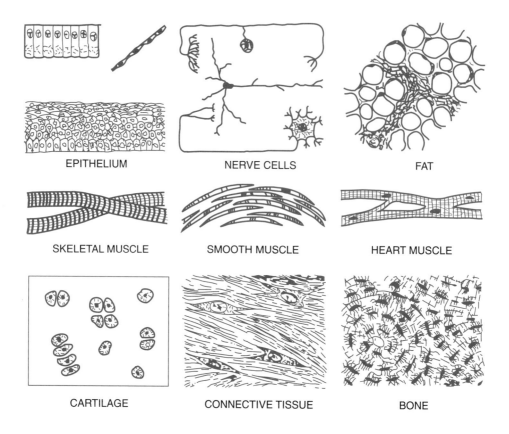

Fig. 4–2. A comparison of the common types of cells and tissues in the human body. The fat droplets within the fat cells, the gristle in which the cartilage cells are embedded, and the hard tissue of the bone are shown unshaded. Bone cells with fibrous processes are in black. (Courtesy University of Chicago Press, Chicago, IL, 1961)

Striped muscle is composed of bundles of long, thin, cylindrical fibers, arranged parallel to one another. Each fiber is an arrangement of several cells that are fused into a single unit; each fiber has many nuclei, figure 4–2. Skeletal muscle is attached to bones, and the contractions of this muscle cause the parts of the skeleton to move.

Smooth muscle is so named because of the absence of stripes. The cells of smooth muscle are positioned with their cells lying parallel to one another, so that a contraction of each cell results in a shortening (and thickening) of the groups of cells in a particular tissue.

The heart (cardiac) muscle somewhat resembles the striped muscle but lacks the elasticity of the skeletal muscle, figure 4–2.

Nerve (Conducting Tissue)

The characteristic structural feature of nerve cells is the extension of long, thin processes from the main body of the cell. Bundles of these extensions make up the nerves of the body and serve as pathways in the brain and spinal cord. Nervous tissue is highly specialized with long hairlike processes and will instantly transmit sensation, depending on the degree of irritability or stimulation causing the response. It may be well to remember that a nervous system that is not irritable (does not respond to irritation) is completely valueless, figure 4–2.

Connecting and Supporting Tissue

Under this heading are grouped a variety of cells of common embryonic origin. These tissues are characterized by the large amount of extra-cellular, or nonliving materials they contain. The *connective tissue* proper is made up of cells some-what resembling smooth muscle cells. These cells have the peculiar property of manufactur-ing long fibrous strands that make up the bulk of the tissue. These fibers are interlaced with one another, giving the tissue a tough, fabriclike consistency. The tissue also possesses a degree of elasticity that varies with the numbers of elas-tic fibers included in it. Connective tissue, as the name implies, connects the cells of the body to one another and binds together the tissues of all the organs. It is found almost everywhere in the body. It binds the nerve and muscle fibers of nerve trunks or muscles into compact bundles and holds together the cells of the internal organs, figure 4–2.

Bone and Cartilage. Bone and **cartilage** (gristle) are living tissues, composed of living cells that are capable of manufacturing the extracellular rigid parts of the tissues. In the case of bone, this consists of calcium and phosphorus com-pounds. It is these cellular products that give bone and cartilage their properties of rigidity and strength, on which depend their more obvi-ous functions, figure 4–2.

Fat Tissue. Fat tissue is composed of specialized cells that have the ability to take up fat and store it—a single droplet within each cell. The bulk of the cell is simply inert fat, which has no ability to move or act, and is compressed into a thin covering wall surrounding the fat droplet. A number of fat cells are bound together in a more

or less structural mass by connective tissue. Fat tissue is found especially under the skin, and much of it is located in and about a number of internal organs, figure 4–2.

WATER AND SALT

The single most important substance in the body is water. An individual can endure hunger for days, but will not survive without water. The water of the body dissolves salts to form electrolytes. An *electrolyte* is a substance that undergoes chemical change to form ions in solu-tion. An ion has a charge of positive or negative electricity through gaining or losing an electron in the chemical process. Because of the formed ions, an electrolyte is capable of conducting elec-tricity within the body.

Electrolytes in the body play an essential role in the workings of the cell and in maintaining balance in the fluids, or acid-base balance. An *acid-base balance* is a state of chemical balance in which the tissues of the body contain the proper proportions of various salts and water. A nor-mal acid-base balance is a state of equilibrium (balance) between acidity and alkalinity of the body fluids. This acid-base balance is referred to as the hydrogen ion (H+) concentration or pH. An optimal pH between 7.35 and 7.45 on a scale of 0 to 10 must be maintained; otherwise, the body will not function properly.

The chief electrolyte ions are formed from sodium, potassium, and calcium salts. *Sodium* is a key regulator in water balance and is also nec-essary to normal function of muscles and nerves. *Potassium* is one of the main components of cell protoplasm. *Calcium* is essential for normal muscle physiology and blood clotting.

Sodium and chloride salts are found in large amounts in the fluid outside the cell (*extracellular fluid*). Potassium, magnesium, and phosphate salts are found in large amounts in the fluid inside the cell (*intracellular fluid*).

BLOOD

Blood is the body's internal transport system from major organs to every living cell. Blood is composed of cells and fluid. *Plasma* is the fluid, a faintly straw-colored substance, that consists of at least 90 percent water, with the balance in cells. Plasma accounts for 55 percent of blood volume, and the cells for 45 percent.

Blood Cells

Erythrocytes. **Erythrocytes** are produced in the red bone marrow and comprise the vast majority of oxygen-carrying cells, figure 4–3. Because of the *hemoglobin* (red color of the blood protein) these cells contain, they are called erythrocytes (eryth-, red; cyt-, cell), or *red blood cells.* Hemoglobin gives the blood its red color and is the principal protein in the erythrocyte. Hemoglobin picks up oxygen from the lungs and releases it to every living cell in the body The blood's most important function is to carry oxygen.

Erythrocytes are biconcave disks, meaning that they have a rounded, hollowed out surface on either side. They are the most numerous of any of the blood cells. During the early stages of formation, before they pass into the circulating blood, the red cells possess a nucleus, but the nucleus is lost before the cell becomes a functioning unit. In view of this, it may be more accurate to refer to these structures not as cells but *corpuscles* or "little bodies," figure 4–4.

Red cells possess remarkable elasticity and tend to bend and twist as they are forced through the smaller blood vessels. However, as soon as a larger channel is reached, they resume their original shape. The cell may reach a fork in the blood vessel and be bent by the stream on either side, then slide on and go back to its original shape, figure 4–5.

The lack of a nucleus in the circulating red cells makes cell division impossible. Actually, the production of new red cells occurs outside the blood stream in the red bone marrow. Red cells are produced at the rate of 200 billion per day. Red cell production depends on a sufficient supply of iron and two main B vitamins, B12 and folic acid, in the body. (Refer to Nutrition, Chapter 30.) Deficiencies in these two vitamins

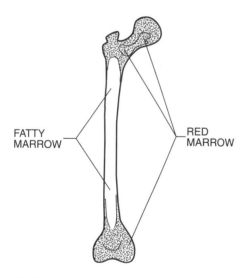

Fig. 4–3. Bone of the leg (femur) split open to show the large space in the shaft filled with fatty marrow and the ends of the bone filled with red bone marrow.

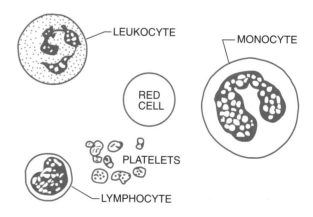

Fig. 4–4. Bone cells in humans vary in size and shape.

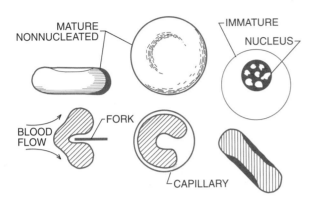

Fig. 4–5. Red blood cells. Note how a red cell may be bent when it strikes a fork in a blood vessel or become twisted as it is forced through a narrow capillary, then resumes its original shape.

occur as a result of poor diet or from failure of the small intestine to absorb them.

Red blood cells remain in circulation for about 110 to 120 days. If so, an individual red blood cell can make more than 40,000 journeys around the body in a month. Based on the average life of a red blood cell, it can be calculated that two million cells are destroyed—and formed—every second of our lives.

Leukocytes. Leukocytes (leuko-, colorless) are semitransparent and contain no hemoglobin; they are referred to as *white cells*, figure 4–4. They are always nucleated (have a nucleus) even in the mature form and when circulating in the blood.

Leukocytes are formed in the red bone marrow, in the same regions from which red cells arise. It is thought by some scientists that in the development of the two different cells, one becomes a red cell while the other results in a white cell. Whether or not this is the case, it is clear that red corpuscles and leukocytes differentiate in the same tissue, the red bone marrow. Although the circulating white cells contain nuclei, white cell division does not occur in the blood stream; they grow and multiply outside the blood stream.

White blood cells are larger than erythrocytes and lack the uniform structure of the red corpuscles. Seventy percent of all leukocytes have numerous small granules in their cytoplasm, and are classified as *granular leukocytes*. Their estimated life span varies from nine to thirteen days. Unlike red cells that are simply carried along in the blood, white cells have freedom of movement. Rapidly activated by infected or injured tissue, leukocytes squeeze their way through the blood vessel walls and engulf foreign particles, such as bacteria.

Because the number of white cells increases three- to fourfold during infection, leukocytes are of major importance in a laboratory diagnosis of disease. White cells provide the body with a line of defense that is second only to the skin. There are several types of white cells, each programmed to perform a specific task.

Lymphocytes. Lymphocytes are termed *agranular white cells* (a-, without) because they lack granules in their cytoplasm. Lymphocytes possess a single nucleus, a thin rim of clear cytoplasm, and a cell membrane, figure 4–4. Lymphocytes are produced in the red bone marrow and develop in the lymphatic tissue, found in many regions of the body, for example, the tonsils and adenoids, figure 4–6.

Lymphocytes are slightly larger than red cells and are concerned with immunity (protection against a particular disease) and combating infection. Lymphocytes are said to be *thymus-dependent*. The *thymus* is a glandlike mass of tissue lying on the midline of the upper chest region, beneath the sternum and over the heart. The thymus manufactures its own characteristic material (thymosin) that it releases directly into the blood and lymph system.

Platelets. Platelets, also called *thrombocytes* (thrombo-, clot), are small platelike structures,

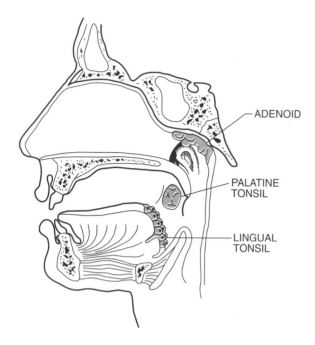

Fig. 4–6. The tonsils and adenoids are composed of lymphatic tissue, found in the upper portions of the nose and throat.

the smallest formed elements of the blood. They are produced in the red bone marrow, have no nucleus, and possess a very thin membrane, figure 4–4. Platelets tend to stick fast to damaged surfaces and help with the clotting of blood.

Blood Vessels

There are three major types of blood vessels in the body: arteries, capillaries, and veins.

Arteries. Arteries are the vessels through which the blood passes away from the heart to various parts of the body. The wall of an artery is well-jacketed, with three coats (layers) to withstand the high pressure of the blood flowing through them. The outer coat is white fibrous connective tissue, covering a middle layer of smooth muscle and elastic tissue. Beneath the middle coat lies an elastic membrane that is lined with a smooth

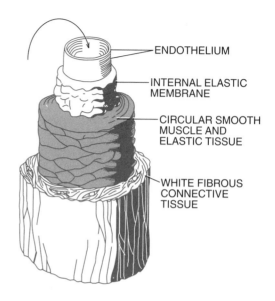

Fig. 4–7. Structure of arteries. Well-jacketed arteries are able to withstand the high pressure of the blood flowing through them and to maintain pressure throughout the arterial system.

endothelium (inner covering). Together, these walls maintain pressure through the arterial system. The muscular and elastic tissues in artery walls ensure that the surges of blood from the heart are converted into a more steady flow, figure 4–7.

Capillaries. Capillaries are the smallest blood vessels in the body. These tiny vessels are the last link in the chain of delivery from the lungs to the cells. The blood stays in the capillaries, while oxygen and other essential substances are exchanged for carbon dioxide and other waste products. This exchange and just how it occurs is one of the miracles of biochemistry (the science of living organisms and of vital processes). It is known that the exchange is made through the capillary walls that are only one cell thick. Capillaries join with tiny veins (venules) that unite to form larger and larger veins.

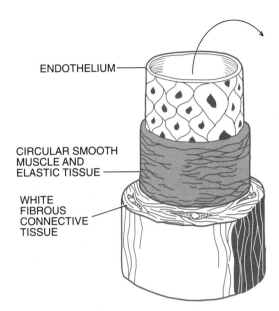

Fig. 4–8. Structure of veins. Veins carry oxygen-depleted blood back to the heart and lungs and do not have to withstand the same pressure as the arteries.

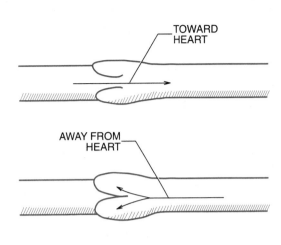

Fig. 4–9. The veins have two-flap valves inside them that provide one-way traffic of the venous blood flow.

Veins. Veins are vessels through which blood passes from various organs to the heart, carrying away blood that has given up most of its oxygen. Veins, like arteries, have three coats: an outer, a middle, and an inner. These coats are not so thick and collapse when the vessel is cut, figure 4–8.

Blood is able to flow uphill through veins because of the valves inside them—two-flap valves—that operate rather like river lock gates. These prevent the blood from flowing backward, figure 4–9. Cell waste is discharged into the veins for excretion through the kidneys or through the lungs. The veins take blood back to the heart, and the heart pumps it to the lungs, where it receives fresh oxygen.

THE CIRCULATORY SYSTEM

The fact misunderstood by physicians and philosophers until some three hundred and fifty years ago was that the body has a double circu-latory system. William Harvey concluded that the blood moves in a continuous onward motion and direction from the heart to the arteries to the veins and back to the heart. But at some point, blood must pick up oxygen from the lungs. This means that blood returning from the body must be pumped to the lungs from the heart, and that is why the heart has four chambers, not two.

From the earliest of times our ancestors have realized the importance of the heart to life itself. It seems appropriate in any review of blood circulation that a brief consideration of the workings of the heart be made.

The *heart* is a hollow, muscular organ whose function is to cause the blood to circulate through the body. The heart lies within the thorax (chest region), enclosed in a sac of fibrous tissue called *pericardium* (peri-, around; cardi-, heart).

Heart Structure

The heart is composed of muscles and valves. It is completely divided by a septum (partition) into two parts, the so-called left heart and right heart. Each part is divided into two chambers. The valves, made up of extraordinary thin membranes, or *endocardium*, also line the heart cavity. Although very thin, the valves prevent even a single drop of blood from leaking through when closed.

On the right side of the heart the *tricuspid valve* divides the chamber into an *atrium* and a *ventricle*, figure 4–10. The tricuspid valve has three segments or parts (tri-, three; cuspid, segment). The atrium receives the venous blood from the body; the venous blood passes through the tricuspid valve into the ventricle. The tricuspid valve prevents any backflow of venous blood. The ventricle sends the impure blood to the lungs by way of the *pulmonary artery* (pulmon, lung.) The mouth of the pulmonary artery is guarded by the *pulmonary valve*.

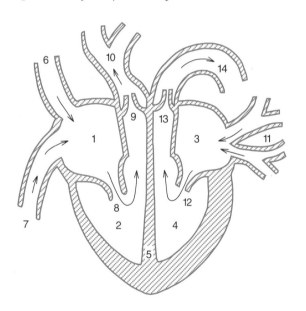

Fig. 4–10. Interior of the heart: (1) right atrium; (2) right ventricle; (3) left atrium; (4) left ventricle; (5) septum; (6) superior vena cava; (7) inferior vena cava; (8) tricuspid valve; (9) pulmonary valve; (10) pulmonary artery; (11) pulmonary veins; (12) mitral valve; (13) aortic valve; (14) aorta. The arrows indicate the direction of blood flow.

The left chamber of the heart is divided by the *mitral valve* which separates the left atrium from the left auricle, and regulates the flow of blood from one chamber to the other. The atrium receives the purified blood from the lungs, and the ventricle sends the blood into the great artery, the *aorta*.

The aorta is the main trunk of the arterial blood system, carrying blood from the left side of the heart to the arteries of all limbs and organs, except the lungs.

Blood Circulation

Leading from the left heart, the aorta branches upward, backward, and then downward; this is referred to as the *aortic arch*. Along its course to the lower abdominal cavity, the aorta gives off *arteries*, that branch into smaller and smaller vessels extending to all parts of the body, figure 4–11. The smallest of the arteries are *capillaries*. Capillaries branch into the very smallest vessels of the arterial system, *arterioles*. Arterioles unite with minute veins, called *venules*, which, in turn, form larger and larger veins. The veins of the lower portion of the body empty into the *inferior vena cava*. The veins of the head and neck flow into the *superior vena cava*. These two venous channels empty into the right heart to complete the *systemic circulation*, figure 4–11.

From the right heart arises the *pulmonary artery* that soon divides into two, one for each lung. Each pulmonary artery divides into smaller and smaller arteries that enter the lung via the *pulmonary capillaries*. These capillaries penetrate all parts of the lung(s), then collect into larger and larger veins, finally forming the *pulmonary veins*, which empty into the left heart. This makes up the *pulmonary circulation*, figure 4–11.

THE LYMPHATIC AND IMMUNE SYSTEMS

The *lymphatic system* makes up the secondary transport system of the human body. This functional unit is composed of lymph vessels, lymph

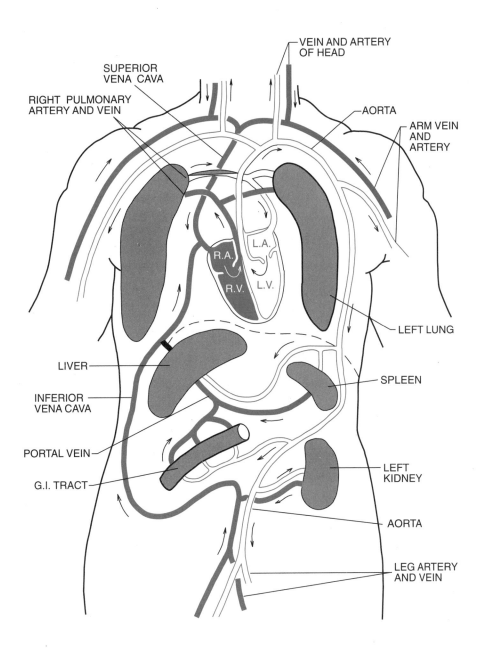

Fig. 4–11. The circulatory system. The aorta and vena cava actually course along the mid-line of the body. Vessels containing oxygen-poor blood are in black. Arrows indicate direction of flow. (Courtesy University of Chicago Press, Chicago, IL, 1961)

fluid, lymph nodes, and spleen. The main function of the lymphatics is to drain the tissue fluids of the body.

As explained, blood carries oxygen and nutrients to the cells and waste products away from them. However, not all the plasma is reabsorbed into circulation. Some is left behind in the tissue fluid and is removed by the lymphatics.

Lymph Vessels

Lymph vessels, like blood vessels, are distributed to all parts of the body. The lymphatic system does not have a continuous closed circulation but appears to have a closed end at the point of origin, figure 4–12.

Lymph Capillaries

Lymph capillaries are thin-walled tubes that carry lymph from the tissue spaces to the larger lymphatic vessels, figure 4–13. Lymph vessels can be compared to veins, in that they conduct

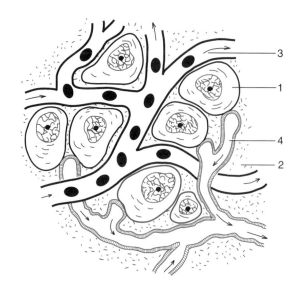

Fig. 4–12.   Tissue fluid bathing body cells: (1) tissue cell; (2) tissue fluid; (3) blood vessel; (4) lymphatic

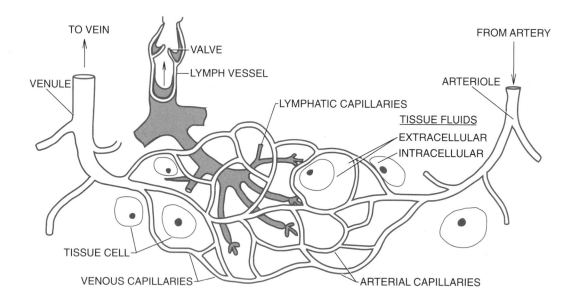

Fig. 4–13. A capillary bed of arterial, venous, and lymphatic flow

the flow toward the thoracic region. As do veins, lymphatic vessels have valves to prevent the backflow of fluid. Small lymph vessels join others lying next to them to form larger channels, figure 4–12.

Lymph Fluid

Lymph fluid is a clear, colorless liquid consisting of about 95 percent water and the remainder plasma. Lymph flows in the spaces between the cells and body tissues. When the plasma seeps through the capillary walls and circulates among body tissues, it is known as *tissue fluid*. When tissue fluid is drained from the tissues and collected by the lymphatic system, it is called *lymph*, figure 4–13.

Since the tissue fluid is constantly being added to, there must be some means of escape. Excess tissue fluid, containing the waste products from the body's living cells, passes through the thin walls of the lymphatics and is carried away as lymph.

Lymph then passes through a series of filters, known as lymphatic glands or *lymph nodes*, figure 4–14. Major lymph nodes are found along the medium-size lymph vessels at the knee, elbow, armpit, groin, neck, chest, and abdomen.

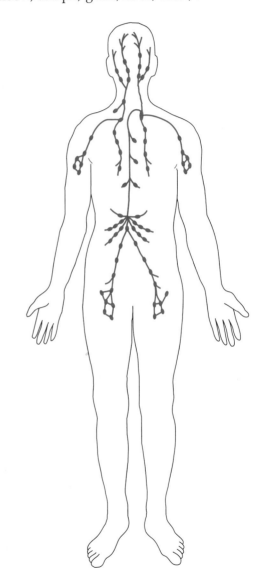

Fig. 4–15. Major lymph nodes are found in the torso, head, neck, and armpits. Lymph nodes that drain infected areas of the body are liable to become inflamed and tender to the touch.

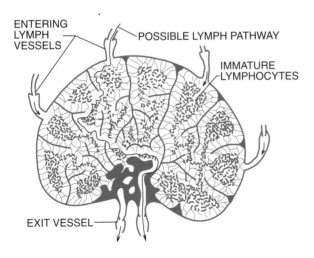

ENTERING LYMPH VESSELS

POSSIBLE LYMPH PATHWAY

IMMATURE LYMPHOCYTES

EXIT VESSEL

Fig. 4–14. Cross-section of a lymph node. Lymph flows slowly through a series of channels within the node. Certain of the white cells (lymphocytes) are formed in the node and added to the lymph as it flows through the node.

Lymph nodes act as filters to trap bacteria and other debris and vary greatly in size, figure 4–15. Normal lymph nodes can be felt in the groin. Swollen lymph nodes may be felt in the armpit of an individual with an infected hand, or in the neck of a person with infected tonsils. It is in the lymph nodes that bacteria and other injurious agents that may have gained access to the tissue fluid are strained out and usually destroyed, figure 4–16. Larger and larger channels join in the left shoulder region in the thorax, near the heart. The lymphatics form one or two main ducts that open into the large veins of the upper body.

The *spleen* is located in the upper left quadrant of the abdomen, just below the diaphragm and behind the stomach, figure 4–11. The spleen produces lymphocytes and monocytes that are important cells in the immune system.

The spleen also filters microorganisms and foreign debris from the blood. Other functions of the spleen include storing red cells, maintaining appropriate balance between blood cells and blood plasma, and destroying and removing worn out red blood cells.

IMMUNE RESPONSES

The mechanisms of **immunity** are concerned with the body's ability to recognize and dispose of substances that it interprets as foreign or harmful to its well-being. When such a substance enters the body, complex mechanical and

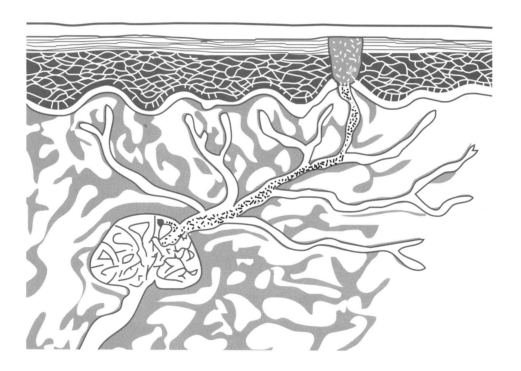

Fig. 4–16. Prevention of the spread of bacteria. Bacteria (black dots) enter the lymph vessels (white channels) and many are filtered out and destroyed in the lymph nodes.

chemical activities are set in motion to protect and defend the body's cells and tissues.

The foreign substance, usually a protein, is called an **antigen**. An antigen may consist of soluble substances, such as toxins (poisons), foreign proteins, or particles of bacteria and tissue cells. The most common response to the antigen is the production of **antibody**. The antigen-antibody reaction is an essential component of the overall immune response.

Antigen-Antibody Reaction

Antigen-antibody reaction occurs as the substance interpreted as a foreign invader gains entrance into the body. Any antigen, be it bacteria or foreign matter, induces the production of antibody that will affect only the specific antigen for which it was created.

Antibodies. Antibodies, also called *immune bodies*, are soluble proteins produced by the white cells. Most all antibodies are proteins. A fraction of the protein consists of gamma globulin. *Gamma globulin* is a specific protein developed in the lymphoid tissues in response to harmful agents. Gamma globulins are essential to the establishment of immunity, because nearly all antibodies contain gamma globulin molecules.

The antigen-specific property of the antibody is the basis of the antigen-antibody reaction that is essential to an immune response.

Cells of the Immune System

Highly specialized cells are involved in the body's immune system. Along with *lymphocytes*, there are *phagocytes, macrophages, monocytes,* and *thrombocytes.*

Lymphocytes. Lymphocytes are cells with a nucleus but no granules in their cytoplasm. Lymphocytes adapt to the functions of the immune system.

T-lymphocytes, also called *T-cells*, originate in the red bone marrow as "stem cells" and are converted by the thymus, figure 4–17. They are stimulated by thymosin, secreted by the thymus, before becoming circulating lymphocytes. Because of this stimulation, T-cells are said to be *thymus-dependent*. T-cells have a dual role; they control immune mechanisms and kill alien cells and organisms. *Helper T-cells* are a type of T-cell that stimulates antibody production in the B-cells.

Lymphokines are potent and biologically active proteins, produced by the T-cells and serve as "signals" for the immune system. Lymphokines can attract macrophages to the site of infection or inflammation, then prepare them to attack.

Interferon, produced by the T-cells, is released by cells that have been invaded by a virus. Interferon influences the noninfected cells to form an antiviral protein that prevents multiplication of the virus. Interferon also assists in antiviral immunity.

B-cells. B-cells, or *B-lymphocytes*, are produced in the red bone marrow and are ordinarily concerned with producing antibodies. B-lymphocytes are *thymus-independent* and migrate to the tissues without passing through or being influenced by the thymus. When faced with a specific antigen, B-cells enlist the helper T-cells who help stimulate antibody production in the B-cells.

Phagocytes. Phagocytes (*phago-*, eating) are white cells, commonly referred to as "cell eaters," and the mechanism involved as *phagocytosis*. The word element, *-osis*, means disease. These cells are found everywhere throughout the tissues. Like leukocytes, they normally collect in great numbers in infected areas. It is a scientific fact that phagocytes circulate through the system and eat diseased and dead cells, figure 4–18.

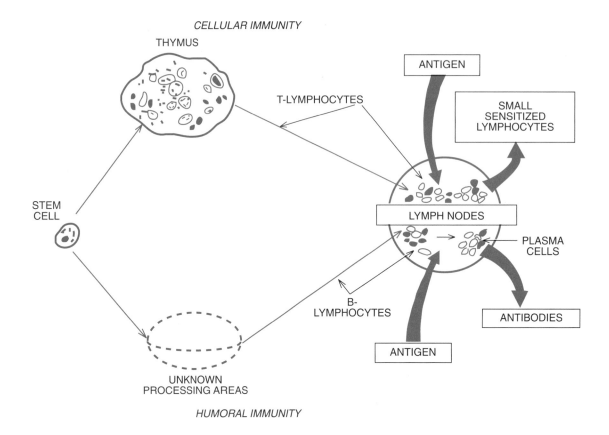

Fig. 4–17. Formation of antibodies and sensitized lymphocytes by a lymph node in response to antigens.

Macrophages. Macrophages (*macro-*, large) are large highly phagocytic cells in the walls of blood vessels and in loose connective tissue. They are usually immobile or *fixed*, but, when stimulated by inflammation, they become actively mobile or *free*. When erythrocytes (red cells) are no longer useful, they are destroyed by macrophages in the spleen and liver. Macrophages are said to provide the janitorial services of the immune system.

Monocytes. Monocytes are phagocytic leukocytes that are formed in the red bone marrow and are carried to other parts of the body, where they mature into macrophages, figure 4–4.

Blood Clotting

Thrombocytes. Thrombocytes (blood platelets) are principally concerned with the clotting of blood and contraction of the blood clot, figure 4–4. The clotting process is complex. The reactions involved in converting the fluid (blood) into a solid (clot) are always set off when blood vessels are ruptured.

When an injury occurs, the blood platelets collect on surfaces of the ruptured vessel, quickly disintegrate, and clotting begins. Apparently, platelets and tissue cells alike yield clot-inducing materials when they are injured. Both cells and platelets release similar substances.

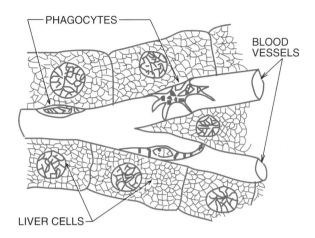

Fig. 4–18. Phagocytic cells in the walls of blood vessels of the liver. These cells engulf and destroy "worn out" red blood cells.

Fibrinogen. Fibrinogen, a protein always present in blood plasma, is necessary for blood clotting. Another agent important to clotting is called thrombin. *Thrombin* (a catalyst) is released by injured tissues or platelet disintegration and reacts with fibrinogen, converting it into *fibrin* (an insoluble protein). Entangled, interlacing threads of fibrin form a meshwork for the basis of the blood clot. Between the meshes, the formed elements (red and white blood cells) become entrapped in a solidifying mass. As it solidifies, the clot also shrinks, squeezing from the small spaces within the mass a straw-colored liquid known as *serum.* The great number of red cells give the clot its color but do not otherwise contribute either to the formation or the final internal structure of the clot. Red cells are simply caught in the fibrin meshwork.

Clotting is a plasma phenomenon rather than a blood mechanism.

Types of Immune Response

Cellular Immunity. Cellular immunity, dependent on T-lymphocytes, is primarily concerned with a delayed type of immune response. These responses may be due to slowly developing bacterial diseases, viral infections, and tumor cells, such as cancer, figure 4–18.

Some of the sensitized T-cells combine with an antigen, causing it to become inactive. Other sensitized T-cells, with the help of lymphokines, destroy the antigen. Another protein, called interferon, is produced by the T-cells following a viral infection. Some of the T-cells are transformed into "killer cells." Killer cells produce a chemical toxin that damages the cell membrane of the antigen, causing it to rupture and lose its contents.

Lymphocytes that have been converted into T-cells but are not used in the immune response may revert back to lymphocytes. If later they are needed to react with an antigen, they can become sensitized again.

Humoral Immunity. Humoral immunity is a broad category of immune response that takes place in the body fluids (humors). *Humor* refers to any fluid or semifluid of the body. Humoral immunity is concerned with antibody and complement activity. *Complement* is a group of enzymatic proteins that are present but inactive in blood serum. During complement action the antigen, antibody, and complement become bound together. The cell membrane of the specific antigen is ruptured, and the cell contents leak into the body fluids. Complement proteins activate the phagocytes and promote phagocytosis.

Most of the B-lymphocytes, activated by the presence of their particular antigen, become plasma cells. These plasma cells then produce and export antibodies. The activated B-cells that do not become plasma cells continue to live in the lymphoid tissue as "memory cells." They stand ready for future encounters with antigens that may enter the body. It is these memory cells that provide continued immunity after initial exposure to an antigen.

Active and Passive Immunity. Individuals whose own tissues have produced the antibodies are said to possess *active immunity*. This immunity may be acquired by a person who had the disease and recovered from it. Immunity can also be induced by the introduction of weakened or dead antigens into the body. The latter is called *vaccination*. The vaccinated individual is said to possess *passive immunity*, because the antibodies of the blood and tissues have not been self-produced.

REVIEW

1. The _____ is referred to as the basis of life.

2. The cells are controlled by units of heredity or _____.

3. Another term for cell division is_____.

4. When cells divide and develop as cells of different shape, size, texture, and function, the process is called _____.

5. The basic structure of a cell includes

    a. _____ b. _____ c. _____

6. The mechanism whereby substances go into and out of a cell is termed _____

    _____.

7. Briefly describe the cytoplasm or cellular fluid. _____

    _____

    _____.

8. The control center of the cell is the nucleus. What influence does the nucleus have in cell development? _____

9. What is a chromosome? _____

    _____.

10. The smallest units of a compound are called _____.

11. What are proteins? What is the function of proteins? _____

   _____

   _____

   _____

   _____

12. Hormones and enzymes are formed from proteins. What are the functions of hormones?_____

   _____.

   What are the functions of enzymes? _____

   _____

   _____

13. Metabolism may be defined as _____

   _____.

14. List the four basic tissues of the human body.

   a._____ b._____ c._____ d._____

15. What is meant by the term *gland*? What is its function? _____

   _____

16. The single most important substance of the body is _____.

17. What is the function of electrolytes in the workings of a cell? _____

   _____

   _____

18. The optimal pH for the body is between _____ and _____.

Blood

19. Another term for erythrocyte is _____.

    What gives the red blood cells their color? _____

20. What is the most important function of blood? _____

    _____

21. Where do red cells form? _____

22. The life span of erythrocytes (red cells) is between _____ and
    _____ days.

23. Briefly describe the structure of a leukocyte (white blood cell). _____

    _____

    _____

24. The estimated life span of a leukocyte varies from _____ to
    _____ days.

25. Briefly describe the structure of a lymphocyte. _____

    _____

    _____

26. What is the function of lymphocytes? _____

    _____

27. Blood platelets help with_____.

Blood Vessels

28. The three major types of blood vessels in the body are:

    a. _____ b. _____ c. _____

29. The vessels through which the blood passes away from the heart to various parts of the body are the _____.

30. The smallest blood vessels of the body are the_____.

31. The vessels through which blood passes from various organs to the heart are the _____.

Immune System

32. List the five specialized cells involved in the immune system.

    a. _____ b. _____ c. _____

    d. _____ e. _____

33. What is meant by the term *phagocytosis*? _____

    _____

34. T-lymphocytes (T-cells) are said to have a dual role. Briefly explain what this means. _____

    _____

35. The primary function of B-lymphocytes is to produce _____.

36. Antigens may be soluble substances such as_____

    _____.

37. Antibodies are soluble proteins produced by the _____ cells.

38. The antigen-specific property of an antibody means that it will _____

    _____.

39. Individuals whose own tissues have produced the antibody are said to possess _____ immunity.

40. Individuals who have been vaccinated against a disease are said to possess _____ immunity.

Chapter 5: The Skull

OBJECTIVES:

After studying this chapter, the student will be able to:
- Name the two parts of the skull.
- Describe the shape and function(s) of the skull.
- Identify the eight bones that form the cranium.
- Identify the movable bone of the skull.
- Associate the terminology as it relates to the bones of the skull.

INTRODUCTION

The skull is divided into two parts: the *cranium* and the *skeleton of the face*. Since we are concerned with the teeth and the tissues that cushion the teeth in the skull, it is necessary to become familiar with the skull in detail.

The skull is the bony framework of the head that rests on the spinal column. It is oval in shape and wider in the back (posterior) than in the front (anterior). The cranium provides protection for the brain and support for the structures attached to it. The twenty-two bones that make up the skull are irregular in shape and, with one exception (the lower jawbone, or *mandible*), are immovably joined. Where two bones are joined with a seam, the line formed is termed a *suture*. Sutures are identified by the region where the bones are joined, such as *coronal suture* (the line formed by the frontal and two parietal bones in the crown; corona, of the head).

The skull consists of two parts:

- The *cranium*, which is composed of eight bones that contain and protect the brain.
- The *face*, which is composed of fourteen bones. These will be discussed in the remaining chapters in this section.

CRANIUM

Eight bones form the cranium, figure 5–1.

- frontal
- parietal (2)
- temporal (2)
- sphenoid
- ethmoid
- occipital

The *frontal* bone forms the forehead, a portion of the roof of the eye sockets, or *orbits*, and part of the nasal cavity. The orbits are the irregular, cone-shaped cavities in which the eyes are located. The arch formed by the frontal bone over the eyes is thick, sharp, and prominent. It protects the eyes and is called the *supraorbital margin* (supra, over; orbital, the eyes; margin, the ridge). The frontal sinuses (large hollow spaces) are located just above the supraorbital margins.

The two *parietal* bones (right and left) form the greater part of the sides and roof of the skull (parietal, forming the walls of a cavity—in this case, the walls of the skull cavity). Each parietal bone is irregularly four-sided in shape with its external surface convex and its internal surface concave.

The *temporal* bones (right and left) form the sides and base of the skull. Each temporal bone

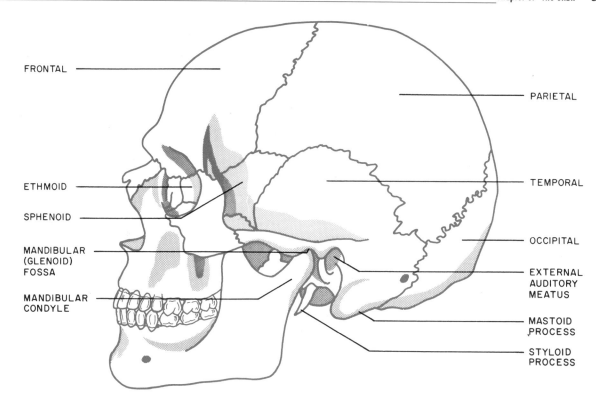

Fig. 5–1. Skull, lateral aspect

is bounded in front by the sphenoid bone; above, by the parietal; and in back by the occipital. Each temporal bone has a pit or depression, called the *mandibular* or *glenoid fossa* (glenoid, shallow or slightly cupped), into which the lower jawbone, or *mandible*, fits, thus allowing movement of the mandible. The sharp projection on the undersurface of the temporal bone is the *styloid process* (styloid, slender and pointed; process, prominence or outgrowth). The rounded projection at the back of the temporal bone is the *mastoid process*, a bony projection behind the external ear. The temporal bone also contains the external auditory canal, or *external auditory meatus*, and the middle and inner ear.

The *sphenoid* bone (sphenoid, wedgeshaped) is situated at the anterior (front) portion of the base of the skull. It is shaped somewhat like a bat with its wings outspread and its body joined to the occipital bone in the back and to the ethmoid bone in the front. Air spaces in the body are the *sphenoid sinuses*, which connect with the nasopharynx, as do the other sinuses of the skull. The wings of the sphenoid bone extend downward and are identified as the *pterygoid process* (pterygoid, wing-shaped; process, projection), figure 5–2.

The *ethmoid* bone is a thin bone at the anterior base of the cranium. It is located between the orbits, and helps form the roof, sides, and septum of the nose. The bone is very light and spongy, or honeycombed. The air spaces in the side (lateral) portions of the bone are the *ethmoid sinuses*.

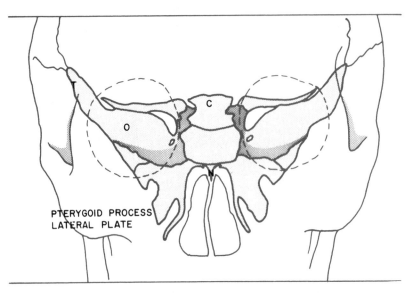

Fig. 5–2. Sphenoid bone, showing pterygoid process and surfaces of bone.
T = temporal; O = orbital; C = cranial; N = nasal.

The *occipital* bone is located at the back and base of the skull (occiput, back part of the head). It is characterized by a large opening called the *foramen magnum* (**foramen**, opening or hole; magnum, large). Through the foramen magnum pass the spinal cord, spinal nerves, and vertebral arteries. If you feel the back of your scalp, you can note a projection or protuberance. This is midway between the top of the occipital bone and the foramen magnum. It is called the *external occipital protuberance* (protuberance, rounded projection), figure 5-3.

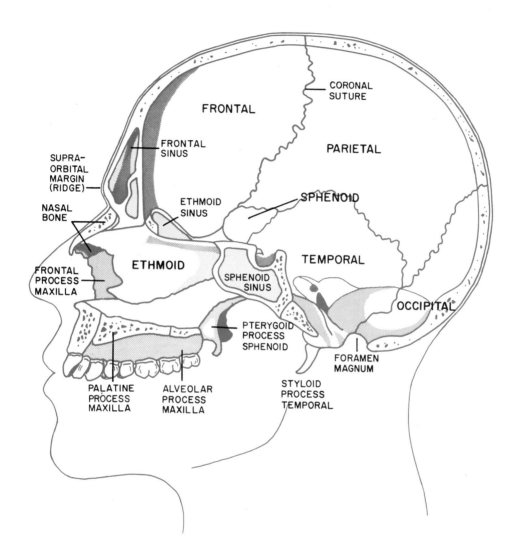

Fig. 5–3. Cranium (cross-section)

REVIEW

1. Identify the lettered parts of the illustration.

   A. _____

   B. _____

   C. _____

   D. _____

   E. _____

   F. _____

   G. _____

   H. _____

   I. _____

   J. _____

   K. _____

2. In your own words, explain the following terms.

   Anterior _____

   _____

   Posterior _____

   _____

   Process _____

   _____

   Suture _____

   _____

3. Define the following terms.

   Supraorbital margin _____

   _____

   Foramen magnum _____

   _____

Mandibular fossa _____

_____

Styloid process _____

_____

Pterygoid process_____

_____

4. Identify the lettered parts of the illustration.

A. _____   M. _____

B. _____   N. _____

C. _____   O. _____

D. _____   P. _____

E. _____   Q. _____

F. _____

G. _____

H. _____

I. _____

J. _____

K. _____

L. _____

5. Complete the following statements.

a. The cranium is composed of _____ bones.

b. _____ are identified by the region where the bones are joined.

c. The _____ suture is formed by the union of the frontal and parietal bones of the skull.

d. The foramen magnum is found in the _____ bone.

e. The mandibular (glenoid) fossa is located on the _____ bone.

f. The temporal bone contains the external _____.

g. The _____ is a projection of the sphenoid bone.

h. Air spaces within the body of the cranial bones are called_____

_____.

Chapter 6: The Face

OBJECTIVES:

After studying this chapter, the student will be able to:
- Identify the bones that form the skeleton of the face.
- Locate the vomer bone.
- Name the smallest and most fragile bones of the face.
- Locate the four processes of the maxilla.
- Describe the function of the alveolar process.

BONES OF THE FACE

There are fourteen bones that form the skeleton of the face:

- nasal bone (2)
- vomer
- inferior nasal conchae (2)
- lacrimal bone (2)
- maxillae (2)
- zygomatic bone (2)
- palatine bone (2)
- mandible

The facial bones are identifiable in figure 6-1.

The *nasal* bone consists of two small, oblong bones, placed side by side to form the bridge of the nose. They are situated at the middle and upper part of the face and lie close to the upper part of the *maxillae*.

The *vomer* is a single bone within the nasal cavity. It is found at the lower and back part of the nasal cavity and forms a part of the nasal septum (the partition between the two nasal chambers). The interior portion is usually bent to one side or another, making the nasal chambers of unequal size.

Situated on the outer wall of each nostril are the *inferior nasal conchae*. Each consists of a thin layer of cancellous bone (cancellous, spongy, having a latticelike structure). This bone appears to be curled on itself to resemble a scroll, or spiral coiled form.

The *lacrimal bones* (lacrimal, pertaining to tears) are found at the front part of the inner wall of each orbit. They are the smallest and most fragile bones of the face. They resemble a fingernail in form, thickness, and size. A part of the tear duct passes through a canal in the lacrimal bone.

The *palatine bones* are L-shaped and are in the back part of the nasal cavity. They help form the roof of the mouth, the floor and outer walls of the nasal cavities, and the floor of each orbit. The vertical portion of the palatine bones extends to the orbit, and the horizontal part helps form the floor of the nasal cavity and the roof of the mouth.

The *maxilla* (maxillary arch) is formed by the union of the two maxillae. It helps to establish the boundaries of the roof of the mouth, the floor and outer walls of the nose, and the floor of each orbit. The maxilla is the largest bone of the upper face and is often referred to as the upper jaw. Each maxilla has a body (the main mass of the bone) and four processes. The body resembles a pyramid, and within its thin walls is a large cavity, the *maxillary sinus* (antrum of Highmore). On the lower part of the posterior surface of the body is the *maxillary tuberosity* (a rounded prominence or projection).

The four processes of the maxilla are named as follows: *zygomatic, palatine, frontal,* and alveolar. The zygomatic process joins the zygomatic bone to form the zygomatic arch, thus making up the cheek bone. The *palatine process* joins the opposing palatine process at the *palatine suture* to form the front part of the floor of the nasal cavity and the roof of the mouth. The *frontal process* extends upward and backward along the side of the nose. The alveolar process extends downward from the body of the maxilla. The sockets for the maxillary teeth are found in the alveolar process of the maxilla.

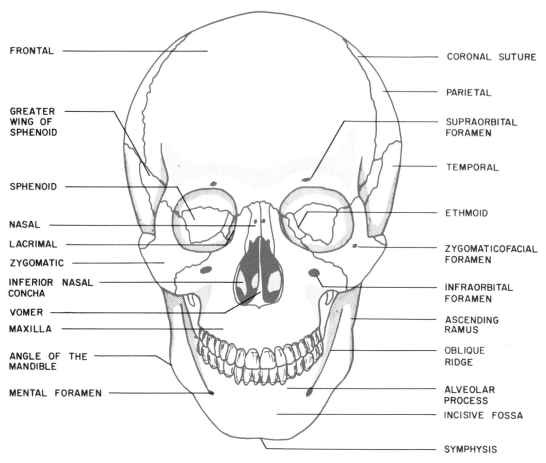

FRONTAL

CORONAL SUTURE

PARIETAL

GREATER WING OF SPHENOID

SUPRAORBITAL FORAMEN

TEMPORAL

SPHENOID

ETHMOID

NASAL

LACRIMAL

ZYGOMATICOFACIAL FORAMEN

ZYGOMATIC

INFERIOR NASAL CONCHA

INFRAORBITAL FORAMEN

VOMER

ASCENDING RAMUS

MAXILLA

OBLIQUE RIDGE

ANGLE OF THE MANDIBLE

ALVEOLAR PROCESS

MENTAL FORAMEN

INCISIVE FOSSA

SYMPHYSIS

Fig. 6–1. Skull, anterior aspect

REVIEW

1. The longest bone of the face is the _____.

2. The four processes of the maxilla are _____, _____, _____, and _____.

3. Another term for the maxillary sinus is _____.

4. The smallest and most fragile bones of the face are the _____ bones.

5. The _____ consist of cancellous bone and are located on the outer wall of each nostril.

6. Identify the lettered parts of the illustration. Select from the following list:

Frontal
Sphenoid
Greater wing of sphenoid
Lacrimal
Nasal
Inferior nasal conchae
Zygomatic
Vomer
Ascending ramus
Maxilla
Mastoid process
Oblique ridge
Mental foramen
Angle of the mandible
Coronal suture
Parietal
Supraorbital foramen
Ethmoid
Temporal
Zygomaticofacial foramen
Infraorbital foramen
Alveolar process
Symphysis
Incisive fossa

A. _____

B. _____

C. _____

D. _____

E. _____

F. _____

G. _____

H. _____

I. _____

J. _____

K. _____

L. _____

M. _____

N. _____

O. _____

P. _____

Q. _____

R. _____

S. _____

T. _____

U. _____

V. _____

W. _____

Chapter 7: The Mandible

OBJECTIVES: After studying this chapter, the student will be able to:
- Describe the anatomy of the mandible.
- Locate and name the three processes of the mandible.
- Define the term *condyle*.
- Locate, then describe the mental protuberance.
- Identify and locate the two sets of foramina found on the mandible.

The *mandible* is the only bone of the skull that is movable; it is the longest and strongest bone of the face. The mandible is sometimes referred to as the *lower jaw*. It consists of a body, a curved horizontal bone, and two perpendicular portions, the *ascending rami* (ramus, branch). The rami unite with the ends of the body, forming the *angle of the mandible*. The upper border of each ramus presents two distinct processes: the *coronoid process* on the anterior, and the *condyloid process* on the posterior. The posterior process is sometimes referred to as the *mandibular condyle* (condyle, a round projection at the end of a bone that fits into a depression on another bone). The condyloid process consists of a *neck* and a condyle. The condyle of the mandible normally rests in the mandibular (glenoid) fossa of the temporal bone. Between the coronoid and the condyloid

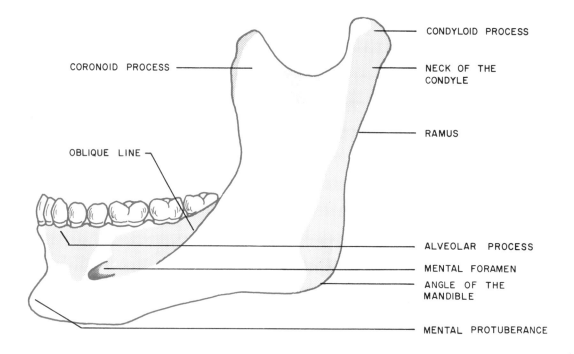

CONDYLOID PROCESS

NECK OF THE CONDYLE

CORONOID PROCESS

RAMUS

OBLIQUE LINE

ALVEOLAR PROCESS

MENTAL FORAMEN

ANGLE OF THE MANDIBLE

MENTAL PROTUBERANCE

Fig. 7–1. Mandible, lateral aspect

62

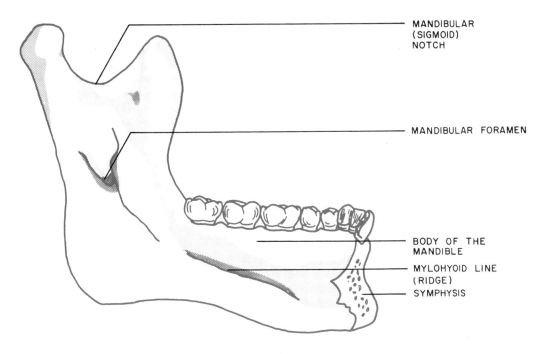

MANDIBULAR
(SIGMOID)
NOTCH

MANDIBULAR FORAMEN

BODY OF THE
MANDIBLE

MYLOHYOID LINE
(RIDGE)

SYMPHYSIS

Fig. 7–2. Mandible, medial aspect

processes is the *sigmoid notch* (or mandibular notch). It is a saddle-like depression in the bone.

The *body* is curved somewhat like a horseshoe with its external surface concave (possessing a curved, depressed surface). There is a thick ridge at the median line. This ridge, or *symphysis*, is the line of fusion where the two distinct bones of the mandible blend together into one. The symphysis divides below and fuses with the lower border of the mandible to enclose a triangular projection called the *mental protuberance* (mental, pertaining to the chin). From either side of the mental protuberance a ridge extends backward and upward and is continuous with the anterior border of the ramus. This ridge is called the *oblique line* (oblique, on a slant, neither perpendicular nor horizontal), figure 7-1.

The superior border of the body contains the **alveoli** (sockets for the teeth) and is called the *alveolar process*. Each alveolar process is composed of two compact bony plates: the external (buccal or labial [buccal, the cheek; labial, the lips]) and internal (lingual), or the surface nearest the tongue. Joining these surfaces are partitions, or septa, that make up the sides of the alveoli.

On the face of the skull are several important foramen. Above the eye orbits are the *supraorbital foramina* (supra, above); under the orbits of the eye on the maxilla are the *infraorbital foramina* (infra, inferior or below). On the zygomatics are the *zygomaticofacial foramina*, figure 6-1. On the lateral surface of the mandible are the *mental foramina*. On the lingual surface of the mandible (next to the tongue) are the *mandibular foramina*, figure 7-2. The *incisive fossae* are found on either side of the symphysis.

REVIEW

1. Name the two surfaces of the body of the mandible.

   a. _____

   b. _____

2. What are the two borders of the mandible?

   a. _____

   b. _____

3. Name the two processes of the ascending ramus.

   a. _____

   b. _____

4. Define the following words.

   a. Foramen _____

   _____

   b. Fossa _____

   _____

5. Identify the lettered parts of the illustration. Select from the following list:

Angle of the mandible   Coronoid process
Oblique line   Condyloid process
Mental foramina   Neck of the condyle
Mental protuberance   Ramus
Alveoli   Alveolar process

A._____

B._____

C._____

D._____

E._____

F._____

G._____

H._____

I._____

6. The only bone of the skull that is movable is the_____.

7. On which bones are the following foramina located?

   a. Infraorbital _____

   b. Supraorbital _____

   c. Zygomaticofacial_____

   d. Mental_____

8. The ascending rami of the mandible unite with the ends of the body to form the _____.

9. The condyloid process consists of a _____and
   a   _____.

10. The line of fusion where the two distinct bones of the mandible blend together into one is called the_____.

11. In the mandible, mental protuberance pertains to the _____.

12. Define the following words:

   a. Condyle _____

   _____

   b. Ramus_____

   _____

   c. Alveoli_____

   _____

13. Identify the lettered parts of the illustration. Select from the following list:

Mylohyoid line (ridge)   Body of the mandible
Mandibular foramina   Mandibular (sigmoid) notch
Alveoli   Symphysis

A. _____

B. _____

C. _____

D. _____

E. _____

14. The foramina under the orbits of the eye are called the _____,
    and those above the eye orbits are called the _____.

15. On the lateral surface of the mandible are the _____,
    and on the lingual surface are the _____.

16. Zygomaticofacial foramina are found on the _____.

OBJECTIVES:
After studying this chapter, the student will be able to:
- Locate and name the four bony parts of the roof of the oral cavity.
- Identify the median palatine suture.
- Identify the transverse palatine suture.
- Locate and describe the anterior palatine foramen.
- Identify the two greater palatine foramina.
- Locate the two lesser palatine foramina.

The oral cavity is only partially surrounded by bones. The lateral and interior walls are formed by the inner surface of the alveolar processes and join at the midline. The inner (lingual) surfaces of the teeth complete these walls.

The roof of the oral cavity, figure 8-1, is formed by the hard palate, which consists of four bony parts. These include the *palatine processes of the maxillae* and the *horizontal plates of the palatine bones*. Between the bones of the right and left halves of the palate is found the *median palatine suture*; between the maxillae and the palatine bones, the transverse palatine suture (transverse, a process that projects across the

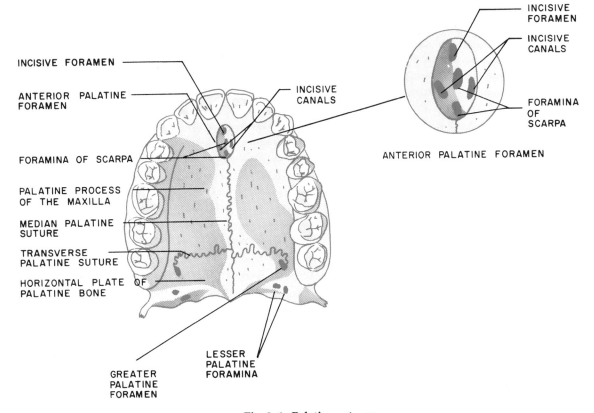

Fig. 8–1. Palatine sutures

palate). The bony processes are joined together by means of this cross-shaped suture.

At the midline, immediately behind the incisors, is the opening of the incisal or *anterior palatine foramen*. It appears to be funnel-shaped and serves as a common opening for the two *incisive* canals, two *foramina of Scarpa*, and the *incisive* foramen. The incisive foramen is the most anterior of the group. Posterior to the incisive foramen are two foramina, situated at the median line, called the foramina of Scarpa. Located laterally to the anterior palatine suture are the incisive canals.

Close to the posterior border of the hard palate and near the transverse palatine suture are other openings in the bone. Each palatine bone has three foramina. Just lingual to the third molar area is the greater palatine foramen. Behind this are found two smaller or lesser palatine foramina.

REVIEW

1. Identify the lettered parts of the illustration. Select from the following list:

Foramina of Scarpa
Palatine process of the maxilla
Transverse palatine suture
Median palatine suture
Horizontal plate of
  palatine bone

Incisive foramen
Anterior palatine foramen
Greater palatine foramen
Lesser palatine foramina
Incisive canals
Alveolar process

A. _____

B. _____

C. _____

D. _____

E. _____

F. _____

G. _____

H. _____

I. _____

J. _____

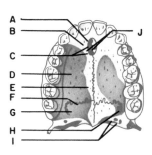

2. The hard palate of the oral cavity consist of four bony parts. Name them.

    a. _____

    b. _____

    c. _____

    d. _____

3. How are the lateral and interior walls of the hard palate formed? _____

_____

_____

Chapter 9: Muscles of Mastication

OBJECTIVES:

After studying this chapter, the student will be able to:
- Define muscle contraction and relaxation.
- Locate the masseter muscle, and determine its insertion.
- Define the word *synergist*, and identify the muscles involved.
- Locate the external pterygoid muscle, and state its function.
- Determine the muscles that control the movements of the mandible and temporomandibular joint.

INTRODUCTION

Movements of the mandible are controlled principally by four pairs of muscles known as the *muscles of mastication* (masticate, chew or grind with the teeth). These muscle *pairs* are the *temporals*, *masseters*, *internal pterygoids*, and *external pterygoids*. Some knowledge of the function and action of these muscles is necessary to fully understand their importance, figure 9-1.

Muscles, generally, have two reactions or reverse movements, termed contraction and relaxation. Contraction is the change in muscles by which they become thickened and shortened. During relaxation, muscles become less tense or rigid. Even when there is no visible movement, not all fibers of the muscles are completely relaxed. Instead, some remain in a slight state of contraction called *muscle tone*, or *tonus*.

Most muscles extend from one bone to another bone, and each is attached to one of these

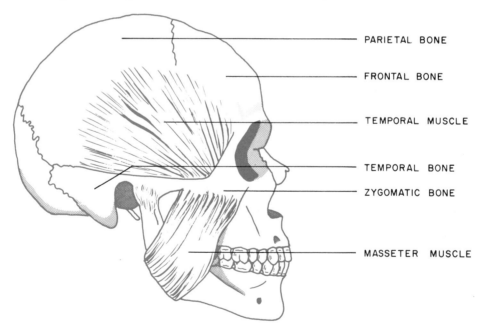

PARIETAL BONE

FRONTAL BONE

TEMPORAL MUSCLE

TEMPORAL BONE

ZYGOMATIC BONE

MASSETER MUSCLE

Fig. 9–1. Mastication muscles

bones by tendons (fibrous cords). The muscles of mastication are found chiefly in the face and are attached at one end to the skin, causing it to move. The point of attachment at the other end of the muscle is more or less stationary and is called the *origin*. The point of attachment that moves is called the *insertion*.

THE TEMPORALS

The *temporal* muscle is a broad, radiating, or fan-shaped muscle. Situated on the lateral surface of the skull, its origin is a wide field that tends to fill the temporal fossa. This field is composed of a narrow strip of the parietal bone, the temporal surface of the greater frontal bone, and the temporal surface of the greater wing of the sphenoid bone. Its fibers converge as they descend and are inserted into the medial surface, the apex (or pointed end) and anterior border of the coronoid process, and the anterior border of the ramus nearly to the third molar area.

The temporal muscle is built for movement rather than power and serves mainly to elevate the mandible and close the jaws. Its posterior fibers have a retracting action because of their slanting direction downward and forward. The zygomatic process acts as a pulley. Below this process, the action of the muscle is very significant, figure 9-2.

THE MASSETERS

The *masseter* muscle is the most superficial (superficial, on or near the *surface*) of the muscles of mastication and stretches as a rectangular plate from the zygomatic arch to the outer surface of the mandible. It consists of two portions that can be separated, although not completely, into a superficial and a deep portion. The superficial portion, the larger of the two, arises by a thick, strong bundle of tendinous fibers from the zygomatic process of the maxilla and from the anterior two-thirds of the lower border of the

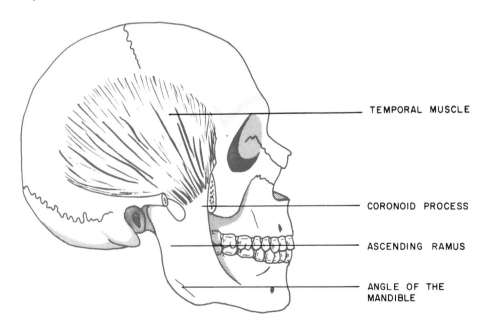

TEMPORAL MUSCLE

CORONOID PROCESS

ASCENDING RAMUS

ANGLE OF THE MANDIBLE

Fig. 9–2. Mastication muscles (view with zygomatic arch removed)

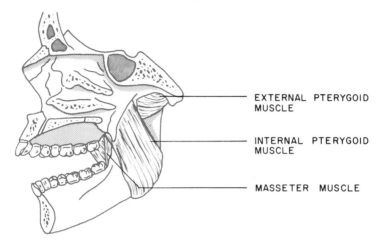

Fig. 9–3. Internal pterygoid muscle, medial aspect

zygomatic arch. The fibers have a general direction downward and backward; their insertion is the angle and lower half of the ramus. The deep portion is smaller and more muscular by nature; its origin is the posterior third of the lower border and the whole of the medial surface of the zygomatic arch. Its fibers pass downward and forward and are inserted in the upper half of the ramus and lateral surface of the coronoid process of the mandible. Refer to Chapter 7.

The masseter is composed of long, parallel fibers and is primarily a muscle of great power and fast contractility. It is capable of exerting much pressure upon the teeth, especially in the molar region. As the superficial fibers protract, or extend, in the closing movement of the jaw, the deep fibers retract.

THE INTERNAL PTERYGOIDS

The *internal pterygoid* muscle (also known as the medial pterygoid muscle) is rectangular in shape, is powerful, and acts as a counterpart to the masseter. It is positioned on the medial side of the ramus of the mandible with its origin in the pterygoid fossa. Three points of origin, or heads, are apparent: one on the medial surface of the lateral pterygoid plate of the sphenoid bone, another at the palatine bone, and a third at the maxillary tuberosity.

The internal structure of the internal pterygoid muscle is an intricate combination of both fleshy and tendinous fibers that arise from one tendon and end on another. These fibers are arranged at an angle to the general direction of the muscle. It is this braided arrangement that tends to increase the power of the muscle.

From the pterygoid fossa, the internal pterygoid muscle runs downward, backward, and outward; its insertion is the medial surface of the angle of the mandible and the medial surface of the ramus, as high as the mandibular foramen. Fibers of the internal pterygoid may meet fibers of the masseter behind and below the angle of the mandible. Its superficial part is a *synergist* of (works with) the masseter muscle and assists in closing the jaws.

Because the main pull of the internal pterygoid is directed upward, this muscle is not able to shift the mandible to one side or the other except in synergism with the masseter muscle. They are so placed that they suspend the angle of the mandible in a sling, which functions in the

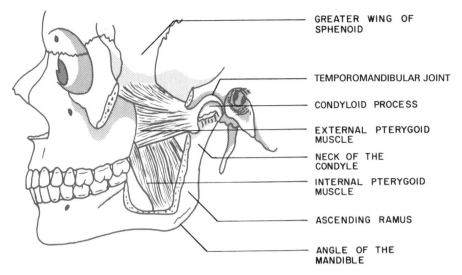

GREATER WING OF SPHENOID

TEMPOROMANDIBULAR JOINT

CONDYLOID PROCESS

EXTERNAL PTERYGOID MUSCLE

NECK OF THE CONDYLE

INTERNAL PTERYGOID MUSCLE

ASCENDING RAMUS

ANGLE OF THE MANDIBLE

**Fig. 9–4. External and internal pterygoid muscle, lateral aspect
(view with zygomatic arch and coronoid process removed)**

articulation of the maxilla and mandible; this is termed the *mandibular sling*, figure 9-3.

THE EXTERNAL PTERYGOIDS

The *external pterygoid* muscle (lateral pterygoid muscle) is a thick, short muscle that arises with two heads. The larger and inferior head arises from the outer surface of the lateral pterygoid plate; the smaller and superior head arises from the lower part of the lateral surface of the greater wing of sphenoid and from the infratemporal fossa. The fibers of the upper head run horizontally backward and outward. The fibers of the lower head converge upward and outward; the upper fibers run more horizontally, and the lower fibers ascend more steeply, figure 9-4. The two heads are separted anteriorly by a gap that varies in width, but they may fuse in front of the temporomandibular joint and can be separated only artificially.

The external pterygoid muscle's action is to open the jaw and protrude it (protrude, to thrust forward).

THE TEMPOROMANDIBULAR JOINT

The *temporomandibular joint* (TMJ) is so named because of the two bones that form the joint—the temporal bone and the mandible. It is located between the mandibular fossa and the *articular tubercle* (tubercle, a small, rounded bone on a bone for attachment of a tendon). On the condyle lies a disc of tough, fibrous tissue called the interarticular disc often referred to as the meniscus (meniscus, a fibrous cartilage within a joint). The thickness and curvature of the disc are varied and conform to the shape of the bones.

Surrounding the meniscus is a dense, fibrous capsule (enclosed sac), the *capsular ligament*, which completely surfaces the TMJ and is attached to the neck of the condyle and to the nearby surfaces of the temporal bone. The disc divides the space between the *glenoid fossa* and the condyle into two cavities. These cavities lie above and below the meniscus and are filled with *synovial fluid* (synovia, a thick, sticky fluid found in joints of bones).

The three *osseus* (osseus, bony) portions making up the TMJ are: (1) the *glenoid fossa*, an oval depression in the temporal bone lying anterior to the ear canal external acoustic meatus; (2) the *articular tubercle*, a raised portion of the temporal bone just anterior to the glenoid fossa, and (3) the *condyloid process* of the mandible. The condyloid process lies in the glenoid fossa with the meniscus separating the bones. The mandible, the only movable bone of the face, is attached to the cranium by the ligaments of the joint.

The majority of the fibers of the capsular ligament are inserted into a depression on the anterior surface of the neck of the condyle. The uppermost fibers of the external pterygoid muscle are attached to the anterior surface of the articular tubercle and the anterior border of the interarticular disc (meniscus). The posterior fibers of the temporal retract the mandible, figure 9–5.

Although supported by ligaments, the temporal, masseter and external and internal pterygoid muscles of mastication control the movements of the mandible and of the TMJ. The left and right TMJs function in unison and are capable of both hinge and gliding actions in mouth opening.

The *hinge action* of the mouth opening uses only the synovial cavity below the meniscus with the head of the condyle rotating around a point on the underside of the meniscus. The body of the mandible drops downward and backward.

The *gliding action* of the mouth opening involves both the upper and lower synovial cavities of the TMJ. This consists of a gliding of the condyle and meniscus forward and downward along the articular disc during protrusion and lateral movements of the mandible during mastication.

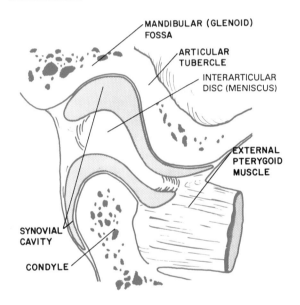

Fig. 9–5. Temporomandibular joint

REVIEW

1. What is the origin of the masseter muscle? _____

   _____

2. Where is the insertion of the masseter muscle?_____

   _____

3. What is the action of the masseter muscle? _____

   _____

4. Identify the lettered parts of the illustration. Select from the following list:

Masseter muscle
Temporal muscle
Coronoid process
Zygomatic bone
Frontal bone
Parietal bone
Temporal bone

A. _____

B. _____

C. _____

D. _____

E. _____

F. _____

5. Identify the lettered parts of the illustration. Select from the following list:

Coronoid process
Zygomatic bone
Angle of mandible
Ascending ramus

A. _____

B. _____

C. _____

6. Identify the lettered parts of the illustration. Select from the following list:

Ascending ramus   Greater wing of sphenoid
Angle of the mandible   Condyloid process
Masseter muscle   Neck of the condyle

A. _____

B. _____

C. _____

D. _____

E. _____

7. Identify the lettered parts of the illustration. Select from the following list:

Internal pterygoid muscle
External pterygoid muscle
Neck of the condyle
Masseter muscle

A. _____

B. _____

C. _____

8. Identify the lettered parts of the illustration. Select from the following list:

Mandibular (glenoid) fossa   Interarticular disc (meniscus)
Synovial cavity   Condyle
Ascending ramus   External pterygoid muscle
Articular tubercle

A. _____

B. _____

C. _____

D. _____

E. _____

F. _____

G. _____

9. The temporal muscle arises from _____

_____.

10. The insertion of the temporalis is _____

_____.

11. The action of the temporal muscle is _____

_____.

12. The larger, inferior head of the external pterygoid muscles arises from _____

_____.

13. The insertion of the external pterygoid is _____

_____.

14. Three main actions of the external pterygoid muscle are:

a. _____

b. _____

c. _____

15. With which muscles does the internal pterygoid act in synergism? _____

_____

16. The internal pterygoid arises from _____

_____.

17. The insertion of the internal pterygoid is _____

_____,

and it acts to_____.

18. Define *muscle tonus.* _____

    _____

19. Define *synovial fluid.* _____

    _____

20. a. Which muscle of mastication is the most superficial? _____

    _____

    b. Which muscle acts as its counterpart? _____

    _____

    c. What is the combination of the two muscles called? What is its function?

    _____

21. Muscles generally remain in a state of _____ contraction.

22. Most muscles are attached to bones by _____.

23. The more or less stationary attachment of muscles is referred to as its_____

    _____.

24. The portion of a muscle attachment that moves is called its_____

    _____.

25. The zygomatic process acts as a pulley for the _____muscle.

26. The main pull of the internal pterygoid is directed_____.

27. The muscles of mastication are all supported by _____.

28. The interarticular disc in the TMJ is separated from the condyle by _____

    _____.

Chapter 10: The Paranasal Sinuses

OBJECTIVES: After studying this chapter, the student will be able to:
- Locate and name the air cells of the anterior group of paranasal sinuses.
- Locate and name the air cells of the posterior group of paranasal sinuses.
- Identify the largest of the paranasal sinuses.
- Discuss the various sizes and shapes of the sinuses.
- List the functions of the paranasal sinuses.

INTRODUCTION

Air cavities in the bones above and on each side of the nasal cavities are termed *paranasal sinuses*. They vary in shape and size in individuals and are normally lined with a mucous membrane that is continuous with that of the nasal cavities, figure 10–1.

Proper ventilation and drainage of the **sinuses** is important because of their close proximity to the roots of the maxillary bicuspids and molars. Any physiological dysfunction may result in serious sinus infection, which is often directly related to the maxillary teeth, sinuses, or both. Maxillary sinus inflammation, or maxillary sinusitis, is frequently accompanied by tenderness of some of the maxillary teeth.

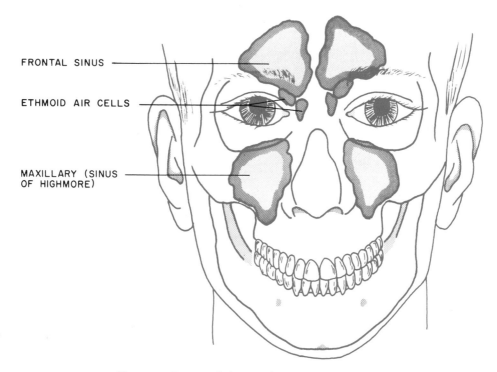

FRONTAL SINUS

ETHMOID AIR CELLS

MAXILLARY (SINUS OF HIGHMORE)

Fig. 10–1. Paranasal sinuses, front cross-sectional view

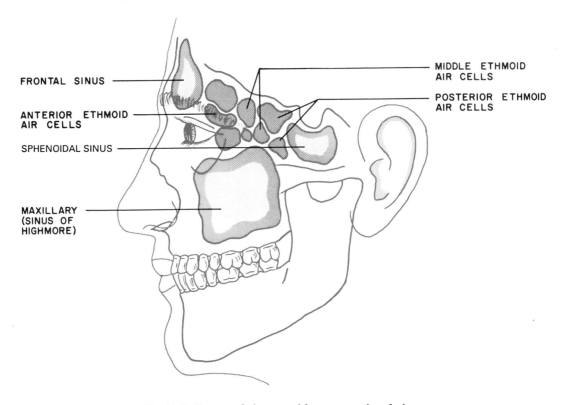

Fig. 10–2. Paranasal sinuses, side cross-sectional view

GROUPS OF SINUSES

The air cells of the nose are the frontal, ethmoidal, sphenoidal, and maxillary. They are named after the bones in which they are located and consist of two groups:

1. *Anterior group* or those opening into the middle meatus (opening or passage) of the nose:
   - maxillary sinus (antrum of Highmore)
   - frontal sinus
   - anterior and middle ethmoid cells
2. *Posterior group*
   - sphenoidal sinus (opens into the sphenoethmoidal recess)
   - posterior ethmoid cells (open into the superior meatus

Anterior Group

Maxillary Sinus. This is a pyramid-shaped cavity in the body of the maxilla and is the largest accessory sinus of the nose. The base is formed by the lateral wall of the nasal cavity, and its apex extends into the zygomatic process. The size of the sinus varies from side to side in the individual but is situated usually below the floor of the nose. In some cases, the floor is perforated with the apical portion of some of the maxillary teeth. The roof of the maxillary sinus is often ridged with elevations of the infraorbital canal, figure 10–2.

Frontal Sinus. The frontal sinus is situated behind the superciliary arch (above the eyebrow). Such a cavity is rarely symmetrical because of the placement of the septum. It drains through the frontonasal duct into the main cavity of the middle meatus and opens from either the right or left, according to its lateral position.

Anterior and Middle Ethmoid Cells. Ethmoid cells consist of a number of thin-walled cavities and are situated between the upper parts of the nasal sinuses and orbits. They are separated from these cavities by thin bony plates.

Posterior Group

Sphenoidal Sinuses. Contained within the body of the sphenoid, the sphenoidal sinuses vary in shape and size and, as in the case of other sinuses, are rarely symmetrical. If they are exceptionally large, they may extend into the great wing of the sphenoid or the roots of the pterygoid process;

they may also enter the base of the occipital bone. An opening is found in the superior part of the anterior wall of sphenoidal sinuses.

Posterior Ethmoid Cells. The posterior ethmoid cells open into the superior meatus under the superior nasal concha. They may, in some cases, connect with the sphenoidal sinus.

FUNCTIONS

1. Reduce the weight of the skull.
2. Give resonance to the voice.
3. Act as reserve chambers for warm air during the physiological process of respiration. During inspiration, the warmed air from the sinuses is drawn into the lungs.*

REVIEW

1. Identify the lettered parts of the illustration. Select from the following list:

   Frontal sinus
   Ethmoid air cells
   Sphenoidal sinus
   Maxillary (sinus of Highmore)

   A. _____

   B. _____

   C. _____

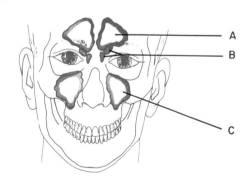

2. The largest paranasal sinus of the skull is the _____.

3. The membrane that lines the paranasal sinuses is the _____.

* Massler, Moury, and Schour, Isaac, *Atlas of the Mouth*, 2nd Ed., American Dental Association, Chicago, IL, 1982.

4. List four symptoms of a sinus infection.

   a. _____

   b. _____

   c. _____

   d. _____

5. What are the three chief characteristics of a dentogenic sinus infection?

   a. _____

   b. _____

   c. _____

6. Another term for nostrils is _____.

7. Identify the lettered parts of the illustration. Select from the following list:

Frontal sinus
Anterior ethmoid air cells
Middle ethmoid air cells
Posterior ethmoid air cells
Sphenoidal sinus
Superciliary arch
Maxillary sinus (antrum of Highmore)

A. _____

B. _____

C. _____

D. _____

E. _____

F. _____

Chapter 11: The Oral Cavity (Mouth)

OBJECTIVES:

After studying this chapter, the student will be able to:
- Describe the basic parts of the mouth cavity.
- Locate and describe the glossopalatine arch.
- Locate and name the two mucosal attachments (frenum) found in the mouth.
- Distinguish the differences of shape and location of the taste buds on the tongue.
- Determine which taste buds are larger in size.

The cavity of the mouth is nearly oval-shaped and consists of two parts: an outer and smaller portion, the *vestibule* (vestibule, an opening, forming an entrance to another cavity), and the inner and larger part, the *mouth cavity* proper.

The vestibule is a slitlike opening, bounded externally by the lips and cheeks and internally by the gums and teeth. The mouth cavity proper is roofed by the *hard palate*, figure 11–1, view A. In the posterior is the *soft palate*, which lacks the bony quality of the hard palate. The greater part of the floor is formed by the tongue. The entire cavity is covered with mucous membrane, or *mucosa*.

The lips are two fleshy folds surrounding the *orifice* (orifice, opening) of the mouth. The inner surface of each lip is connected at the medial line by a fold of mucous membrane, the *frenulum* or *labial frenum*, to the gum tissue (**gingivae**). The upper attachment, or frenum, is larger and stronger than the lower attachment, figure 11–2, view B.

The *cheeks* (buccae) form the sides of the face and are continuous in front with the lips.

The soft palate, in a relaxed state and with its lower border free, appears to hang as a curtain-like partition and is referred to as the *palatine velum* (velum, veil-like). It is continuous with the *glossopalatine arch* (glosso, tongue; palatine, pertaining to palate). Suspended from the middle of its lower border is a small, conical, fleshy body, the *palatine uvula*. Posterior to the glossopalatine arch is the *pharyngopalatine arch* (pharyngo refers to pharynx, the cavity that connects the mouth and nasal passages with the esophagus and stomach).

The palatine tonsils are two prominent masses located on either side of the oral cavity between the glossopalatine and pharyngopalatine arches. The tonsils consist basically of lymphatic tissue, figure 4–6.

The *tongue* (lingua) lies on the floor of the mouth, within the curve of the mandible. The tongue is the principal organ of taste and an important organ of speech. It assists in mastication (the act of chewing) and deglutition (the act of swallowing) of food. The *dorsum* (the upper surface) of the tongue is marked by a *median sulcus* that divides it into symmetrical halves (corresponding parts in size and form) on either side of the sulcus. Thickly distributed over the anterior two-thirds of the dorsum are projections, or *papillae* filiform (filiform, cone-shaped). Scattered irregularly and sparingly over the dorsum are large, round projections of a deep red color called *papillae fungiform* (fungiform, mushroom-shaped). They are narrow at their attachment to the tongue and broad and rounded at their free edges; they are covered with secondary papillae, figure 11–2, view B.

At the back of the tongue are the *papillae vallate* (vallate, cup-shape), large in size and varying in

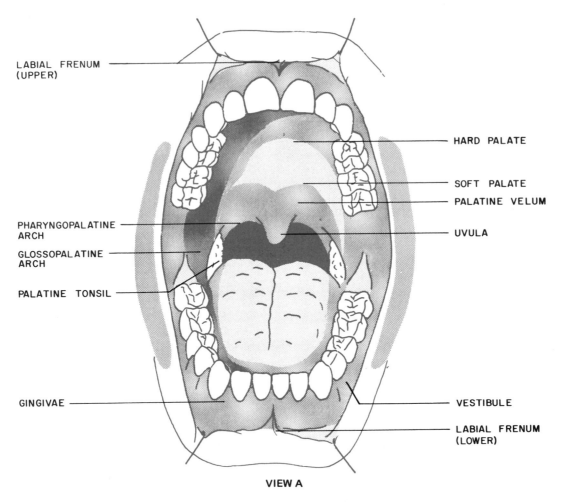

LABIAL FRENUM
(UPPER)

HARD PALATE

SOFT PALATE
PALATINE VELUM

PHARYNGOPALATINE
ARCH

UVULA

GLOSSOPALATINE
ARCH

PALATINE TONSIL

GINGIVAE

VESTIBULE

LABIAL FRENUM
(LOWER)

VIEW A

Fig. 11–1. The mouth—view A

number from eight to twelve. Usually found in two rows, the papillae form a *V* (inverted form) at the median line. Each papilla is in the form of a truncated cone (a cone-shaped object appearing to have its apex cut off) from 1 to 2 millimeters (mm) wide with the smaller end directed downward and attached to the tongue. The *taste buds* are scattered over the mucous membrane of the mouth and tongue at irregular intervals. They are found especially in the sides of the papillae vallate.

For a substance to have a taste, it must be soluble; that is, the substance must be dissolved in the saliva and must come in contact with the taste buds. The four primary tastes are sweet, sour, salty, and bitter. Although a specific taste bud transmits only one of the primary taste sensations, most of them respond to a lesser extent to substances that produce one or two of the other primary tastes. It is probably the combination of response on the part of two or three types of taste buds that characterizes the specific taste sensation associated with a particular substance.

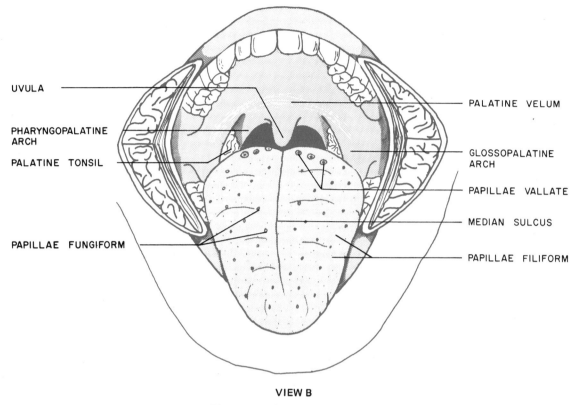

UVULA

PHARYNGOPALATINE ARCH

PALATINE TONSIL

PAPILLAE FUNGIFORM

PALATINE VELUM

GLOSSOPALATINE ARCH

PAPILLAE VALLATE

MEDIAN SULCUS

PAPILLAE FILIFORM

VIEW B

Fig. 11–2. The mouth—view B

The acid taste is usually transmitted through the taste buds on the anterior half of the tongue toward the midline; sweet and salty are on the lateral borders of the tongue in the anterior portion. The bitter taste is transmitted through receptors in the posterior third of the tongue.

REVIEW

1. Without referring to the preceding pages, identify the lettered parts of the illustration. Select from the following list:

Palatine tonsil   Papillae filiform
Gingivae   Hard palate
Labial frenum   Soft palate
Glossopalatine arch   Palatine velum
Pharyngopalatine arch   Uvula
Vestibule

A. _____

B. _____

C. _____

D. _____

E. _____

F. _____

G. _____

H. _____

I. _____

J. _____

K. _____

2. Match the facts in Column I with the right response from Column II.

Column I

_____1. Continuous with palatine velum

_____2. Covers entire mouth cavity

_____3. Larger of the taste buds

_____4. Anterior portion of roof of mouth

_____5. Middle anterior of the tongue

_____6. Is location of frenum attachment

_____7. Transmits bitter taste sensations

_____8. Smaller and weaker frenum

Column II

A. Mucosa
B. Uvula
C. Papilla fungiform
D. Papillae vallate
E. Hard palate
F. Lower frenum
G. Upper frenum
H. Posterior third of tongue
I.   Median line of inner lip surface

3. Identify the lettered parts of the illustration. Select from the following list:

Pharyngopalatine arch   Glossopalatine arch
Palatine tonsil   Papillae vallate
Uvula   Median sulcus
Papillae fungiform   Papillae filiform
Palatine velum   Hard palate

A. _____

B. _____

C. _____

D. _____

E. _____

F. _____

G. _____

H. _____

I. _____

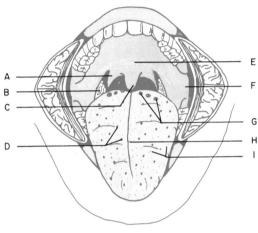

Chapter 12: Salivary Glands

INTRODUCTION

The mucous membrane that lines the oral cavity is called the *oral mucosa*. Under the oral mucosa in certain areas, such as the lips, the cheeks, and the palate, are the *minor salivary glands*. In addition, there are *major salivary glands* that supply secretions to the oral cavity. Some of the salivary glands are serous glands; i.e., they secrete *serum* (serous pertains to serum, a clear liquid). Others are *mucous glands* (mucous, or mucin, a slimy, gluelike secretion). Some are *mixed glands* that secrete both serum and **mucus**. Secretions of the major and minor salivary glands become mixed or blended to form *saliva*. In this chapter the importance of the major salivary glands is stressed, figure 12–1.

Secretion is defined as the biological expulsion of material that has been chemically modified by

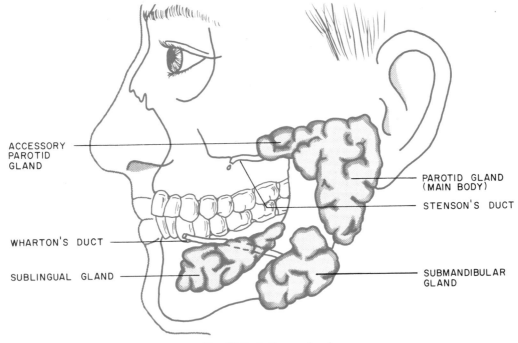

Fig. 12–1. Salivary glands

a cell to serve a purpose elsewhere in the body or in some body process. Saliva protects the lining of the mouth (mucous membrane) against drying and aids in *expectoration* (the act of ejecting or spitting out) of injurious or distasteful substances. Saliva makes speech easier through the continuous moistening of the oral tissues and the teeth. Saliva lubricates food, aiding its passage to the stomach. In man, as in some other mammals, saliva contains a digestive enzyme called *salivary amylase* (ptyalin). The suffix "-ase" designates an enzyme (enzyme, a secretion of living cells capable of causing or accelerating a chemical reaction). Amylase refers to enzyme action on *amylon* (from the Greek word for starch).

Salivary amylase is an enzyme that splits cooked starches. It breaks down the complex molecule to simple components. Although this action happens rather quickly, salivary digestion is usually incomplete by the time the food is swallowed, even though the chewing process has been conscientiously prolonged. Most of the enzyme action occurs within the saliva-saturated mass of food during the passage of the food from the mouth to the stomach before the gastric juice of the stomach has been mixed with the food.

It is remarkable to note that salivary amylase cannot split starches into simple sugars; and double sugars taken by mouth as such (e.g., ordinary cane sugar) are unaffected by this enzyme. The reason for this is unknown but acceptable when it is realized that double sugars (disaccharides) cannot be absorbed by the body as such. Further enzyme action is necessary for the breakdown of double sugars into absorbable simple sugars; this occurs later in the small intestine.

The salivary glands lie just outside the oral cavity proper and are connected to the cavity by ducts (duct, a canal or passage for fluids). Their secretions are controlled under normal conditions by various stimuli, such as touching the oral mucosa and the smell, sight, or thought of food.

Many tiny mucous glands lie under the mucosa of the hard and soft palates, see Chapter 8. Some of the largest mucous glands of the palate are found near the base of the uvula (see figure 11–1). The buccal areas also have tiny mucous glands that secrete constantly into the vestibule.

Of the many glands that supply the oral cavity, there are three pairs of major salivary glands: the *parotid*, *submandibular*, and *sublingual*.

PAROTID GLANDS

The *parotid* (parotid, near the ear) is a serum-secreting gland and lies in front of and below the ear, one on either side of the face; it is the largest salivary gland. It is positioned between the external ear and the angle of the mandible. Above, it is broad and reaches nearly to the zygomatic arch. A small projection of the parotid gland passes over the upper portion of the masseter muscle (refer to Chapter 9). This small part, separated from the main body of the gland by a slight groove, is often referred to as the *accessory parotid gland* (accessory, a subordinate or added part). The lower part of the main body is somewhat tapered and reaches below the level of a line joining the tip of the mastoid process and the angle of the mandible. The remainder of the gland is irregularly wedge-shaped and extends deeply inward toward the styloid process and the muscles arising from it. The *parotid duct* (also called Stenson's duct) enters the mouth opposite the buccal surface of the maxillary second molar tooth. The location of the opening of the duct in the oral cavity is marked by a small flap of tissue, the *parotid papilla*, which varies greatly in size and shape. The secretion of the parotid is almost entirely *ptyalin*, or *amylase*.

SUBMANDIBULAR GLANDS

One *submandibular gland* is located on each side of the face. The gland is irregular in shape and about the size of a walnut. It is a mixed salivary gland, one that contains both serum- and mucus-secreting cells and that secretes both ptyalin and mucin. The serous cells contribute the major part of the secretion. The submandibular gland lies beneath the lower jaw and discharges its secretion into the oral cavity through the *submandibular duct* (Wharton's duct) at the anterior base of the tongue and on either side of the lingual frenum. The opening is marked by an elevation, the sublingual caruncle (a small fleshy elevation). Occasionally, the duct may become closed due to the formation of salivary calculus (a hard mass containing lime salts and found in saliva). This partial or complete closure of the duct produces swelling of the floor of the mouth. On the other hand, stimulation of the gland may induce secretion so forcefully that the liquid is released in tiny streams that spurt completely out of the oral cavity.

SUBLINGUAL GLANDS

The *sublingual gland* is the smallest of the major salivary glands. It is situated beneath the mucous membrane of the floor of the mouth and is primarily mucus-secreting; its secretion does not contain ptyalin. It is situated on either side of the base of the tongue and is shaped somewhat like an almond. The ducts number from eight to twenty. The numerous small ducts (ducts of Rivinus) and the single larger duct (duct of Bartholin) either join the mandibular duct or open directly onto the floor of the mouth. Any infection of the sublingual gland results in swelling of the floor of the mouth and pain during movement of the tongue.

REVIEW

1. Identify the lettered parts of the illustration. Select from the following list:

Sublingual gland
Submandibular gland
Wharton's duct
Ducts of Rivinus
Accessory parotid gland
Parotid gland (main body)
Stenson's duct

A. _____

B. _____

C. _____

D. _____

E. _____

F. _____

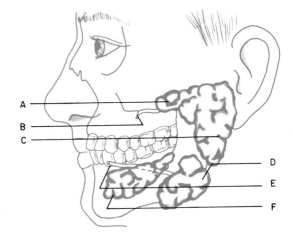

2. Define *gland*. _____

_____

3. Define *duct*. _____

_____

4. Another term for the parotid duct is _____.

   Another term for the opening of the parotid duct is _____.

5. Name the four functions of the salivary glands *not* related to chemical digestion.

   a. _____

   b. _____

   c. _____

   d. _____

6. What stimuli normally control the flow of secretion of the salivary glands?

_____

_____

7. Which of the sublingual ducts are smaller? _____

_____

8. What is the major duct of the sublingual gland called? _____

_____

9. Which of the salivary glands is the largest? The smallest? ____

_____

10. What salivary glands secrete ptyalin? What salivary glands do not secrete ptyalin? _____

_____

11. What is meant by digestion? _____

_____

12. What part does saliva play in digestion? _____

_____

_____

_____

13. What is meant by the phrase "a mixed salivary gland"?_____

_____

OBJECTIVES:

After studying this chapter, the student will be able to:
- Name the three divisions of the trigeminal nerve.
- Discuss the areas of the face and head supplied by the ophthalmic division of the trigeminal nerve.
- Locate the maxillary division of the trigeminal nerve, and determine its branches and the areas it supplies.
- Locate the mandibular division of the trigeminal nerve, and discuss how it differs with the two other nerve divisions.
- Locate and discuss the four ganglions found with the cranial nervous system of the trigeminal nerve.

INTRODUCTION

The nerves that supply the region of the oral cavity and face are called *cranial nerves*. There are three kinds of nerves: *sensory* (those concerned with sensation), *motor* (those that stimulate movement of muscles), and *mixed* (those possessing both sensory and motor nerve fibers).

This chapter is concerned with the *trigeminal nerve* (tri-, three; geminal, paired, or in twos), largest of the twelve cranial nerves. All cranial nerves come in pairs (a right and a left); the trigeminal nerve is paired and has three main branches, or divisions. The trigeminal nerve is called the *fifth cranial nerve*, the number corresponding to its position on the brain in relation to the other cranial nerves.

TRIGEMINAL NERVE

The fifth cranial, or trigeminal nerve, emerges from the midbrain and passes forward for a short distance. It then spreads fanlike to form a *ganglion* (ganglion, a mass of nerve cells found outside the brain or spinal canal). This mass is called the *gasserian*, or *semilunar ganglion* (semi, half; lunar, moon; i.e., it is half-moon or crescent-shaped). The small motor portion of the trigeminal nerve passes along a course below the semi-lunar ganglion and joins the mandibular branch, continuing on, beside the *otic ganglion* (otic, ear). The sensory portion that forms the gasserian ganglion receives fibers from three main divisions: the *ophthalmic* (ophthalmic, eye), *maxillary*, and *mandibular* nerves.

Ophthalmic Division

The *ophthalmic division* (first division) of the trigeminal nerve is the smallest branch from the gasserian ganglion. It passes forward and leaves the cranium through an opening in the posterior wall of the orbit, called the *superior orbital fissure* (fissure, or natural groove, found in the orbit). Before this division leaves the cranium, it divides into three branches: the *frontal*, *lacrimal* (lacrimal, tears), and *nasal* (nasociliary) nerves, figure 13–1.

This division of the trigeminal nerve supplies: (1) the lacrimal gland; (2) the skin of the eyelids, eyebrows, forehead and nose; (3) part of the mucous membrane of the nasal cavity; (4) the cornea (the "window" of the eye) and conjunctiva (delicate membrane lining the eyelids and covering the eyeball); (5) the ciliary body (muscle attached to the lens of the eye that helps to focus the eye); and (6) the iris (pigmented membrane surrounding the pupil), which gives the eye its color and controls the amount of light entering the eye.

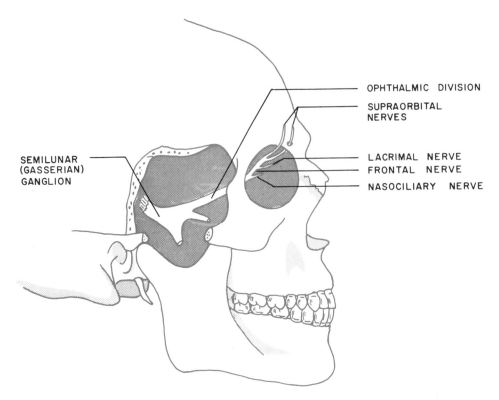

Fig. 13–1. Trigeminal nerve, ophthalmic division

The *frontal* nerve is the largest branch of the ophthalmic nerve and appears to be a direct continuation of it. It passes into the superior orbital fissure and eventually divides into the *supraorbital* and *supratrochlear* nerves, which supply the anterior part of the scalp. The supraorbital nerve leaves the orbit through the supraorbital foramen, ascends up the frontal bone, and divides into a middle (medial) and lateral branch. It is distributed to the upper eyelids, the covering of the forehead, and the scalp. The supratrochlear nerve passes over the *trochlea* (the pulley-shaped muscle that controls the superior oblique muscle of the eye). The supratrochlear nerve, a branch of the trigeminal (ophthalmic division), is purely sensory.

The *lacrimal* nerve sends branches to the lacrimal gland and the tissues of the upper eyelid.

The *nasociliary branch* passes below the *superior rectus muscle* of the eye (its fibers are connected to the eyeball). A branch of the nasociliary nerve, the *posterior ethmoidal*, passes through the posterior ethmoidal foramen and continues downward to supply the posterior ethmoidal sinuses and the sphenoidal sinus (refer to Chapter 5, figure 5–3). The *infratrochlear* nerve of the nasociliary branch passes forward and below the trochlea of the superior oblique muscle of the eye; its small branches end in the tissues at the corner of the eye and supply the tissues of this region.

Maxillary Division

The *maxillary division* (second division) of the trigeminal, a sensory nerve, leaves the cranial vault by way of the *foramen rotundum* (rotundum, or round; i.e., a large round, natural opening in

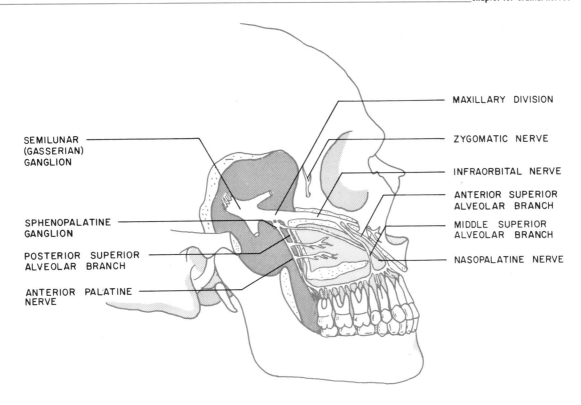

Fig. 13–2. Trigeminal nerve, maxillary division

the bone of the greater wing of sphenoid through which the superior maxillary nerve passes). It then enters the pterygopalatine fossa and divides into three main branches: the *infraorbital*, *zygomatic*, and *sphenopalatine* nerves.

Infraorbital Nerve. The *infraorbital branch* is the largest branch of the maxillary nerve. It passes through the infraorbital canal, emerges from the bone through the infraorbital foramen, and branches into three superior alveolar nerves: the *anterior superior alveolar, middle superior alveolar,* and *posterior superior alveolar.* The terminal fibers of these branches supply the tissues below the orbit, the lateral tissues of the nose, and the upper lip, figure 13–2.

The *anterior superior alveolar branch* travels forward and downward through the bone beneath the infraorbital foramen and sends its fibers into the pulp chambers of the maxillary central incisor, lateral incisor, and cuspid teeth, the periodontal membrane, and the gingivae of this area. Some fibers pass forward to innervate the mucous membrane of the oral cavity just below the nose.

The *middle superior alveolar branch* moves in a forward direction through the bone and slightly behind the anterior superior branch. Its fibers supply the maxillary first and second bicuspid teeth and the mesiobuccal root of the maxillary first molar. Other small fibers of this branch innervate the periodontal membrane and gingivae surrounding these teeth.

The *posterior superior alveolar branch* is composed of two or three branches, coursing down the posterior surface of the maxilla to enter one or several posterior superior dental foramina.

This nerve supplies all the roots of the maxillary second and third molar teeth and two roots of the maxillary first molar tooth. (As previously stated, in the majority of cases, the mesiobuccal root of the maxillary first molar is supplied by the middle superior alveolar nerve.)

Zygomatic Nerve. The *zygomatic nerve* is situated in the lower fissure of the orbit, along with part of the infraorbital branch. The zygomatic sends branches along the orbital surface and pierces the zygomatic bone; it emerges to form the *zygomaticofacial branch* (so called because of its location). A second small branch, the *zygomatic temporal*, emerges from a small foramen on the temporal surface to innervate tissues of that region.

Sphenopalatine Nerves. The *sphenopalatine nerves* branch from the maxillary nerve in a downward direction. A body of nerve tissue found suspended by two short nerves from the maxillary nerve is the *sphenopalatine ganglion* (*Meckel's ganglion*). This ganglion lies just below the maxillary nerve in the sphenopalatine fossa. Two nerves of interest here are the *nasopalatine nerve* and the *anterior palatine nerve*. The nasopalatine courses from Meckel's ganglion along the septum of the nose, through the palatine canal, and terminates in the foramina of Scarpa located on the median line and palatally to the maxillary central teeth. This nerve innervates the maxillary anterior mucosal tissues and the *palatal mucoperiosteum* (the fibrous sheath covering the hard palate) and is directly related to the anterior palatine nerves. The anterior palatine nerve arises from Meckel's ganglion, descends through the *posterior palatine canal* (in the palatine bone), and emerges on the palate from the *posterior palatine foramen*. It passes forward on the palate and intermingles with the nasopalatine nerve, opposite the cuspid tooth. It innervates the maxillary molar and bicuspid mucosal tissues and the palatal mucoperiosteum in that area.

Mandibular Division

The *mandibular division* (third division) of the trigeminal, a mixed nerve, is the largest branch given off from the gasserian ganglion. It exits from the cranium through the foramen ovale (ovale, egg-shaped) and is made up of two roots, a large sensory root, and a small motor root (the motor part of the trigeminal). It differs from the other two divisions of the trigeminal, because it is both sensory and motor. The mandibular nerve supplies the teeth and gums of the mandible, the skin of the temporal region, the lower lip, the muscles of mastication, and the anterior two-thirds of the tongue.

The *anterior portion*, a branch of the mandibular nerve, is basically motor in character. It innervates the temporal, masseter, internal pterygoid, and external pterygoid muscles, as well as the anterior surface of the temporomandibular joint; refer to figures 9–3 to 9–5 and 13–3.

The *buccal nerve*, a continuation of the anterior portion, is sensory only. It passes forward and toward the side, and divides into many small fibers that supply the mucous membrane of the cheek. Although this nerve passes through the buccinator muscle, it does not supply the motor stimulation for that muscle.

The *lingual nerve* branches just below the buccal nerve and from the posterior portion of the mandibular nerve. It travels forward and downward to the lingual surface of the mandible. As it nears the area, lingual to the mandibular second or third molar roots, it attaches itself to the *submandibular ganglion*. The attachments are usually two short nerves by which the ganglion appears to be suspended. This small mass of nerve tissues is self-controlling (autonomic) in its work with involuntary nerve impulses that innervate the sublingual and tongue glands. The fiber ends of the lingual nerve supply the lateral and superior surface tissues of the tongue and record sensations of touch and taste and promotes glandular function.

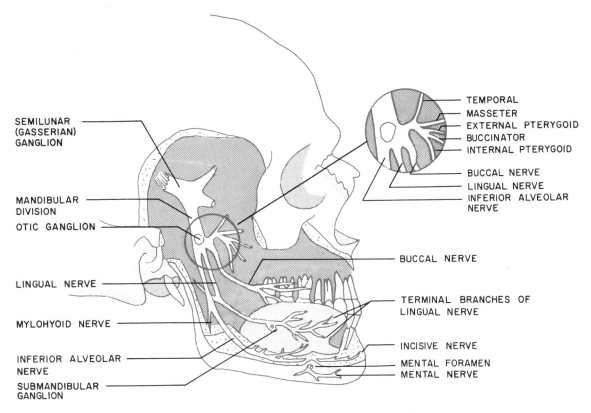

Fig. 13–3. Trigeminal nerve, mandibular division

The inferior alveolar nerve is a continuation of the mandibular nerve and is the largest branch of the mandible. It gives off a branch called the mylohyoid nerve, just above the point where it enters the mandibular foramen. The fibers of this branch are motor in character. The inferior alveolar nerve passes through the mandibular foramen and follows the mandibular canal; it sends sensory branches to all the molar and biscupid teeth. At a point, approximately between the apices of the first and second bicuspids, the interior alveolar divides into the mental and incisive branches. These branches pass through the mental foramen; the mental branch innervates the chin and lower lip, and the incisive branch supplies the mandibular anterior teeth.

REVIEW

1. Name the three types of cranial nerves.

a. _____

b. _____

c. _____

2. Another term for the trigeminal nerve is _____.

3. Identify the lettered parts of the illustrations. Select from the following list:

Otic ganglion
Ophthalmic division
Semilunar (gasserian) ganglion
Nasociliary nerve
Frontal nerve
Lacrimal nerve
Supraorbital nerves

A. _____

B. _____

C. _____

D. _____

E. _____

F. _____

4. Identify the lettered parts of the illustration. Select from the following list:

Frontal nerve
Maxillary division
Semilunar (gasserian) ganglion
Anterior superior alveolar branch
Middle superior alveolar branch
Posterior superior alveolar branch
Anterior palatine nerve
Infraorbital nerve
Zygomatic nerve
Sphenopalatine ganglion
Nasopalatine nerve

A. _____

B. _____

C. _____

D. _____

E. _____

F. _____

G. _____

H. _____

I. _____

J. _____

5. Define the term *ganglion*. _____

   _____

6. Another term for the semilunar ganglion is _____.

7. Three main divisions of the trigeminal nerve are _____,

   _____, and _____.

8. The smallest branch or division is _____.

9. The largest branch of the ophthalmic division is _____.

10. The two branches of the nerve indicated above are _____

    and _____.

11. Why is the supratrochlear nerve called a sensory nerve? _____

    _____

12. Which of the maxillary nerves innervates the pulp, periodontal membrane,
    and gingival tissues of the maxillary central incisor, lateral incisor, and cuspid
    teeth? _____

13. What nerve innervates the maxillary first and second biscuspid teeth? _____

    _____

14. What nerve innervates the mesiobuccal root of the maxillary first molar? _____

    _____

15. Another term for the sphenopalatine ganglion is _____.

16. That branch of the mandibular division that is basically motor in character is

    _____.

17. The largest branch of the mandibular nerve is_____.

18. Identify the lettered parts of the illustration. Select from the following list:

> Mandibular division
> Semilunar (gasserian) ganglion
> Lingual nerve
> Buccal nerve
> Mylohyoid nerve
> Submandibular ganglion
> Mental nerve
> Incisive nerve
> Terminal branches of lingual nerve
> Otic ganglion
> Mental foramen
> Inferior alveolar nerve
> Frontal nerve

A. _____

B. _____

C. _____

D. _____

E. _____

F. _____

G. _____

H. _____

I. _____

J. _____

K. _____

L. _____

19. Are the fibers of the mylohyoid nerve sensory or motor in character?_____

_____

20. Two additional branches of the inferior alveolar nerve are_____

and_____.

21. Match the cranial nerves listed in Column I with the correct description in Column II.

Column I

_____ Nasopalatine

_____ Anterior superior alveolar

_____ Mandibular

_____ Mental and incisive

_____ Maxillary

_____ Posterior superior alveolar

_____ Infraorbital

_____ Inferior alveolar

_____ Ophthalmic

_____ Middle superior alveolar

Column II

A. Largest branch of the maxillary nerve
B. Innervates the lingual and distobuccal roots of the maxillary first, second, and third molars
C. First division of the trigeminal nerve
D. Innervates the maxillary first and second bicuspids and the mesiobuccal root of the maxillary first molar
E. Innervates the chin and lower lip
F. Sensory branch of all mandibular molar and bicuspid teeth
G. Third division of the trigeminal nerve
H. Innervates maxillary centrals, laterals, cuspids, and supporting tissues of this area
I. Second division of the trigeminal nerve
J. Innervates the maxillary teeth, palatine nerves, and the palatal mucoperiosteum

22. The inferior alveolar nerve passes through the_____ and follows the_____.

23. The fiber ends of the lingual nerve record sensations of _____, _____ and _____.

24. The lingual nerve attaches itself to the_____ganglion.

OBJECTIVES:

After studying this chapter, the student will be able to:
- Locate the lingual artery, a branch of the internal carotid, and discuss its importance to the oral cavity.
- Locate the internal maxillary artery, and determine its importance to the field of dentistry.
- Locate the three branches of the internal maxillary artery, and discuss the areas supplied by each.
- Locate the pterygoid plexus, and trace the venous flow to the internal jugular vein.
- Determine the importance of the maxillary vein.

INTRODUCTION

Many individuals take for granted the fact that blood circulates, and the concept is implied rather than expressly stated, even when the gross anatomy of the circulatory system is discussed. About 300 years ago, however, although much was known about the heart and the blood vessels and their distribution, the nature of blood was unknown. At that time William Harvey demonstrated that the blood moves in a continuous double circulation.

The organs of the blood-vascular (vaso, blood vessel) system are the heart and blood vessels (arteries, capillaries, and veins). These organs form a closed passageway of tubes through which the blood circulates. The heart is a muscular pump that propels the blood through the blood vessels. The arteries are elastic tubes that carry the blood away from the heart to the tissues of the body. Capillaries are microscopic, hairlike vessels through which blood passes from arteries to veins. Veins are less muscular than arteries; their walls are thinner, and most have paired valves that prevent the backward flow of blood.

The arteries carry oxygenated blood from the heart to all regions of the body. Because of this high-pressure delivery system, blood flows rapidly. The arteries expand and contract with the pumping beat of the heart. A rupture of the arterial system can be readily detected by the rhythmic spurting of bright red blood. If the blood spurts from a wound as in a severed artery, pressure should be applied against the artery on the side of the wound toward the heart. This helps to control bleeding.

Veins, although similar in form to arteries, serve as the low-pressure system that returns the blood to the heart. Veins are equipped with valves that open in the direction of the flow of blood. This valve arrangement is effective in preventing a reverse flow as the blood is carried to the heart. Venous flow can be detected when blood runs slowly but steadily from a wound. When a vein is severed, pressure should be applied to the vein on the side of the wound away from the heart.

ARTERIES

The common *carotid arteries* (right and left) supply arterial blood to the head. Each divides in the neck (at the upper border of the thyroid cartilage) to form two branches: *external* and *internal arteries*. The internal carotid arteries lie deep and supply branches to the brain and the

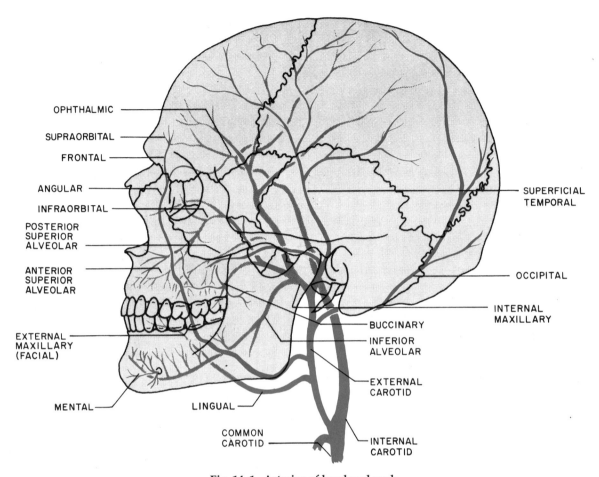

OPHTHALMIC

SUPRAORBITAL

FRONTAL

ANGULAR

INFRAORBITAL

POSTERIOR
SUPERIOR
ALVEOLAR

ANTERIOR
SUPERIOR
ALVEOLAR

EXTERNAL
MAXILLARY
(FACIAL)

MENTAL

LINGUAL

COMMON
CAROTID

SUPERFICIAL
TEMPORAL

OCCIPITAL

INTERNAL
MAXILLARY

BUCCINARY

INFERIOR
ALVEOLAR

EXTERNAL
CAROTID

INTERNAL
CAROTID

Fig. 14–1. Arteries of head and neck

eyes. The external carotid arteries are more superficial (situated nearer the surface) and have branches that go to the throat, tongue, face, ears, and to the wall of the cranium, figure 14–1.

The branches of the external carotid artery are named according to the area they supply. The *external maxillary (facial) artery* arises from the external carotid artery and enters the face at the lower border of the masseter muscle, where it is comparatively superficial. This artery is easily compressed against the lower border of the mandible. At this point, the external maxillary artery passes forward and upward to the angle of

the mouth, where it takes a more vertical course to become the *angular artery.* It travels upward to the middle of the eyelid and terminates.

The *lingual artery* is the second major branch of the external carotid and is directly related to the oral cavity. From the anterior of the external carotid, the lingual branches in archlike fashion, then travels in a straight course and passes under the mandible. It again divides into four branches. One branch supplies the mucous membrane of the top surface of the tongue, the glossopalatine arch, the tonsil, and the soft palate. Others supply muscles, the alveolar process of the

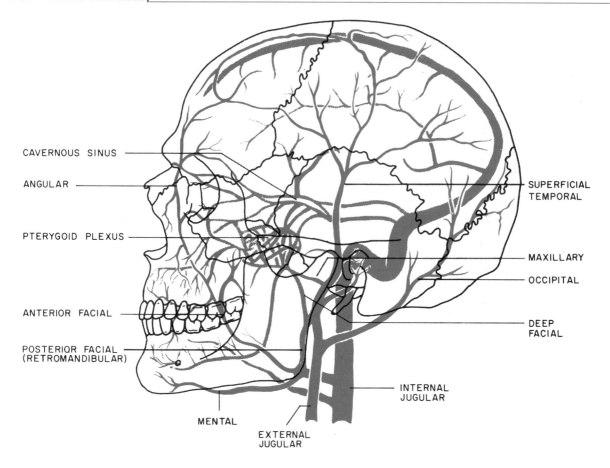

CAVERNOUS SINUS

ANGULAR

PTERYGOID PLEXUS

ANTERIOR FACIAL

POSTERIOR FACIAL
(RETROMANDIBULAR)

MENTAL

EXTERNAL
JUGULAR

SUPERFICIAL
TEMPORAL

MAXILLARY

OCCIPITAL

DEEP
FACIAL

INTERNAL
JUGULAR

Fig. 14–2. Veins of head and neck

mandible, and the mucosa. Yet another, the *deep lingual artery*, runs along the under surface of the tongue, ending at the tip.

The *superficial temporal artery* is the smaller of the two terminal branches of the external carotid artery. It travels behind the neck of the condyle and travels upward in front of the ear. There it branches to supply the frontal and parietal areas of the scalp.

The *occipital artery* arises from the posterior part of the external carotid, opposite the external maxillary (facial) artery. It runs along the occipital bone and ends in the posterior part of the scalp.

Other arteries of the face are the buccinator and *infraorbital arteries* from the internal maxillary artery. The *ophthalmic artery* branches to form the *frontal* and *supraorbital arteries*.

The *internal maxillary artery* (sometimes referred to as maxillary artery) is the largest of the two terminal branches of the external carotid. Its three branches provide the blood supply for the teeth. The *inferior alveolar artery* supplies the mandibular teeth; the *posterior superior alveolar artery* supplies the maxillary bicuspids and molars; and the *anterior superior alveolar artery*, a branch of the infraorbital artery, supplies the maxillary central and lateral incisors and cuspids.

VEINS OF THE HEAD

Blood drains from the head and the interior of the skull into venous channels situated between two layers of the *dura mater* (the outermost membrane) of the brain. These are called *venous sinuses*. In relation to dentistry, the most important of these sinuses are the two *cavernous sinuses* that are connected with veins of the face (through veins of the orbits). Because of this direct association, infection in and about the nose and cheeks can easily enter the sinuses.

Major veins of the area are the *facial vein*, the *superficial* and *deep temporal veins*, the *maxillary vein*, the tributaries (those that flow into the larger veins), the *internal jugular vein*, and the *external jugular vein*, figure 14–2.

The facial vein is divided into sections according to the structures over or through which it courses. At the inner canthus of the eye (where the upper and lower eyelids fuse), it arises as the *angular vein*. It follows a course similar to that of the external maxillary artery. Near its point of origin, it receives blood from the infratrochlear and infraorbital veins. At the root of the nose, and as a continuation of the angular vein, the *anterior facial vein* runs downward and backward across the face, crossing the border of the mandible at the anterior border of the masseter muscle. Beneath the angle of the mandible, it unites with the *posterior facial vein* to form the common facial vein. The anterior facial vein unites with the deep facial vein, one of considerable size, from

the *pterygoid plexus* (a network of veins). This plexus forms a rather dense network around the external pterygoid muscle. The facial vein carries the blood collected from the facial region to the *internal jugular vein*. This large blood vessel is found running parallel to the common carotid artery, figure 14–2.

The *superficial* and *deep temporal veins* join together in the region anterior to the external acoustic meatus and bring blood from the superficial tissue of the skull and the temporal fossa. At a point just below the junction of the temporal vessels, the *maxillary vein* connects to the main tributary to form a complex union of *occipital, posterior facial*, and *external jugular vessels*. The maxillary vein receives blood from the maxillary and mandibular alveolar systems, including all the teeth.

The *posterior facial vein* is normally a short vessel. The vein is an auxiliary vessel to the external jugular at the junction of the maxillary vein and the common facial vein. It is attached to the common facial vein just behind and below the angle of the mandible. This vessel is otherwise referred to as the *retromandibular vein* because of its location.

The *external jugular vein* usually takes a course posterior and superficial to the internal jugular vein. From its junction with the superficial temporal, maxillary, and retromandibular vessels, the external jugular travels downward to join the internal jugular vein under the clavicle (collarbone).

REVIEW

1. What blood vessel causes blood to spurt from a wound? _____

_____

2. What blood vessel would cause blood to run slowly but steadily from a wound? _____

3. Where would you apply pressure to control arterial bleeding? _____

   _____

4. Where would you apply pressure to control venous bleeding? _____

   _____

5. The source of the blood supply for the tongue is _____

   _____.

6. Identify the lettered parts of the illustration. Select from the following list:

   Internal jugular vein   Cavernous sinus
   Superficial temporal vein   Angular vein
   Maxillary vein   Anterior facial vein
   Occipital vein   Deep facial vein
   Posterior facial   Pterygoid plexus
      (retromandibular) vein   Mental vein
   External jugular vein   Common carotid

   A. _____

   B. _____

   C. _____

   D. _____

   E. _____

   F. _____

   G. _____

   H. _____

   I. _____

   J. _____

   K. _____

   L. _____

7. Where does the common carotid artery divide? _____

   _____

8. What blood vessel supplies the mandibular teeth? _____

   _____

   The maxillary biscuspids and molars? _____

   _____

   The maxillary central and lateral incisors? _____

   _____

9. Name the vein which receives the blood collected and carried by the facial veins. _____

10. Which of the veins receive blood from both the maxillary and mandibular alveolar systems (including all the teeth)? _____

    _____

11. Name the junction of the external and internal jugular veins. _____

    _____

(review questions continued)

12. Identify the lettered parts of the illustration. Select from the following list:

Inferior alveolar artery
Posterior superior artery
Infraorbital arteries
Anterior superior alveolar artery
Buccinator arteries
Ophthalmic artery
Frontal artery
Supraorbital artery
External maxillary (facial) artery
Common carotid artery
External carotid artery
Internal cartoid artery
Mental arteries
Angular artery
Lingual artery
Superficial temporal artery
Occipital artery
Internal maxillary
Pterygoid plexus

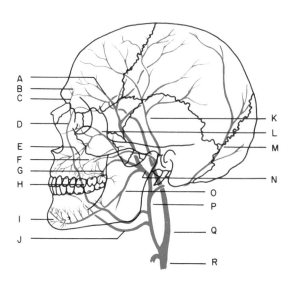

A. _____   J. _____

B. _____   K. _____

C. _____   L. _____

D. _____   M. _____

E. _____   N. _____

F. _____   O. _____

G. _____   P. _____

H. _____   Q. _____

I. _____   R. _____

Chapter 15: Development of the Face and Nose

OBJECTIVES: After studying this chapter, the student will be able to:
- Discuss the process of cell division.
- Discuss the specialization process of tissue differentiation.
- List the three distinct cell layers that form in the developing human embryo.
- Distinguish epithelial cells from connective cells with respect to their structure and function.
- Discuss the chronological stages of development of the face and associated structures.

INTRODUCTION

The human body is formed from the division of the fertilized *ovum* (ovum, the female reproductive or germ cell that after fertilization is capable of developing into a new member of the same species). The process of division, *mitosis*, results in the formation of two daughter cells, each of which resembles the original. As division follows division, the daughter cells may exhibit new or altered structures and functions. This process is called *differentiation* (when the original cells take on the duty of forming a particular type of tissue). The first evidence of differentiation in the mass of cells of the developing human embryo (embryo, a young organism up to the end of the second month of intrauterine life) is the formation of three distinct cell (germ) layers. An outer layer of cells forms the **ectoderm** (ecto, outer) while a tube develops within the mass and the cells lining it form the **endoderm** (endo, within). This tube forms the basis of the future alimentary canal and the organs that arise from it—lungs, liver, pancreas.

The **mesoderm** (meso, middle) consists of cells lying between the ectoderm and the endoderm of the primary germ layers.

The primitive cells of each germ layer can differentiate along two separate lines to form either epithelium or connective tissue.

Epithelial cells cover surfaces (e.g., skin) or line cavities (e.g., the mouth). In these situations, they are essentially protective in function, figure 15–1.

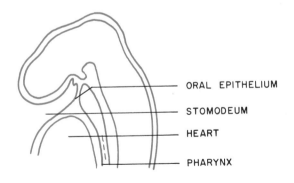

— ORAL EPITHELIUM

— STOMODEUM

— HEART

— PHARYNX

Fig. 15–1. Head end of human embryo (three to four weeks)

109

A secondary function that may be performed by covering epithelia, such as the intestinal and respiratory epithelia, is secretion of mucus. A feature common to all epithelial cells is that they are closely contiguous (touching along a boundary or at a point) with one another.

Connective tissue cells are the other cell type present in the body. They are usually widely separated from each other by a zone containing a substance in which fibers are embedded. *Collagen fibers* (collagen, a vital crystalline, protein substance present in all connective tissue) are the most abundant, but in some areas (e.g., the walls of the large arteries), *elastic fibers* are also present. This type of connective tissue (tendon, bone, cartilage, and fibrous tissue) is primarily supportive in function. Other connective tissue cells have the capability of *contraction* (muscle fibers) or *conduction* (nerve cells).

The cells of the body show considerable diversity of structure and function, yet each is remarkably independent. Each receives a supply of oxygen and food stuffs from the bloodstream with which it will produce its own structural components and secretions. Each cell will also release the energy required for chemical, electrical, or mechanical work.

Histology is the study of plant and animal tissues and involves the internal structure of organisms and their parts. Their structures are so minute that they must be studied under a microscope. This chapter describes the tissues and internal structure of the teeth and closely related parts of the oral cavity. The development of the face, its associated structures, and the masses of tissue that are directly involved are discussed.

STAGES OF DEVELOPMENT

During the chronological development (chronology, accepted order of past events) of single systems or parts of systems, it must be remembered that these systems do not arise independently of one another. To simplify the study, we describe the development of isolated structures and their relationships in detail.

An examination of a human embryo reveals, as early as the third or fourth week, the *pharynx* (upper portion of the digestive tract) and a large cavity known as the *stomodeum* (stomodeum, a depression at the head end of the embryo that becomes the front part of the mouth), figures 15–1 and 15–2. This completes the first important step in the development of the face. During the same period, two paired structures are evident, the maxillary and mandibular processes; these form the lateral walls of the *primitive oral cavity* (primitive, first in time, original). A lateral view of the embryo shows the relation of these two processes and the line of union between them.

In the sixth week of development, two additional structures originate; these are known as the nasal processes (comprised of the frontal and lateral portions). By the end of the seventh week, an inverted U-shaped elevation of tissue surrounds each process and forms the *primitive external nares* (nares, nostrils). As the nasal processes develop, the maxillary processes increase in size and grow toward the midline of the face. At the same time, they tend to push the

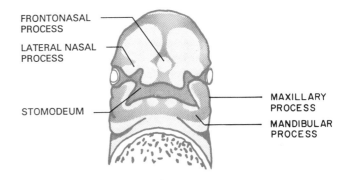

Fig. 15–2. Head of human embryo (three to four weeks)

nasal processes closer together, figure 15–3. By the tenth week, the maxillary arch is formed and its parts aligned (aligned, arranged in a line) from side to side. The two nasal processes migrate medially, meet, and fuse, and the *primitive nasal septum* is established (septu, dividing wall, or partition).

In the meantime, the mandible has continued to develop. As these processes migrate from their lateral position, they fuse at a point in the midline.

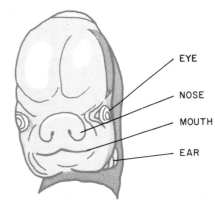

EYE

NOSE

MOUTH

EAR

Fig. 15–3. Head of human embryo (about eight weeks)

REVIEW

1. The process of cell division is termed _____.

2. Define the term *differentiation*. _____

_____

3. The three distinct cell layers are _____,

_____ and _____.

4. Primitive cells of each germ layer can differentiate to form either_____

_____ or _____tissue.

5. Collagen may be defined as _____.

6. Epithelial cells are said to be essentially_____
in function and are found closely contiguous with one another.

7. Connective tissue cells are primarily _____
in function and are usually widely separated from each other.

8. Connective tissue cells of the heart have the capability of _____;
nerve cells have the capability of _____.

9. Define the term *histology*. _____

_____

10. Define the term *embryo*. _____

_____

11. When does the digestive tract develop in the embryo? _____

_____

12. What is another term for the digestive tract? _____

_____

13. What two processes form the lateral walls of the primitive oral cavity?

    a. _____

    b. _____

14. The period of development for the nasal process is _____.

15. The period of development for the primitive external nares is _____

    _____.

16. The period of fusion of the maxillary arch is _____.

17. The period of fusion of the mandible is _____.

18. The period when the primitive nasal septum is established is _____.

19. Identify the lettered parts of the illustration. Select from the following list:

Frontonasal process   Maxillary process
Eye   Mandibular process
Lateral nasal process   Stomodeum
Pharynx

A. _____

B. _____

C. _____

D. _____

E. _____

20. Identify the lettered parts of the illustration. Select from the following list:

Nose   Ear
Eye   Mouth
Pharynx

A. _____

B. _____

C. _____

D. _____

Chapter 16: Development of the Tongue and Palate

OBJECTIVES:

After studying this chapter, the student will be able to:
- Determine the time at which the embryonic development of the tongue occurs.
- Determine the time at which the embryonic development of the palate occurs.
- Describe the development stages of the tongue.
- Describe the development stages of the palate.
- Discuss the reasons for the occurrences of an anomaly.

INTRODUCTION

As the external structures of the face develop, other important developments occur internally. The tongue and palate, for example, appear during this time and are discussed in this chapter.

TONGUE

The tongue develops from mucous membrane composed principally of epithelium and connective tissue. Mucous membrane coverings of the tongue consist of a swelling along the median floor of the pharynx and can be recognized during the fifth week of embryonic life.

Later development of the tongue is involved in a rapid proliferation, or multiplication, of the cells. By the seventh week, the tongue becomes fairly well separated from the mandible. It becomes elevated from the floor of the mouth because of the infiltration of the muscle as it builds up internally.

PALATE

In the sixth week, the beginning of the palate appears. There are several processes, one of which originates from the medial nasal process. The others, which are located laterally, develop from the maxillary tissue. There are two important stages of development. The first is known as the *open palate stage*. During this stage, the medial migration of the nasal processes and the fusing of the primitive septum occur. The cavity of the palate is H-shaped. The upper half of the *H* represents the future nasal cavity; the lower half, the oral cavity, figure 16–1.

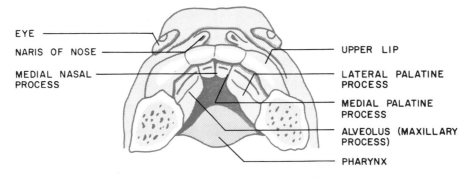

EYE
NARIS OF NOSE
MEDIAL NASAL PROCESS
UPPER LIP
LATERAL PALATINE PROCESS
MEDIAL PALATINE PROCESS
ALVEOLUS (MAXILLARY PROCESS)
PHARYNX

Fig. 16–1. Palatal view of human embryo (about ten weeks)

In the lower (oral) part of the cavity, the position of the tongue is largely responsible for the shape of the opening. Its superior surface projects above the mandibular tissue to such an extent that it lies just below the nasal septum.

The second stage of development is the *closed palate stage* and consists of two important changes. First, the tongue drops to a lower position in the oral cavity, which permits the fusion of the palatal processes at the medial surface of the palate. This fusion occurs first in the anterior region. The palate fuses posteriorly sometime during the nineteenth week.

Second, during this fusion process, ossification (conversion into bone) of the anterior part of the palate begins. This eventually results in the formation of the hard palate. See Chapter 8.

It is important to remember that the processes forming the framework of the primitive nose comprise the central core around which the later development of the soft part of the face is laid down.

At times, anomalies (anomaly, any deviation from the normal) occur. Failure of the lateral palatine processes to unite or fuse at the midline is a condition termed *cleft palate* (cleft, an opening or crevice). Variations of this condition are many: clefts in the palatine process usually are evidenced at the midline, and those involving the hard palate may occur on one or both sides of the midline in close proximity to the nares. A condition known as *harelip* (imperfect fusion of the upper lip) is frequently associated with cleft palate and is also a congenital defect.

REVIEW

1. Mucous membrane coverings of the tongue begin to develop during the_____
   _____week of embryonic life.

2. The palate originates from two different processes. Name them.

   a. _____

   b. _____

3. The palate begins to develop during the _____week of embryonic life.

4. Name the two stages of development of the palate.

   a. _____

   b. _____

5. Where does the fusion of the palatal process begin? _____

   _____

6. When does this fusion process begin? _____

   _____

7. What two biological developments occur during the fusion process?

   a. _____

   b. _____

8. Define the term *anomaly*. _____

   _____

9. Cleft palate is the result of what failure? _____

   _____

10. Define the term *harelip*. _____

    _____

11. Both cleft palate and harelip are termed _____defects.

12. How does a cleft of the palatine process and one of the hard palate differ?

    _____

    _____

13. Identify the lettered parts of the illustration. Select from the following list:

Naris of nose	Upper lip
Eye	Alveolus (maxillary process)
Medial nasal process	Lateral palatine process
Medial palatine process	Pharynx
Ear	

    A. _____

    B. _____

    C. _____

    D. _____

    E. _____

    F. _____

    G. _____

14. Before each statement indicate whether it is true (T) or false (F).

_____ A. The earliest sign of development of the human face usually occurs during the third week in utero with the formation of the stomodeum.

_____ B. The nasal cavity, the pharynx, and the hard palate all develop from the depression known as the stomodeum.

_____ C. Mucous membrane coverings of the tongue can be recognized during the fifth week of embryonic life.

_____ D. The frontonasal process of the early embryo gives rise to the center of the nose, the sides, the nasal septum, the maxillary process, and the center of the upper lip.

_____ E. In the development of the oral cavity, fusions of the embryonic processes that form the roof of the mouth are usually completed by the end of the third month.

_____ F. Mucous membrane is composed of epithelium and connective tissue.

_____ G. Mucosa lining the oral cavity includes the areas of the under-surface of the tongue, lips, cheeks, soft palate, and floor of the mouth.

Chapter 17: Early Development of the Teeth and Tooth Buds

OBJECTIVES:

After studying this chapter, the student will be able to:

- Describe the early (embryonic) development of tooth tissues and the beginning formation of tooth buds.
- Discuss the periods of cell development from initiation through morphodifferentiation.
- Define the terminology used in the chapter.
- Describe the stages of development of the tooth buds, including the formation of dentin, enamel, and roots.
- Discuss the order or sequence of organic tissue development.

INTRODUCTION

In the study of the structure and development of the teeth, it is appropriate to point out that the teeth are formed by two distinct embryonic tissues: (1) *ectoderm*, the origin of the **enamel organ** (crown) portion of the tooth (ectoderm is the outermost of the three primitive germ layers of the embryo) and (2) **mesenchyme**, from which all the other parts of the tooth and the associated supporting structures develop. Mesenchyme, a layer of specialized cells of the mesoderm (connective tissue), forms a spongework of cells out of which the dentin, the cementum, and the periodontal ligament originate.

The formation of the teeth begins during the embryonic stage and extends through the *fetal period* (from the second month to full term) and after birth to age 21 (age of complete maturation). At birth there are normally forty-four teeth in various stages of development. The *deciduous* (primary) teeth number twenty and advance in development to the point of eruption. Soon after birth, about the sixth month, they begin to erupt; the majority of teeth erupt by age 2 to 3 years. The twenty-four remaining buds are *permanent* (secondary) teeth, which continue their formation through childhood. It must be emphasized that all eruption schedules are approximations, because no two individuals are alike in their development.

PERIODS OF DEVELOPMENT

The development and beginning formation of the tooth buds (at about the sixth week) arise from the **oral epithelium** tissue, which lines the primitive cavity of the stomodeum. This period of development is termed **initiation**. At first, these dental tissues consist of a continuous ridge of tissue, one for each jaw, and appear as solid **proliferations** (multiplications of cells) of the oral epithelium extending into the underlying mesenchyme. However, these *laminae* (thin layers or plates) are found to be in a position at about right angles to the surface epithelium. They extend around the arch of each jaw and are known as the *labiodental laminae* (labiodental, pertaining to the areas of the lips and teeth).

Differentiation (when the original cells take on the duty of forming each type of tooth tissue) is the second period of development and one that may be further separated into two phases: (1) **histodifferentiation** occurs when the cells of the inner epithelium of the ectoderm prepare to form enamel and become ameloblasts (enamel-forming cells) and the peripheral cells become *odontoblasts* (dentin-forming cells); and (2) **morpho-differentiation** occurs when the formative cells are arranged to establish the future shape and size of the organ. Their formation along the future dentinoenamel (and dentinocemental) junction serves to outline the future crown and root portions of the tooth.

As soon as the *labiodental lamina* is differentiated, it can be seen as two distinct parts. One part consists of a vertical labial ingrowth, marking off the future lip and vestibule. This structure is termed the *labial lamina* (a thin layer of tissue that forms the lips). The second part continues as an extension toward the tongue. This epithelium gives rise to the enamel organs and is termed the *dental lamina* (thin layer of tooth-producing cells).

Tooth buds form as outgrowths of the dental laminae. Ten of these buds are normally present in each jaw at sites corresponding to the location of the future deciduous teeth. As the jaw develops, the dental lamina and the ten separate tooth buds can be distinguished. At first, these buds appear as solid structures; they then become hollowed out by the further development of the underlying mesenchyme. In this form they serve as molds to fashion the developing crowns of the teeth.

Tooth development begins, as previously mentioned, at about the fifth to sixth week of intrauterine (embryonic) life. Within a short time, the development of all the deciduous teeth is initiated. Development of the permanent teeth begins about the seventeenth week of prenatal life. However, initiation and growth of the various tissues are spread over a period of several years.

STAGES OF DEVELOPMENT

During the first stage of development, the tooth bud enlarges to become the embryonic *enamel organ*. This organ subsequently develops the enamel of the tooth. A shallow, indented area appears along the lower margin of the enamel organ; the enamel organ assumes the shape of a cap. This stage of tooth development is called the *cap stage*.

The connective tissue within the cap becomes more cellular, because of the proliferation of the cells, and forms what is termed the *dental papilla*. This connective tissue eventually forms the dental pulp and dentin. As the dental papilla becomes further enveloped by the enamel organ, the structure of the enamel organ assumes the shape of a bell. This period of development is called the *bell stage*. During this stage, the cells of the enamel organ differentiate and become four separate and distinct layers.

During the bell stage, the cells that have been joined to the oral epithelium begin to disintegrate. At the same time, connective tissue surrounds the enamel organ, and the dental papilla forms a rather dense band of tissue, called the *dental sac*. Development of the cementum, the periodontal ligament (formerly referred to as "periodontal membrane"), and the lamina dura of the alveolus occurs within the dental sac.

Formation of the Dentin

The development of the dentin occurs just prior to that of the embryonic enamel. The first step is the formation of a reticular membrane (reticular, netlike), the fibers of which appear in a fan-shaped arrangement as they approach the crown area. At the same time, other reticular fibers are developing in the crown area; these pass between the cells arranged on the periphery of the pulp. These specialized cells develop from the outer surface of the dental papilla and are called *odontoblasts*. They become dentin-forming cells. The process of the formation of dentin is termed dentinogenesis (beginning of dentin). **Dentin** is first differentiated on the tip of the developing crown and gradually envelops the entire pulp cavity, figure 17–1.

Dentin forms in the shape of small tubes, referred to as *dentinal tubules*. During formation, the dentinal tubules retain a small amount of organic tissues, or *collagen* (a vital, crystalline,

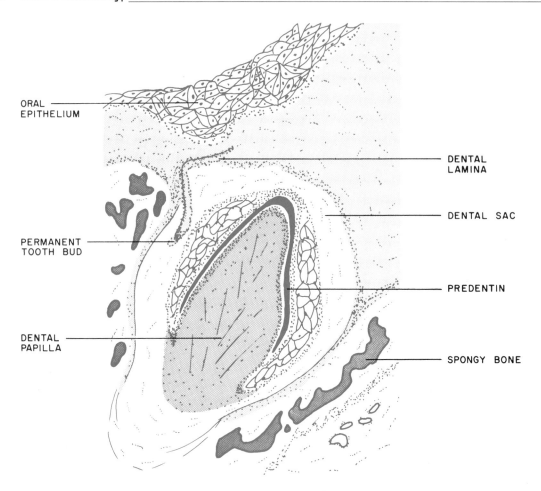

ORAL EPITHELIUM

DENTAL LAMINA

DENTAL SAC

PERMANENT TOOTH BUD

PREDENTIN

DENTAL PAPILLA

SPONGY BONE

Fig. 17–1. Formation of dentin

protein substance present in all connective tissue), in their **lumen** (canal of the tubule). These collagenous tissues are called *odontoblastic processes*, or *Tomes' dentinal fibrils*. The area these fibrils occupy during this stage of development is known as *predentin*, an uncalcified layer of material. Once the predentin has been established, the organic framework receives inorganic salts, principally of calcium and phosphorus; this stage is called **apposition** (adding together). The predentin becomes calcified (hard) and is converted to dentin. The growth of dentin is incremental; i.e., the dentin increases layer upon layer. As each additional layer is deposited, the former layer becomes calcified. **Calcification** continues until the entire dentin of the crown has been formed.

In the calcification of dentin, Tomes' dentinal fibrils do not calcify but maintain a metabolic pathway (for the exchange of nutrients and energy, which keep the organ vital) between the pulp and the dentin.

Formation of the Enamel

Immediately after the first layer of dentin is laid down, special epithelial cells (called *ameloblasts*) begin to form enamel. The process of enamel formation is called amelogenesis (beginning of enamel). Many details with regard to enamel formation are uncertain, but it is generally believed that the ameloblasts play approximately the same role as that of the odontoblasts.

Enamel formation takes place in two distinct phases: the *formative phase* and the *maturation phase*. The first or formative phase involves the formation of an enamel matrix (matrix, a layer of cells that gives form to the crown). The enamel matrix is the detailed development of a wide protoplasmic process (protoplasm, the essential constituent of a living cell). These are called *Tomes' enamel* processes and arise in the region of the future dentinoenamel junction at growth centers corresponding to the location and the number of tips of the cusps. The centers of

development are often called **lobes** because they have marked fissures, or divisions. Calcification of Tomes' enamel processes is from the tip of each cusp toward the cervical portion of the tooth (cervix, necklike). It is believed that the thickness of enamel is completed in a matrix state before final calcification starts, figure 17–2.

During the second or maturation phase in the development of enamel, the matrix undergoes calcification. With calcification, many-sided columns of enamel form; these are called *enamel rods*, or prisms. Separating each prism is a calcified substance called *interprismatic substance*.

The ameloblasts retain their structural characteristics until the crown appears, or erupts, in the oral cavity. However, during the later phase of development, the ameloblasts have a horny

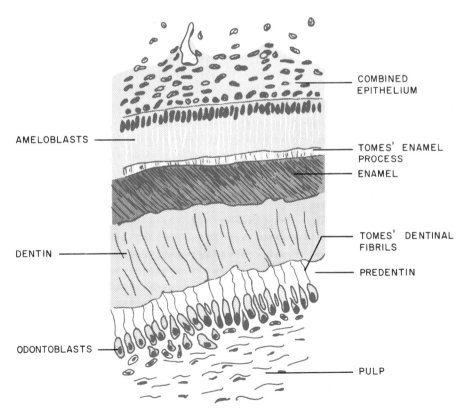

Fig. 17–2. Increments of dentin and enamel (highly magnified)

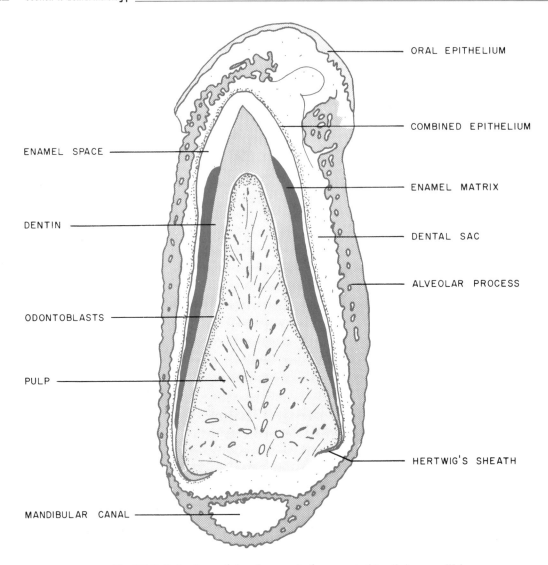

Fig. 17–3. Late stage of development of unerupted tooth in mandible

covering that is firmly attached to the outer enamel surface. The covering, or *cuticle*, is called **Nasmyth's membrane**. Although some authorities believe this to be a protective covering for the crown, positive function of the membrane is questionable. When the enamel has completely formed, layers of the enamel organ merge and form the reduced (less vital) enamel epithelium or Nasmyth's membrane. As the tooth erupts, the part that remains on the crown proper is soon lost. The remaining reduced enamel epithelium fuses with the epithelial lining of the oral cavity, forming the epithelial attachment.

Root Formation

During morphodifferentiation, the enamel epithelium in the apical portion of the tooth, together with the dental papilla, form the outline of the root. At this time, the innermost cell layer, or *inner enamel epithelium*, and the outermost cell layer, or *outer enamel epithelium*, merge in a loop at the site of the cervix of the tooth. This is called the *cervical loop*. The layers then grow downward for a short distance as a double row of cells termed *Hertwig's epithelial root sheath*, figure 17–3. The sheath acts as a limiting membrane for shaping the root of the tooth and is responsible for the formation of root dentin. Under the influence of the inner layer of cells, the cells of the dental papilla become odontoblasts, and the formation of the root begins. As the root dentin forms, the tooth moves toward the surface and erupts. Soon after the root dentin begins to form, Hertwig's sheath in that area begins to disintegrate, and the connective tissue of the dental sac grows through the disintegrating sheath and contacts the dentin. As the connective tissues contact the dentin, they become cementoblasts and deposit a layer of cementum on the surface of the dentin.

There is an order to the sequence of events in root formation: (1) the dentin forms, (2) the root lengthens; and (3) cementum is deposited. This sequence is repeated until the root is fully formed.

REVIEW

1. Name the origin of the enamel portion of the tooth. _____

2. The origin of parts of the tooth (other than the enamel) and its supporting structures is called _____.

3. The specialized cells that produce enamel are _____.

4. The specialized cells that produce dentin are_____.

5. The period of development when the tooth bud formation begins is called

   _____

6. Another term for multiplication of cells is _____.

7. The period of develoment when the cells prepare to form enamel and dentin is called_____.

8. The period when the formative-cell arrangement establishes the future shape and size of the organ is_____.

9. The number of deciduous tooth buds normally present is _____.

10. The number of permanent tooth buds normally present is _____.

11. Without referring to the preceding pages, identify the lettered parts of the illustration. Select from the following list:

Oral epithelium
Dental lamina
Dental sac
Predentin
Spongy bone of mandible
Dental papilla
Permanent tooth bud
Cervical loop

A. _____

B. _____

C. _____

D. _____

E. _____

F. _____

G. _____

12. After the tooth bud has developed, what is the next stage of development?

_____

13. What type of tissue forms the dental papilla? _____

14. Name the parts of the tooth that form the dental papilla. _____

_____

15. The dense band of tissue surrounding the enamel organ is called _____

_____.

16. What tooth structures develop within the dental sac? _____

_____

17. What are the specialized cells that develop from the outer surface of the dental papilla called? _____

18. Describe the function of the above-named cells._____

_____

19. The organic tissues found in Tomes' dentinal fibrils are called _____

_____

20. The stage when the predentin receives mineral salts, which leads to calcification, is _____.

21. Identify the lettered parts of the illustration. Select from the following list:

Combined epithelium   Pulp
Ameloblasts   Dental sac
Tomes' enamel process   Tomes' dentinal fibril
Enamel   Predentin
Odontoblasts   Dentin

A. _____

B. _____

C. _____

D. _____

E. _____

F. _____

G. _____

H. _____

I. _____

22. Identify the lettered parts of the illustration. Select from the following list:

Oral epithelium
Combined epithelium
Enamel space
Enamel matrix
Dentin
Dental sac
Alveolar process
Odontoblasts
Pulp
Hertwig's sheath
Mandibular canal
Permanent tooth bud

A. _____

B. _____

C. _____

D. _____

E. _____

F. _____

G. _____

H. _____

I. _____

J. _____

K. _____

23. What is the function of Tomes' fibrils? _____

_____

24. The enamel-forming cells are called _____.

25. The two stages of enamel formation are _____
and _____.

26. What is involved in the first phase? _____

    _____

27. What is involved in the second phase?_____

    _____

28. Another term for "reduced enamel epithelium" is _____.

29. Another term for a double row of enamel epithelium that helps to shape the root of the tooth is_____.

30. The classification of Tomes' enamel processes occurs directionally from _____

    _____.

Chapter 18: Composition and Formation of the Teeth

INTRODUCTION

A tooth consists of three parts: the **anatomic crown**, the anatomic root, and the **pulp** cavity. The *anatomic crown* is that portion that is covered by enamel and is exposed in the oral cavity. The *anatomic root* is that portion of the root covered by cementum; the root is embedded in a bony socket within the maxillae or mandible and surrounded by soft tissue. The narrowed portion, or cervix, and the line denoting the junction of the anatomical crown and the anatomic root are known as the **cementoenamel junction**, or *cervical line*. The tip of the root is called the **apex**.

Both the crown and the root consist of two layers of hard substance (tissue) surrounding the dental pulp. The crown's outer layer is *enamel*, and its inner layer is *dentin*. The root's outer

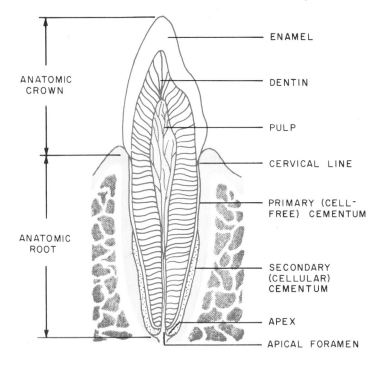

Fig. 18–1. Tissues of teeth

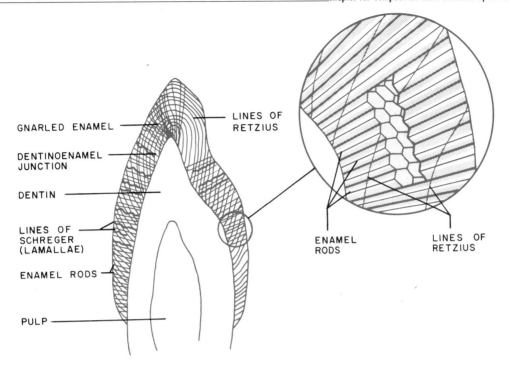

Fig. 18–2. Structure of enamel

layer is cementum, and its inner layer is dentin, figure 18–1.

The *pulp cavity* is a space in the central portion of the crowns and roots of teeth that is surrounded by dentin and normally filled with *pulp tissue*. That portion of the pulp cavity found mainly in the coronal portion is termed the *pulp chamber*. It is always a single cavity. The remaining portion confined within the root is known as the *pulp canal*, or *root canal*. The pulp chamber is comparatively large, and the root canals are small, tapering from the pulp chamber to a minute opening at the apex of the root, which is known as the *apical foramen*.

From a histological point of view, the teeth are made up of four main tissues: enamel, dentin, cementum, and dental pulp. This chapter describes these tissues and the internal structures of the teeth in detail.

ENAMEL

Enamel is the hardest tissue in the human body and consists of approximately 96 percent inorganic material and 4 percent organic material. Calcium and phosphorus are its main inorganic components. Designated carbon compounds are the organic components. (Refer to Chapter 17.) Made of this calcified substance, enamel is the hard tissue that covers the entire crown of the tooth and protects the dentin.

The morphological structure of enamel is known as the enamel rod or prism (morphology, the science of organic form and structure). The enamel rods are continuous structures that originate at the dentinoenamel junction and terminate at the free enamel surface. In a transverse section, human enamel rods are roughly polygonal (having many sides) in shape. One or more of the surfaces may be convex or concave. These highly

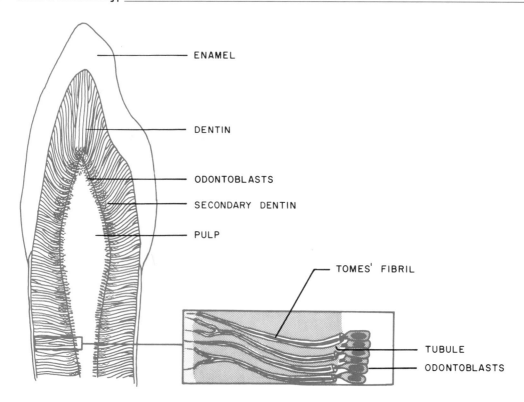

Fig. 18–3. Structure of dentin

calcified rods are separated by a minute inter-prismatic space, which is also calcified in mature enamel, figure 18–2.

The direction of the rods varies in different teeth. In general, they are arranged radially, in a fan-like arrangement, from the tip of the cusp to the dentinoenamel junction. They gradually assume a more acute (sharp) angle in the direction of the dentinal tubules as the cemento-enamel junction is approached.

Lines of Retzius

In a longitudinal tooth section (lengthwise cut through the tooth), a number of brown lines may be observed that represent the contour lines of the enamel. These are known as the *lines of Retzius*, or incremental lines. They are areas of diminished calcification caused by brief pauses in the development of the enamel. The lines of Retzius are similar in appearance to the annual developmental rings seen in the trunk of a tree, and they indicate stages of tooth development in much the same way, figure 18–2.

Lines of Schreger

The so-called *lines of Schreger*, or enamel lamellae, are narrow cracks that become filled with organic matter during the formation period. They are the result of the wavy direction of the enamel rods caused by stretching or twisting the enamel as it develops. These lamellae extend from the surface of the tooth toward the dentinoenamel junction. Some are known to reach the junction and even penetrate the dentin. Some authorities believe the lamellae provide an entry for bacteria and make teeth more susceptible to decay. Through transillumination (passing a light through the crown of the tooth), these areas appear as alternating light and dark bands and are sometimes mistaken for fractures.

A further variation in the direction of the rods also appears in enamel. This consists of an inter-twining of the rods, giving rise to what is termed _gnarled enamel_, figure 18–2. This structure apparently increases the strength of the enamel.

Enamel is formed by epithelial cells that lose their functional ability once the tooth has been completed. Mature enamel has no power of further growth or repair and is an inert substance.

DENTIN

Dentin is the hard, dense, light yellow substance that makes up the bulk of the tooth. It is harder than bone but softer than enamel. Dentin consists of approximately 70 percent inorganic matter. The chief inorganic components are calcium and phosphorus.

Structure of Dentin

Morphologically, dentin consists of a calcified matrix and _dentinal tubules_, figure 18–3. In the living state, there is no unoccupied space in the dentinal tubule, except for a minute capillary area that allows for the circulation of tissue fluid. Variations in the structure of dentin are numerous.

Generally, the dentinal tubules follow a somewhat S-shaped course, beginning at the surface of the pulp and ending at the dentinoenamel junction. These hollow structures are known as _Tomes' dentinal tubules_. Each tubule contains a fiber called a _Tomes' dentinal fibril_, which is a protoplasmic extension of an _odontoblast_ (dentin-forming cell) on the surface of the pulp. Some of the dentinal fibrils pass across the dentino-enamel junction and terminate in the enamel.

The cell bodies of the odontoblasts appear as a layer of columnar cells between the pulp and the dentin. They are considered to be part of the pulp.

Formation and calcification of the dentin begin at the tip of the cusp(s) and proceed inward toward the pulp. Brief pauses between the deposited layers (increments) are marked by fine lines that are at right angles to the dentinal tubules.

Secondary Dentin

All the dentin in a newly formed tooth is called _primary dentin_. Soon after eruption, a layer of dentin adjacent to the pulp cavity forms. This may appear somewhat different in form from the dentin near the periphery and is classified as _regular secondary dentin_. When the dental pulp is irritated as a result of caries (dental decay), cavity preparation, abrasion (wearing away), or erosion (disintegration of tooth surfaces other than those used in mastication), a layer of secondary dentin begins to form directly under the site of the structural change. This formation, which is a direct result of the irritation or stimulation, is called _irregular secondary dentin_.

Sensitivity

Dentin is sensitive to various stimuli. It reacts to tactile (touch), thermal (temperature), and chemical stimulation. Sensitivity is not uniform in all teeth; it varies greatly from person to person. The mechanism transmitting the sensation through the dentin to the pulp is not thoroughly understood in spite of numerous studies that have been made. It is generally agreed that dentin does not have nerve fibers and that the sensitivity may be due to changes in the dentinal fibrils.

Age Changes

It may be noted that layers of dentin form in locations beneath areas of the tooth that have been heavily worn through **attrition** (wearing away by continued friction and chewing). As long as pulp tissue remains sound and unaltered, the apposition of dentin may continue. This causes the pulp chamber to become reduced in size—a condition generally found in the teeth of people in their later years of life.

CEMENTUM

Cementum is the bonelike tissue that covers the roots of the teeth in a thin layer. Its composition is approximately 55 percent inorganic and 45 percent organic. The inorganic components are mainly calcium salts. The chief constituent of the organic material is collagen.

Cementum originates in a manner similar to bone. The cells concerned with *cementogenesis* (beginning of cementum) arise from embryonic connective tissue and develop from the dental sac. They differentiate and enlarge to become fairly large round cells that lie adjacent to the root of the tooth. Cementum is deposited in layers. The end product of this deposition is a thin layer of calcified tissue that is deposited on, and firmly attached to, the entire root surface. Embedded in the cementum are the *principal* (collagenous) *fibers* of the periodontal membrane. The opposite ends of these fibers are embedded in the alveolar bone and are called *Sharpey's fibers*. These fibers are responsible for supporting the tooth in the socket.

The cementum joins the enamel near the cervix of the tooth; the cementoenamel junction is somewhat variable. It may extend precisely to the termination of the enamel; it may extend beyond the cervical termination of the enamel; or, it may fail to extend to the enamel. In a few teeth, a break is present between the enamel and the cementum, exposing a narrow area of root dentin. Such areas are very sensitive to thermal, chemical, or mechanical stimuli.

Histologically, two types of cementum are recognized: cell-free (*primary*) and cellular (*secondary*). *Primary cementum* does not contain cells and is usually distributed quite uniformly over the surface of the root. *Secondary cementum* contains cells similar to bone, or *cementocytes*, and is usually confined to the apical third of the root.

Functions of Cementum

The main function of cementum is mechanical. It anchors the tooth to the bony wall of the socket.

In addition to the important function performed by cementum in anchoring the fibers to the root of the tooth, there is another process in which it may take part. Frequently, the root undergoes resorption; i.e., both cementum and dentin are destroyed. When this happens, new cementum may replace the lost tissue of the root and bring about a functional repair. This situation may arise in cases in which a fracture of the root takes place.

Cementum is formed throughout the life of the tooth. This compensates for the loss of tooth substance due to wear on the occlusal (biting and chewing) surfaces of the teeth. This process allows for the attachment of new fibers of the periodontal membrane to the surface of the root. This is discussed in Chapter 19, Tissues Surrounding the Teeth.

DENTAL PULP

Blood Supply

The blood supply of the pulp enters through the apical foramen and is accompanied by a lymphatic draining system, figure 18–4. (*Lymph* is a clear, colorless fluid that is derived from and closely resembles blood. It is carried by an independent system of vessels, called the lymph system, from the tissues to the heart.) The arteries have narrow lumina with some smooth muscle fibers in their walls. The veins are often more numerous, have exceedingly thin walls and relatively wide lumina. In young teeth, the pulp is filled with blood vessels. In older teeth, some of these blood vessels are replaced with other tissue.

Sensitivity

The nerve supply of the pulp consists of one type of fiber that ends in a dense network below

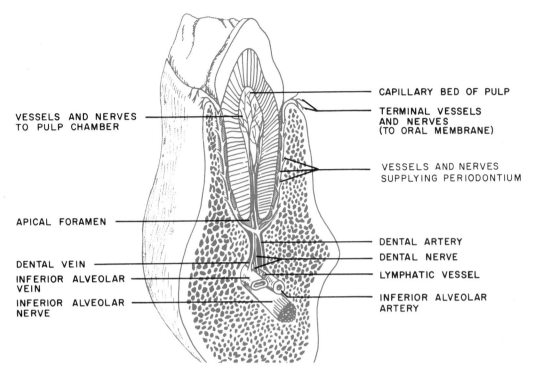

VESSELS AND NERVES
TO PULP CHAMBER

CAPILLARY BED OF PULP

TERMINAL VESSELS
AND NERVES
(TO ORAL MEMBRANE)

VESSELS AND NERVES
SUPPLYING PERIODONTIUM

APICAL FORAMEN

DENTAL VEIN

INFERIOR ALVEOLAR
VEIN

INFERIOR ALVEOLAR
NERVE

DENTAL ARTERY

DENTAL NERVE

LYMPHATIC VESSEL

INFERIOR ALVEOLAR
ARTERY

Fig. 18–4. Blood and nerve supply to tooth and surrounding structures

the odontoblast layer. Another type of fiber terminates as fine nerve endings on the surface of the odontoblasts. Depending on their structure and function, these nerve endings transmit sensations of either pain or touch.

Functions of Dental Pulp

The chief function of the pulp is the formation of dentin. However, it also provides nourishment to the dentin, provides sensation to the tooth, and responds to irritation either by forming secondary dentin or by becoming inflamed.

Dental pulp is enclosed within the hard walls of the pulp chamber, which permits no expansion of the pulp tissue. Swelling of the pulp tissue due to inflammation compresses the blood vessels against the walls of the chamber. This results in thrombosis (clotting of the blood within the vessels) and may result in strangulation and necrosis (death of cells due to disease or injury). These dead cells are referred to as necrotic tissue.

Age Changes in the Pulp

Other facts concerning the pulp are important to recognize. Pulp tissue is more extensive in young teeth than in the teeth of the mature individual. Furthermore, thickness of dentin in the coronal (crown) part of the deciduous or young permanent tooth is less than in the tooth of the mature individual.

REVIEW

1. Identify the lettered parts of the illustration. Select from the following list:

Lines of Retzius (shown in both views)   Dentinoenamel junction
Lines of Schreger (lamellae)   Dentin
Enamel rods   Pulp
Gnarled enamel   Apical foramen

A. _____

B. _____

C. _____

D. _____

E. _____

F. _____

G. _____

H. _____

I. _____

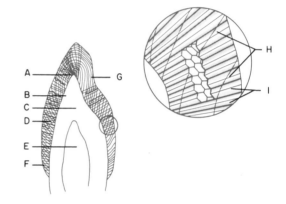

2. As a self-review and without referring to previous information, identify the lettered parts of the illustration. Select from the following list:

Anatomic crown
Anatomic root
Enamel
Dentin
Pulp
Secondary (cellular) cementum
Apex
Apical foramen
Cervical line
Primary (cell-free) cementum
Gnarled enamel

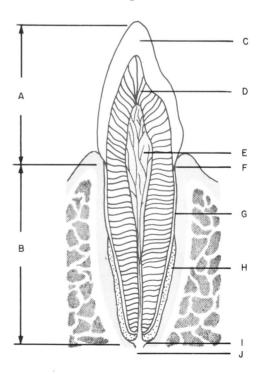

A. _____   F. _____

B. _____   G. _____

C. _____   H. _____

D. _____   I. _____

E. _____   J. _____

3. Identify the lettered parts of the illustration. Select from the following list:

Enamel   Dentinal tubule
Dentin   Tomes' fibril
Odontoblasts (shown in both views)   Apical foramen
Secondary dentin
Pulp

A. _____

B. _____

C. _____

D. _____

E. _____

F. _____

G. _____

H. _____

4. Another term for the cementoenamel junction is _____.

5. The hard tissues of the crown are_____and
   _____.

6. The hard tissues of the root are_____and
   _____.

7. The portion of the pulp cavity found in the crown of the tooth is the_____
   _____.

8. The portion of the pulp cavity found in the root of a tooth is_____
   _____.

9. The natural opening at the apex of the root is _____.

10. The hardest tissue in the human body is_____.

11. The lines that indicate the stages of development in tooth enamel are called

    _____.

12. Narrow lines in enamel that may be mistaken for fractures are called

    _____.

13. Identify the lettered parts of the illustration. Select from the following list:

Vessels and nerves to pulp chamber   Terminal vessels and nerves
Apical foramen   (to oral membrane)
Dental vein   Vessels and nerves supplying
Inferior alveolar vein   periodontium
Inferior alveolar nerve   Dental artery
Capillary bed of pulp   Lymphatic vessel
Inferior alveolar artery   Tomes' fibril

A. _____

B. _____

C. _____

D. _____

E. _____

F. _____

G. _____

H. _____

I. _____

J. _____

K. _____

L. _____

14. Mature enamel is referred to as an "inert substance." This means that _____

    _____.

15. The tissue that makes up the bulk of the tooth is_____.

16. The cell bodies that appear as a layer of columnar cells between the pulp and the dentin are_____.
    They are considered a part of the _____.

17. All the dentin in a newly formed tooth is called _____.

18. Dentin that may appear somewhat different in form than primary dentin is termed _____.

19. What type of dentin forms as a direct result of irritation or stimulation?_____

    _____

20. Some examples of the common irritants of dentin-forming cells are _____

    _____.

21. Cementum joins the enamel near the _____of the tooth.

22. Name two types of cementum formation.

    a. _____

    b. _____

23. Which type of cementum forms and is usually confined to the apical third of the root?_____

24. From what type of tissue does dental pulp tissue develop? _____

    _____

25. Name the functions of the dental pulp. _____

    _____

26. Death of cell tissue due to disease or injury is called _____.

27. Why should dental caries progress more rapidly in dentin than in enamel?

    _____

28. Two tooth tissues that are formed continuously throughout the life of the tooth are _____ and _____.

29. In a mature tooth, is the dental pulp more or less extensive? _____

Chapter 19: Tissues Surrounding the Teeth

OBJECTIVES:

After studying this chapter, the student will be able to:

- Determine the supporting tissues of human teeth.
- Discuss the structure and function of the alveolar process(es).
- Discuss the structure, functions, and importance of the periodontal ligament.
- Identify the types of gingiva and their function.
- Discuss the radical changes that may occur in the gingiva(e) and the contributing reasons for the change.

INTRODUCTION

In the first chapters of this section, histology has been limited to the development and structure of teeth. However, it must be realized that without the presence and function of a group of structures that immediately surround the cervical part of the crown and root, these teeth would be nonfunctional. Although these structures are closely related and often blend together, it is helpful to consider them separately.

The tissues that surround and support the teeth are the *alveolar process*, the **periodontal ligament** (membrane), and the gingivae. Collectively, they are called the *periodontium*.

ALVEOLAR PROCESS

The alveolar process as such develops in connection with the growth of the jaw and the eruption of the teeth. The alveolar processes are not structures separate from the maxilla and mandible but are parts of them that are especially

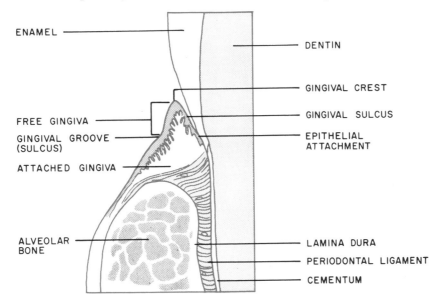

Fig. 19–1. **Structure of periodontium**

139

designed to provide sockets and supports for the teeth. To understand the relationships of the teeth, mandible, and maxilla, it will be helpful to review the structure of these bones. Refer to Chapters 5 and 7.

Histologically, the alveolus is made up of compact bone with an inner (lingual) and outer (facial) plate called the *cortical plate*. Between these two plates, the bone is spongy (cancellous). Both the inner and outer cortical plates are continuous with a thin layer of compact bone, the alveolar process proper, or **lamina dura**. This dense bone lines the root socket and affords attachment for the principal fibers of the periodontal ligament. In some areas of the jaw, the lamina dura and cortical plates are interrupted by perforations (small openings) through which pass blood, lymph vessels, and nerves, figure 19–1.

The cortical plate provides strength and protection for the supporting bone (maxilla and mandible) and also acts as a site for attachment of skeletal muscles. The cortical plate is covered by periosteum (fibrous sheath) and varies slightly in the different regions of the arches. In the labial sections, the cortical plate is attached directly to the alveolar process proper (lamina dura). Because of this arrangement, the bone overlying the roots of the anterior teeth is of a brittle nature. The cortical plate is more dense in the mandible than in the maxilla and has fewer perforations for passage of vessels and nerves.

PERIODONTAL LIGAMENT

The periodontal ligament (membrane) is a term used for a group of connective fibers that suspend the tooth in the socket and support the

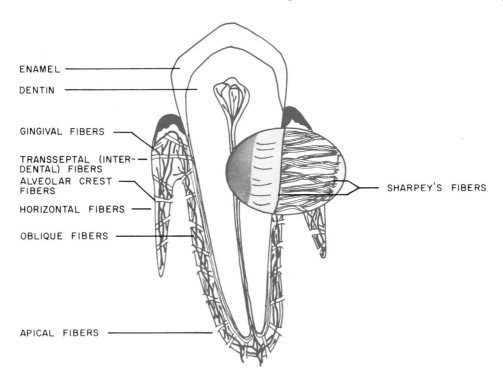

Fig. 19–2. Structure of periodontal membrane, principal fibers

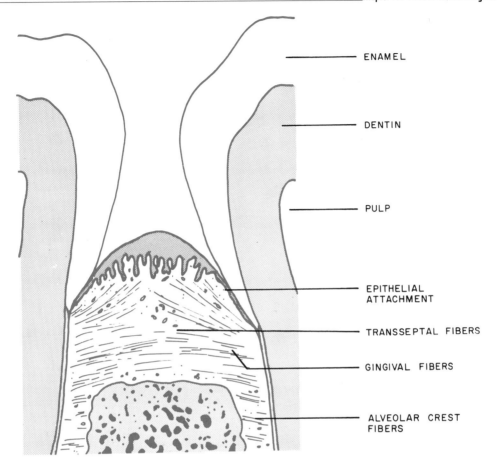

ENAMEL

DENTIN

PULP

EPITHELIAL
ATTACHMENT

TRANSSEPTAL FIBERS

GINGIVAL FIBERS

ALVEOLAR CREST
FIBERS

Fig. 19–3. Fibers of periodontal ligament

gingiva. Note: Previously, some references have used the term *peridontal membrane*. However, the term *periodontal ligament* is widely accepted, because it is more descriptive when reviewing its function. This ligament is made up primarily of *Sharpey's fibers* and *principal fibers*, figure 19–2. *Sharpey's fibers* are bundles of principal fibers anchored in the cementum on one end and in bone on the other. They form bundles of fibers that are arranged so as to withstand the functional stresses of the tooth after it has fully erupted. The fibers are not elastic but owing to the wavy direction of their course, some slight tooth movement is permitted.

In the erupted tooth, several groups of fibers can be distinguished. The principal fibers are concerned with the support of the gingival tissues and the tooth. They are white collagenous fibers and are arranged as follows: (1) *gingival fibers*—radiate in the gingiva and are attached to the tooth in the region of the cementoenamel junction; (2) *transseptal (interdental) fibers*—connect cervical portions and cementum of adjacent teeth; and (3) *alveolar group fibers*—attached to the alveolar process and to the tooth, figure 19–3. The alveolar group may be further divided into four subdivisions: (a) *cervical crest fibers*—extend from the cervical cementum to the crest of alveolar bone; (b) *horizontal fibers*—extend from the cementum to the alveolar process at right angles to the root of the tooth; (c) *oblique fibers*—extend obliquely (in a slanting direction) from the cementum to the apical two-thirds of the root to the alveolar process; and (d) *apical fibers*—radiate from the cementum surrounding the apex of the root to the alveolar process.

The principal fibers support the gingival tissue and suspend the tooth in the socket. This type of attachment is termed *gomphosis*.

The blood supply of the periodontal ligament is derived from the vessels in the alveolus. These vessels may enter the ligament by three different routes: (1) some accompany the vessels that supply the pulp and branch just before the pulpal vessels enter the apical foramen; (2) some are extensions of vessels that supply the alveolus; and (3) some are from the deep vessels that supply the gingiva. An adequate lymphatic drainage accompanies the blood vessels. Refer to figure 18–4.

Within the ligaments are cementoblasts that form cementum, osteoblasts that build bone, and fibroblasts that form fibrous tissues. The presence of small nests of slightly modified epithelial cells may be observed in the periodontal ligament. These cells are remnants of the enamel organ and are known as *epithelial rests*.

The functions of the periodontal ligament are formative (cementoblasts and osteoblasts), supportive (principal fibers), and sensory and nutritive (nerves and blood vessels).

GINGIVA

The surface of the gingiva consists of various layers of epithelium. The gingiva consists of **free gingiva** and **attached gingiva**. The free gingiva (so-called because it is movable) fits snugly around the crown of the tooth just above the cervical part (cervix). The edge, or lip, of the free gingiva is the *gingival crest* (**gingival margin**). Between the tooth and the free gingiva is the space called the *gingival sulcus* (sulcus, groove) that extends to the point at which the gingiva is attached to the tooth. Below the sulcus, the attachment of the tooth and gingiva is a marked line separating the free gingiva and the attached gingiva; this is called the *free gingival groove*. Triangular folds of gingival tissue between the teeth consist of both free and attached gingiva; these are called *interdental papillae* (papilla, cone-shaped projection). The chief function of this tissue is protection—it prevents injury and infection to the deeper tissues.

Changes in the Gingiva

Radical changes can and do occur in both the composition making up the gingiva and in the relation of the gingiva to the tooth. These changes may be referred to as *gingival recession*. As the term implies, the gingivae recede rootward, and, as a result, the gingival crest recedes from its original position to a more rootward position. Such changes may be the result of advancing age, improper oral hygiene, malocclusion, and physiological or pathological disturbances.

Epithelial downgrowth is accompanied by detachment of the periodontal fibers from this portion of the root. Recession may proceed to the degree that the crest of the gingiva may recede to a point below the cementoenamel junction. This type of gingival recession occurs in the absence of any known pathological disturbance (alterations produced by disease). It results in the exposure of more of the crown in the tooth cavity, and because it is accompanied by a detachment of the gingiva, an extremely wide and deep space in the gingival crevice, it is called a *periodontal pocket*.

REVIEW

1. Identify the lettered parts of the illustration. Select from the following list:

Enamel
Dentin
Gingival fibers
Transseptal (interdental) fibers
Cementum
Horizontal fibers

Oblique fibers
Apical fibers
Alveolar crest fibers
Sharpey's fibers

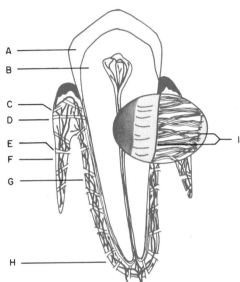

A. _____

B. _____

C. _____

D. _____

E. _____

F. _____

G. _____

H. _____

I. _____

2. To review this chapter, identify the lettered parts of the illustration.

Enamel
Dentin
Gingival crest
Gingival sulcus
Epithelial attachment
Lamina dura
Apical fibers
Periodontal ligament
Cementum
Free gingiva
Gingival groove (sulcus)
Attached gingiva
Alveolar process

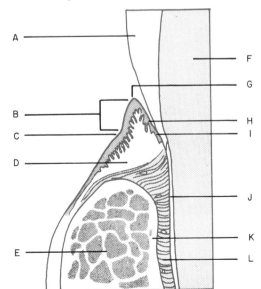

A. _____

B. _____

C. _____

D. _____

E. _____

F. _____

G. _____

H. _____

I. _____

J. _____

K. _____

L. _____

3. The three supporting structures of the teeth are _____,
_____, and _____.

4. Collectively, these tissues are called _____.

5. A thin layer of compact bone, continuous with the cortical plate and lining
the alveolus is the _____.

6. What type of fibers are those that suspend the tooth in the socket and support
the gingiva? _____

7. The two terms used when referring to these fibers are _____
and _____.

8. What are the three groups of principal fibers?

a. _____

b. _____

c. _____

9. What are the four subdivisions of the alveolar group?

    a. _____

    b. _____

    c. _____

    d. _____

10. The attachment of the principal fibers to cementum or bone is called

    _____.

11. Three functions of the periodontal ligament are _____,
    _____, and _____.

12. Two types of gingival tissue are _____
    and _____.

13. The edge of the free gingiva is called_____.

14. The space between the tooth and free gingiva is called the _____
    _____.

15. The attachment of the tooth and the gingiva is the _____.

16. A biological change in gingival tissue not due to a pathological disturbance is
    called_____.

Chapter 20: Eruption of the Teeth

After studying this chapter, the student will be able to:
- Discuss the events that occur prior to the tooth-eruption process.
- Determine some of the physiological symptoms leading to the eruption of deciduous (primary) teeth.
- Explain the sequence and usual times of eruption of deciduous teeth.
- Explain the sequence and usual eruption times of permanent teeth.
- Discuss the progressive changes that occur in the dental pulp of a tooth.

INTRODUCTION

The eruption of the teeth is a normal physiological process—a result of growth—during which the crown of the developing tooth and the root are formed. All the factors that allow crowns to escape from their bony surrounding and appear in the oral cavity are not fully understood. Growth results in the enlargement and elongation of the tooth, accompanied by the positioning of the tooth in the oral cavity. Some authorities have speculated that the process is a result of pressure exerted by the roots as they elongate during development. Only recently has it been concluded that the teeth of human beings are in a state of continuous eruption.

PROCESS OF ERUPTION

A review of the events that occur prior to or that accompany **eruption** may give us a better understanding of this process. In the enamel organ stage of development, the tooth is enclosed in a fibrous sheath (the dental sac) that lies within a crypt (space within the alveolar bone). Differentiation of the cells results in the formation of the permanent tooth bud. Fibers from the dental sac position themselves in the root of the tooth, and since the crown is virtually complete just preceding eruption, the result is

the *occlusal movement* of the tooth, also referred to as *active eruption* (occlusal, the contacting surfaces of opposing teeth, upper and lower arch).

When the crown emerges through the oral epithelium, a union of the oral and combined epithelia occurs. The portion made up of the oral mucosa is altered somewhat and forms the gingiva. The combined epithelium on the cervical part of the crown is retained and becomes the epithelial attachment. (Refer to figure 19–1.)

At the time of eruption, the fibers of the peridontal ligaments are not fully formed or attached; this occurs when the teeth are formed sufficiently to occlude (biting surfaces of maxillary and mandibular teeth meet).

There are normally ten deciduous (primary) teeth and sixteen permanent teeth in each jaw. During early childhood and before all the deciduous teeth have erupted, the child is said to have *incomplete deciduous dentition*. Later on, when the child has a full complement of deciduous teeth, the term used is *complete deciduous dentition*. Loss of the deciduous anterior teeth, and replacement by permanent teeth at about the age of 5 or 6 years, is called *mixed dentition*.

Some deciduous teeth erupt entirely uneventfully, and others erupt with some incident. A study of the **symptoms** (evident disorder in the functions of the body) of deciduous tooth eruption reveals excessive *salivation* (secretion of saliva), or drooling. This is followed by periods of

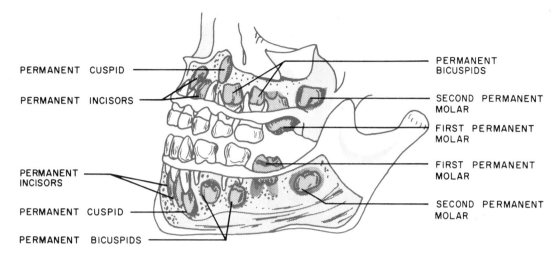

PERMANENT CUSPID

PERMANENT INCISORS

PERMANENT INCISORS

PERMANENT CUSPID

PERMANENT BICUSPIDS

PERMANENT BICUSPIDS

SECOND PERMANENT MOLAR

FIRST PERMANENT MOLAR

FIRST PERMANENT MOLAR

SECOND PERMANENT MOLAR

Fig. 20–1. Mixed dentition (approximately age 7)

fretfulness and biting, accompanied by a loss of appetite. In the event that body resistance is lowered, a rise in body temperature, coughing, sneezing, and diarrhea may be evidenced.

Ordinarily, the permanent teeth develop to replace and assume the position of the deciduous teeth after **exfoliation** (involved in the process of shedding the primary teeth); such teeth are called _succedaneous teeth_. They develop in close proximity to the root(s) of the deciduous teeth, figure 20–1. As the permanent tooth crown develops, the root of the deciduous tooth undergoes the physiological process of **resorption** (resorption, a loss of substance and reduction of the volume and size of tissues). This results in a loss of attachment, and the tooth is exfoliated. In the areas where the permanent tooth buds do not replace the primary teeth, the permanent tooth buds arise independently.

Eruption of the permanent teeth, although somewhat less dramatic, often presents problems not present in the eruption of deciduous dentition. Tooth buds of the permanent teeth develop in the jaw during the time the deciduous teeth are in their normal positions; they are not situated so that their lengthwise movement alone will bring them into position in the dental arch. They must erupt to pierce the oral epithelium and at the same time assume the relative position of other teeth in the arch. Consequently, these teeth must, and often do, undergo movements in several directions in addition to the occlusal movement.

ERUPTION OF DECIDUOUS (PRIMARY) TEETH

The eruption of deciduous (primary) teeth commences about the seventh month after birth and is completed about the end of the second year. In some individuals there may be considerable variation from the schedule. In most instances, the mandibular teeth erupt before the maxillary teeth; i.e., generally, a mandibular incisor erupts shortly before the incisor of the maxillary arch with which it occludes. The anterior group consists of two central incisors, two lateral incisors, and two cuspids in each arch. Posterior dentition consists of two first molars and two second molars in each arch.

Authorities agree that the explanations of extremes in the eruption sequence cannot be given in every case. However, they have noted

TABLE 20–1

DECIDUOUS TEETH: APPROXIMATE AGES AND MOST USUAL TIMES OF ERUPTION

Deciduous Teeth	Normal Span in Months	Average Age in Months
Mandibular central incisor	3–9	6
Maxillary central incisor	5–9	7
Mandibular lateral incisor	5–9	7
Maxillary lateral incisor	7–11	9
Mandibular first molar	10–14	12
Maxillary first molar	12–16	14
Mandibular cuspid	13–18	16
Maxillary cuspid	15–20	18
Mandibular second molar	18–22	20
Maxillary second molar	22–26	24

TABLE 20–2

PERMANENT TEETH: APPROXIMATE AGES AND MOST USUAL TIMES OF ERUPTION

Permanent Teeth	Normal Span in Years	Average Age in Years
Mandibular first molar	5–7	6
Maxillary first molar	5–7	6
Mandibular central incisor	5–7	6
Maxillary central incisor	6–8	7
Mandibular lateral incisor	6–8	7
Maxillary lateral incisor	7–9	8
Mandibular cuspid	8–10	9
Maxillary first bicuspid	9–11	10
Mandibular first bicuspid	9–12	10
Maxillary second bicuspid	9–12	10
Maxillary cuspid	10–12	11
Mandibular second bicuspid	10–12	11
Mandibular second molar	10–13	11
Maxillary second molar	11–13	12
Mandibular third molar	16–25	17
Maxillary third molar	16–25	17

that the positions of erupting teeth and the time period involved follow a relatively uniform plan, table 20–1.

ERUPTION OF PERMANENT TEETH

The permanent dentition, or teeth that erupt to take the place of the deciduous teeth and those that erupt posterior to the space occupied by the deciduous teeth, should total thirty-two teeth when fully erupted and complete. These are divided into two groups (maxillary and mandibular) consisting of sixteen teeth each. The anterior group consists of two central incisors, two lateral incisors, and two cuspids in each arch. The posterior dentition is composed of two first bicuspids (premolars), two second bicuspids (premolars), two first molars, two second molars, and two third molars in each arch.

Eruption of the permanent teeth is dependent to some extent on the exfoliation of the deciduous teeth. There is great variation in the sequence of eruption. Table 20–2 is meant as a guide to normal eruption.

CHANGES IN DENTAL PULP

After the crown and part of the root are formed, the tooth penetrates the mucous membrane and becomes evident in the mouth. Further formation of the root is thought to be an active factor in pushing the crown toward its final position. Eruption of the tooth is said to be complete when most of the crown is apparent and when it has made contact with a tooth or teeth in the opposing arch.

Actually, eruption continues as more of the crown is exposed; root dentin and cementum continue to form after the tooth is in use. Formation of the root is about half–finished when the tooth emerges. Cementum covers the root. Ultimately, the root is completed.

The pulp tissue continues to function with its blood and nerve supply after the tooth is formed. By this time, the pulp cavity within the tooth has become small in comparison to the tooth size. Its outline is similar to the outline of the crown and the root, with the opening of the pulp cavity constricted at the apex. This opening is called the *apical foramen*. The pulp continues in its tissue-forming function; it may form *secondary dentin* as a protection to itself.

The dental pulp is a connective-tissue organ containing a number of structures. Among these structures are veins, arteries, a lymphatic system, and nerves. The primary function of the pulp is to form the dentin structure of the tooth. When the tooth is newly erupted, the dental pulp is large. It becomes progressively smaller as the tooth formation is completed. The pulp is relatively large in deciduous teeth and in newly erupted permanent teeth. For this reason, the teeth of children and young people are more sensitive than the teeth of older persons when exposed to changes in temperature and to dental operative procedures.

As a person ages, the pulp cavity becomes more constricted and smaller in size. Sometimes the pulp chamber within the crown is completely obliterated; in some rare instances, the entire pulp chamber has been found to be filled with secondary deposit. Although deciduous teeth are not usually affected by this process, they may show secondary dentin in the pulp chambers as a result of irritation produced by caries or excessive wear.

REVIEW

1. Identify the lettered parts of the illustration. Select from the following list:

Mandibular	**Maxillary**
Permanent incisors	Permanent incisors
Permanent cuspid	Permanent cuspid
Permanent biscuspids (premolars)	Permanent biscuspids (premolars)
First permanent molar	First permanent molar
Second permanent molar	Second permanent molar

A. _____

B. _____

C. _____

D. _____

E. _____

F. _____

G. _____

H. _____

I. _____

J. _____

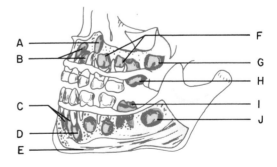

2. Occlusal movement of the teeth is also called _____.

3. When all the permanent teeth have erupted, the condition may be described as _____.

4. The presence of some deciduous teeth and some permanent teeth is described as _____.

5. The process of shedding the primary teeth is called _____.

6. Teeth that replace and assume the relative position of the deciduous teeth are called _____.

7. A loss of substance and reduction in the volume and size of the tissues at the root of the tooth is termed _____.

8. Eruption of the permanent teeth is dependent to some extent on what factor?

   _____

9. What would be the normal span of months involved in the eruption sequence of deciduous teeth? _____

10. What would be the normal span of years involved in the eruption sequence of permanent teeth? _____

11. The apical foramen is the opening of the _____ at the _____.

12. The primary function of dental pulp is to form the _____.

Chapter 21: Resorption of the Deciduous Roots

OBJECTIVES:

After studying this chapter, the student will be able to:
- Review and determine the usual positions of the succedaneous teeth in relation to the permanent teeth.
- Explain the area of greatest resorption of the deciduous teeth.
- Explain why deciduous roots may be retained and unresorbed as permanent (succedaneous) teeth erupt.
- Discuss the specialized cells involved in the process of root resorption.

The resorption (shedding) of deciduous roots is a natural phenomenon. The smaller teeth, even though they are well suited for the growing jaw, are replaced with larger teeth that are better able to perform the work of more mature jaws. Because the jaws have become larger, the pressure of mastication has increased, and stronger structures are needed to withstand the stress.

By the time the deciduous teeth have erupted, the permanent teeth are left to occupy a position near the apices of the deciduous anterior teeth and between the roots of the deciduous molars. If the succedaneous tooth is lingual to the root of the deciduous tooth, resorption will be greatest in the area of the root that lies next to the permanent tooth organ; i.e., the lingual surface (refer to figure 20–1). When the deciduous roots surround the permanent tooth bud, as in molars, the root surfaces of the tooth nearest the permanent (succedaneous) tooth are the first to experience resorption.

In cases where the permanent successor is not in alignment with the deciduous roots, eruption may be along a path that permits a portion of the deciduous root to be retained and unresorbed. This can be revealed by means of a radiographic (x-ray) examination. The deciduous root should be physically extracted to make room for the proper development of the permanent tooth. On the other hand, deciduous roots tend to resorb even when no permanent successor is present. A deciduous tooth may remain in position far beyond its natural shedding time, and resorption occurs because the deciduous tooth is unable to withstand the forces of mastication. In this case, the root is resorbed by traumatic stimulation (trauma, damage produced by external force).

The process of shedding (exfoliating) deciduous teeth can be summarized by saying that it is the result of progressive destruction of the roots. Pressure created during growth and eruption of permanent teeth stimulate activity of the **osteoclasts**, **cementoclasts**, and **dentinoclasts**. Osteoclasts are specialized cells that destroy the bone between the deciduous tooth and its permanent successor. The cementoclasts and dentinoclasts then cause general resorption of the roots of the deciduous (primary) teeth until only the crowns remain. As this takes place, the permanent tooth is moving into position. When the deciduous tooth crowns are shed, this space is occupied by the permanent tooth. Permanent molars erupt in the space posterior to the deciduous teeth that have developed during the forward growth of the maxillae and mandible.

SUGGESTED ACTIVITY

- Study a cut-away typodont containing both primary and permanent tooth buds (mixed dentition).

Chapter 22: External Features of the Teeth

INTRODUCTION

The section entitled *Dental Histology* described the tissues of the teeth, their surrounding structures, and development. This section deals with the description of the teeth.

Odontology is the study of the descriptive anatomy of teeth; i.e., the external form and relationship of the teeth. *Teeth* are appendages (added parts) usually found in the mouth and attached to but not forming a part of the skeleton. The main purposes of teeth are to seize and masticate food and to act as "weapons of defense."

We learned from Section 4 that man has two series of teeth: (1) deciduous, or sets that are exfoliated (shed); and (2) permanent (succedaneous) teeth that replace deciduous teeth and permanent molars.

To become familiar with terms generally used in describing the external appearance of the teeth is the objective of this chapter. Some of these terms have been used in previous chapters and may be familiar, but they will be repeated to make this chapter complete.

NOMENCLATURE OF TEETH

A scientific system and terms for the several parts of the teeth, as well as their names and locations in the skull, is called *nomenclature*. The dental assistant can be of great help to the dentist by becoming well acquainted with all these terms, figure 22–1.

Maxillary teeth are located in the upper arch of the mouth (bones forming the upper arch are the maxillae), in the **maxillary arch**, and their roots are embedded in the alveolar processes of the maxillae. They are sometimes referred to as "upper teeth."

The lower arch (formed by the mandible) is called the **mandibular arch**. Teeth of the lower arch are called mandibular teeth rather than "lower teeth."

The teeth of human dentition are divided into certain groups, according to their function. They are: **incisors** (incise, to divide or cut) called *central* and *lateral incisors* respectively, and **cuspids** (or **canine**, so named because they are similar in appearance and development with a *Canidae*—Latin: family of dogs), used for tearing, piercing,

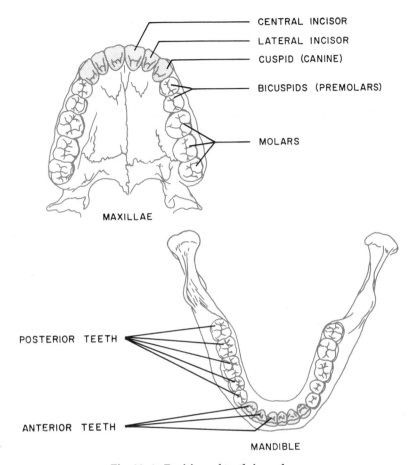

CENTRAL INCISOR
LATERAL INCISOR
CUSPID (CANINE)
BICUSPIDS (PREMOLARS)
MOLARS
MAXILLAE
POSTERIOR TEETH
ANTERIOR TEETH
MANDIBLE

Fig. 22–1. Position of teeth in arch

and holding food. These six teeth are collectively called *anterior teeth* (anterior, toward the front).

Bicuspids (or **premolars**, so named because they take an anatomical position in front of the molars) are used to pierce and crush food; **molars** (derived from the word *molaris*—Latin: grindstone), are the grinding teeth. These teeth (a total of ten in each arch) are called the *posterior teeth* (posterior, toward the rear).

Crown Surfaces

There is really only one surface on the crown— the *coronal* surface of a tooth (derived from the Latin *corona dentis*, the crown of a tooth). How-

ever, because this surface bends over in several directions, areas result that face different directions. These areas receive their names from the direction in which they face. An imaginary line is drawn from the most prominent part of the forehead (the *glabella*) to a point on the alveolar margin and then between the two central incisors in each arch. This is commonly known as the *median line*, figure 22–2. Those surfaces that face this line are called **mesial** surfaces; those facing away from it are known as **distal** surfaces.

Collectively, **facial** surfaces are: (1) the surfaces of the anterior teeth that face toward the

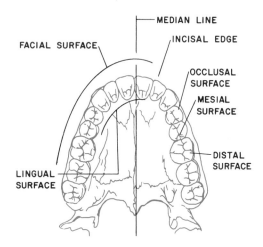

Fig. 22–2. Median line and surfaces of teeth

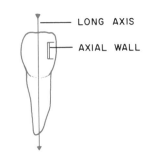

Fig. 22–3. Long axis of tooth

lips (**labial** surfaces); and (2) the surfaces of the posterior teeth that face toward the cheeks (**buccal** surfaces). The facial surfaces of the anterior teeth are generally seen when a person smiles; depending on the breadth of the smile, some of the posterior facial surfaces may also be evident.

Lingual surfaces are the surfaces of both the anterior and posterior teeth that face toward the tongue (lingua, tongue). A term sometimes used to denote those surfaces of the maxillary teeth is **palatal**, since they face the hard palate.

Occlusal surfaces are the horizontal surfaces of the posterior teeth used for masticating food. They derive their name from occlusion (the relationship between the masticating surfaces of the maxillary and mandibular teeth when they are in contact).

Incisal edges are the cutting edges of the anterior teeth. After these surfaces become flattened from wear, they are called incisal surfaces.

The *long axis* of a tooth is the imaginary line (axial line) around which the structures of the teeth are more or less symmetrically arrranged. The amount of deviation from the axial line differs in every individual and in every tooth of the individual. However, any surface of a tooth that is parallel to the long axis of the tooth is called an

axial surface. The mesial, distal, facial, and lingual surfaces are axial surfaces. The boundary of a cavity lying within the tooth and parallel to the long axis is termed the *axial wall*, figure 22–3.

Proximal surfaces are tooth surfaces that lie adjacent to one another in the same arch. Mesial and distal surfaces of adjacent teeth are proximal surfaces. Areas on the proximal surfaces that actually touch each other are called *contact areas*. The space between proximal surfaces is called **interproximal** space. Part of the interproximal space is occupied by the interdental papilla. The part that is not so occupied is referred to as the **embrasure** (the V-shaped space radiating from the contact areas of the teeth). Embrasures may extend in different directions from the proximal surfaces and are distinguished by their direction: (1) occlusal; (2) facial; (3) lingual; and (4) gingival, figure 22–4.

Embrasures (1) serve as escapeways for food during mastication, (2) tend to promote "self-cleaning" of the interproximal surfaces by allowing the free passage of food from between the teeth during mastication, and (3) a well-formed contact protects the underlying soft tissues in the gingival embrasure by preventing the wedging of fibrous food between the teeth.

Division into Thirds

For descriptive purposes when teeth are discussed, each axial surface of the crown and root

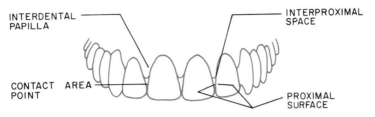

Fig. 22–4. Proximal surfaces and contact areas

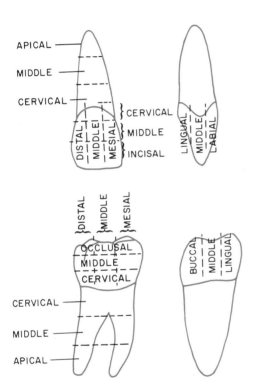

Fig. 22–5. Division into thirds

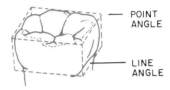

Fig. 22–6. Line angle and point angle, shown on molar tooth

off in thirds when viewing or studying any aspect. There is one middle third and two other thirds that are named according to the area they approach, such as cervical, occlusal, mesial, or lingual. In addition, each axial surface may be divided longitudinally (lengthwise) into thirds; i.e., each mesial and distal surface may be divided into a facial (labial or buccal), a middle, and a lingual third.

Angles of the Teeth

A **line angle** is formed by the junction of any two surfaces of a tooth crown, and its name is derived by combining the names of the two surfaces. A **point angle** is formed by the junction of any three surfaces of a tooth, and its name is derived by combining the names of the three surfaces, figure 22–6.

It should be noted here that in combining names to denote line angles, the "al" ending of the first name is dropped and the letter *o* is substituted (as in mesiobuccal or mesiocclusal). In the case of point angles, the letter *o* is substituted

of the tooth is divided horizontally into thirds, with each third being named in accordance with the area in which it lies, figure 22–5. When looking at the tooth from the labial or buccal aspect, one sees that the crown and root may be divided into thirds from the incisal or occlusal surface of the crown to the apex of the tooth. Each of the five surfaces (aspects) of a crown may be marked

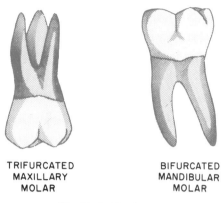

TRIFURCATED
MAXILLARY
MOLAR

BIFURCATED
MANDIBULAR
MOLAR

Fig. 22–7. Tooth roots

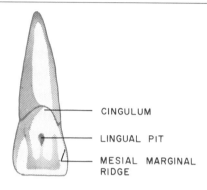

CINGULUM

LINGUAL PIT

MESIAL MARGINAL
RIDGE

Fig. 22–8. Lingual aspect of maxillary central incisor

in the first two names, as in mesiobuccocclusal. Line angles and point angles are used only as descriptive terms to indicate location.

OTHER LANDMARKS OF TEETH

To briefly review the subject, each tooth has a crown and a root portion. The *anatomic crown* is that part of the tooth covered with enamel. The **anatomic** root is that part covered with cementum. The **clinical crown** is the part of the tooth that is exposed in the oral cavity. The *cervix*, or neck, of the tooth is the constricted portion at which the anatomic crown and the root meet. The *cervical line* (cementoenamel junction) is the slight indentation that encircles the tooth at the cervix and marks the junction of the enamel with the cementum.

A tooth may have a single root, or it may have two or three roots. When a tooth has two roots, the root portion is said to be **bifurcated** (divided into two branches). When it has three roots, the root portion is said to be **trifurcated** (divided into three branches), figure 22–7.

To intelligently study each tooth, the dental assistant must be able to recognize the following important landmarks:

A **cusp** is a rounded elevation, or mound on the working surface of a cuspid, bicuspid, or molar tooth. Each cusp is representative of a center of calcification (a lobe) in the developing tooth.

A **cingulum** is the lingual lobe of an anterior tooth and appears on the cervical third of the tooth, figure 22–8.

A **mamelon** is one of the three prominences at the incisal edge of a newly erupted incisor. These prominences will wear away during use, leaving a flattened surface to the incisal portion.

A **ridge** is any linear elevation on the surface of a tooth that is named according to its location and form, such as *buccal* ridge, *incisal* ridge, and *marginal* ridge.

Marginal ridges are those rounded borders of the enamel that form the **margins** of the occlusal surfaces of the bicuspids (premolars) and molars mesially and distally, and the mesial and distal margins of the incisors and cuspids lingually, figure 22–9.

Triangular ridges are the ridges that descend from the tips of the cusps of bicuspids and molars toward the center part of the occlusal surfaces.

A *transverse ridge* is formed by two triangular ridges that join and cross the occlusal surface of the posterior tooth.

An *oblique ridge* runs diagonally across the occlusal surface of maxillary molars.

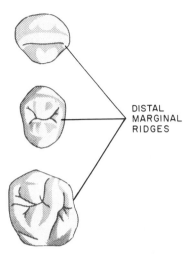

DISTAL
MARGINAL
RIDGES

Fig. 22–9. Marginal ridges

A **sulcus** is a notably long depression or valley in the surface of a tooth between ridges and cusps. It has a developmental groove at the junction of its inclines.

A *developmental groove* is a shallow **groove** or line on the surface of a tooth. It represents the junction of two or more developmental lobes. A supplemental groove is also a shallow linear depression on the surface of the tooth, but it does not mark the junction of primary parts.

Buccal and *lingual grooves* are developmental grooves found on the lingual surfaces of posterior teeth.

A **fissure** is a *linear* fault occurring along a developmental groove. It is caused by failure of the enamel of the separate lobes to become properly fused, or joined.

A **fossa** is an irregular depression on the surface of a tooth.

A **pit** is a small pinpoint depression on the surface of a tooth, usually located at the end of a groove or where two or more grooves join (i.e., the *central* pit of the mandibular first molar is located where the developmental grooves join in the central fossa).

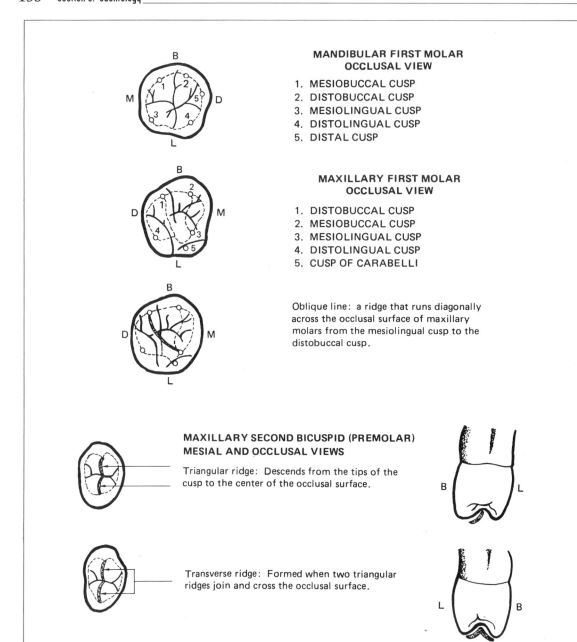

MANDIBULAR FIRST MOLAR OCCLUSAL VIEW

1. MESIOBUCCAL CUSP
2. DISTOBUCCAL CUSP
3. MESIOLINGUAL CUSP
4. DISTOLINGUAL CUSP
5. DISTAL CUSP

MAXILLARY FIRST MOLAR OCCLUSAL VIEW

1. DISTOBUCCAL CUSP
2. MESIOBUCCAL CUSP
3. MESIOLINGUAL CUSP
4. DISTOLINGUAL CUSP
5. CUSP OF CARABELLI

Oblique line: a ridge that runs diagonally across the occlusal surface of maxillary molars from the mesiolingual cusp to the distobuccal cusp.

MAXILLARY SECOND BICUSPID (PREMOLAR) MESIAL AND OCCLUSAL VIEWS

Triangular ridge: Descends from the tips of the cusp to the center of the occlusal surface.

Transverse ridge: Formed when two triangular ridges join and cross the occlusal surface.

Fig. 22–10. Cusps and ridges of teeth (occlusal views)

REVIEW

1. The groups that make up the anterior teeth are _____.

2. The groups that make up the posterior teeth are _____.

3. Surfaces facing the median line are called _____ surfaces.

4. Tooth surfaces of the anterior teeth that face the lips are called _____ surfaces; the surfaces of the posterior teeth that face the cheeks are called _____ surfaces. Collectively, these surfaces are classed as _____ surfaces.

5. What is the difference between an occlusal and an incisal surface? _____

   _____

   _____

6. When we speak of the long axis of a tooth, what do we mean? _____

   _____

7. Name the axial surfaces of a tooth. _____

   _____

8. What do we call a boundary of a cavity lying within the tooth that is parallel to the long axis? _____

9. If proximal surfaces of teeth lie adjacent to one another in the arches, which surfaces become the proximal surfaces? _____

10. The areas where proximal surfaces actually touch one another are called

    _____.

11. What is an embrasure? _____

    _____

12. What are three functions of embrasures?

    a. _____

    b. _____

    c. _____

13. What are pits? What are fissures?_____

    _____

14. What are marginal ridges? _____

    _____

15. Which teeth make up the succedaneous teeth?_____

    _____

16. Name the point angles of an incisor, considering the incisal as a surface.

    _____

17. Name the line angles of the incisal surface of a maxillary central incisor.

    _____

18. On which teeth are oblique ridges likely to be most pronounced? _____

    _____

19. Which teeth have triangular ridges?_____

    _____

20. If the root portion of a tooth has two branches, it is _____.
    If the root portion of a tooth has three branches, it is _____.

Chapter 23: Descriptions of Individual Teeth

OBJECTIVES:

After studying this chapter, the student will be able to:

- Describe individual variations in size, shape, and other characteristics of teeth as well as their basic design and function.
- Compare cusps, roots, and the occlusal aspects of anterior and posterior teeth.
- Define terms and identify anatomical landmarks of individual teeth.
- List the prominent characteristics of each permanent tooth.

INTRODUCTION

In this chapter each tooth in the permanent dentition will be described and illustrated. It is well to remember that teeth show considerable variations in size, shape, and other characteristics. Certain teeth show a greater tendency to deviate from the normal. The descriptions that follow are of normal teeth.

To make it easier for the dental assistant to relate these descriptions to his or her work in assisting the doctor to chart the mouth of the patient, detailed sketches of all aspects of the teeth are included.

MAXILLARY CENTRAL INCISOR

The maxillary central incisor looks like a wedge when viewed mesially or distally with the point of the wedge at the incisal (cutting) edge of the tooth, figure 23–1.

The *labial surface* resembles a thumbnail in outline. The mesial margin is nearly straight and meets the incisal edge at almost a 90° angle, but the distal margin meets the incisal edge in a curve. The incisal edge is straight, but the cervical margin is curved in the shape of a half moon. There are two developmental grooves on the labial surface.

The *lingual surface* is quite similar to the labial surface in outline, but it is smaller in all dimensions. There are marginal ridges at the mesial

and distal margins. Generally, there is a cingulum at the junction of the lingual surface and the cervical line, figure 22–8. Sometimes a deep pit (the lingual pit) is found in conjunction with the cingulum. As the dental assistant assists the

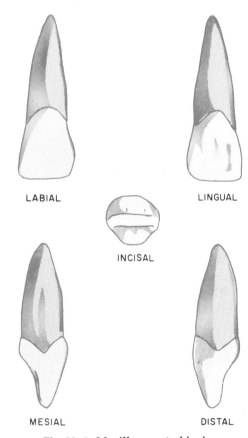

LABIAL LINGUAL

INCISAL

MESIAL DISTAL

Fig. 23–1. Maxillary central incisor

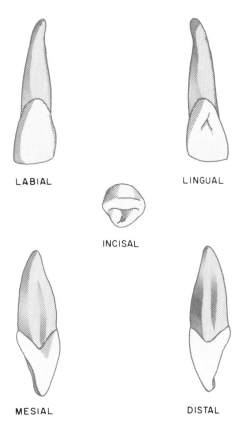

LABIAL   LINGUAL

INCISAL

MESIAL   DISTAL

Fig. 23–2. Maxillary lateral incisor

doctor in a root canal procedure (which includes removing the pulp tissue and refilling the hollow length of the root), the assistant may see the doctor make an external opening through this pit and drill into the root canal.

As with all anterior teeth, the *root* of the maxillary central incisor is single. This root is from one and one-fourth to one and one-half times the length of the crown. Usually, the apex of the root is inclined distally to a slight degree. The line angles of this tooth are well rounded.

MAXILLARY LATERAL INCISOR

The maxillary lateral incisor is much like the maxillary central incisor, but it is shorter, narrower, and thinner, figure 23–2.

The developmental grooves on the *labial surface* are not so evident as those of the central incisor. More significant, however, is the disto-incisal edge, which is well rounded with the curvature continuing to the cervical line. The mesiolabial angle is nearly straight, paralleling the long axis of the tooth for half its length. Then it turns inward as it approaches the cervical line.

The shape of the *lingual surface* varies with the individual. In some persons it is markedly concave (almost spoonlike in appearance), and in others it is flat. The lingual surface is the same width as the facial surface. The *root* is cone-shaped but sometimes flattened mesiodistally.

MAXILLARY CUSPID

The maxillary cuspid is said to be the longest and strongest tooth in human dentition, figure 23–3.

The *labial surface* of the crown differs considerably from that of the maxillary central or lateral incisors. By comparison, the incisal edges of the central and lateral incisors are nearly straight, and the cuspid has a definite point, or cusp. The distoincisal cutting edge is the longer of the two. Therefore, the tip of the cusp is closer to the mesial surface than to the distal surface. The curvature of the labial surface is more prominent by the *labial ridge*, which extends from the tip of the cusp to the cervical line. The developmental grooves, which are so prominent on the labial surface of the central incisor, are present here, extending two-thirds of the distance from the tip of the cusp to the cervical line.

The *lingual surface* has the same general outline as the labial surface but is somewhat smaller because the mesial and distal surfaces of the crown tend to move toward each other as they meet the lingual surface. The lingual surface is concave, with very prominent mesial and distal marginal ridges, and a *lingual ridge* that, like the labial ridge, extends from the tip of the cusp

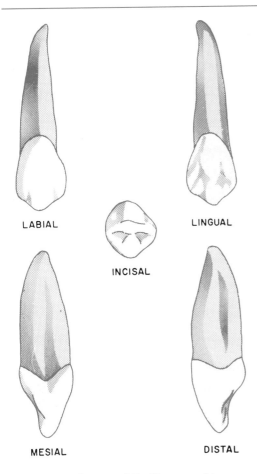

LABIAL   INCISAL   LINGUAL

MESIAL   DISTAL

Fig. 23–3. Maxillary cuspid

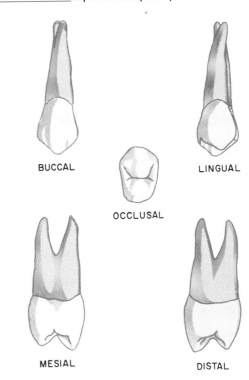

BUCCAL   OCCLUSAL   LINGUAL

MESIAL   DISTAL

Fig. 23–4. Maxillary first bicuspid (premolar)

toward the cervical line. There is generally a cingulum in the cervical portion of the lingual surface of the crown.

The *root* is single and is the longest root in the arch. It is usually twice the length of the crown—because the cuspid is designed for seizing and holding. Progressing into a dental health career, the dental assistant will notice the frequent use of cuspids as abutment teeth (teeth that anchor a bridge).

MAXILLARY FIRST BICUSPID (PREMOLAR)

The maxillary first bicuspid (premolar) is the fourth tooth from the median line. It is con-sidered to be the typical bicuspid ("bicuspid" means having two cusps). However, as has been mentioned before, they are currently called premolars because they are just in front of the molar teeth, figure 23–4.

The *buccal surface* is somewhat similar to the labial surface of the cuspid. In the case of the bicuspid (premolar), however, the tip of the buccal cusp is located in the center of the "biting" edge; this is called the *occlusal edge*, or occlusal margin. Therefore, the mesiocclusal and distocclusal edges appear to be of equal length. From the cusp tip to the cervical margin there is a slight ridge, the *buccal ridge*, which is similar to the labial ridge found in cuspid teeth.

The *lingual surface* is narrower and shorter than the buccal surface and is smoothly convex in all directions. The cusp tip is in the middle of the occlusal edge.

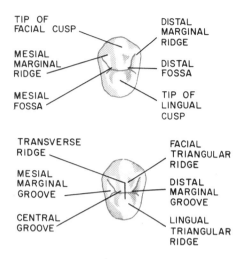

Fig. 23–5. Occlusal surface of maxillary first bicuspid (premolar)

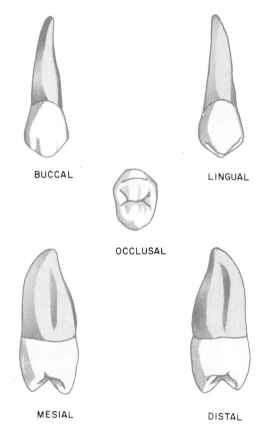

Fig. 23–6. Maxillary second bicuspid (premolar)

The *contact areas* are normally located in the occlusal third or at the junction of the occlusal and middle thirds, see figure 22–5.

The *occlusal surface* has a buccal cusp and a lingual cusp, figure 23–5. There is also a mesial marginal ridge and a distal marginal ridge. These correspond to the marginal ridge on the lingual surfaces of anterior teeth. There are two fossae on the occlusal surface. The one near the mesial marginal ridge is called the *mesial fossa*, and the one near the distal marginal ridge is called the *distal fossa*. The two cusps are separated by a groove, known as the *central groove*, and a triangular ridge extends downward from the tip of each cusp toward the central groove. One is called the *buccal triangular ridge* and the other the *lingual triangular ridge*.

The root is quite flat on the mesial and distal surfaces. In approximately half of the maxillary first bicuspids, the root is divided at the apical third. When it is so divided, the tips are slender and finely tapered.

MAXILLARY SECOND BICUSPID [PREMOLAR]

The maxillary second bicuspid (premolar) resembles the first bicuspid (premolar) very closely, but it is smaller in all dimensions. It has a *single root*, figure 23–6.

MAXILLARY FIRST MOLAR

The maxillary first molar is the sixth tooth from the median line, figure 23–7. The first molars are often called "6-year molars," because they erupt when the child is about six years of age.

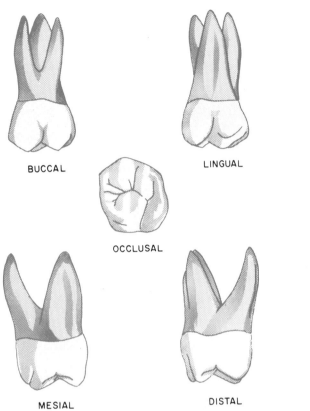

Fig. 23–7. **Maxillary first molar**

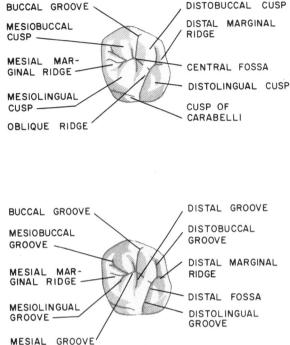

Fig. 23–8. Occlusal surface of maxillary first molar

The *buccal surface* is convex in all directions. The *buccal groove*, which continues over from the occlusal surface, is quite prominent and terminates in the middle third of the buccal surface.

The *lingual surface* resembles the buccal surface but is somewhat smaller. The *distolingual groove* of the occlusal surface continues over onto the lingual surface, where it fades out in the middle third. In a great many instances there is a prominent lobe, or cusp, on the lingual surface of the mesiolingual cusp. There is a fifth cusp in addition to the four cusps on the occlusal surface. This is called the **cusp of Carabelli**.

In all molars the pattern of the *occlusal surface* is quite different from that of the bicuspids, figure 23–8. The cusps are large and prominent, and the broad grinding surfaces are broken up into rugged-appearing ridges and well-defined grooves. By the nature of these physical characteristics of the occlusal surfaces, it can be seen why most mastication (chewing and grinding) takes place on the molar teeth. The occlusal surface has four cusps—the mesiobuccal, the mesiolingual, the distobuccal, and the distolingual. The cusp of Carabelli can be seen when the tooth is viewed occlusally, but it does not form part of the occlusal surface. All the cusps are prominent, the mesiolingual being the highest. The mesial and distal margins differ from those of the bicuspids in that they are broader and appear stronger. An *oblique ridge*, which is not present on the bicuspids (premolars), appears here. (It should be noted that it also appears on the maxillary second and third molars but often is not so pronounced.) The oblique ridge runs from the mesiolingual cusp to the distobuccal

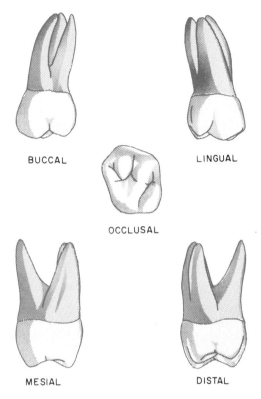

Fig. 23–9. Maxillary second molar

molars are often called "12-year molars," because they erupt when the child is about 12 years of age.

Because it has the same function as the maxillary first molar, its physical characteristics are the same, except that it is smaller, and the cusp of Carabelli does not appear. There is a marked reduction in the size of the distolingual cusp.

MAXILLARY THIRD MOLAR

The maxillary third molar is the eighth tooth from the median line, figure 23–10. Third molars are often called "wisdom teeth," because they erupt when the young adult is passing into manhood or womanhood. This tooth is much smaller than either the maxillary first or second

cusp and is marked in its midsection by the passage of the *distal groove*. On the mesial side of the oblique ridge is the *central fossa*: on the distal side is the *distal fossa*, which is smaller than the central fossa. In the distal fossa the most prominent feature is the *distolingual groove*; it parallels the course of the oblique ridge.

The *roots* of the first molar are widespread, which tends to give the tooth strength and firm anchorage. The maxillary first molar has three roots, which are named according to their location—mesiobuccal, distobuccal, and lingual. The lingual root is the largest.

MAXILLARY SECOND MOLAR

The maxillary second molar is the seventh from the median line, figure 23–9. The second

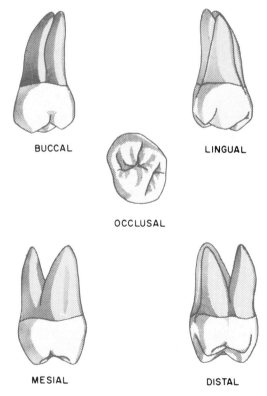

Fig. 23–10. Maxillary third molar

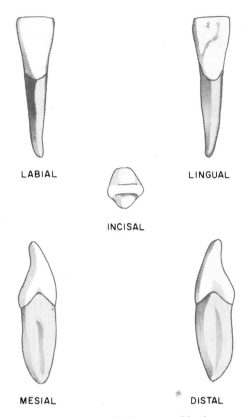

Fig. 23–11. **Mandibular central incisor**

molar, and the occlusal outline is almost circular, owing to the nearly complete disappearance of the distolingual cusp.

The *occlusal surface* is generally covered with numerous fissures and grooves.

The *root* may have from one to as many as eight divisions. These divisions are usually fused and are often curved distally.

MANDIBULAR CENTRAL INCISOR

The mandibular central incisors are, as a general rule, the first permanent (succedaneous) teeth to erupt, replacing deciduous teeth, figure 23–11. They are the smallest teeth in either arch.

The *labial surface* of the mandibular central incisor is widest at the incisal edge. Both the

mesial and the distal surfaces join the incisal surface at almost a 90° angle. Although these two surfaces are nearly parallel at the incisal edge, they move toward one another at the cervical margin. The developmental grooves may or may not be apparent. When present, they appear as very faint furrows.

The *lingual* surface is concave from the incisal edge to the cervical margin.

The *root* is slender and much flattened on its mesial and distal surfaces.

MANDIBULAR LATERAL INCISOR

The mandibular lateral incisor is a little wider mesiodistally than the mandibular central incisor, and the crown is slightly longer from the incisal edge to the cervical line, figure 23–12.

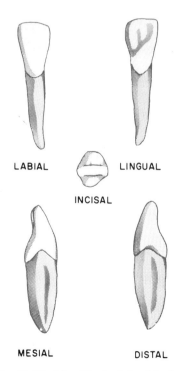

Fig. 23–12. **Mandibular lateral incisor**

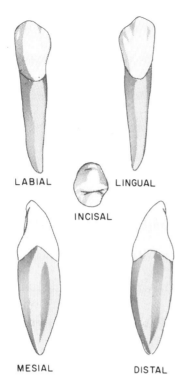

Fig. 23–13. Mandibular cuspid

The *root* is not so long as the maxillary cuspid root and is flatter mesiodistally.

MANIDBULAR FIRST BICUSPID (PREMOLAR)

A mandibular first bicuspid (premolar) is the fourth tooth from the median line. It is the smallest of the four bicuspids, figure 23–14. Viewed from its buccal aspect, it shows a marked constriction at the cervical line; the term "bell-crowned" is used to describe this characteristic appearance. The mandibular first bicuspid differs greatly from the maxillary first bicuspid. Although there are two cusps—a buccal and a lingual, the latter has little prominence (in most cases) and might be compared to the cingulum on the lingual surface of the maxillary cuspid. The buccal cusp is long and sharp and resembles the cusp of the mandibular cuspid.

The *incisal edge* is not at right angles to the mesial and distal edges as it is in the mandibular central incisor.

The *root* is single and much flattened on its mesial and distal surfaces.

MANDIBULAR CUSPID

The mandibular cuspids, like the mandibular incisors, are smaller and more slender than the opposing teeth in the maxillary arch, figure 23–13.

The *labial surface* of a mandibular cuspid is much the same as that of a maxillary cuspid, except that the distoincisal cutting edge is almost twice the length of the mesioincisal edge.

The *lingual surface*, as a rule, is very smooth, and a cingulum is rarely present.

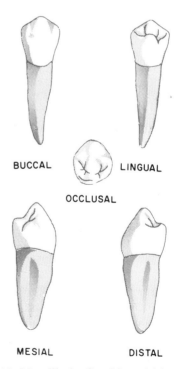

Fig. 23–14. Mandibular first bicuspid (premolar)

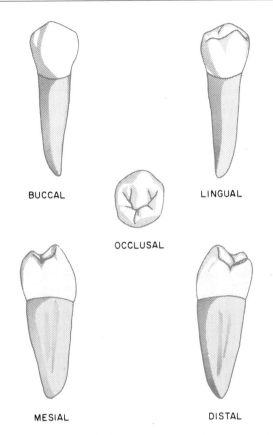

Fig. 23–15. **Mandibular second bicuspid (premolar)**

The *buccal surface* is very convex in all directions.

The *mesial surface* is distinctly convex in the occlusal third but is concave in the other two thirds.

The *distal surface* is shaped like the mesial surface.

The *lingual surface* is small and very convex and appears to overhang the lingual surface of the root.

MANDIBULAR SECOND BICUSPID (PREMOLAR)

The mandibular second bicuspid (premolar) is the fifth tooth from the median line, figure 23–15.

Its *buccal surface* characteristics are the same as the first bicuspid (premolar), with a prominent buccal ridge.

The *lingual surface* is similar to that of the mandibular first bicuspid (premolar), with the exception that there may be two lingual cusps.

The *occlusal surface* of the tooth occurs in different patterns. The first is the three-cusp type, in which the lingual groove divides the lingual marginal ridge into two distinct parts. This type of occlusal surface takes the shape of a Y. In the Y-form the buccal, the mesiolingual, and the distolingual cusps are evident. A less common two-cusp type has no lingual groove, but the central groove forms a half circle; there are only two prominent cusps—the buccal and the lingual.

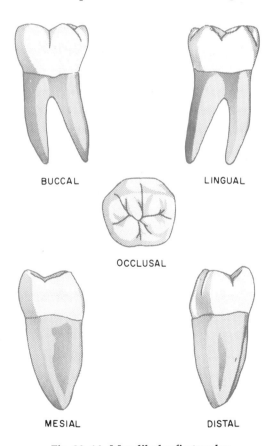

Fig. 23–16. **Mandibular first molar**

The root of the tooth is single, and in many instances the apical region is quite curved.

MANDIBULAR FIRST MOLAR

The mandibular first molar is the sixth tooth from the median line. It is the first permanent tooth to erupt, figure 23–16.

The *buccal surface* of this tooth is more convex than its counterpart in the maxillary arch. There are two grooves on the buccal surface—the *buccal groove*, which is an extension of the buccal groove from the occlusal surface, and the *distobuccal groove*, and extension of the distobuccal groove from the occlusal surface.

The *lingual surface* is smaller in area than the buccal surface and is marked by an occlusal margin. The margin shows two distinct cusps created by a sharply defined lingual groove that ends in the middle third of the surface.

There are five cusps on the occlusal surface, figure 23–17. This is in contrast to the maxillary first molar, in which the fifth cusp is on the lingual surface of the mesiolingual cusp, figure 23–8. On the mandibular first molar, this fifth cusp is called the distal cusp. It is between the distobuccal and the distolingual cusps but nearer to the buccal surface than to the distal surface. The other two cusps are the mesiobuccal and mesiolingual. The mesiolingual cusp is the highest cusp.

Three main grooves on the *occlusal surface* have already been mentioned: the *buccal groove*, which helps to distinguish the mesiobuccal and the distobuccal cusps; the *distobuccal groove*, which likewise extends over the facial margin and separates the distobuccal cusp from the distal cusp; and the *lingual groove*, which divides the lingual margin into two portions and thus creates the distolingual cusp and the mesiolingual cusp. The remaining two grooves that should be noted are the mesial groove and the distal groove. The *mesial groove* runs from the

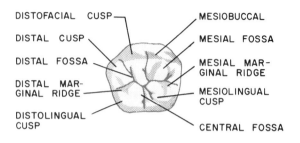

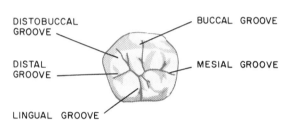

Fig. 23–17. Occlusal surface of mandibular first molar

central fossa over the mesial marginal ridge. The *distal groove* also originates in the central fossa and runs over the distal marginal ridge, where it separates the distal cusp from the distolingual cusp.

The tooth has two *roots*, a mesial and a distal.

MANDIBULAR SECOND MOLAR

The mandibular second molar is the seventh tooth from the median line, figure 23–18.

The *buccal surface* has only one groove, the *buccal groove*, which originates in the occlusal surface and extends over the buccal margin onto the buccal surface; it usually ends in a deep fossa, the *buccal fossa*.

The *lingual surface* resembles that of the mandibular first molar in that it has a lingual groove. However, in this tooth the area of this surface is almost as great as that of the buccal surface.

The *mesial* and *distal surfaces* are more convex than those of the first molar.

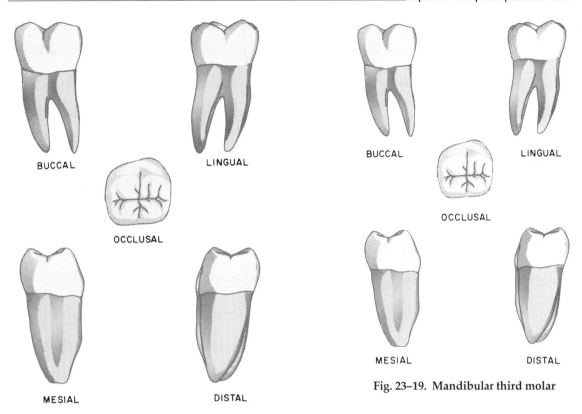

BUCCAL   LINGUAL

OCCLUSAL

MESIAL   DISTAL

Fig. 23–18. Mandibular second molar

BUCCAL   LINGUAL

OCCLUSAL

MESIAL   DISTAL

Fig. 23–19. Mandibular third molar

The greatest difference between the *occlusal surfaces* of the mandibular first and second molars is that the occlusal surface of the second molar has no fifth cusp. Four cusps—the mesiobuccal, the mesiolingual, the distobuccal, and the distolingual—are outlined by the buccal, lingual, mesial, and distal grooves. A *central fossa* is present and appears in the geometric center of this surface.

There are two *roots* and they are smaller than those of the first molar.

MANDIBULAR THIRD MOLAR

The mandibular third molar appears in many shapes, forms, and sizes, figure 23–19. Its general appearance is similar to the two other mandibular molars, but it has smaller surfaces, more supplemental grooves, and four or five cusps, which are not so sharply differentiated as those of the first two molars.

The roots, usually two in number, often show a distinct distal curvature.

All third molars, whether maxillary or mandibular, often vary widely from the usual pattern.

REVIEW

1. How many permanent teeth should appear in the maxillary arch? In the mandibular arch? _____

2. The labial surface of a maxillary central incisor could be compared to a

   _____ in outline.

3. Where is the lingual lobe of a maxillary central incisor located? _____

   _____

4. How many of the anterior maxillary teeth usually have more than one root?

   _____

5. Which tooth is usually the longest in human dentition? _____

6. Compare the incisal edge of the maxillary central incisor with that of the maxillary cuspid. _____

   _____

7. Does the maxillary cuspid have a cingulum? _____

   _____

8. Where are the contact areas generally located in most teeth? _____

   _____

9. How many cusps does the maxillary first molar usually have? Are all of them found on the occlusal surface? _____

10. Give the location of the cusp of Carabelli. _____

    _____

11. Name the four occlusal surface cusps of a maxillary first molar.

    a. _____

    b. _____

    c. _____

    d. _____

12. Locate the oblique ridge on a maxillary molar. _____

_____

13. Which of the mandibular incisors are wider mesiodistally? _____

_____

14. Compare the maxillary and mandibular cuspids. _____

_____

_____

15. Which of the bicuspids (premolars) is the smallest? _____

16. Compare the occlusal aspect of a maxillary first bicuspid (premolar) with that of a mandibular first bicuspid. _____

_____

_____

17. Which of the maxillary and mandibular first bicuspids (premolars) may have two roots? _____

18. Which of the bicuspids may be found to have two lingual cusps? _____

_____

19. How many cusps does a mandibular first molar have? Do they all appear on the occlusal surface? _____

20. Which of the cusps of a mandibular first molar is the highest? _____

_____

21. How many roots does a maxillary first molar have? Name them. _____

_____

_____

22. Name the longest root of the maxillary first molar. _____

23. How many roots does a mandibular first molar have? Name them. _____

_____

_____

Chapter 24: Infectious Diseases in the Dental Environment

OBJECTIVES:	After studying this chapter, the student will be able to: • Define the meaning of disease. • Discuss the etiological factors of disease. • Identify the diseases that most often spread from person to person in the dental environment. • Discuss the means by which indirect transmission of infectious disease may occur. • Discuss the means by which direct transmission of infectious disease may occur. • State the precautionary measures of control for the various infectious diseases.

INTRODUCTION

Infectious diseases that can be transmitted from one person to another have proven to spread to and from the patient in the dental environment. The patient health questionnaire, though valuable, cannot be relied upon to identify infectious patients. In fact, many patients do not realize they have been exposed and are potential disease carriers; for example, only one of five persons who has had hepatitis B is aware of it.

The patient with a disease at the incubation stage may be more infectious than one with the active disease, as with hepatitis and measles. The **incubation period** of an infectious disease is measured by the time of its entry into an organism up to the time of the first appearance of signs or symptoms. Patients may not appreciate the importance of informing the dental office of their health status, past or current, because they regard the mouth as being separate from the rest of the body! Others may deliberately conceal information for fear they might be denied treatment.

Adding to public health anxiety is the emergence of acquired immunodeficiency syndrome (AIDS). This has generated a great deal of interest about the impact of viral infections on the practice of dentistry. Of major concern to all dental practitioners are tuberculosis, herpes simplex, serum hepatitis B, and AIDS. The onset and residual effects of these diseases vary greatly. They do, however, have one aspect in common—their potential to be spread in the dental office.

WHAT IS DISEASE?

Before entering on a discussion of the possible causes of disease, it may be well to ask ourselves, What is disease? This is a question that is a great deal easier to ask than to answer. To the patient it means dis-comfort, dis-ease, dis-harmony with his or her environment; to a dentist or physician, it means a variety of signs and symptoms with one or more structural changes or lesions.

Disease may be defined as the *pattern of response of a living organism to some form of injury.* With the presence of disease, there is usually some altered or disordered cell function. Thus, disease is a response to all kinds of injury, ranging from infection with bacteria or virus, to stress or depression.

The presence of **lesions** (disease-related or external injury-induced tissue damage) may bear an obvious relation to symptoms. Lesion is a broad term and includes wounds, sores, ulcers, tumors, cataracts, and other tissue damage.

Etiology

The relationship of cause, origin, reason for something, and effect is known as the **etiology** of a disease. It might be supposed that the relation of the etiological agent to disease, of cause to effect, was a relatively simple matter. The reverse is the case. Perhaps, we are misled into imagining that only one cause is responsible. We say that the cause of tuberculosis is the tubercle bacillus, but we know that many people may inhale these bacilli, yet only one may develop the disease. The bacilli may lurk in the body for years and only become active as a result of factors such as an existing infection, prolonged strain (stress), and starvation. In determining the cause of a disease, such elements as heredity, sex, environment, immunity, allergy, and other agents must be considered.

Infections

By far, the most common cause of disease is **bacteria**. These, together with molds or fungi, properly belong to the animal kingdom. Certain lowly forms of animal life, known as animal *parasites*, may live in the body and produce disease. Finally, there are *filterable **viruses***, forms of living matter so minute they pass through the pores of filters fine enough to hold back bacteria, so tiny that they cannot be seen by the most powerful light microscope and are said to be *ultramicroscopic*. They can be made visible with the electron microscope. This last group has attracted a great deal of attention in recent years.

TUBERCULOSIS

Tuberculosis was considered the number one killer in the United States at the turn of the century. Since the 1930s it has been on the decline, and by the 1980s was no longer considered a major health threat.

Of late, tuberculosis cases have grown in number. In 1990 it increased by 5 percent, along with the dramatic increases in HIV- (Human Immunodeficiency Virus) infected persons. Estimates of Americans infected with tuberculosis now near the 10-million mark.

Tuberculosis is a chronic inflammation caused by human bacillus tuberculosis (*Myobacterium tuberculosis*). There is evidence that the natural defensive power of the body against tuberculosis is sufficiently great to hold it in check in the majority of cases. This defense may be broken down by an infection such as influenza, which undermines health, by overwork, poor hygienic conditions, insufficient food, and such. This bacillus may live outside the body for six months if not exposed to sunlight and is an exceptionally resistant germ.

Transmission of Infection

Tuberculosis infection may spread from one person to another by inhalation. When an infected person coughs, the discharged droplets infect the air in the immediate area with millions of tubercule bacilli contained in tiny droplets of moisture. Transmission occurs in the dental office through handling of unclean objects and used, contaminated dental instruments, a very good reason for following the universal guidelines for infection control when treating *all* patients.

Hospital-grade disinfectants approved by the Environmental Protection Agency (EPA) and used in the dental office *do* kill the tuberculosis bacterium. However, to be totally effective, they must be used according to the manufacturer's instructions. It is heartening to realize that in healthy persons the probability of a tuberculosis infection developing into an active tuberculosis that is infectious is remote.

HERPES SIMPLEX VIRUS

Two types of **herpes simplex** virus have been identified: HSV-1 and HSV-2. HSV-1 is more common in children between 1 and 3 years of age, whereas HSV-2 is transmitted after puberty usually through sexual contact. Both HSV-1 and HSV-2 can produce lesions around the mouth. These lesions are painful and affect the exposed pink or reddish border, called the **vermilion border** of the extraoral lip. Regardless of the location, the lesions begin as either a single or multiple vesicular (a serum-filled blister) eruption. The vesicles burst, ulcerate, and scab within five to ten days. The lesions of herpes infections shed virus and are infective until healing is complete.

A primary herpetic infection usually is self-limiting, and complications are rare. Unfortunately, there presently is no antiviral therapy for herpes. Treatment is neither specific nor very satisfactory. Tincture of benzoin and camphorated lip ice may help to dry the lesions around the mouth.

Secondary or recurrent herpetic lesions may affect oral tissues as well as the human genitalia (external sex organs).

According to the Occupational Safety and Health Administration (OSHA), a splatter of herpes in saliva can cause blindness within forty-eight hours. Eye protection for the dental operatory personnel and the patient is a must!

VIRAL HEPATITIS

The term *hepatitis* means inflammation of the liver (hepat(o), liver; -itis, inflammation). This inflammation can occur from a variety of injurious or harmful agents, including recognized viral forms of the disease.

Hepatitis A (HAV)

Hepatitis A, known as *infectious hepatitis*, usually occurs in children and young adults. It is frequently transmitted from person to person by way of contaminated foods and liquids or by the oral-fecal route, as, for example, when someone who is carrying the virus does not wash hands after using the restroom and then handles food.

Hepatitis A is a virus that multiplies in the intestinal tract and invades the blood stream, localizing in the liver. It has an incubation time of two to six weeks and is most infectious a week *before* the onset of any clinical symptoms. At this time, large amounts of the virus can be found in the stools and urine of the infected individual. Clinical symptoms are an acute onset accompanied by a high fever and sometimes jaundice.

Most hepatitis A infections are without severe complications and are treated with bedrest and high-protein and -carbohydrate diets. Recovery takes six to eight weeks.

Hepatitis B (HBV)

It is estimated that 600,000 to 1 million carriers of the **hepatitis B** virus (HBV) live in the United States. According to the Centers for Disease Control (CDS), the number of new cases increases by approximately 200,000 each year. Surveys show that the incidence of hepatitis B resulting from work-related accidents decreased by 75 percent between October 1981 and September 1988. No doubt the decline is due to hepatitis B immunization and to following standardized precautions. It is obvious that hepatitis B, because of its tendency to spread, is a real problem for individuals in the dental profession.

Hepatitis B, referred to as **serum hepatitis**, was once thought to be transmitted only by contaminated needles during transfusion of blood or blood products. Sexual contact, needle sharing among drug addicts, mother to fetus transmission, and infected blood or blood products remain the principal avenues for spreading the virus.

The hepatitis B virus can be found in all body fluids and may spread from one person to another in a variety of ways, including household contact through sharing utensils, food, razors, and the like. The CDC has shown that HBV can be transmitted by a splatter of any body fluid into the eye. The CDC projects that a health worker stands a one-third of 1 percent chance of contracting the disease of an AIDS patient from a splatter, but a 30 percent chance from a hepatitis patient. Hepatitis B can spread in the dental environment through patient debris on contaminated instruments, surfaces, and dental charts.

The incubation period for HBV is from two to six months. The onset of hepatitis B spreads in a harmful but not easily detected manner, making it difficult to diagnose. Symptoms may mimic the flu: headache, malaise (feeling of illness or depression), mild stomach upset, flitting joint pain. Infection with HBV increases the risk of developing liver cancer.

Should a needle prick or other wound occur while a staff member is performing a procedure on a member of any high-risk group, the person should receive an injection of Hepatitis B Immune Globulin (HBIG) as soon as possible if he or she has not been immunized against the virus already. HBIG will provide passive immunity for two to three months.

Protection. The best protection against any disease is immunity to that disease. The American Dental Association (ADA) and OSHA recommend that all dental professionals receive the hepatitis B vaccine. The OSHA guidelines state that the employer-dentist make available the vaccine for his employees and that vaccination be kept up-to-date!

Three different vaccines used to immunize against HBV are Heptavax-B (a plasma-derived vaccine), Recombivax-HB, and Energix-B (both are genetically engineered products). Energix-B has recently been approved for immunization against all known subtitles of hepatitis virus. Each of the vaccines requires a series of three injections and can be administered by either an intramuscular or intradermal method.

There is one very important part of the vaccination process that many individuals do not complete. Three months after you complete your last injection, have a titer for antibodies to the hepatitis B surface antigen. This titer will tell you if you developed antibodies (protection) and what your protection level is at that time. The chart below should be used to determine your level of protection.

0.0 to 2.0	Neg. (no immunity)
2.1 to 9.9	Borderline
10.0 and above	Immunity

If your titer indicates a level below 10.0, you should have an additional booster and recheck your titer again. If you completed your vaccination process sometime ago and never had a titer, you should proceed with it now to determine if you ever developed antibodies.

The average individual probably will need a booster vaccination somewhere between five to seven years after their initial series. However, some studies indicate that a booster requirement is based on the original titer and age of the individual and will vary from person to person.

On April 14, 1991, the National AIDS Network reported that most people, including health care workers, do not consider hepatitis B as great a threat as the AIDS virus. Furthermore, even health care workers, who should know better, have a problem taking hepatitis B seriously. Sullivan cited a CDC survey of hospitals with established vaccination programs that found only 30 percent of their health care workers were vaccinated against hepatitis B.

Hepatitis B is a major health risk in dentistry, responsible for many lost weeks or months of work, as well as the inability to continue in dental practice, permanent disability, or death.

Hepatitis C (HCV)

Hepatitis C, a chronic disease of the liver, is considered to be the major cause of posttransfusion hepatitis. Like hepatitis B, hepatitis C is transmitted through blood transfusions, contaminated water, infected drug needles, and sexual body fluids. Health care personnel risk the possibility of exposure through accidental needle stick injuries.

In May 1990, the Food and Drug Administration (FDA) approved a test that detects antibodies to the hepatitis C virus. This currently used test screens blood donations and reduces the risks of transmission through transfusions. The test identifies carriers of the virus. Presently, it is effective in detecting chronic infections of six months or longer. However, it may not be as effective in detecting acute cases.

There is no effective treatment for hepatitis C nor a vaccine against it at this time.

Hepatitis D (HDV)

Hepatitis D has been determined to occur simultaneously with hepatitis B. The ability to spread rapidly and extensively among many individuals in a given area and its clinical course are similar. Fortunately, immunization against HBV will provide protection against HDV.

AIDS

Acquired Immunodeficiency Syndrome (AIDS), now a worldwide epidemic, is one of the most serious health problems that has faced the American public. An *epidemic* may be defined as a contagious disease that spreads rapidly and extensively among many individuals in any geographic area. The hysteria created by this disease is unfounded and has resulted in misunderstanding and intolerance. Individuals have been denied access to schools, fired from jobs, harassed, evicted, and refused medical and dental treatment. It is important that everyone, regardless of who they might be, understand this disease.

Acquired Immunodeficiency Syndrome is a disease caused by the **Human Immunodeficiency Virus (HIV)**, the AIDS virus. As of May 1989, more than 94,000 cases of AIDS had been reported to the CDC and 58 percent of those diagnosed had already died. Projections indicate that in 1993 there will be 365,000 reported cases of AIDS and 263,000 AIDS-related deaths. As of January 1992, CDC reports indicated that there were 206,000 HIV-infected persons in the United States.

The CDC and medical research teams in the United States have projected a sizeable increase in the number of both HIV and AIDS cases, with a comparable increase in AIDS related deaths throughout the decade.

The HIV virus enters the body and attaches itself to particular target cells. T-lymphocytes (helper T-cells) are the virus's main, but not exclusive, targets. As the widespread invasion continues, the virus seems to target more and more types of cells and to present itself in different ways. The HIV virus has been known to infect nerve cells, travel to the brain, and cause *dementia* (loss of thought processes and memory).

Contrary to theory, AIDS *cannot* be transmitted by casual contact, such as sharing of household items, drinking glasses, toothbrushes, sharing a bed or clothing, and such. The virus is not specific to any particular group of individuals. It is most important to realize that a person can be infected with HIV without showing any symptoms at all. It is possible for her or him to be infected for years, feel fine, and have no way of knowing if he or she is infected.

It can be said that HIV is no longer considered a virus of *high-risk groups*, but a virus of *high-risk behaviors*. Transmission of AIDS occurs by any of the following routes.

The AIDS virus can spread from one person to another through sexual activity. Any person engaging in *unprotected* sexual intercourse with a HIV carrier is at risk. Many experts indicate that the only "safe sexual intercourse" can occur between two individuals who have been in an absolutely monogamous relationship for at least seven to eight years, who have both been tested, and have no other risk behavior or sexual contacts.

The male homosexual population was the first in the country to feel the effects of AIDS. However, the number of heterosexuals is growing. Risky sex behavior and lack of standards for selection of sex partners place those persons in a high-risk group.

The second route of transmission of HIV is through blood and blood products. In many communities, the sharing of drug needles and syringes by those who shoot drugs is the fastest route by which HIV spreads. Sharing needles, even once, is an extremely easy way to become infected with HIV. Blood from an infected person can be trapped in the needle or syringe, then injected directly into the blood stream of the next person who uses the needle.

Other behaviors involving needles increase the risk of HIV infection. Many young people pierce each other's ear lobes, using the same needle to puncture the ears of several friends. Some young athletes inject themselves with steroids, then pass the needle and syringe on to others. Studies show that over half of all high school seniors have used illegal drugs, some of which were injected intravenously.

Numerous young people are taking risks that can lead to AIDS. Although 13- to 19-year-olds account for only 1 percent of the recognized AIDS cases, the 20 to 29 age group now accounts for 21 percent of the diagnosed cases. In less than five years, AIDS is projected to be the leading killer of this age group. Since there is a long (an average of 9.8 years) incubation period between infection with HIV and the onset of AIDS symptoms, researchers believe that many young adults diagnosed with AIDS contracted the virus during their adolescent years.

Testing for the HIV antibody in all donated blood has been occurring for the past several years and has drastically reduced the numbers of people who contract the disease through transfusions of blood and blood products. A test developed by Abbott Laboratories can determine the presence of the virus itself and should make blood supplies safer for the transfusion recipient. Bear in mind that, although there is still a risk factor connected with transfusions, most recipients are in a life-threatening situation and may well die without the transfusion.

A third mode of transmission, and one that is increasing, is the passing on of the virus from an infected mother to her infant, either before birth or at the time of delivery.

Detection of AIDS

The *HIV Antibody Test*, or so-called AIDS test, does *not* determine the presence of the AIDS disease. It *does* show if a person has been *infected* with the HIV, or AIDS, virus. The test looks for changes in blood that occur after being infected. It is very reliable when testing is conducted by a reputable laboratory and the results checked are by a knowledgeable physician.

When the HIV Antibody Test became available in 1985, most AIDS agencies remained neutral on its use. Because of complex political, ethical, and public health issues surrounding the test, it was left as a matter of personal choice. It was viewed more as an educational tool than a medical determination, and there were few treatment options to offer someone who tested positive.

According to the CDC, spring 1993, a more recently developed blood test, the ELISA, may indicate a negative or positive result. If the test indicates positive, the patient should submit to the _Western Blot_, to make a determination and verify whether a false-positive or true-positive result has occurred. The Western Blot is a more highly involved blood test than is the ELISA and requires a series of laboratory testing and study over a period of time prior to reaching a conclusion.

Since the spring of 1989, community AIDS Foundations have run advertisements in local newspapers encouraging people at risk to "seriously consider voluntary, anonymous testing." In the spring of 1991, the National AIDS Network urged dental health care providers to "know their risks, and help police their own." To date, the number of recorded cases where patients have visited the dental office and were later found to be infected with HIV are few. However, health professionals and federal health officials are calling for persons at high risk to volunteer for testing.

The psychological stress involved in deciding to be tested is significant, and there still exists a real risk of housing, insurance, and job-related discrimination resulting from a breach of confidentiality. With new treatment options, most AIDS organizations are coming to feel the benefits of knowing antibody status outweigh the risks and burdens. They are reconsidering their attitudes on advocated testing. The gradual development of a medical model of disease management emphasizes early detection of infection and immune system monitoring.

AIDS Management

Presently, there is no vaccine and no cure for AIDS. _AZT_, a highly toxic (poisonous) drug approved by the FDA, is now used in antiviral therapy for the AIDS virus. This drug prevents the reproduction of HIV cells and has been shown in clinical studies to prolong the lives of some AIDS victims. AZT has been administered to those diagnosed with full-blown AIDS, but a few prelininary studies have indicated possible benefits from prescribing it earlier in the course of HIV infection.

A 1991 report of the San Francisco AIDS Foundation (SFAF) notes that researchers are now mixing AZT with other antiviral drugs in an attempt to find a combination of chemicals that will destroy HIV. In October 1991, the FDA approved the drug DDI for AIDS treatment. DDI may be used in conjunction with AZT when AZT proves too toxic for a particular patient.

The _New England Journal of Medicine_ reports that doctors from Walter Reed Army Institute of Research presented evidence of the encouraging results of an experiment by the vaccine pioneer, Jonas Salk. Salk's notion was to base his vaccine on a deactivated (no longer active) version of the AIDS virus, much like the polio vaccine he developed in the 1950s. Salk's approach uses a vaccine to boost the body's immune system after the AIDS virus has already become established. Thus, the body will be better armed to stop the harmful destruction of white blood cells. In the past, vaccines have been used solely to prevent an initial infection from occurring.

Aerosolized pentamidine, officially approved by the FDA in mid-June 1989, has proven effective in slowing or preventing **Pneumocystis carinii** pneumonia (PCP). A diagnosis of this particular type of pneumonia depends on a laboratory culture of lung tissue. Termed an "opportunistic" disease, it occurs in people suffering from AIDS, whose natural defenses have been reduced by the AIDS disease itself. Studies indicate that in over one-half of AIDS deaths PCP was determined as the cause.

The ability to prevent, delay, or treat the complications accompanying HIV infection has lent optimism to the future of the disease. Project Inform, a San Francisco organization, provides information about therapeutic options and access to treatment.

Promising drug therapies and greater understanding of the course of HIV infection have fundamentally changed prevailing attitudes towards AIDS.

For the present, the best way to slow AIDS is through worldwide education and prevention. These efforts will fight not only the epidemic of the disease but also the "second epidemic" of fear and mistrust that AIDS often generates.

Dental Care for the AIDS Patient

Like other patients with chronic diseases, AIDS patients need ongoing routine dental care. Oral findings in the AIDS patient include infections of the mucosa (mucous membranes of the mouth): **thrush**, characterized by white patches on a red, moist, inflamed surface; *recurrent herpes simplex virus*; and *progressive disease of the periodontal tissues*. Some of these disorders require treatment that can be provided in the dental office. HIV-related periodontal problems is a case in point.

Human Immunodeficiency virus infections may appear in many ways, and the dental professional should become familiar with the oral evidence, because this is often the first sign of the presence of the disease. For instance, a herpes simplex ulcer that persists longer than one month is particularly significant as an indicator of AIDS. Periodontal lesions of HIV periodontitis, or *AIDS virus–associated periodontitis (AVAP)*, are marked by swelling and intense *erythema* (redness of the tissue caused by congestion of the capillaries in the lower layers of that tissue) of the free and attached gingiva. AVAP is a rapidly progressive gingivitis with symptoms of intense pain, spontaneous bleeding, and bad breath.

Often, AIDS patients display a high incidence of **Kaposi's sarcoma** (a purplish, localized malignant cancer of the skin), which spreads from the original site to one or more sites elsewhere in the body. *Squamous* (scaly) *carcinoma* is a malignant new growth or tumor that appears on the skin surface, and has a potential to infiltrate (penetrate) surrounding tissues and to spread.

If the individual with AIDS is a regular patient, a dentist must be particularly careful if he or she wishes to assist the patient in obtaining care through other sources. Referral to clinics or hospitals equipped to treat those with infectious diseases is one means of assisting these patients to receive the necessary dental care. Each patient must be evaluated individually, and in some cases referral may be the best action for that patient. The ADA recommends that local dental societies attempt to set up a referral system for patients with AIDS and other infectious diseases to enable all patients to receive quality dental care when it is needed.

REVIEW

1. Define the term disease. _____

_____

_____

2. Lesions are _____.

3. The incubation stage of disease is measured by _____

_____.

4. Which four diseases are of major concern to all dental practice?

   a. _____ b._____ c. _____

   d. _____

5. State the definition of the *etiology* of a disease. _____

_____

6. Infections are caused by _____ and _____.

7. Tuberculosis, a chronic inflammation, is spread by the _____

_____.

8. The herpes simplex virus usually produces a lesion on the_____.

9. The term *hepatitis* means _____.

10. Infectious hepatitis (HAV) usually occurs in which two age groups?

_____

11. How can an individual contract HAV? _____

_____

12. What are some of the symptoms of a HAV infection? _____

_____

13. The incubation period for HAV is _____ weeks. Recovery usually
    takes _____ weeks.

14. Serum hepatitis (HBV) may be directly spread from person to person through four principal avenues. What are they?

   a. _____ b._____ c._____

   d. _____

15. HBV can spread in the household environment through _____

   _____.

16. What are some of the symptoms of HBV? _____

   _____

17. HBV can spread in the dental environment through _____

   _____.

18. The best protection against any disease is _____ to that disease.

19. The vaccination process for hepatitis consists of _____ injections. The average individual will need a booster vaccination somewhere between _____ and _____ years after their initial series.

20. The recommended titer test determines if you have developed _____

   _____.

21. Define the word epidemic. _____

   _____

22. AIDS is caused by infection by the _____,

   otherwise referred to as _____.

23. State three ways by which the AIDS virus can spread from one person to another.

   a. _____

   b. _____

   c. _____

24. What is meant by an "opportunistic" disease? _____

_____

_____

25. The HIV Antibody Test shows the following conditions

a. _____

b. _____

26. The average incubation period between infection with HIV and the onset of AIDS symptoms is _____ years _____ months.

27. Along with the usual symptoms of pneumonia, how can the presence of PCP be determined?_____

_____

Chapter 25: Principles of Personal Protection in Dentistry

OBJECTIVES:

After studying this chapter, the student will be able to:
- Discuss the principles of personal grooming for the conscientious chairside assistant.
- Cite the steps for disinfecting the hands and forearms.
- Demonstrate the accepted handwashing technique.
- Compare the types of gloves used in the practice of dentistry.
- Explain the rationale for wearing gloves in dentistry.
- Demonstrate the proper method(s) for donning and removing dental treatment gloves.
- Discuss the protection provided by a face mask.
- Describe the recommended eyewear for dental operatory procedures.

INTRODUCTION

The nature of dental assisting leads to the possibility of spreading infectious organisms from patient to chairside assistant, and from chairside assistant to family and coworkers as well as to other patients. For the sake of the assistant, patients, coworkers, and the assistant's family, it is necessary to break the chain of infection wherever possible, figure 25–1.

At least, a person should think about what is carried home to family members on clothing or being transmitted to fellow commuters. More than one spouse or child have become ill from microorganisms brought home on soiled clothing of a health care worker.

PERSONAL GROOMING

The conscientious chairside assistant will strictly follow several principles of good grooming in the prevention of cross-contamination.

Nails. Short, clean, with smooth tips and cuticles. Long fingernails increase the possibility of puncturing a dental glove. Nail polish is not acceptable due to microscopic chips and crevices that harbor organisms.

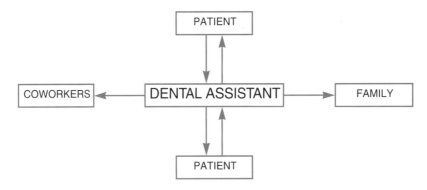

Fig. 25–1. Potential chain of infection

Uniform. Professional uniforms should be washable and bleachable, whether white or of a color. The uniform should be free of frills and other catchalls. Sleeves should be short to allow washing of the forearms. Uniform should be removed *before* leaving the office at the end of the workday and laundered separately from other clothes. Studies from Centers for Disease Control (CDC) report that professional uniforms may be laundered in a normal laundry cycle, should be given a high-temperature (140º–160ºF) wash cycle with normal bleach concentration, followed by machine drying (212ºF or more).

Hair. Short, clean, off the face and neck, or tied back and firmly secured to keep loose strands from falling forward or down.

Jewelry. Inappropriate items, such as rings, watches, bracelets should be removed at the beginning of the workday. It is impossible to scrub them free of organisms that are constantly working their way from deeper layers to the surface of the skin.

Tobacco. Odor is offensive to patients and fellow workers. Nicotine stains are unsightly and objectionable.

WASHING HANDS

Assisting with or performing intraoral procedures demands that hands be as free as possible from impurities and microorganisms that contribute to infection and disease. There are no chemicals that can be depended on to kill all organisms on the skin; therefore, hand cleansing is vital. Mechanical removal (rubbing, rinsing, drying) with the use of germicidal cleansing agents helps to prevent cross-contamination.

Supplies

Germicidal Soap Preparations. Current research indicates that the antimicrobial agents proven to be most effective against a broad range of microorganisms are chlorhexidine gluconate and providone-iodine preparations. These may be irritating to the skin of some persons; in such cases, bactericidal lotion-type cleansers containing triclosan or trilocarbon may be preferable. *Accepted Dental Therapeutics*, a publication of the American Dental Association (ADA), should be consulted for brand names.

Hand Towels. Use absorbent, disposable hand towels for complete drying. *Never* reuse any hand towel.

Procedure for Washing Hands

Effective steps must be developed for disinfection of the hands and forearms. Ideally, antimicrobial preparations should be available for use from a dispensing device, and the water source operated by a foot or forearm control. Most dental offices are furnished with hand-activated water faucets. Paper hand towels should be dispensed one at a time.

- Turn on and adjust the flow of *cool* water.
- Wet both hands, then apply sufficient amount of antimicrobial soap to work into a lather.
- Wash hands for 15 seconds by rubbing lather over all surfaces of forearms and hands. Include the palms, knuckles, and especially tips of all fingers and under the nails. Make certain both hands are cleaned.
- Using an orangewood stick, clean debris from under nails. Discard after use.
- Thoroughly rinse hands in *cold* water to close pores.

- Dry with hand towel, beginning with the fingers. Use the towel to thoroughly dry the cuticles of the nails, then run the edge of the towel under the tip of each nail. Proceed to dry hands and forearms.
- Turn off hand-activated faucet with hand towel. Discard towel in trash container.
- Apply antimicrobial lotion to hands. *Note:* Keeping the hands from cracking and drying is most important. Lotion should be applied at least three to four times a day, especially before lunch and at the end of the day.
- Prepare to don gloves.

It is advisable that front-office staff wash with antimicrobial soap several times during the workday to remove the number of pathogens from the hands. An ADA report, published September, 1985 in the *Journal of the American Dental Association*, showed that contaminated debris on dental charts can remain active for as long as five days. Although front-office staff do not wear gloves, it seems reasonable that they should take precautions for their own protection. Handwashing is a *must* for all dental personnel prior to lunch and before leaving the office at the end of the day.

PROTECTIVE GLOVES

Gloves should always be worn for protection during intraoral procedures or when handling objects that have become contaminated with saliva or blood. Bear in mind that gloves offer the best, although not perfect, barrier to organisms to and from the hands.

Gloves minimize the risk of cross-infection from patient to patient, from patient to dentist and chairside assistant, and from the dental operatory personnel to patient. Routine handwashing procedures and germicidal handwashing agents are very important, as they reduce the number of pathogens on the hands. However, these procedures alone have proved inadequate in eliminating pathogenic organisms from the hands.

In the dental situation, saliva contacted by dental personnel may become contaminated with blood. It is wise to assume that where blood and saliva are mixed, there is a potential for transmission. Dental professionals can contract infectious agents, such as herpes, HIV, hepatitis B, tuberculosis, and common respiratory viruses, through microscopic cuts and skin punctures, even hangnails. Refer to Chapter 24, *Infectious Diseases in the Dental Environment*. Patients may not be aware they have contracted an infectious disease and may seek dental care before diagnostic symptoms develop.

Use of Gloves

For years, dentistry personnel used gloves almost exclusively for surgical procedures. Today, they are used for every patient, under the guidelines of the CDC and the mandate of the Occupational Safety and Health Administration (OSHA). Although CDC can only recommend the use of gloves, OSHA has the power to enforce the guidelines.

According to the CDC, "universal precautions" must be taken. This is interpreted to mean "treat every patient as though he or she has an infectious disease that is deadly."

Types of Gloves

Dentistry uses several types of gloves: vinyl or latex examination gloves, latex treatment gloves, latex surgical gloves, cotton undergloves, plastic over-gloves, and heavy utility gloves.

Examination gloves. *Examination gloves* may be made of vinyl or latex and are dispensed unsterilized. Vinyl is used in procedures where a tight fit is not absolutely necessary. Vinyl lacks the elasticity of latex and may tear when stretched. Gloves made of vinyl easily adapt to either the left or right hand. In some cases, the choice of vinyl or latex is due to skin irritations caused by the latex material.

Treatment Gloves. *Treatment gloves* are made of latex, the preferred material. Latex is strong, tough, and elastic, capable of stretching then returning to its molded shape to fit snugly over the hand. Latex affords an ideal sense of touch during a dental procedure. Latex gloves are designed for the left or right hand and are dispensed in sizes ranging from small to large. Nonsterile latex treatment gloves can be purchased in quantities, and are adequate for most dental operatory procedures. The manufacturer treats treatment gloves with cornstarch powder, making the process of donning them much easier.

Treatment gloves are to be worn during direct patient care. They should be worn while handling radiograph films that have been in the patient's mouth, as well as dentures, dental appliances, impressions, or other items that could contribute to disease transmission.

Surgical Gloves. *Surgical gloves* are made of latex, have been sterilized and are required when dental procedures involve extensive surgical manipulation.

Over-gloves. *Plastic over-gloves* are very inexpensive; they are not a suitable replacement for latex or vinyl. Made of clear plastic, they are acceptable as an over-glove for treatment gloves. For instance, the chairside assistant needs to contact a surface that cannot be covered with a barrier and cannot be disinfected. The assistant may dry his or her gloved hands, don the plastic gloves—for this short procedure only—then simply remove and discard the over-gloves before returning to the patient. An example of

such a situation might be the need to look for information on the patient chart, or reach for supplies in a cabinet or drawer. Careful planning can reduce situations such as these.

Should gloves become sticky after washing, a small amount of cornstarch, in a disposable dappen dish placed on the corner of the instrument tray or countertop will be ready for use. *Lightly* dip a gloved finger tip into the cornstarch, rub the fingers together, then return to the patient.

Heavy Utility Gloves. *Heavy utility gloves* are used for operatory disinfection and instrument clean-up. Utility gloves are made of nitrile plastic chemically bonded with rubber. These protective gloves are puncture resistant, and not to be confused with household gloves sold in grocery or hardware stores. Utility gloves should be thoroughly washed and dried while still on the hands. Remove and spray with a disinfectant. Hang to dry.

Contaminated utility gloves should be washed, dried, and placed in the autoclave for sterilization, along with other disposables, before being discarded. Repeat handwashing and drying.

Allergic Reaction to Latex Gloves

There has been some misunderstanding about cornstarch powder on latex gloves being the sole cause of skin irritation for the wearer. It is a well-known fact that there are only three sources of cornstarch in the world. Most manufacturers use the same source for their cornstarch. Cornstarch powder is biodegradable and non-irritating.

Where the glove of one manufacturer causes irritation, that of another will not. This occurs because there are different qualities of latex material as well as variations in the manufacturing process.

Latex rubber, like maple sap, seeps from the rubber tree. Many chemical additives are used in the latex solution before it is molded. The glove is removed from the mold and washed in water to remove the residual chemicals; otherwise, the chemicals remain in the glove. Lack of this important step, rather than the cornstarch powder, probably contributes to skin irritations.

Powder-Free Gloves. A *powder-free latex glove* is chemically washed with chlorine to remove 100 percent of all the chemicals and the cornstarch powder. Powder-free or hypoallergenic (hypo-, below; or below the level to cause an allergic reaction) gloves are available. Powder-free gloves are considerably more costly than other latex gloves.

Under-gloves. Thin *cotton under-gloves* are available for use under latex and vinyl gloves and help to avoid skin surface reactions. Some dental personnel are inclined to perspire under their gloves. Under-gloves help in such situations, without the loss of any tactile (touch) sensations. A light dusting of cornstarch on the hands prior to gloving enables the glove to slip over the hand without difficulty.

Double Gloving

Double gloving is a precautionary measure taken by dental personnel during an operative procedure, when the patient is known to have an infectious disease (herpes, HIV, hepatitis B) and dental treatment is necessary. In case a small hole or tear develops during treatment, double gloving will help to avoid transmission of the disease.

Should gloves be punctured during treatment, it is always better to take the time, if possible, to immediately change them. Thus, the microorganisms trapped inside the glove will be eliminated and the likelihood of disease transmission decreased. Of course, handwashing must be repeated before donning fresh gloves.

Storage of Treatment Gloves

Latex or vinyl treatment gloves should be stored in a cool, dark place, within easy access of the dental operatory personnel. Prolonged exposure to heat and light increases the tendency to develop minute perforations. The shelf life of treatment gloves is reasonably long, but the expiration date on the container should always be checked. Manufacturers offer a variety of glove dispensers, either with a wall mount or countertop fitting.

Posttreatment Care of Gloves

Upon completion of a dental procedure:

- Wash gloved hands with a generous amount of antimicrobial soap, water, and friction.
- Rinse under running cool water tap. Dry.
- Remove gloves, turning them inside out, as they are pulled free of the fingers.
- Tuck one glove inside the other. Discard gloves in plastic disposal bag.
- In cases in which gloves are known to be contaminated, they should be sterilized, preferably by autoclaving along with other disposable materials and before they are placed in an appropriate disposal bag.
- Repeat handwashing and drying.

DISPOSABLE GOWNS

A disposable *cover-up gown*, worn over the professional uniform is now required during dental procedures. According to OSHA regulations, traditional professional uniforms are not intended to function as protection against any hazard. Refer to Chapter 27 for stated regulations.

Cover-up gowns are available in a fabric that "breathes," resists absorption, and provides an effective barrier. They protect against splatter and splash in aerosol-type environments, figure 25–2. Disposable gowns, made in hip-length

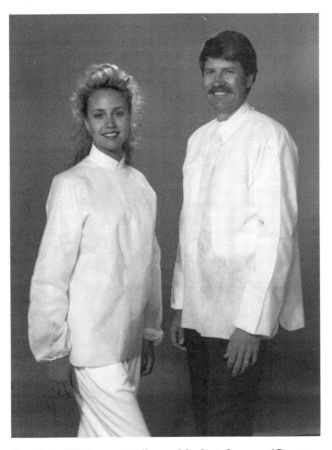

Fig. 25–2. Clinicovers™ disposable dental gowns (Courtesy Clinetex, Inc., Montrose, CO)

and thigh-length styles, can be changed at the discretion of the operator and chairside assistant. Changes are more frequent when the cover-up is visibly spattered with debris or after working with the high-risk patient. Unisex sizes range from extra small to extra large.

FACE MASKS

The choice of masks may be dictated by comfort, fit, and price. To be effective, the mask should filter out at least 95 percent of all larger particles of aerosol debris. Traditional types are the multifolded tie-on and the dome-type. Both create a problem, because the wearer will often remove the mask from the face, then allow it to hang around the neck after treatment is completed. A more recently developed face mask is multifolded with slender straps that hook over the ears. Impossible to hang around the neck!

Choose the mask, and change it at least every hour during operative procedures, or after each patient, whichever comes first. After an hour, the mask becomes moistened from the breath of the wearer and aerosol spray, gets splattered, and no longer serves its purpose. Thus, it becomes a "nest" for bacterial growth rather than a barrier. Refer to Chapter 1, figures 1–1, 1–3.

PROTECTIVE EYEWEAR

Now OSHA requires the use of eyewear with sideshields. Refer to Chapter 27 for stated regulations. This type of eyewear offers maximum protection, resists scratching and fogging, and does not cause visual distortion. For those who already wear corrective lens eyewear, the newer protective eyewear will fit over existing glasses.

Each member of the dental operatory team *must* wear appropriate eye protection. Refer to Chapter 1, figure 1–4.

SUGGESTED ACTIVITIES

- Using the recommended steps, practice handwashing, rinsing, and drying.
- Practice donning and removing treatment gloves.
- Orally explain the method(s) of disposal for treatment gloves.

REVIEW

1. Personal grooming for the dental assistant involves the following aspects

   a. _____

   b. _____

   c. _____

   d. _____

2. Handwashing involves the use of cool water and_____.

3. Front-office staff do not wear gloves but should practice handwashing for ___

   _____.

4. The two principal agencies that establish guidelines for the use of gloves in dentistry are

   a. _____

   b. _____

5. The types of gloves used in dentistry are

   a. _____

   b. _____

   c. _____

   d. _____

   e. _____

   f. _____

6. The difference between latex treatment gloves and surgical gloves is that _____

_____.

7. Cotton under-gloves are used by those dental personnel who_____

_____.

8. Double gloving is advocated for treating the patient who_____.

9. Plastic over-gloves are worn over treatment gloves when it becomes neces-sary to _____.

10. Heavy utility gloves are used for

   a. _____

   b. _____

11. Disposable gowns are worn over professional uniforms to provide_____

_____.

12. A disposable gown should be changed when

   a. _____

   b. _____

13. A face mask should be changed

   a. _____

   b. _____

14. OSHA now requires that protective eyewear have _____.

OBJECTIVES:

After studying this chapter, the student will be able to:

- Determine the two best-known chemical hazards in dental practice and their routes of entry into the human body.
- Cite the most common respiratory irritants used in the dental office.
- State the prime concern of OSHA regarding the dental staff.
- Discuss the procedures manual and its importance in controlling the use of chemicals in dentistry.
- Discuss the MSDS procedure with regard to hazardous materials.
- Determine the standards for infectious waste control and the identification of contaminated materials.
- Discuss the guidelines for infection control in the practice of dentistry.
- Determine the various immersion chemicals used in dentistry, their advantages, and disadvantages.
- Determine the chemicals used for hard-surface disinfection, their advantages, and disadvantages.
- Discuss the difference between disinfection and sterilization.
- Describe the steps involved in preparing and packaging dental instruments for sterilization.
- Compare the steam autoclave with the chemical vapor sterilizer.
- Discuss special precautions to take for instruments used on high-risk patients.

CHEMICAL HAZARDS IN THE DENTAL OFFICE

Several hazardous chemicals are found in the dental environment. Some will be addressed in this chapter.

Mercury (Hg) is perhaps the best known of the chemical hazards in dentistry. Because mercury is odorless and vaporizes at 10°F, its vapors can easily be inhaled and not be detected. The American Dental Association (ADA)'s Council on Dental Materials and Devices offers guidelines for achieving good mercury hygiene in the dental office.

Because the most serious hazard associated with mercury in dental practice is accidental spills from bulk containers of mercury, employers should consider changing to premeasured amalgam capsules. Rubber treatment gloves should be worn when handling mercury or amalgam, because it can be absorbed through the pores of the skin.

Formaldehyde is one of the chemical substances in solutions used in chemical vapor sterilizers. Routes of entry for the vapors of this chemical are inhalation, ingestion (swallowing), and skin contact. It is classified by the Occupational Safety and Health Administration (OSHA) as a human carcinogen and should be handled with care. The area where formaldehyde is used *should be well ventilated*. Rubber treatment gloves should be worn if skin contact is likely to occur, when pouring solution into a sterilizer. Should the solution come into contact with the skin, immediately wash with soap and water.

195

Manufacturers' instructions for chemical vaporizer sterilizer use must be closely followed to reduce the possibility of vapors escaping into the dental environment. Ideally, these sterilizers should be placed under hoods that are vented to the outside.

Dentistry uses many respiratory irritants. Methyl methacrylate, alcohol-based preparations, and photographic chemicals used to develop radiographs are some of the most common.

OSHA STANDARDS FOR BIOLOGICAL HAZARDS

The Occupational Safety and Health Administration has spelled out requirements for infection control in the dental office. Among these are written procedures for the proper handling of chemicals.

A loose-leaf procedures manual will provide the basis for policy and training of dental personnel. Such a manual can be easily revised to meet the dental office needs.

The Procedures Manual

A procedures manual can be in either printed or computerized form. Both are available, thus eliminating the necessity of writing one.

A manual contains the procedures needed to meet OSHA rules that cover labeling, chemical handling, containers, storage, and ordering chemicals. The manual can also include documented Material Safety Data Sheets (MSDSs) required by OSHA. These help in the event of an OSHA inspection, to prove that OSHA-required procedures and practices are in place.

Standard procedures for sterilization, surface disinfection, and ordering supplies should be included in the manual.

OSHA's prime concern is that of safe chemical handling, and how staff is protected from bloodborne diseases. Both OSHA and the Environmental Protection Agency (EPA) require safe disposal techniques for infectious wastes.

The Material Safety Data Sheets

Basically, OSHA requires an MSDS for any chemical that is supplied in a bottle, can, or bag.

Items requiring an MSDS can be listed in alphabetical order. The list should include the product name, manufacturer's name and telephone number, and the work area where the product is used. The list can be easily updated if new hazardous materials are introduced or can result in the disposal of materials that are no longer useful.

If a manufacturer fails to provide an MSDS for a hazardous product, it is the responsibility of the employer to request it. The vendor is required by law to provide the latest MSDS for that substance.

As the MSDSs are collected, a checkmark is made in the appropriate box to indicate the MSDS is on file. OSHA requires an MSDS for each substance listed.

When the MSDS arrives, the name of the material and any first-aid instructions should be highlighted with a colored felt-tipped pen. The pages are then inserted in the appropriate section of the procedures manual. Should an emergency occur, that particular MSDS should be easily found.

It is well to remember that MSDSs need to be kept only for materials that are biologically hazardous, not for regular household cleansers and detergents.

OSHA REGULATIONS FOR INFECTIOUS WASTE MATERIALS

OSHA has requirements for infectious waste materials. These regulations are designed to protect employees from accidentally or mistakenly coming in contact with HBV or HIV. Refer to Chapter 24, *Infectious Diseases in the Dental Environment*.

Biohazard Labeling

Requirements set down by OSHA cover labeling when removing hazardous materials from

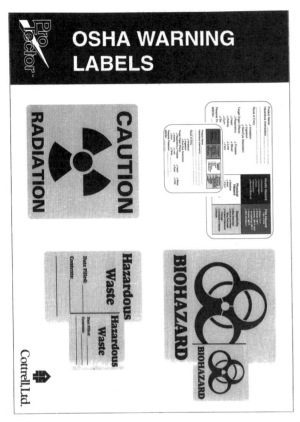

Fig. 26–1. OSHA warning labels (Courtesy Cottrell Ltd.)

original containers and placing them in a more convenient dispenser. For instance, a surface disinfectant bottle must be labeled with the MSDS number, the contents of the bottle, and the major health hazards the disinfectant may present, figure 26–1.

In addition to the requirements of the Department of Health Services, OSHA has regulations for infectious materials. The OSHA standards for infectious waste control emphasize identification of contaminated materials.

- Biohazard warning tags or labels are used as a means to prevent accidental injury or illness to employees who are exposed to hazardous or potentially hazardous conditions, equipment, or operations that are out of the ordinary, unexpected, or not readily apparent. Tags or labels are not necessary when signs or other means of protection are used.

- All warning tags or labels contain a signal word or a major message. The signal word shall be *BIOHAZARD* or the biological hazard symbol, and the major message shall indicate the specific hazardous condition or the instruction to be communicated to the employee. Bags or other receptacles contaminated with potentially infectious material, including contaminated disposable items, are tagged or otherwise identified, figure 26–1. If warning tags or labels are not used, other equally effective means of identification shall be used (e.g., red bagging).

GUIDELINES FOR INFECTION CONTROL

1. Sterilize everything that can be sterilized.
2. Use disposables wherever possible to eliminate microbial life from the area and prevent additional handling during cleanup. It takes far less time to discard disposables than to completely disinfect an operatory.
3. Use barriers wherever possible to prevent contamination of surfaces. It is easier to dispose of them rather than disinfect or sterilize surfaces.
   Dental staff barriers
   - disposable treatment gloves
   - disposable face masks
   - protective eyewear, with sideshields
   - professional uniform, covered with a disposable gown
   Patient barriers
   - protective eyewear
   - rubber dam
   - patient drape/napkin
   - high-volume evacuation

TABLE 26—1
DISINFECTION AGENTS

Immersion Chemicals
(for instrument holding)

Gluteraldehyde liquid 2%*	Relatively expensive; recommended
Synthetic phenolic compounds*	Relatively nontoxic, nonirritating; recommended
Sodium hypochlorite 1%	Bleaches, corrodes

Surface Disinfection Chemicals
(not to be rinsed off)

Iodophors EPA-registered*	Relatively inexpensive; residual action; recommended
Sodium hypochlorite 1%	Odorous, irritating

Not Recommended for Immersion or Surface Disinfection
  alcohol
  quaternary ammonium compounds

* Refer to *Accepted Dental Therapeutics* for brand names.

Disposable surface barriers (clear plastic)
- full chair covers
- lamp handle covers
- air/water syringe covers
- tray and cabinet covers
- tubing covers/sleeves
- perforated barrier wrap material—to wrap x-ray tubehead and control, drawer handles, and cover countertops

Biohazardous waste disposal
- Includes contaminated materials, such as gauze square sponges, cotton rolls and pellets, dental floss, or any disposable item that has touched blood and/or saliva.
- Tape a paper or plastic refuse bag to a cabinet surface, to use during the dental treatment. Upon completion of the treatment, this bag must be sealed and disposed of in a labeled *BIOHAZARD* receptacle.
- Needles and surgical blades must be discarded in a sharps container.

General waste disposal
  Includes disposables such as gowns, masks, disposable eyewear, patient bib, paper towels, plastic covers, and such. Discard in a refuse bag, labeled *HAZARDOUS WASTE*, figure 26–1.

CHEMICAL DISINFECTION

Disinfection is accomplished by applying a chemical substance that cleans and frees an object from pathogenic (disease-producing) **microorganisms**. Disinfectants are usually applied to surfaces and objects that cannot tolerate heat or live steam sterilization.

Immersion Chemicals

All immersion chemicals are more or less toxic (poisonous), emit (release) odor, and must be registered with the EPA. The one exception is sodium hypochlorite (regular household bleach), refer to table 26–1.

Substances accepted by the EPA are used in dilute form as a holding medium until time permits preparation of items for sterilization. Immersion chemicals also function as a disinfectant for items that will receive no further treatment before reuse. Glass slabs, plastic protective eyewear, plastic syringes used for impression materials, and other nondisposable items that cannot withstand heat will tolerate this method of disinfection.

A holding solution will: (1) prevent debris from remaining on the instrument; (2) prevent the spread of airborne microorganisms; (3) begin the process of killing microorganisms that remain on soiled instruments; and (4) minimize the necessity for handling contaminated instruments.

Heavy utility gloves should always be worn during all disinfection procedures. Disinfection agents will leave a yellow stain on the skin and, in some cases, create a chemical burn.

Contaminated items must be dry before being immersed. The chemical balance (**pH**) and level of a dilute immersion solution must be maintained. Therefore, wet objects must not be placed in the solution, because any added moisture will dilute and destroy the solution's effectiveness. The immersion chemical must be sufficient in volume to completely cover the items. Immersion time is specified by the manufacturer.

- *Alkaline gluteraldehyde 2% solution.* Diluted chemical in a ratio of 2:100 water. Should not be used as a surface disinfectant, because of odor and toxicity. May cause eye and nasal passage irritation or damage. Corrosive to some metals. Gluteraldehyde immersion will corrode aluminum (temporary crowns), aluminum instrument handles, and impression material syringes (if they contain aluminum) because of the effect of the chemical on the metal.
- *Synthetic phenol compounds.* Relatively new, they consist of phenol combined with a soap or detergent in a liquid medium. By comparison with gluteraldehyde, they are less corrosive, will not stain, and are less irritating to the skin. Effects on plastic, glass, and painted surfaces should be noted before application. Manufacturers suggest a test be performed prior to use, to determine compatibility. The compound should be mixed according to the manufacturer's recommendations, and discarded daily. It is biodegradable, which tends to be an asset as use becomes more widely accepted. Immersion time is set by the manufacturer.
- *Sodium hypochlorite 1% solution.* Diluted household bleach in a ratio of 1:100 water. Must be prepared and discarded daily. Emits odor. Irritating to eyes and skin. Causes corrosion of some metals, particularly aluminum.

When the dental procedure is complete, soiled instruments are removed from the operatory in the container of holding solution or tray insert and taken to the sterilization area.

ULTRASONIC CLEANING

To minimize the amount of handling of instruments, an ultrasonic cleaner is used. This cleaning process involves the use of sound waves, causing the formation of minute bubbles in the special solution. The mechanical action (bursting) of the bubbles in solution, and the chemical action of the specialized solution, produce the necessary process that removes debris from the instrument surface. The ultrasonic cleaner is capable of reaching areas that hand scrubbing cannot.

Soiled instruments are transferred from the holding solution and placed into the insert basket of the ultrasonic cleaner, rinsed thoroughly, and drained. The basket is then gradually lowered into the ultrasonic solution, to prevent

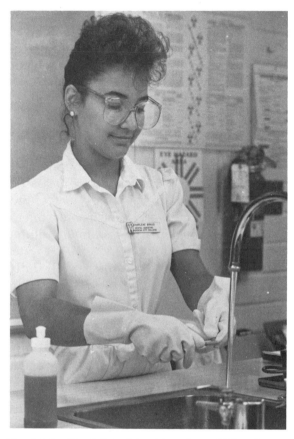

Fig. 26–2. Dental assistant hand-scrubbing instruments, wearing heavy utility gloves

splash. The level of the solution must be enough to completely submerge the instruments. With the cover closed, the cleaner unit is run for five minutes.

Following ultrasonic cleaning, the basket, with instruments still in it, is thoroughly rinsed under cold running tap water. Roll instruments from the ultrasonic basket onto a disposable paper towel. Pat dry with a second towel. If any debris remains on the instruments, further hand scrubbing may be necessary.

Frequent changing of the cleaner solution is an absolute necessity. The inside of the container

and cover are wiped with a disinfecting agent, when the solution is changed.

HAND SCRUBBING

Wearing heavy utility gloves,

- Thoroughly scrub instruments with a stiff brush and antimicrobial soap, figure 26–2.
- Rinse under cold running tap water. Cold water easily removes the soap residue.
- Pat dry with disposable paper towels. Prepare for sterilization.

SURFACE DISINFECTION

Chemicals

Chemicals used for hard-surface disinfection should be suitable for wiping all surfaces in the treatment operatory, table 26–1.

- *Iodofor hard-surface disinfectants.* **Iodofors** are EPA-registered, with an EPA number on the label and consist of certain other chemicals in combination with iodine and a surface-active agent that is continuously released after the surface appears to be dry. This remaining action provides continued protection throughout patient treatment. Dilute according to manufacturer's instructions. Color change, from amber to light yellow, signals loss of potency.
- *Sodium hypochlorite 1% solution.* It is inexpensive but useful, highly irritating to eyes and skin, and damaging to clothing. It has an objectionable odor and is not to be used in areas where space is limited and ventilation restricted.
- *Not recommended as disinfectants* are alcohol and quaternary ammonium compounds.

For accepted brand names, refer to Accepted Dental Therapeutics, a publication of the ADA.

Procedure

Surface disinfection requires the application of an EPA-approved surface disinfectant to equipment or working surfaces of the dental operatory. Chemicals used for surface disinfection constitute only a portion of the process. Friction created during vigorous wiping results in reduction of numbers of microorganisms.

Effective surface disinfection is accomplished by using 4″ by 4″ gauze or 4″ square sponges, open-cell plastic foam sponges, or disposable paper towels. The 2″ by 2″ or 2″ square gauze sponges are not large enough to accommodate the wiping process. Gauze sponges and disposable paper towels should be discarded with hazardous waste. Plastic sponges used on contaminated objects must be thoroughly rinsed with cold water, squeezed dry, sprayed with surface disinfectant, and set aside to dry.

Spray-Wipe-Spray Technique

- Surface clean with a spray bottle of aqueous iodofor solution to remove gross debris.
- Vigorously wipe with a 4″ x 4″ gauze sponge, plastic sponge, or disposable paper towel.
- Saturate a fresh sponge or paper towel with the disinfecting solution. Apply to surface. Allow to dry from two to ten minutes.

STERILIZATION

Sterilization is the process of destroying all microorganisms and their pathogenic products. It is accomplished by moist heat (steam) under pressure or by dry heat.

Methods of Sterilization

- steam under pressure (autoclave)
- chemical vapor under pressure (Chemiclave)
- dry heat (oven)
- hot bead

Packaging Instruments/Objects

Instruments should be wrapped and packed loosely enough to allow steam penetration of all surfaces during autoclaving. It is recommended that all instruments be prepackaged before sterilizing. Inexpensive one-use sterilization bags, figure 26–3, and perforated plastic wraps are available. Paper bags are used for small items, and plastic wraps that can be folded around larger items are used. Bags and wraps must be carefully sealed, with the contents indicated on the packet and the date of sterilization clearly marked. A soft lead, dull pencil should be used rather than a pen. Care must be taken in labeling a paper packet; a sharp pencil may perforate the paper. Ink used in pens may be dissolved by the vapor and the residue deposited on the instruments and walls of the autoclave chamber.

It is advisable not to mix differing metals in a packet, since a strong galvanic action tends to increase corrosion (i.e., high-carbon steel and chromium plated handles on instruments).

Hinged instruments (forceps, scissors) or those with movable parts need to be opened

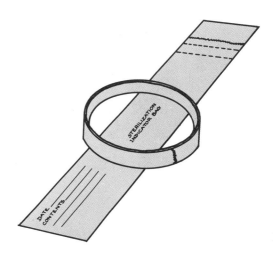

Fig. 26–3. Sensitized tape and sterilization bag

during sterilization. Autoclavable contra-angles and handpieces should be sterilized in a chemical vapor sterilizer. Refer to Chapter 33, *Dental Handpieces*.

1. Prepare the disposable sterilizing bag or wrap, figure 26–4.
2. Indicate the contents and date of sterilization, figure 26–4.
3. Insert sharp surfaces of small instruments into paper coin envelopes (with the gummed flap removed) then into the paper wrapper.
4. Seal packet with sensitized tape. Double-fold ends of the bag, figure 26–5, then with the tape, seal over the fold and around reverse side of bag, figure 26–6. Plastic wraps are sealed over the outside fold and around the entire packet.

Steam Autoclave Sterilization

The steam **autoclave** was invented in 1873 by a pupil of Louis Pasteur, a French chemist. Pasteur is known for his discoveries in immunology and microbiology. The autoclave remains the oldest and most widely accepted dental sterilization method, figure 26–7. The high temperatures that can be obtained (250–270ºF, 121–132ºC) and 15 pounds per square inch (psi) pressure for thirty to forty minutes are commonly accepted. Shorter periods of time for flash emergencies, when a fast instrument turnaround is necessary, may be used.

This shortened sterilization time is not intended for routine practice but is limited to emergencies only, table 26–2.

When operating the autoclave, be certain that (1) an adequate distilled water supply is present; (2) all air is allowed to escape and is replaced by steam; (3) the pressure of the steam reaches at least 15 psi and remains there; and (4) the thermometer reads at least 250ºF (121ºC) without fluctuating downward. It is important to remember that this is the optimum combination of temperature and pressure for sterilization. At 15 psi and 250ºF (121ºC) *saturated steam* is generated. If too little water is used, the steam will become superheated rather than saturated, and

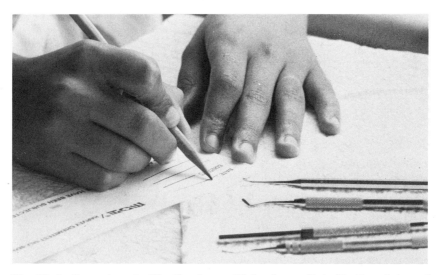

Fig. 26–4. Preparing sterilization bag with lead pencil, indicating date and contents

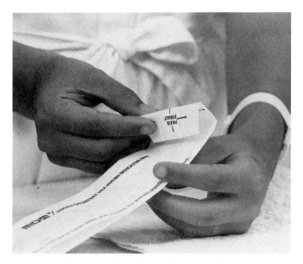

Fig. 26–5. Double fold ends of bag

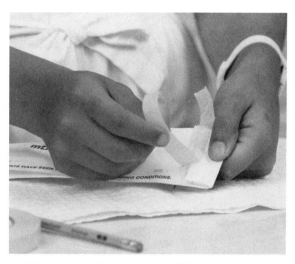

Fig. 26–6. Affixing tape to seal instrument bag

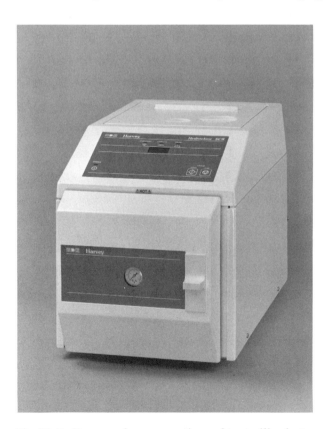

Fig. 26–7. Steam under pressure is used to sterilize instruments. (Courtesy MDT Corporation, Torrance, CA)

TABLE 26—2
STERILIZATION FACTORS

Steam Autoclave (routine)			Flash Emergency
Temperature	250ºF (121ºC)		270ºF (132ºC)
Pressure	15 psi (pounds per sq. in.)		30 psi
Time	30–40 min.	Unwrapped: 30 min. / Wrapped: 40 min.	5 min

Chemical Vapor Sterilizer	
MDT/Harvey Chemiclave	
Temperature	260ºF (127ºC)
Pressure	20 psi.
Time	30 min.

Dry Heat			
Temperature	320ºF (160ºC)	or	250ºF (121ºC)
Time	2 hours		4 hours

Hot Bead	
Temperature	425ºF–475ºF (218ºC–246ºC)
Time	15–30 seconds

its action is the same as hot air. Saturated steam is on the boundary between the liquid and the vapor phase. As this steam strikes colder objects, it condenses to water. This condensation causes a shrinking of volume and local reduction of pressure that draws in more surrounding steam. As objects are heated, the temperatures are equalized, and condensed water returns to the vapor phase.

Steam displaces all air. The increase in temperature from 212 to 250ºF (100 to 121ºC) gives the added destructive power that will kill spores. Air pockets must be eliminated by the pistonlike action of steam itself. In other words, steam must enter the chamber at one end and drive out air at the lower side of the opposite end.

Factors adversely influencing the efficiency of autoclave sterilization are:

- *Superheated Steam.* This condition occurs in office autoclaves if there is insufficient water in the sterilizer to retain some water in liquid state at the temperature the autoclave is used. Superheating may be caused by carrying a higher pressure in the outer jacket than in the chamber or by placing moist items in the autoclave.
- *Trapped Air.* Air becomes trapped in the chamber by an improper air-ejecting device or by faulty packing and improper loading of objects in the autoclave. Air reduces the penetrating power of steam into the depth of packets and prevents contact between steam and microorganisms.

Steam autoclaves create the need to dry the "load" after completion of the cycle. The following steps may be followed:

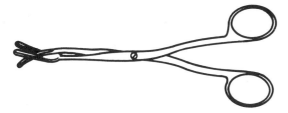

Fig. 26–8. Transfer forcep used in handling sterile instruments

1. Allow pressure gauge to return to zero.
2. Open door slightly to release any steam remaining in the chamber.
3. Remove packets from autoclave tray with sterile transfer forcep, figure 26–8.
4. Place packets on a clean, dry, sterile towel without touching the packets. Excess moisture is driven off by the heat of the instruments.
5. When dry, store packets in an appropriate clean, dry drawer or cabinet until ready to use.
6. Exact technique calls for resterilization of instruments that will penetrate soft tissue just before using.

The transfer forcep is often the weakest link in the sterilization process. Therefore, several pairs of large transfer forceps should be sterilized with each load of instruments. A sterile forcep should be used not only for sterilized instruments but also for such items as plastic saliva ejectors when they are removed from a bulk package. This practice will minimize the contamination of the other items remaining in the package. Transfer forceps should not be stored in a gluteraldehyde solution; only dry, sterile forceps are acceptable.

Sterilizers must be listed by Underwriters Laboratories, Incorporated. A manual is provided by the manufacturer with illustrations to explain proper operation and loading. All instructions are written in easily understood language.

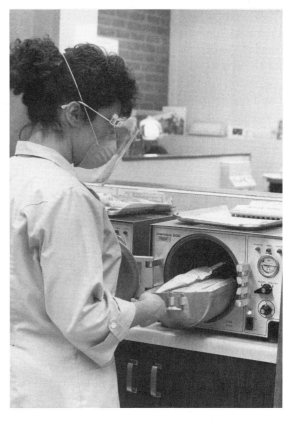

Fig. 26–9. Using chemical vapor sterilizer to sterilize instruments (Courtesy Registered Dental Hygiene Program, Pasadena City College, Pasadena, CA)

Chemical Vapor Sterilizer

The system used for chemical vapor sterilization depends on heat, water and chemicals working in synergy (substances acting to achieve an effect of which each is individually incapable), figure 26–9. The solution in the system is comprised of specific amounts of alcohol, organic solvents, chemical disinfectants, and water. The water is kept below the level (approximately 15%) at which rust, corrosion, and dulling of metals occur. Pressure is used to evacuate air pockets and to raise the internal temperature to the point at which the liquid solution turns to chemical vapor.

Since the solution used in the sterilizer produces a chemical odor, the manufacturer of the chemical vapor sterilizer offers a filtration unit that removes most of the chemical odor after the cycle is completed. The area should be well ventilated and, if possible, placed under a hood that is vented to the outside.

The fact that chemical vapor sterilization does not harm metals is of utmost importance, as this method offers more protection to carbon steel instruments, burs, knives, and other sharp-edged instruments than does a steam autoclave. It can be said that the chemical vapor sterilizer offers a practical method for sterilization, thus eliminating any cross-contamination of instruments and other items that may have been only disinfected.

After sterilization is complete, and when the pressure gauge has returned to zero, the door is opened slightly to evaporate all remaining vapor. Objects should be dry and ready for removal after three to four minutes.

Unloading and storing of sterile packets does not vary from that of the steam autoclave.

Dry-Heat (Oven) Sterilization

Dry-heat sterilization is a low-cost device. The units are of simple construction, with few moving parts; maintenance is minimal. In offices where patient load is such that instrument turnaround time is not of primary concern, dry heat may be used in some instances. However, an alternative method of sterilization should be used for high-heat sensitive items, such as instruments.

Dry-heat sterilizers require two hours at 350°F (160°C) for a complete cycle. Temperatures above 300°F begin to damage metals and other materials; cutting edges on instruments are destroyed with repeated cycling in dry heat.

Added to the limits of time and temperature, heat distribution tends to be irregular. Dry-heat sterilizers must be loaded loosely and carefully to achieve maximum penetration around instruments. Instruments must be clean, dry, and placed on a metal oven tray or wrapped in a sealed foil bag. Inexpensive paper wraps will scorch and char. Definite procedures for loading and unloading must be observed.

Because of the dry-heat sterilizer's limited use, of glassware and dry chemicals, it is recommended that the manufacturer's manual be used as a guide and reference.

Hot Bead Sterilization

The device used for hot bead sterilization consists of an electrically heated cup containing glass beads or table salt granules. The cup must be preheated for twenty minutes before use.

Burs, reamers, broaches, absorbent points and other instruments used in the practice of endodontia are sterilized by submersion into such a medium. Burs and root canal instruments require fifteen to twenty seconds. Surfaces of absorbent points require from five to ten seconds and will change from white to a slight yellowish color when they are sterile. The hot bead sterilizer is not intended for other than limited use.

Storage of Sterile Packets

Taped-seal sterile bags, wraps, and trays should be stored unopened, preferably in a closed drawer or cabinet, until ready to use. Tightly sealed paper packets, if well-protected, will remain sterile for as long as three months, and for about two months, even though storage is in a drawer or cabinet that is frequently opened and closed. In either case, the seal must remain unbroken. Sealed foil bags will remain sterile longer than paper packets because of the resistance of the packaging material.

MONITORING

From time to time, equipment can malfunction and human errors occur. It is advisable to periodically monitor sterilization methods. A record of monitoring should be kept for legal purposes.

There are three methods of monitoring: (1) *Process indicators*, which confirm that the indicator has been exposed to a certain temperature of heat and steam or chemical vapor, as occurs with the stripe on the paper sterilizer bag and sensitized tape. The color change does not guarantee that the items are sterile but only that the load was processed. (2) *Biological monitoring*, the more reliable method, consists of a strip of paper on which resistant spores have been applied. The strip is encased in a sealed bag that is opened and placed in the sterilizer just prior to beginning the sterilizing cycle. Strips are placed throughout the chamber and in the center of the load. On completion of the sterilizing cycle, the strips of spores are cultured to determine if the spores are still vital. Although this simple procedure can be done in the dental office, several companies and institutions (dental schools) will provide the strips, culture them and keep legal records for a reasonable fee. Ideally, biological monitoring should be performed on a weekly basis in a large-practice office or institution. Once a month is probably sufficient for a private office. (3) *Control indicators* determine if the time, temperature, and pressure were appropriate during the cycle. These vary from the process indicator and biological monitor.

THE HIGH-RISK PATIENT

High-risk patients may be classified into two groups: (1) the *suspected high-risk patients*, who may have had or are presently a carrier of a disease; and (2) the *known high-risk patients*, who are either a carrier or in an active stage of a disease. Infection-control procedures must be followed in the treatment of either category.

Emergency Patients

Patients not on record should be screened most carefully, as many high-risk groups, including drug users, neglect any preventive care of their teeth and seek help only on an emergency basis.

New emergency patients must be considered high risk; therefore, special precautions must be taken, and only procedures to relieve pain should be performed on the initial visit. Radiographs necessary for diagnosis may be completed. Further treatment should be postponed until the dentist's medical questionnaire is completed and medical laboratory blood test results have been evaluated. Always obtain medical clearance from the patient's physician.

The high-risk patient is scheduled for the last appointment of the day to allow for a longer posttreatment disinfection and sterilization time.

SUGGESTED ACTIVITIES

- Practice the spray-wipe-spray technique for disinfection.
- Practice placing barriers, including wrap materials, on the operatory equipment.
- Select a mouth mirror, explorer, and cotton pliers; assume the instruments are contaminated. Follow the steps of procedure for disinfection. Include placing them in holding solution, then into the ultrasonic cleaner.
- Using all the precautionary measures, package the instruments for sterilization.
- Study the manufacturer's instruction booklet for using a high-heat sterilizer.
- Under the supervision of the instructor, complete a sterilization cycle.
- Maintain proper storage for the sterile instruments.

REVIEW

1. The two best-known chemical hazards in the practice of dentistry are

   a. _____

   b. _____

2. The three most common respiratory irritants used in the dental office are

   a. _____

   b. _____

   c. _____

3. The prime concern of OSHA for dental personnel is _____

   _____.

4. A procedures manual should contain

   a. _____

   _____

   b. _____

   c. _____

5. Bags or receptacles contaminated with potentially infectious material must be tagged with one of two signal words

   a. _____

   b. _____

6. The three principal guidelines for the control of infection are

   a. _____

   b. _____

   c. _____

7. Chemical disinfection procedures are used on those surfaces that _____

   _____.

8. The four purposes of a holding solution are to

   a. _____

   b. _____

   c. _____

   d. _____

9. The three chemicals used for immersion disinfection are

   a. _____

   b. _____

   c. _____

10. The purpose of the ultrasonic cleaner is_____

    _____.

11. Chemicals used for hard-surface disinfection should be suitable for _____

    _____.

12. Three steps in the spray-wipe-spray technique used for surface disinfection
    are

    a. _____

    b. _____

    c. _____

13. Why is friction an important factor in the process of cleaning and disinfecting
    when using the spray-wipe-spray technique? _____

    _____

    _____

14. What are the fundamental reasons for surface disinfection even though protective barriers will be used?

   a. _____

   b. _____

15. Sterilization may be defined as the process of_____

   _____.

16. List the four methods of sterilization.

   a. _____

   b. _____

   c. _____

   d. _____

17. When operating an autoclave, it is important to have an adequate supply of

   _____.

18. What causes the steam created in the autoclave to become superheated rather than saturated?_____

   _____

   _____

19. Why is high heat the preferred method of sterilization? _____

   _____

   _____

20. Why are spore strips more useful than process indicators in monitoring results of sterilization procedures? _____

   _____

   _____

Chapter 27: Occupational Safety and Health Administration (OSHA) Regulations

OBJECTIVES:

After studying this chapter, the student will be able to:
- Cite the health agencies involved in establishing the infection-control standards for dentistry.
- Discuss the principal requirements of the revised regulations determined by OSHA.
- Cite the agency that approves the disposal of infectious waste materials.
- Determine the necessary documentation for a dental office to be in compliance with OSHA regulations.
- Discuss the primary reasons for a complaint-generated OSHA inspection.
- Discuss the means by which an OSHA inspection may be avoided.

INTRODUCTION

The OSHA General Duty Clause requires an employer to furnish employees with "employment and a place of employment which are free from recognized hazards that are causing or likely to cause death or serious physical harm."

Some time ago, dentists were notified by OSHA that "health care employers must provide their staff members with the materials and information they need to comply with the infection-control guidelines recommended by the Centers for Disease Control (CDC) and the American Dental Association (ADA)."

Further, an OSHA spokesperson is credited with saying, "Health care professionals are obliged under the law to provide staff members with a safe, sanitary workplace." OSHA interprets its responsibility in that area as ensuring that dental practices are in compliance with CDC and ADA guidelines.

Recently, OSHA issued a new and revised set of regulations aimed at protecting the more than 316,000 employees in dental offices from the risks of bloodborne disease, including hepatitis B and the virus that causes AIDS.

OSHA described the action of the requirements as "necessary and appropriate" to prevent transmission of disease in the workplace. A timetable for the new standards was published in 1991 in the *Federal Register*, an official record of government business. Individual states must adopt comparable plans within six months of publication of the regulation.

The ADA has been very active working with OSHA in bringing the regulations affecting dentistry into perspective. The ADA advises employers to follow the existing regulations, which took effect in toto July 6, 1992.

OSHA, a U.S. Department of Labor agency, issued the rules with the backing of the Bush administration budget and health agencies and under considerable pressure from Congress to enforce CDC guidelines.

Included in the plan of new regulations are:

- One of the first requirements to take effect, and the one OSHA inspectors will be checking on, is that every employer have a written exposure control plan, identifying workers with occupational exposure and other potentially infectious materials, and specifying means to protect and train them.

- The plan must also include the barrier techniques, sterilization, and disinfection, hepatitis vaccination, handling of office accidents, postexposure evaluation and follow-up, communication of hazards to employees, and record keeping.
- The plan must be reviewed and updated at least annually, and it must be acceptable to the employees.
- The standard requires such engineering controls as puncture-resistant containers for used needles, handwashing when gloves are changed, and appropriate protective equipment.
- The standard requires the use of disposable cover-up gowns, to be worn over the professional uniform during dental procedures.
- The standard prohibits recapping of sharps, unless the employer can demonstrate that no alternative is feasible or that such action is required by a specific procedure. OSHA cites administration of an anesthetic as an example of a procedure that may require recapping; this was urged and supported by the ADA. In this case, only a one-handed or mechanical device may be used to recap.
- Employees are required to wear disposable gowns and gloves when there is reasonably anticipated skin contact with blood, body fluids, or saliva in dental procedures. The standard states that traditional professional uniforms are not intended to function as protection against any hazard. Disposable gloves may not be washed for reuse.
- Employees are required to wear masks and protective eyewear or a face shield when splashes, spray, splatter, or droplets of blood, body tissue, or saliva may be generated and eye, nose, or mouth contamination can be reasonably anticipated. Protective eyewear must have solid sideshields.
- OSHA requires employers not only to pay for necessary personal protective equipment, such as disposable gowns, gloves, masks, and eyewear, but also to ensure that employees wear such equipment.
- Sharps containers are required to be labeled, easily accessible, and as close as feasible to the immediate area where sharps are used.
- Employers must offer the hepatitis B vaccination without charge to employees after they have been trained, and within ten days of assignment to a position with occupational exposure. Employers must also pay for recommended boosters.
- The new standard also imposes certain record-keeping, labeling, training, and waste-handling requirements that oblige employers to ensure that all employees with occupational exposure participate in a training program at no cost to the employee during working hours. The training program shall be on a continued basis, at least once annually. Detailed records of training must be maintained for three years.
- Waste-handling requirements oblige employers to handle certain waste as infectious:
  - blood and body fluid
  - items that release blood, body fluid, or saliva when compressed
  - items caked with dried blood, body fluid, or saliva if they are capable of releasing these materials during handling
  - sharps
  - pathological waste

For disposal of dental waste materials, contact the local Environmental Protection Agency (EPA), who will direct the dentist in how to obtain an EPA-approved system.

OSHA INSPECTION

OSHA has indicated that they would respond to complaints immediately, now that the guidelines are known to health care professionals. The strong OSHA position on the matter takes the guidelines out of the voluntary realm and makes compliance mandatory. The responsibility for instructing employees and ensuring that infection-control procedures are followed, rests with the employer. Dentists who fail to educate their office employees risk the possibility of an OSHA inspection.

An OSHA inspection of a dental office most generally occurs as the result of an employee complaint.

What to expect during a complaint-generated inspection?

- The OSHA representative would request infection-control records from the employer. If documentation of needle sticks and injury or illness records are available, these would also be requested.
- Following review of the records, the OSHA representative would interview employees, then inspect the dental office. Areas of concern would be those of direct patient care, such as the dental operatory and x-ray area. When the inspection visit to the dental office is complaint-generated, the area of complaint is also inspected.
- In addition to inspection of records, employee interviews, and site inspections, the compliance officer would also evaluate the hazard communication program in the office. Areas

of concern would include the presence of Material Safety Data Sheets (MSDS) for all chemicals used in the office, a written program of identification of hazardous materials, and verification of employee training in the use of materials and of provisions for continual training of employees.

To minimize the chance of an OSHA inspection,

- Follow CDC and ADA infection-control guidelines.
- Document current infection-control practices.
- Make certain that all employees are informed, trained, and follow all precautionary measures of infection control.
- Establish open communication among all dental personnel. This will encourage employees to discuss and address complaints and problems with the employer, thus eliminating the necessity for OSHA to become involved.

There is no one in the dental field today who is not aware of OSHA. This four-letter word has become a part of our daily lives and vocabulary. However, how to deal with it still is a mystery to most dental offices. Information is coming from all directions and sources, each with its own interpretation. It may be some time before revisions will complete the legislative process and become law. As one official from the EPA said, *"The 90s is the age of enforcement. It will be more expensive not to comply than to comply."*

REVIEW

1. The health agencies that establish infection-control standards for dentistry are

    a. _____

    b. _____

    c. _____

2. OSHA is an agency of _____.

3. The first requirement of the plan of new regulations is that _____

    _____.

4. Other methods of control that must be included in the plan are

    a. _____

    b. _____

    c. _____

    d. _____

    e. _____

    f. _____

    g. _____

5. The plan must be reviewed and updated on an _____ basis.

6. Required engineering controls include

    a. _____

    b. _____

    c. _____

7. Personal protection requirements include

   a. _____

   b. _____

   c. _____

   d. _____

8. Requirements for sharps containers are that they be _____ and _____.

9. Hepatitis B vaccinations and boosters are to be offered and paid for by _____ _____.

10. Training for personnel is to include requirements such as

    a. _____

    b. _____

    c. _____

11. Infectious waste materials include

    a. _____

    b. _____

    c. _____ _____

    d. _____

    e. _____

12. Disposal of infectious waste materials must be approved by the _____ _____.

13. An OSHA inspection of a dental office generally occurs as the result of _____

_____.

14. The hazard-communication program of a dental office must include

a. _____

b. _____

c. _____

d. _____

15. To minimize the chance of an OSHA inspection, the dental office should

a. _____

b. _____

c. _____

d. _____

Chapter 28: Dental and Medical Emergencies

After studying this chapter, the student will be able to:
- List the purposes of a health history.
- Take and record vital signs.
- Recognize medical emergencies, their symptoms, and treatment.
- Use good judgment and prompt action in responding to medical emergencies.
- Describe the legal aspect of medical emergencies in the dental office.

INTRODUCTION

With more and more individuals seeking dental treatment, the chance of a medical emergency arising in the dental office also increases. Advances in medical technology present situations unknown just a few decades ago. Patients who have organ transplants or implants, or who may be undergoing extensive drug therapy bring the dental team a wide variety of challenges. Are you prepared to recognize emergency situations that may arise and assist in promptly and responsibly caring for the patient?

HEALTH HISTORY

Knowing the dental and medical history of a patient provides valuable information for the dentist, figure 28–1. Most often, the new patient is asked to complete the history form in the reception area. Once in the operatory, the dental assistant can review the health history with the patient and explain the importance of an accurate patient history. The purposes of the health history are fourfold: (1) to determine if there are any chronic health conditions or illnesses that may interfere with dental treatment; (2) to determine if any medications that the patient is currently taking will have a potential drug interaction with the local anesthetic; (3) to have a list of the patient's allergies; and (4) to be familiar with the patient in case of a medical emergency.

VITAL SIGNS

Prior to the start of treatment, the patient's vital signs should be taken and recorded for the dentist to evaluate. These include blood pressure, pulse (heart rate), respirations, and temperature.

Blood Pressure

Blood pressure is the pressure created by the force of the blood on the artery walls. The *systolic blood pressure* arises from the contraction of the ventricle that pushes oxygen-rich blood through the arteries. The *diastolic blood pressure* occurs when the heart is relaxing and the ventricles begin to fill with more blood. Blood pressure is measured in millimeters of mercury (mm Hg). When recording blood pressure, systolic pressure is written over diastolic pressure, much like a fraction. Normal blood pressure ranges for an adult are a systolic pressure of 100 to 140 and a diastolic pressure of 60 to 90.

Materials Needed

- stethoscope
- aneroid or mercury-type manometer, figures 28–2 and 28–3
- patient's chart
- pen
- gauze
- disinfectant

Medical History Form

Date _____

Name _____
       Last   First   Middle

Home Phone (____) _____

Address _____
         Number, Street

Business Phone (_____) _____

City _____ State _____ Zip Code _____

Occupation _____ Social Security No. _____

Date of Birth __/__/__ Sex M F Height _____ Weight _____ Single _____ Married _____
        mo. day yr.

Name of Spouse _____ Closest Relative _____ Phone (____) _____

If you are completing this form for another person, what is your relationship to that person? _____

Referred by _____

For the following questions, *circle yes or no*, whichever applies. Your answers are for our records only and will be considered confidential. Please note that during your initial visit you will be asked some questions about your responses to this questionnaire and there may be additional questions concerning your health.

1. Are you in good health?	Yes	No
2. Has there been any change in your general health within the past year?	Yes	No
3. My last physical examination was on _____		
4. Are you now under the care of a physician?	Yes	No
If so, what is the condition being treated? _____		
5. The name and address of my physician(s) is _____		
6. Have you had any serious illness, operation, or been hospitalized in the past 5 years?	Yes	No
If so, what was the illness or problem? _____		
7. Are you taking any medicine(s) including non-prescription medicine?	Yes	No
If so, what medicine(s) are you taking? _____		

8. Do you have or have you had any of the following diseases or problems?

a. Damaged heart valves or artificial heart valves, including heart murmur or rheumatic heart disease	Yes	No
b. Cardiovascular disease (heart trouble, heart attack, angina, coronary insufficiency, coronary occlusion, high blood pressure, arteriosclerosis, stroke)	Yes	No
1. Do you have chest pain upon exertion?	Yes	No
2. Are you ever short of breath after mild exercise or when lying down?	Yes	No
3. Do your ankles swell?	Yes	No
4. Do you have inborn heart defects?	Yes	No
5. Do you have a cardiac pacemaker?	Yes	No
c. Allergy	Yes	No
d. Sinus trouble	Yes	No
e. Asthma or hay fever	Yes	No
f. Fainting spells or seizures	Yes	No
g. Persistent diarrhea or recent weight loss	Yes	No
h. Diabetes	Yes	No
i. Hepatitis, jaundice or liver disease	Yes	No
j. AIDS or HIV infection	Yes	No
k. Thyroid problems	Yes	No
l. Respiratory problems, emphysema, bronchitis, etc.	Yes	No
m. Arthritis or painful swollen joints	Yes	No
n. Stomach ulcer or hyperacidity	Yes	No
o. Kidney trouble	Yes	No
p. Tuberculosis	Yes	No
q. Persistent cough or cough that produces blood	Yes	No
r. Persistent swollen glands in neck	Yes	No
s. Low blood pressure	Yes	No
t. Sexually transmitted disease	Yes	No
u. Epilepsy or other neurological disease	Yes	No
v. Problems with mental health	Yes	No
w. Cancer	Yes	No
x. Problems of the immune system	Yes	No

(over)

Fig. 28–1. Medical history questionnaire, long form (Courtesy American Dental Association, Chicago, IL)

9. Have you had abnormal bleeding?. . . . .   Yes   No
   a. Have you ever required a blood transfusion? . . . .   Yes   No

10. Do you have any blood disorder such as anemia? . . . .   Yes   No

11. Have you ever had any treatment for a tumor or growth? . . . .   Yes   No

12. Are you allergic or have you had a reaction to:
    a. Local anesthetics   . . . .   Yes   No
    b. Penicillin or other antibiotics   . . . .   Yes   No
    c. Sulfa drugs . . . .   Yes   No
    d. Barbiturates, sedatives, or sleeping pills . . . .   Yes   No
    e. Aspirin   . . . .   Yes   No
    f. Iodine   . . . .   Yes   No
    g. Codeine or other narcotics . . . .   Yes   No
    h. Other _____

13. Have you had any serious trouble associated with any previous dental treatment?   . . . .   Yes   No
    If so, explain _____
    _____

14. Do you have any disease, condition, or problem not listed above that you think I should know about? . . . .   Yes   No
    If so, explain _____
    _____

15. Are you wearing contact lenses? . . . .   Yes   No

16. Are you wearing removable dental appliances? . . . .   Yes   No

Women

17. Are you pregnant? . . . .   Yes   No

18. Do you have any problems associated with your menstrual period? . . . .   Yes   No

19. Are you nursing? . . . .   Yes   No

20. Are you taking birth control pills? . . . .   Yes   No

Chief Dental Complaint _____
_____

I certify that I have read and understand the above. I acknowledge that my questions, if any, about the inquiries set forth above have been answered to my satisfaction. I will not hold my dentist, or any other member of his/her staff, responsible for any errors or omissions that I may have made in the completion of this form.

_____
Signature of Patient

For completion by the dentist.
Comments on patient interview concerning medical history: _____
_____
_____

Significant findings from questionnaire or oral interview: _____
_____
_____

Dental management considerations: _____
_____
_____
_____

_____   _____
(Date)   Signature of Dentist

Medical history update:

Date	Comments	Signature

S500 © American Dental Association 1988

Fig. 28–1 (con't). Medical history questionnaire, long form (Courtesy American Dental Association, Chicago, IL)

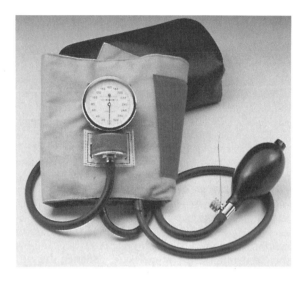

Fig. 28–2. Aneroid-type manometer (Courtesy Omron Healthcare, Inc.)

Instructions

1. The patient should be comfortably seated in an upright or supine position in the dental chair and allowed to relax for a minimum of five minutes. Because many patients may be apprehensive and thus have higher blood pressure than normal, this gives them time to calm down. During this time, the assistant can explain the purpose for taking vital signs.

2. Place the patient's arm at the level of the heart, slightly flexed, palm upward, and supported on the arm of the chair. If the patient has a tight-cuffed sleeve, it should be loosened and rolled above the elbow.

3. The center of the inflatable portion of the deflated cuff should be placed over the brachial artery approximately 1 inch above the *antecubital fossa* (small depression on the inner arm). The rubber tubing will follow along the inside of the arm (figure 28–4.)

4. Wrap the cuff around the arm, and fasten it snugly. Two fingertips should fit under

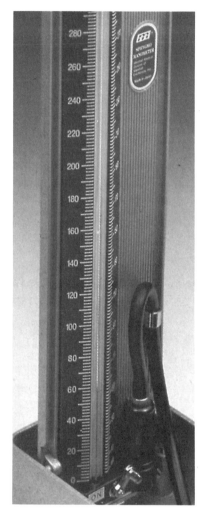

Fig. 28–3. Mercury-type manometer (Courtesy Keir, Wise, and Krebs, *Medical Assisting: Administrative and Clinical Competencies*, 3rd ed., Delmar, Albany, NY, 1993)

the lower edge of the deflated cuff. It is important that the cuff is neither too tight nor too loose.

5. With the fingertips of your left hand, locate the patient's radial artery to find the pulse.

6. Make sure that the valve on the rubber bulb is closed.

7. With your right hand, pump the rubber bulb to inflate the cuff until you can no longer feel the pulse.

8. Slowly open the valve, and allow the mercury to drop at 2 mm per second (2 millimeters equals 1 notch on the gauge). Note the reading when the radial pulse returns. This is the *palpatory systolic pressure*. Now the valve can be opened completely.

9. Place the stethoscope into your ears with the earpieces facing anteriorly, figure 28–5.

10. Position the diaphragm of the stethoscope over the brachial artery, below the blood pressure cuff.

11. Close the valve. Inflate the cuff to 30 mm Hg above the palpatory systolic pressure.

12. Release the pressure on the cuff gradually. Listen for the first sound heard, this is the systolic pressure.

13. Continue to deflate the cuff. When the sounds become muffled or you can no longer hear any sounds, this is the diastolic pressure.

14. Release the pressure in the cuff completely.

15. Record the blood pressure in the patient's chart. Indicate if it was taken on the left arm or right arm. A reading on the left arm is generally higher.

16. Remove the blood pressure cuff. Clean the earpieces and diaphragm of the stethoscope with gauze sponge moistened in suitable disinfectant. *Important:* If the blood pressure needs to be retaken, wait at least 15 seconds before reinflating the cuff. Blood may be trapped in the arm and cause an inaccurate reading.

Pulse

The *pulse* or *heart rate* is the rhythmic expansion of the artery when the blood is pushed

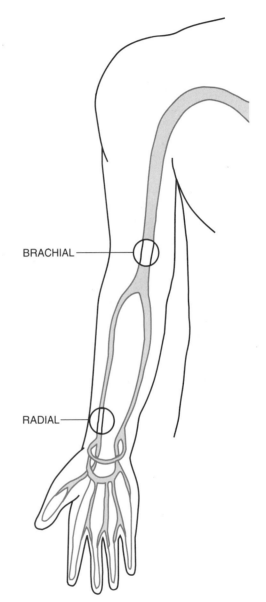

Fig. 28–4. The sites for locating radial and brachial pulses (Courtesy White, *Basic Clinical Lab Competencies for Respiratory Care*, 2nd ed., Delmar, Albany, NY, 1993)

through with each heart beat. Generally, the pulse is taken at the radial artery on the thumb side of the arm. In an emergency, however, it is

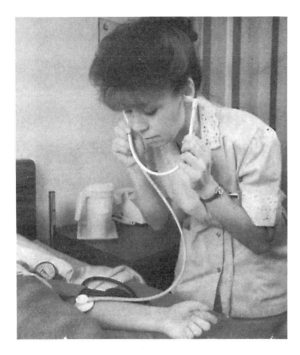

Fig. 28–5. Stethoscope earpieces are inserted facing inward. (Courtesy Hegner and Caldwell, *Auxiliar de Enfermeria: Introduccion al Proceso de Enfermia*, 6th ed., Delmar, Albany, NY, 1993)

best to use the carotid artery in the neck. The assistant should check for three conditions of the pulse: (1) *heart rate* (beats per minute); (2) *heart rhythm* (regular or irregular); and (3) *quality of the beats* (strong, thready, or weak).

Materials needed
- watch with a second hand
- patient's chart
- pen

Instructions
1. Locate the radial artery.
2. Use the index and middle fingers and place them over the artery. (*Note:* Do not use the thumb, as it has its own pulsing artery and may cause an inaccurate reading.)

3. Once the pulse is located, count the beats for one minute. Note the regularity and quality of the pulse.
4. Record the pulse in beats per minute (bpm) in the patient's chart. Normal pulse rate for an adult is between 60 and 80 bpm.

Respirations

Respirations or *respiratory rate* indicate how fast the patient is breathing in and out. Patients should not be aware that their respirations are being counted, because they may alter the normal pattern of breathing. The respiratory rate is often observed immediately after the pulse rate. The assistant watches the chest rise and fall for one minute and records the result as breaths per minute. Normal respiratory rate in an adult is between 14 to 18 breaths per minute.

Temperature

The patient's temperature is usually not taken prior to dental treatment; however, the assistant should be prepared to take a patient's temperature if the need arises.

Materials needed
- oral thermometer
- watch with a second hand
- patient's chart
- pen
- suitable disinfectant
- gauze sponge

Instructions
1. Moisten the gauze sponge with disinfectant.
2. Wipe the thermometer, going from the stem end to the mercury-filled bulb in one motion. Discard the gauze.
3. Rinse the thermometer under cool water to remove the taste of the disinfectant.
4. Holding the thermometer firmly, shake it until the reading is below 96°F.

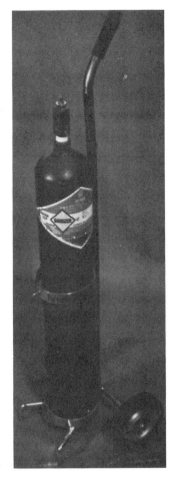

A

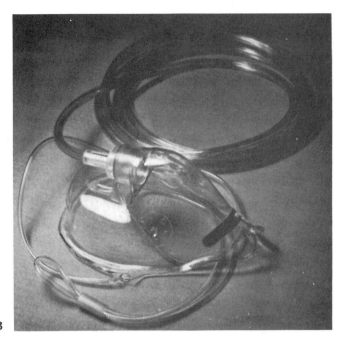

B

Fig. 28–6. E. cylinder of oxygen with delivery system (A). An oxygen mask (B). (Courtesy White, *Basic Clinical Lab Competencies for Respiratory Care***, 2nd ed., Delmar, Albany, NY, 1993)**

7. Record the temperature. Normal temperature is 98.6°F, or 37°C.

8. Disinfect the thermometer.

EMERGENCY EQUIPMENT AND PREPARATION

Every dental office should have some form of emergency kit and oxygen-delivery system, figure 28–6, on hand. Keep the emergency kit stocked at all times. It is useless to have a kit in an emergency without the necessary drugs. Important information for each drug such as indications for use, standard dosages, adverse reactions, and the expiration date can be kept handy on a notecard.

Having the necessary equipment in an emergency and knowing how to react are the keys to avoiding a crisis. The rule of thumb in any emergency is not to panic! Emergency numbers

5. Ask the patient if he or she had anything to eat, drink, or smoke within the past fifteen minutes. If so, wait until fifteen minutes have elapsed so that the reading will be closer to normal. Instruct the patient to lift his or her tongue, insert the bulb of the thermometer sublingually, and ask the patient to close his or her lips around it. Tell the patient to remove the thermometer if he or she has to cough or sneeze.

6. After three minutes, remove the thermometer and read it.

should be posted near all telephones. Every member of the dental team should be currently certified in basic life support procedures, and each office member should know their role in an emergency. Above all, never leave the patient alone.

MEDICAL EMERGENCIES

Syncope

Perhaps the most frequent medical emergency in the dental office is **syncope** or *fainting*. *Syncope* is defined as a momentary loss of consciousness due to a decrease in blood flow to the brain. Patients who are anxious, upset, or in pain are susceptible to fainting. Symptoms include a feeling of warmth, pale skin, perspiration, and clamminess. At these first signs, the chair should be put into the *Trendelenburg* position (supine position with feet above the head) to increase blood flow to the brain. Loosen any tight clothing. Aromatic spirits of ammonia can be passed underneath the nostrils. (*Note:* do not hold the ampule directly under the nostrils, as the odor is very strong.) Following these steps, the patient should respond within a few minutes.

Shock

Shock is a condition that occurs when there is a considerable reduction of blood to the brain and an increase of blood in the extremities. The patient's pupils are dilated; breathing is labored; the pulse is rapid, weak, or nonexistent; and the skin is pale, moist, and cool. Frequently, the patient becomes nauseous. If the patient is able to breathe, maintain the airway and place him or her in a comfortable position. Treatment for more severe shock cases includes oxygen administration.

Orthostatic Hypotension

Orthostatic, or *postural*, *hypotension* (decrease in blood pressure when returned to a seated position after reclining) is often seen in patients who have been in a supine position for a lengthy period of time. When the chair is returned to the upright position, the patient's blood pressure drops suddenly, and he or she becomes light-headed. The chair should be quickly returned to the supine position. In order to prevent cases of orthostatic hypotension, raise the chair slowly, pausing for a short period of time between elevations.

Angina Pectoris

Angina pectoris (acute constriction surrounding the heart) is characterized by a sharp pain that occurs in the chest. It is often associated with physical or emotional stress. The coronary artery narrows, causing decreased blood flow to the heart. If the patient experiences an angina attack during treatment, he or she should be moved to an upright position. This will alleviate pressure on the chest. A nitroglycerin tablet is placed sublingually and 100% oxygen can be given.

Myocardial Infarction

A *heart attack*, or *myocardial infarction*, is the death of a part of the heart muscle. This occurs because clogged coronary blood vessels are unable to provide sufficient blood to the heart. Symptoms of a heart attack include intense substernal pain, cold perspiration, shortness of breath, **cyanotic** (bluish) lips, and anxiety. The patient should be raised to a sitting position to lessen the strain on the heart, and tight clothing should be loosened. Oxygen can be given if necessary, and an ambulance should be called.

Cardiac Arrest

Cardiac arrest, or *clinical death*, occurs when the heart stops beating. The patient will lose consciousness; become cold and clammy; have an absence of breathing, heart beat, and pulse in the large arteries; exhibit dilated pupils; and become _cyanotic_ (of bluish-gray appearance). An ambulance should be summoned immediately, and cardiopulmonary resuscitation (CPR) should be started.

Stroke

A _stroke_, or _cerebrovascular_ (cerebro, brain; vascular, blood vessel) _accident_, is caused by an abrupt change in blood flow to the brain tissues. In older patients it is caused by a change in the blood vessels brought on by age or hypertension. The affected blood vessels cause hemorrhaging in the cerebral tissues. If the stroke is slight, the symptoms may include dizziness, headache, or confusion. The patient should be seated comfortably and reassured. Oxygen can be administered if necessary and an ambulance should be called.

Hyperventilation

Hyperventilation (hyper, excessive; ventilation, respiration) can be characterized by rapid breathing brought on by a stressful situation. The patient becomes nervous and takes rapid and deep breaths, causing excessive elimination of carbon dioxide from the blood. Raise the chair to an upright position, and instruct the patient to take slow breaths, usually four to six per minute. If the patient is unable to slow his or her breathing, then a paper bag or headrest cover is placed over the mouth and nose. Tell the patient to breathe into the bag. The exhaled air contains additional carbon dioxide to aid in recovery.

Airway Obstruction

Aspiration (_inhalation_) of objects is the leading cause of _airway obstruction_ in a dental office. These objects may include burs, endodontic files, large pieces of tooth or amalgam, crowns, or cotton rolls. An obstruction may cause partial or complete blockage. The patient may grab at his throat while gasping for air, or he or she may cough to try and dislodge the foreign object. If he or she cannot cought or speak and is wheezing, then abdominal thrusts are recommended. If the patient can breathe and speak, _do not_ perform abdominal thrusts!

Prevention is the best way to avoid airway obstruction. When performing restorative procedures, use a rubber dam. Make sure that the rubber dam clamp has several inches of floss attached so that it can be easily retrieved in case it breaks or slips off of the tooth. A throat pack should be used during surgery or whenever a rubber dam is contraindicated. Simply open a 2″ by 2″ gauze square and lay it toward the back of the throat.

Convulsive Seizure

A central nervous system disorder called _epilepsy_ may lead to a _convulsive seizure_. _Epilepsy_ is an interrupted flow of messages to the brain, causing unexpected behavior. Epileptic seizures may be either _petit mal_ or _grand mal_. In _petit mal_ seizures, the patient may become disoriented and stop talking for a few seconds. Seizures of this type are mild and need no treatment. _Grand mal_ seizures are more intense. The patient may experience an _aura_, or warning, of an impending seizure. Involuntary muscle contractions occur along with unconsciousness lasting three minutes or more. Although a seizure cannot be stopped or treated, the assistant should protect the patient from injury. Assist the patient out of the chair and onto the floor. Move any large objects so that the patient does not injury him- or herself. A cloth towel should be placed between the patient's teeth so that no biting of the tongue or lip occurs. _Never_ use a mouth prop or put your fingers between the teeth during a seizure.

Allergic Reactions

An **_allergic_** _reaction_ occurs when the body has developed a sensitivity to a foreign substance (allergen). With each exposure to the **allergen**, the response is more intense. Symptoms include **edema** (swelling), *urticaria* (rash), *wheals* (large welts), and *erythema* (red rash). A more immediate reaction includes swollen and watery eyes, runny nose, and respiratory distress. Epinephrine should be given immediately. Keep the airway open to assist the patient's breathing. Antihistamines should be prescribed as a follow-up measure. If the patient is conscious, oxygen can be provided. Medical assistance should be called immediately.

Hyperglycemia—Diabetic Coma

Hyperglycemia (hyper, increase; glycemia, blood sugar) is a condition that occurs when there is excessive sugar in the blood and urine, causing an increase in the body's demand for insulin. If left untreated, the patient may progress to a *diabetic coma*. Symptoms of diabetic coma are dry mouth and excessive thirst; red lips; flushed and dry skin; rapid and weak pulse; "acetone" (sweet) breath odor; drowsiness; and weakness. If the patient is left untreated, unconsciousness ensues. If the patient is conscious, the assistant needs to determine (1) when the patient last ate; and (2) if he or she took insulin. Whether the patient is conscious or not, his or her physician should be notified immediately.

Hypoglycemia—Insulin Shock

Hypoglycemia (hypo, decrease; glycemia, blood sugar) or *insulin shock* is low blood sugar. The patient may have taken his regular dose of insulin but either did not eat or ate later than usual. A patient who is hypoglycemic appears nervous and hungry. There is an increase in perspiration, causing the skin to be moist. The pupils are dilated, and the patient is pale and weak. Candy or a sugar cube can be given to the patient, and his physician should be called immediately.

LEGAL RAMIFICATIONS OF MEDICAL EMERGENCIES

It has been shown that 7 to 8 percent of dentists are sued annually. If a lawsuit is served against the dentist, the patient (plaintiff) must prove the following: (1) that the dentist was at fault; (2) that the dentist's fault caused injuries to the patient; and (3) that damages (financial compensation) must be paid to the patient. An *expert witness* is called in on behalf of the plaintiff to describe the appropriate standard of care and to determine whether the dentist followed that course of treatment. If the jury decides that the standard of care was less than what was to be expected, then it claims that the dentist was *negligent* (failed to use ordinary care).

Res Ipsa Loquitur

This Latin phrase means "the thing speaks for itself." Applied to the dentist, this means that the dentist must have performed an injustice to the patient for the result to occur or the patient would not have been harmed.

Good Samaritan Law

The Good Samaritan Law states that health care workers cannot be held liable for death or injury if they acted in good faith when treating someone other than their patient. In other words, if the patient's elderly neighbor is in the waiting room to drive the patient home, suffers a heart attack, and the office staff tries unsuccessfully to resuscitate the individual using standard CPR, liability on the part of the dental team will be difficult to prove.

Respondeat Superior

Respondeat superior means "let the master answer." In this case, the dentist is responsible for any actions that are performed by his or her staff during their employment.

Prevention

There are several ways to avoid a **malpractice** suit in the dental office. (1) The dentist should have a complete medical/dental history and update it at each visit. (2) Make sure that the patient (or patient's legal guardian if underage) is aware of the diagnosis, treatment, and subsequent results if the patient does not follow proper home care procedures or follow the doctor's orders. (3) Document everything completely in the patient's chart. Include any unusual situations and treatment. Leave *nothing* to memory. (4) Train the office staff for their roles in an office emergency and practice periodically. (5) Attend continuing education seminars to stay abreast of current trends in dentistry.

REVIEW

1. List the four purposes of a health history.

   a. _____

   _____

   b. _____

   _____

   c. _____

   d. _____

2. What are the four vital signs that can be taken prior to dental treatment? _____

   _____

3. Blood pressure is_____.

4. Blood pressure is measured in _____.

5. Normal blood pressure for an adult is _____

   _____.

6. Another name for the pulse is_____.

7. The pulse is most commonly measured at the _____ artery.

8. Normal adult heart rate ranges from _____beats per minute.

9. Respiration rate for a normal adult is between _____ breaths per minute.

10. A temperature of _____ degrees Fahrenheit and _____ degrees Celsius is considered normal.

11. Every dental office should have a complete _____ and _____.

12. Fainting is the common term for _____. The patient who is faint should be put into the_____ position.

13. A patient who has difficulty breathing, skin that is cool and moist, a rapid and weak pulse, and dilated pupils may be experiencing _____.

14. An elderly patient who has been lying in the chair and has undergone lengthy dental treatment is returned to the sitting position. He complains of feeling "lightheaded." This condition is _____.

15. _____ is a sharp pain in the chest and is treated with a tablet of _____.

16. Symptoms of a heart attack include _____ _____.

17. _____ or _____ death occurs when the heart stops beating.

18. When blood vessels cause hemorrhaging into the brain, a _____ occurs.

19. Hyperventilation occurs because of a lack of _____ in the blood.

20. Two ways to prevent airway obstruction include the use of _____ and _____.

21. A convulsive seizure is often seen in a patient with _____.

22. A _____ seizure is more severe than a _____ seizure.

23. Define the following terms indicative of an allergic reaction:

    a. Edema _____

    b. Urticaria _____

    c. Wheals _____

    d. Erythema _____

24. Compare hyperglycemia and hypoglycemia.

    a. _____

    _____

    _____

    b. _____

    _____

    _____

25. In a malpractice suit, an _____ establishes a standard of care that the dentist should follow in an emergency.

26. Match the three word phrases to their description:

    a. _____ Res Ipsa Loquitur   1. "let the master answer"

    b. _____ Good Samaritan   2. "the thing speaks for itself"

    c. _____ Respondeat Superior   3. treatment provided in good faith for an individual who is not the dentist's regular patient

27. List five ways that the dentist can prevent a malpractice suit from being filed against his or her office.

    a. _____

    b. _____

    _____

    _____

    c. _____

    d. _____

    e. _____

OBJECTIVES:

After studying this chapter, the student will be able to:
- Describe dental plaque and its relationship to tooth decay and periodontal disease.
- Explain the role of diet and caries susceptibility tests in preventive dentistry.
- Discuss the use of fluoride and of pit and fissure sealants.
- Differentiate between methods of toothbrushing.
- List and describe auxiliary aids in preventive dentistry.
- Outline a plan for patient education in preventive dentistry.

INTRODUCTION

Unlike early beliefs that tooth loss was part of the aging process, it is now an accepted fact that the teeth were designed to last a lifetime. Prevention of any problems is a key in order to fulfill that goal. To avoid destruction of the teeth and supporting structures, the patient must understand how to maintain optimum oral health. For this reason, the dental assistant must have a thorough knowledge of the fundamentals of preventive dentistry—the *etiology* (cause) of dental decay and periodontal disease and the measures that preserve the oral cavity.

DENTAL PLAQUE

Dental **plaque** is a soft, sticky accumulation of bacteria and products of saliva. It is responsible for the development of tooth decay and periodontal disease. Plaque formation occurs in four stages. Initially, a thin, bacteria-free, translucent film called *acquired pellicle* forms on the teeth. Second, microorganisms that inhabit the oral cavity adhere to the acquired pellicle. The bacteria then begin to multiply and grow in layers forming *colonies* (clusters of bacteria). By the end of three weeks, the plaque has become a completely developed mass of microorganisms.

Plaque and Tooth Decay

Figure 29–1 shows a simplified diagram of the development of tooth decay.

One of the first microorganisms to attach to the acquired pellicle is *Streptococcus mutans*. These bacteria grow and multiply by consuming carbohydrates, especially sugars, from the foods that are eaten. Acids are then produced as a waste product. The acid begins decalcification of the tooth. As the plaque thickens, the acid is trapped against the tooth and cannot be neutralized by saliva. Decalcification of the tooth continues and another microorganism called *Lactobacillus* begins to form inside the carious area.

Plaque and Periodontal Disease

As plaque develops, the highest concentration occurs at the cervical third of the tooth along the gingival margin. Bacteria invades the gingival sulcus and attacks the gingiva. These bacteria cannot be easily removed. Left undisturbed, **calculus** (mineralized layers of plaque) forms and acts as a further irritant to the tissue.

> **Bacteria + Sugar = Acid**
> **Acid + Tooth = Decay**

Fig. 29–1. The process of tooth decay

Dietary Control

The effect of diet in preventive dentistry is twofold. As the tooth grows and develops, it needs several vitamins and minerals that promote resistance to tooth decay. Of particular importance are vitamins A, C, and D and the minerals fluoride and calcium. In addition, certain foods promote caries development and gingival destruction. Sticky foods, which are predominantly carbohydrates, adhere to the tooth and provide sugar for the bacteria. Soft diets that lack fibrous foods helpful in stimulating the gingiva encourage the production of plaque and the deterioration of the periodontal structures. For this reason, it is important that the patient understand the significance of diet and nutrition in order to maintain a healthy oral cavity.

Caries Susceptibility

There is no single cause of dental caries, but it can be identified by the decalcification of the inorganic salts of the tooth. Bacterial infection caused by acid-producing organisms results in fermentation of refined carbohydrates retained in the mouth as food debris in undisturbed areas around the teeth. The organic acids formed by the organisms attack the enamel and give bacteria the opportunity to work unmolested, with no danger of the acids produced being washed away by the saliva.

The tendency to develop a carious condition may be caused by faulty diet. To inhibit the development of dental caries, proper home care procedures should be reinforced, such as toothbrushing and flossing, with emphasis on an adequate diet.

FLUORIDE

One of the best preventive methods for tooth decay, fluoride has significantly reduced the amount of caries in school-age children. Fluoride works by causing the crystal structure of the enamel to become more resistant to acids produced by bacteria and by preventing the acid-producing bacteria from developing. Fluoride intake occurs during three stages of tooth development: the mineralization stage, after mineralization and before eruption, and after eruption. It is normally ingested in drinking water in 1 ppm (1 part fluoride for every million parts of water), and fluoride supplements can also be given from birth to age 14. These can be in liquid or tablet form. Excessive fluoride, however, is detrimental to the teeth. Both **fluorosis** (brown staining) and _mottling_ (pitted enamel surfaces) have been seen in such instances.

Types of Fluoride

There are two types of topical fluoride used in dental offices: _stannous fluoride_ and _acidulated phosphate fluoride._

Fluoride gels and solutions for topical application are preparations of stannous fluoride and acidulated phosphate. Because stannous fluoride solution is unstable, a combination of acidulated phosphate and stannous fluoride is commercially prepared and is available in gel form.

Depending on the carious condition of the patient's mouth, the doctor may prescribe a stannous fluoride application or a topical fluoride gel application. Stannous fluoride treatments are completed in a single application and may be repeated every six months.

Topical Fluoride Application

Materials

    basic tray setup

    cotton rolls

    HVE tip

    prophylaxis angle with rubber cup

    prophylaxis paste stannous fluoride commercial gel

    dental floss

preformed commercial trays, either two single trays placed separately or two trays connected as one

liners for trays

fluoride gel

saliva ejector tip

Procedure

1. Perform a *rubber cup prophylaxis* (procedure in which the coronal surfaces of the tooth are polished).
2. Floss the teeth.
3. Rinse the teeth well.
4. Dispense the fluoride solution into the tray.
5. Dry the teeth well. When doing both arches simultaneously, dry the maxillary arch first.
6. Insert the tray into the mouth. Instruct the patient to close down so that all surfaces are adequately covered.
7. Use the saliva ejector inside the mouth to remove the excess fluoride.
8. After four minutes, remove the tray. Do not rinse the mouth. Use the HVE to suction out any excess fluoride.
9. Instruct the patient not to eat or drink for 30 minutes to allow the fluoride to be absorbed into the teeth.

PIT AND FISSURE SEALANTS

Pit and fissure sealants are indicated when there are deep pits and fissures in the occlusal surfaces of the teeth that may be difficult to clean. The sealant bonds to the surface and protects the tooth from an accumulation of bacteria that produce acids. Chapter 53 discusses pit and fissure sealants in more detail.

TOOTHBRUSHES AND TOOTHBRUSHING

The single most important instrument in plaque control is the toothbrush. Because of the variety of toothbrushes, it is necessary to be familiar with each patient's needs. Sizes, shapes, and type of bristles are just a few characteristics of toothbrushes. Generally accepted toothbrushes vary from pedodontic (small) to adult sizes. Bristles may be in two or three rows and range from soft to medium-hard. In addition, the toothbrush should be sturdy, easily cleaned, economically priced, and easy to use. Because of the microorganisms existing in the oral cavity, toothbrushes should be discarded after two to three months of use. In the event of a heavy cold or viral infection, a more frequent replacement will help to prevent recurrent disease.

To make the best selection, several factors should be considered. These include the (1) patient's current oral hygiene conditions; (2) recommended brushing technique; (3) personal and professional preferences; (4) patient"s manipulative ability; and (5) the desire to follow suggested methods.

Battery-powered or electrical toothbrushes can be used for all patients, but they are especially helpful for those who are unable to use a manual toothbrush. Geriatric patients and the physically and mentally compromised have been successful in cleaning the teeth with such a brush. The same principles apply in using a powered toothbrush as a manual toothbrush for each brushing technique.

Toothbrushing

There are several methods of toothbrushing that can be used for plaque control. In order to decide which technique to recommend to the patient, one must take into account two considerations: (1) the specific technique should remove plaque; and (2) there should be no detrimental effects to the gingivae.

Bass or Sulcular Method. The *Bass* or *Sulcular* method is recognized as one of the most efficient techniques, because it advocates cleaning along the gingival margin and interproximal areas

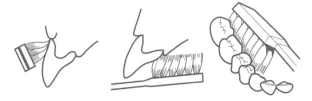

Fig. 29–2. Bass method of brushing. (A) Bristles are placed in the gingival sulcus at 45° to the long axis of the tooth. (B) Position of brush for the maxillary anterior teeth, lingual surface. (C) Position of brush for the mandibular posterior teeth, lingual surface

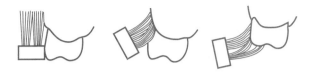

Fig. 29–3. Rolling stroke brushing method. (A) Brush handle is even with occlusal plane, and bristles are pointing apically. (B) Push against both tooth and gingiva to flex bristles. (C) Roll brush over the teeth.

where periodontal disease is likely to begin. It is also recommended for patients who have had periodontal surgery.

A soft bristle brush is used to avoid damage to the gingiva by overzealous or incorrect brushing.

Procedure (figure 29–2)

1. Place the brush on the last two or three teeth in the arch.
2. Position the brush at a 45° angle to the long axis of the tooth, figure 29–2A.
3. Gently guide the bristles into the gingival sulcus.
4. Move the brush in short strokes back and forth at least ten times without moving the tips of the bristles away from the sulcus.
5. Move the brush anteriorly over the next two or three teeth. Be sure to overlap on the previous area.
6. Repeat Steps 2 through 5 continuing along the entire facial surface.
7. Move the brush to the lingual surface, fibure 29–2B. Follow steps 1 through 5.
8. When cleaning the maxillary and mandibular anterior lingual areas, hold the brush vertically and push the bristles into the sulcus.
9. Finish each arch by brushing the occlusal surfaces, figure 29–2C.

Roll or Rolling Stroke Method. The *Roll* or *Rolling Stroke* method is recommended when

concentration on cleaning the gingival sulcus is not of primary concern. Young children and adults with healthy gingiva use this technique.

Procedure (figure 29–3)

1. Hold the brush with the bristles pointing apically, figure 29–3A.
2. Position the side of the brush (bristles) on the gingiva and the brush handle even with the occlusal plane of the teeth.
3. Flex the bristles by pressing against the side of the teeth and gingiva, figure 29–3B.
4. Roll the brush over the teeth by turning the wrist, figure 29–4C.
5. Repeat this five times.
6. Move to the next area. Be sure to overlap the previous area.
7. Continue along the facial surfaces.
8. Move to the lingual surfaces and repeat Steps 1 through 5.
9. To clean the maxillary and mandibular anterior lingual surfaces, hold the brush lengthwise.
10. Press the bristles against the teeth and gingiva.
11. Roll down for maxillary teeth and up for mandibular teeth. Do this five times in each area.
12. Clean the occlusal surfaces. (*Note:* Brushing too high on the gingivae during initial placement can lacerate the gingival mucosa.)

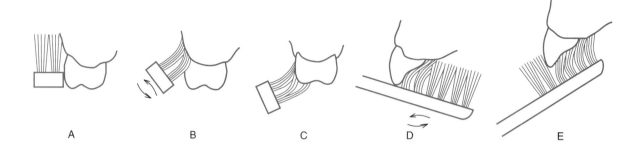

A   B   C   D   E

Fig. 29–4. Modified Stillman brushing method. (A) Position handle even with occlusal surface, and point bristles apically. (B) Angle the bristles at 45° to the long axis, and vibrate the brush. (C) Roll the brush over the crown. (D) Mandibular anterior lingual toothbrush placement. Press the brush and vibrate. (E) Roll the brush over the crown.

Modified Stillman Method. The *modified Stillman* technique is used to stimulate and massage the gingiva in addition to cleaning the cervical third of the tooth.

Procedure (figure 29–4)
1. Hold the brush with the bristles pointed apically, figure 29–4A.
2. Place the brush against the tooth, pushing lightly against both tooth and gingiva. This will cause the tissue to *blanch* (turn pale in color).
3. Angle the bristles of the brush at 45° to the long axis, figure 29–4B.
4. Vibrate the brush to the count of ten then roll it along the crown of the tooth, figure 29–4C.
5. Do this five times before moving to the next area.
6. In the anterior lingual region, hold the brush lengthwise, figure 29–4D.
7. Press and vibrate the brush, roll, then repeat.
8. Clean the occlusal surfaces as in the sulcular method, figure 29–4E. (*Note:* without careful brush placement, tissue lacerations can result. Choose a soft-bristle brush rather than one with hard bristles.)

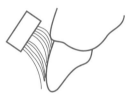

Fig. 29–5. Charters brushing method. Angle the toothbrush at 45° to the long axis with the tips of the bristles directed toward the incisal or occlusal surface.

Charters Method. The *Charters* method stresses cleaning and massaging of the gingiva, especially in patients who have had periodontal surgery. It is not used when the interdental papilla is normal.

Procedure (figure 29–5)
1. Place the brush against the tooth with the bristles pointing toward the occlusal surface.
2. Place the brush at the neck of the tooth, and angle the brush at 45° to the occlusal surface.
3. Press the bristles lightly against the margin of the gingiva.

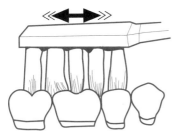

Fig. 29–6. Occlusal brushing. Use a back-and-forth motion while pushing the bristles into the occlusal surface.

4. Vibrate the brush slowly while counting to ten.
5. Because the Charters method is difficult to perform on the lingual surfaces, the modified Stillman toothbrushing method is often employed for these areas.

General Information Regarding Toothbrushing

Regardless of the type of toothbrushing method used, certain general considerations apply.

1. *Cleaning occlusal surfaces.* Press the bristles firmly into the pits and fissures. Use the back-and-forth method to scrub these areas, figure 29–6.
2. *Overlapping.* As the brush is moved to an unclean area, it should overlap partially onto the previously cleaned area. This reduces the possibility of missing any teeth during brushing.
3. *Counting strokes.* Patients can count the number of strokes (such as five or ten) or use a timer to encourage concentration on a thorough cleaning.
4. *Cleaning sequence.* The patient should begin by focusing on areas where problems in cleaning may exist. In this way, if time is limited, the critical areas are cleaned well. Generally, the patient should begin on the facial surface and proceed

from one side to the other then continue to the lingual surface. The occlusal surface is cleaned prior to moving on to the opposing arch.

5. *Timing routine of brushing.* As in all instances, the frequency of brushing and the time of day depend on the individual patient's needs. It is recommended that most patients brush at least twice daily with a thorough cleaning prior to bedtime.

DENTIFRICE

A *dentifrice* is used in conjunction with a toothbrush to clean the teeth. Most commonly known as *toothpaste*, it can be either a paste or powder. Ingredients may include *fluoride* (to inhibit tooth decay), *flavorings* (to provide an agreeable taste), *abrasives* (to clean and polish), *coloring agents* (to enhance appearance), and *detergents* (to produce a foaming action). Other chemicals may lessen sensitivity to the cementum of the tooth, reduce mouth odors, or chemically aid in plaque removal. Professional recommendations are geared to the patient's gingival condition, caries susceptibility, and need for desensitization of the cementum. It is the method of toothbrushing and flossing, however, not necessarily the type of dentifrice used, that should be of primary concern in home care.

DENTAL FLOSS

Toothbrushing can only clean three tooth surfaces well—facial, occlusal, and lingual. In order to reach the interproximal surfaces—mesial and distal—dental floss or dental tape is used.

Dental floss is round and can be either waxed or unwaxed. Waxed floss is used for tight contacts, since it will not fray as unwaxed floss does. Unwaxed floss is recommended for easy-to-clean tooth surfaces, smooth restorations, and areas without calculus. Dental tape is flat and

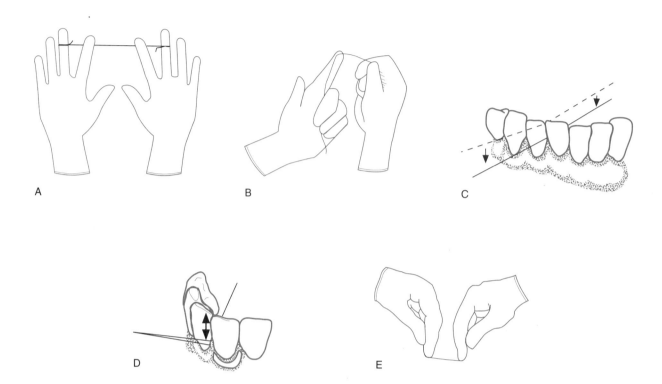

A   B   C   D   E

Fig. 29–7. Use of dental floss. **(A)** Wrap floss around the middle two fingers. **(B)** The floss can be guided in one of two ways for the maxillary arch: with thumb and forefinger or with both thumbs. **(C)** See-saw the floss interproximally. **(D)** Be sure to floss into the sulcus. **(E)** When flossing in the mandibular arch, guide the floss with both index fingers.

has sharp edges. It can be used for the same purpose as waxed floss.

Flossing can be performed either before or after brushing. When flossing is done first, the fluoride in the toothpaste will cover the interproximal areas where plaque was removed. Flossing should be performed at least once a day and preferably before retiring to bed.

Procedure (figure 29–7)

1. Use a piece of floss approximately 15 to 18 inches in length. Wrap most of the floss around the middle finger on one hand and just a small amount on the middle finger of the other hand. When moving from tooth to tooth, floss can be unwrapped from one finger and onto the other, figure 29–7A.

2. Begin in the maxillary right quadrant on the most distal surface. With no more than 2 inches of floss between the fingers, guide the floss with both thumbs or thumb and index finger, figure 29–7B.

3. Pull the floss around the distal surface of the tooth. Starting at the sulcus, move the floss up and down several times.

4. Before moving to the next area, use a clean piece of floss. Unwrap the floss from one finger and onto the other.

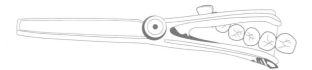

Fig. 29–8. Floss holder

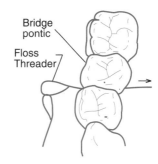

Bridge
pontic

Floss
Threader

Fig. 29–10. Use of floss threader with a fixed bridge

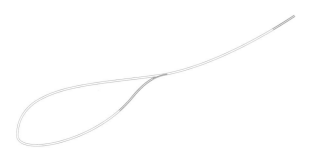

Fig. 29–9. Floss threader

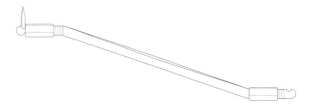

Fig. 29–11. Perio-aid

5. See-saw the floss between the contact areas. Do not force or snap the floss as the interdental papilla may be injured in the process, figure 29–7C.

6. Pull the floss around the mesial surface of the tooth. Starting at the sulcus, move the floss up and down several times. Cross the interdental papilla, and wrap the floss around the distal surface of the neighboring tooth. Slide the floss up and down several times, figure 29–7D.

7. Remove the floss using a see-saw motion. If the contact is too tight or the floss begins to shred, hold it against the proximal surface and pull the floss through, unwrapping it from the opposite finger.

8. Move to the mandibular arch. Guide the floss with both forefingers, figure 29–7E. Continue with Steps 3 through 7.

9. Move from tooth to tooth until all teeth have been flossed.

INTERPROXIMAL AIDS

If a patient experiences difficulty flossing, a *floss holder* may be used, figure 29–8. Patients who lack the manual dexterity to floss will benefit most from using a holder. In the event that the patient has a fixed bridge, a *floss threader* is a convenient way to guide the floss under the *pontic* (an artificial tooth that replaces a missing tooth) to clean the space and the cervical portion of the crown. It resembles a needle with a large eye, figures 29–9 and 29–10.

A *perio-aid* is a device that has two angled ends and round toothpick tips inserted into either end, figure 29–11. It is recommended for removing plaque in furcation-involved (division in multirooted tooth where supporting bone has been lost) teeth or at the gingival margin.

A 2-inch triangular wooden tip known as a *Stim-U-Dent* is suggested for use when there is lack of interdental papilla. The Stim-U-Dent is inserted interproximally with the base of the

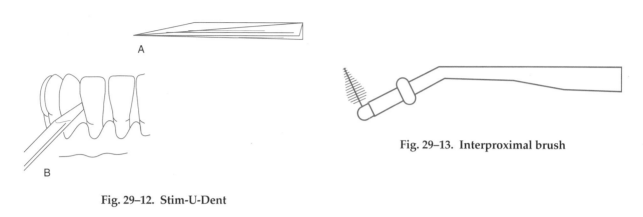

Fig. 29–13. Interproximal brush

Fig. 29–12. Stim-U-Dent

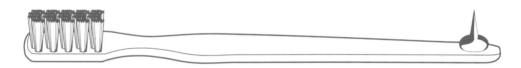

Fig. 29–14. Rubber-tipped stimulator

triangle positioned on the gingiva. By moving it back and forth, the proximal tooth surfaces are cleaned simultaneously, figure 29–12.

When areas of the mouth are inaccessible or where there are open contacts or bridgework, it is advisable to use an *interproximal brush*. Consisting of a handle that is straight or curved and a minibrush that may be tapered or straight, the interproximal brush is inserted and moved back and forth, figure 29–13.

To revive unhealthy gingivae, a *rubber-tipped stimulator* is available. By massaging the diseased area, blood flow is increased. A rubber-tipped stimulator should *never* be used on healthy gingiva to avoid damaging the existing interdental papilla and disturbing the periodontal ligament attachment, figure 29–14.

OTHER ORAL HYGIENE AIDS

Because dental plaque is usually colorless, a *disclosing solution* or *disclosing tablet* is used to identify the deposits, figure 29–15. The disclosing agent can be either a liquid mixture or tablet that contains a dye or coloring chemical. Solutions are used most often in dental offices, because they are too messy to use at home. The solution is swabbed directly onto the teeth. The advantage of using disclosing solutions is that they stain plaque deposits more readily. Tablets are recommended for home use. They are chewed and mixed with the saliva by swishing them around in the mouth. The main disadvantage of using these agents is that they stain not only the teeth but the lips, tongue, and gingiva. For this reason, patients are encouraged to disclose, floss, and brush before bedtime. The stain will disappear by morning.

Oral irrigation is a process whereby water is forced continuously or periodically through an irrigation tip, figure 29–16, into the interproximal areas to eliminate debris. Most systems used at home are either power-driven pumps or attached to a water faucet. The unit is turned

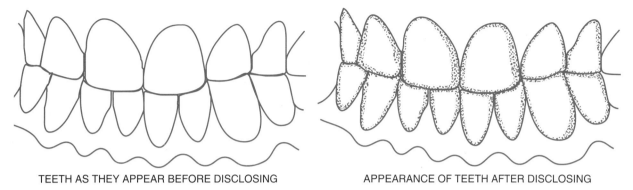

TEETH AS THEY APPEAR BEFORE DISCLOSING   APPEARANCE OF TEETH AFTER DISCLOSING

Fig. 29–15. Disclosing agent

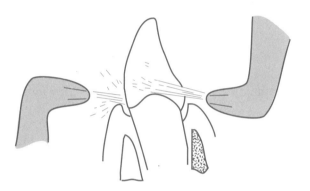

Fig. 29–16. Oral irrigation tips.

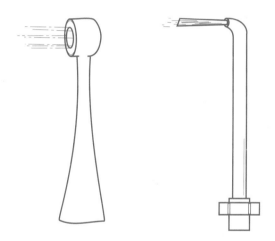

Fig. 29–17. Water irrigation. Note horizontal spray to avoid forcing bacteria into the sulcus.

on, and the water flow is adjusted. The irrigation tip is directed at the interproximal space and not into the gingival sulcus, figure 29–17. If a high pressure is used, damage to the gingival tissues may occur, or bacteria may be forced into the gingival sulcus. Other chemical agents such as mouthwashes, sanguinarine, or _chlorhexidine gluconate_ (an antiinfective agent used topically) can be used in lieu of water to reduce the number of bacteria in the oral cavity. Oral irrigation is advantageous for patients undergoing orthodontic treatment or those who have fixed bridges to clean hard-to-reach areas. It should be stressed in all situations, however, that oral physiotherapy is not a replacement for daily toothbrushing and flossing.

ORAL RINSES OR MOUTHWASHES

Oral rinses or _mouthwashes_ can be categorized as either breath fresheners (cosmetic) or as an aid in reducing bacteria (therapeutic). They can be prepared at home or purchased in a store. Mixtures prepared at home usually consist of plain water, saline (salt) solutions, or bicarbonate of soda (baking soda). Commercial rinses contain water, sweetener, alcohol, flavoring, and coloring. Mouthwash is often used as a rinse before dental procedures to reduce microorganisms. Patients use mouthwash at home for a "quick cleaning" when they do not have the time to brush and floss, for care following surgery, for reduction in decay-producing bacteria, or just to eliminate breath odors. Therapeutic mouthwashes that contain chlorhexidine gluconate or sanguinarine aid in controlling plaque and mouth odors. Unfortunately, chlorhexidine gluconate may alter the taste of some foods or stain the teeth. Patients using these rinses should have regular prophylaxis appointments.

PATIENT EDUCATION AS A PART OF PREVENTIVE DENTISTRY

No matter how much time and money are invested in restoring an unhealthy mouth, if the patient does not understand the need for adequate home care, then all is lost. During the initial patient education counseling session, the role of plaque and diet should be discussed. The patient should then be given a plan of personal oral hygiene based on his or her needs. Once the patient understands the first two steps, he or she should be encouraged to return for recall appointments in order to monitor home care.

The patient education plan is divided into three sections: motivation, education, and reinforcement.

In order to develop a patient education program, the patient must show the desire to learn. This includes being made aware of the problem and subsequently being willing to change behavior.

After the patient is motivated to learn, he or she needs to be educated. Always encourage the patient, correcting mistakes in a positive manner. Involve as many of the senses as possible. This is more stimulating to the patient than just hearing a lecture. Pamphlets with pictures or videotapes can be excellent tools when they address the patient's individual needs. Actively engaging the patient in participation is by far the best method for learning. The patient learns faster and retains the information longer.

Once learning is complete, the patient must practice these skills. Reinforcement is essential in making these activities a habit.

REVIEW

1. Define plaque. _____

2. Plaque causes two dental diseases: _____.

3. List the four steps of plaque formation.

   a. _____

   b. _____

   c. _____

   d. _____

4. Write out the two steps of decay formation.

   _____

   _____

5. What are the two bacteria that contribute to tooth decay? _____

   _____

6. If bacteria remains in the gingival sulcus, layers of plaque build up. This is called_____.

7. List the vitamins and minerals that increase resistance to tooth decay.

   _____

8. Which foods stimulate the gingiva—soft foods or fibrous foods? _____

   _____

9. Caries susceptibility may be attributed to two major causes:

   a. _____

   b. _____

10. Two problems cause by excessive fluoride are _____

    _____.

11. Three types of fluoride used for topical application are _____

    _____.

12. Why are pit and fissure sealants used?_____

    _____

13. Match the toothbrushing method to the correct description.

    a. _____ Bass

                      1. Stimulates and massages gingiva as well as cleans the cervical third of the tooth.

    b. _____ Rolling Stroke

                      2. Cleans the gingival margin, recommended in post-surgical patients.

    c. _____ Modified Stillman

                      3. Used when gingiva is healthy.

    d. _____ Charters

                      4. Cleans the gingival area; not recommended when the interdental papilla is intact. Bristles are pointed occlusally.

14. Another name for toothpaste is _____.

15. Floss used for tight contacts is _____.

16. Why is a floss holder used? _____

17. A _____ guides floss under the pontic of a bridge.

18. A device which uses toothpicks at either end of a handle to clean interproximally is a _____.

19. _____are wooden sticks which clean areas where interdental papilla is missing.

20. An _____ cleans inaccessible areas or areas where bridgework is in place.

21. A _____ is used to massage unhealthy gingivae.

22. Because plaque is translucent, _____ can be used to stain the teeth.

23. _____uses water to free interproximal areas of debris.

24. Mouthwashes can be categorized as either_____.

Chapter 30: Nutrition

After studying this chapter, the student will be able to:

- Make a distinction between mechanical and chemical digestions.
- Describe the digestive changes that occur in the mouth, stomach, small intestine, and large intestine.
- State the site where most nutrients are absorbed into the body.
- Make a distinction between anabolism and catabolism in the metabolic process.
- Name the six key nutrients required by the body for total health.
- Discuss the meaning of RDAs and how they are established.
- Explain the importance of protein in the diet.
- Explain the difference between essential and nonessential amino acids.
- Determine what carbohydrates are, their source, and why they are essential to body functions.
- Explain the importance of fats in the diet.
- Name the two types of fatty acids, and give the source for each type.
- State three conditions or health problems associated with too much fat in the diet.
- Compare the two types of vitamins and the sources of each.
- Describe the functions of vitamins in human nutrition.
- Name the vitamin essential for the proper assimilation of calcium and phosphorus.
- Name the three minerals that have a direct relationship in the formation of teeth.
- Give the two minerals most prominent in bone and tooth structures and the functions of each.
- Discuss the difference between macrominerals and microminerals.
- Give the five main functions of water in maintaining proper body water balance.
- Describe the deficiency signs (symptoms) of excessive water loss.
- Establish a diet plan.

INTRODUCTION

Nutrition is a complex and often debated subject. Theories without scientific basis continue to prevail. Much information tends to confuse the public rather than present proven principles.

Dentistry retains a respected tradition for providing patients with sound nutrition advice. Consider the fact that dentists routinely see many more healthy persons than do physicians. As a result, dental personnel have more time to discuss reliable nutritional information.

To better understand what happens to the food we eat, a review of the human digestive system is in order.

THE DIGESTIVE SYSTEM

Digestion involves both mechanical and chemical processes. *Mechanical processes* include the chewing of food, the churning actions of the stomach, and the muscular contractions of the intestinal tract. This regulated pattern of contractions is known as **peristalsis**. Peristalsis breaks up food into smaller and smaller particles, mixes them with digestive juices, and continually moves the food mass through the intestinal tract.

Chemical processes involve substances affecting the organs of the body, the *enzymes*. An enzyme is usually a protein that initiates and accelerates a chemical reaction. Enzymes are responsible for chemical changes that break down foods into simpler forms that can be absorbed. Enzymes bring about these changes without having their own composition changed in the process, i.e., as **catalysts**. Enzymes have a specific action. A particular enzyme will act only on one kind of foodstuff and will react with no other. For instance, an enzyme that digests starch will not digest fat.

Digestive Process

Mouth. In the mouth begins the mechanical and some chemical breakdown of foods, figure 30–1.

- Teeth grind food.
- Saliva adds moisture to food, acts as a lubricant, and forms a small, round ball of food (bolus).
- The tongue helps food bolus along the way and to cross the trachea (windpipe).
- The epiglottis, a trapdoor that closes the windpipe, forcing the food into the esophagus.

Digestion of some carbohydrates begins because of the chemical action of the enzyme *salivary amylase*, formerly called ptyalin.

Pharynx (throat). A tube leading to the stomach, the pharynx is connected to the esophagus and moves food finely chopped as puree to the stomach.

- Nerve endings along the esophagus cause waves of constriction (unusual narrowing), or *peristalsis*, as food moves to the stomach.
- The brain alerts the stomach to start the release of gastric juices, hydrochloric acid (HCl) and pepsin, a protein-specific enzyme.

Stomach. Food in the stomach is churned and mixed with gastric juices (HCl and pepsin) until it reaches a liquid consistency. The food will spend approximately one-half hour in the stomach. Partial digestion of some nutrients occurs:

- carbohydrates—minor action
- fats—minor action
- protein—action of HCl forms *polypeptides* (two or more amino acids combined with water)

Intestines. In the stomach HCl stimulates intestinal hormones from the liver and pancreas; the liver releases bile that has been stored in the gallbladder; the pancreas releases pancreatic juice. Both juices are alkaline and will neutralize the HCl remaining in the food mass.

- The *small intestine* (duodenum). In the first 10 inches of small intestine, where nutrients are absorbed into the body system, food, having been churned and bathed in digestive juices, is now sent on a four- to eight-hour journey through the small intestine. Peristalsis waves twist and wrench the intestine and swish food solution back and forth. Millions of nearly microscopic fingers, called villi, in the intestine stir the solution and transfer the usable nutrients into the blood and lymph systems.

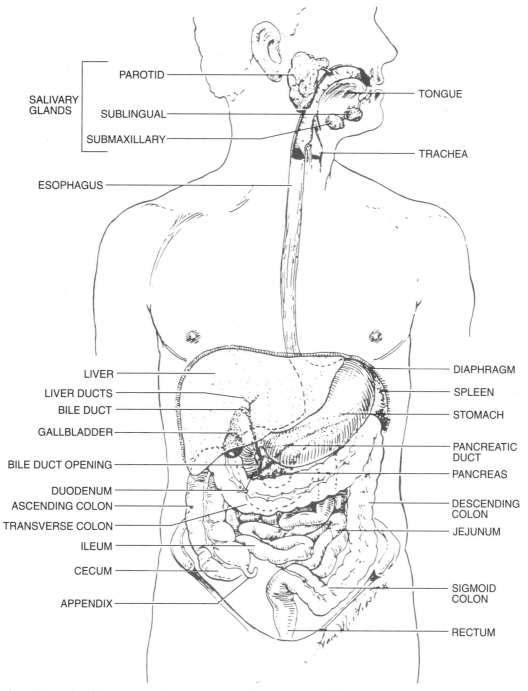

Fig. 30–1. The digestive system (Courtesy Kinn, M. *Medical Terminology—Review Challenge,* Delmar, Albany, NY, 1987)

Chemical Reactions in Digestion/Absorption of Nutrients

- All *carbohydrates* convert to monosaccharides (simple sugar that cannot be broken down to a simpler substance).
- All *fats* are emulsified by bile (combined with glycerin). Emulsified fats are further converted to monoglycerides (glycerol) and fatty acids.
- All *proteins* convert to amino acids. Cellulose, fiber, some fats resist digestion and move on!
- In the *large intestine* (colon), remains of food solution will spend approximately ten to twelve hours. Large quantities of water and some nutrients wait here to be absorbed into the system.
- Food solution remaining in colon is fed by colonies of bacteria to decay remains; intestinal contents take on solid consistency.
- Fecal matter is excreted as body waste.

Therefore, orange juice, buttered toast, egg and milk for breakfast will leave the body as heat, carbon dioxide (CO_2), water (H_2O), and nitrogenous waste!

Liver and Its Function

The liver is the first station through which blood passes after leaving the small intestine, where it has picked up absorbed compounds (nutrients).

Carbohydrates

- Carbohydrates come from the intestine and reach the liver in the form of monosaccharides.
- Liver transforms monosaccharides to glycogen (for storage).
- From glycogen the liver produces glucose; glucose is sent in a steady amount to all cells of the body via blood circulation.

- Liver keeps blood glucose (sugar) level constant; liver may convert more glycogen into blood glucose as needed—should there be too much glucose, it will convert back to glycogen.
- Liver is responsible for keeping glycogen and glucose in chemical equilibrium.
- Excess glycogen is stored as *fat.*

Fatty Acids and Glycerin (Glycerol)

- Fatty acids and glycerin reach the liver from the intestine.
- Liver recombines fatty acids and glycerin into fats.
- Liver fats may be sent via the blood system to all cells of the body.
- Fats may be stored under the skin, along membranes of the abdomen, around the heart, kidneys, and other organs.
- Liver and fat deposits communicate via the blood system; if too much fat is in the liver, remaining fat is deposited elsewhere; if there is too little fat in the liver, fats from other areas of the body can replenish the reduced fat in the liver.

Protein

Any amino acids not passed to the body cells via blood are chemically removed as carbon dioxide (CO2) during respiration (breathing); nitrogen that is left is removed in the urine.

Metabolism

Metabolism is the sum total of the physical and chemical processes and reactions taking place among the ions, atoms, and molecules of the body. Metabolism involves the way nutrients are absorbed into the blood following digestion. Refer to Chapter 4, *Human Cell Structure and Function.*

Chemical Reactions. The chemical reactions in metabolism require the activity of *enzymes.*

Many of these enzymes require other substances, or *coenzymes*. Where an enzyme substance is usually made of protein, a coenzyme is an organic substance that is *not protein*. It is one that can unite with a given protein to form an active enzyme system. One of the important functions of vitamins, certain minerals and hormones is to act as coenzymes.

The Two Phases of Metabolism

1. *Anabolism*. The constructive phase; the conversion of compounds derived from nutrients into living, organized substances that the body can use. Example: the formation of body tissues.

2. *Catabolism*. The destructive phase; the substances are reconverted into simpler compounds with the release of energy for the proper functioning of body cells. Example: breakdown of tissue associated with surgery, burns, or other trauma.

Basic Metabolic Rate (BMR). The *basic metabolic rate* is the minimal rate at which the body must produce energy to continue its essential life processes. It is the measure of how quickly an individual converts food into energy.

The BMR is calculated from the person's rate of metabolism while at complete rest and in a fasting state. The rate expressed is in a percentage that indicates how far it varies from the norm, or from the average range for a person of the same age, sex, and size.

Basic Metabolic Need. Basic metabolic need is the amount of energy required to carry on the involuntary work of the body and to maintain the body temperature.

- One-third of energy is maintained in functional activities of various organs—heart, kidneys, and lungs.
- Two-thirds of energy is needed for oxidation in the resting tissues, especially the maintenance of muscle tone.

KEY NUTRIENTS

Nutrients are substances that supply the body with essential nourishment. The key nutrients are described in figure 30–2.

Key nutrients are necessary for

- growth, maintenance, and repair of tissues
- energy requirements
- regulating body processes
- maintaining a constant internal environment

Good nutrition depends on an ample supply of all the essential nutrients found in the food of a well-balanced diet. *Diet* is the total of all food taken into the body and includes both liquid and solid forms. Each nutrient has a key role to play, but it is important to remember that all the nutrients work together in an intricate metabolic balance. An extra supply of one nutrient cannot make up for the shortage of another. In fact, a deficiency of one nutrient may interfere with maximum use of others.

Proteins. Proteins furnish energy and are the only nutrients capable of building body tissues. Their sources are from both animal and plant life.

Carbohydrates. Carbohydrates are "energy" nutrients. Their source is primarily plants.

Fats. Fats are the highest calorie nutrient. Fats provide energy and other nutritional needs. Their source is from both animal and plant life.

Vitamins. Vitamins are obtained from organic (living) substances. They are necessary in minute amounts for growth, development, and optimum health.

Minerals. Minerals are inorganic substances whose origin is neither organic life nor any product of organic life. Minerals are necessary in very small amounts for growth, development, and optimum health.

Water. Water is the principal constituent of the body and an important nutrient.

Fig. 30–2. Key nutrients

RECOMMENDED DIETARY ALLOWANCES (RDAS)

Recommendations for the average daily amounts of nutrients that population groups (by age and sex) should consume over a period of time are termed *Recommended Dietary Allowances* (RDAs) and are established by the Food and Nutrition Board of the National Academy of Sciences–National Research Council.

They are guidelines established on available scientific knowledge. They are adequate to meet the known needs of practically all healthy persons. However, the intake recommended for one nutrient assumes that the requirements for energy and all other nutrients are fully met.

Recommended Dietary Allowances are a guide to determine the nutritional adequacy of a diet. They do not take into consideration the additional needs that occur from disease, trauma, or other special conditions.

CALORIES

One calorie (spelled with a small *c*) is the amount of heat required to raise the temperature of 1 gram of water by 1°C. A Calorie (spelled with a capital C) is 1,000 times larger than the calorie and is used in metabolic studies.

In common usage, a *calorie* pertains to the amount of energy contained in food required for activity and growth in daily life. The term *energy* is used interchangeably with *calorie*.

Body requirements mainly depend on body size, basal metabolic rate, activity, age, sex, and environmental temperature. Calories come from carbohydrates, protein, fat, and alcohol.

1 gram of protein = 4 calories
1 gram of carbohydrate = 4 calories
1 gram of fat = 9 calories
1 gram of alcohol = 7 calories (and no nutritional value)

Basal metabolic need is based on 1 Calorie per hour, per kilogram of body weight (1 kilogram = 2.2 pounds).

FOOD GROUPS

Food can be classified into *food groups* that provide essential nutrients in about the same quantities. Systems for dividing food into groups may vary. For the purposes of this chapter, four essential food groups plus a nonessential group will be discussed.

Major Nutrient Contributions
Calcium
Phosphorus
Protein
Riboflavin
Vitamin A
Vitamin D

Recommended Servings Per Day
Children under 9: 2 to 3 cups
Children 9 to 12: 3 or more cups
Teenagers: 4 or more cups
Adults: 2 or more cups
Pregnant women: 3 or more cups
Nursing mothers: 4 or more cups

Serving Size
1 cup = 8 ounces fluid milk (whole, skim, buttermilk, nonfat, and lowfat) or designated milk equivalent

Designated equivalents (based on equal content of calcium)
1 1/2 ounces cheddar or swiss cheese
1 1/2 to 2 cups cottage cheese
1/4 cup dry skimmed milk powder
1 1/2 cups ice cream
1/2 cup evaporated milk

Foods Found in the Group
Fluid milk (whole, skim, nonfat, lowfat, buttermilk)
Condensed, evaporated, and powdered milk
Cheeses
Ice cream
Yogurt
Dishes made with milk products

Fig. 30–3. The milk group

Major Nutrient Contributions
Protein
Iron
Thiamin
Riboflavin
Vitamin B_{12} (animal products only)

Recommended Servings Per Day
2 or more servings

Serving Size
2 to 3 ounces lean, boneless, cooked meat, poultry, or fish
2 eggs
1 cup cooked dry beans or peas
4 tablespoons peanut butter
$^{1}/_{2}$ to 1 cup nuts, sesame, or sunflower seeds

Foods Found in the Group
Beef
Lamb
Veal
Pork, except bacon
Organ meats (such as liver or sweetbreads)
Poultry (chicken, turkey, goose, duck)
Fish, shellfish
Lunch meats (bologna, liverwurst)

Meat Alternatives
Eggs
Dried beans, peas, and lentils
Nuts
Peanuts and peanut butter
Soybeans and soybean flour

Fig. 30–4. The meat group

All the food from each of the four food groups work together to supply the necessary energy and nutrients for growth, maintenance, and health. It is recommended that a wide variety of foods from each group be selected. Adjustment in size and number of servings should be based on individual RDA needs. A description of the four groups is presented in figures 30–3, 30–4, 30–5, and 30–6.

The Nonessential Group

Because these foods are not included in any other official group, they are classified as the

Major Nutrient Contributions
Carbohydrates
Vitamin A
Vitamin C

Recommended Servings Per Day
4 or more servings

Serving Size
$^{1}/_{2}$ cup vegetable or fruit
1 medium apple, banana, orange, potato
$^{1}/_{2}$ medium grapefruit or melon
1 small salad

Foods Found in the Group
All fruits and vegetables (either cooked or raw)

Fig. 30–5. The vegetable and fruit group

Major Nutrient Contributions
Carbohydrates
Thiamin
Niacin
Iron
Riboflavin

Recommended Servings Per Day
4 or more servings of whole-grain, enriched, or restored

Serving Size
1 slice of bread
1 roll
1 biscuit
1 cup ready-to-eat cereal, flake or puff varieties
$^{1}/_{2}$ to $^{3}/_{4}$ cup cooked cereal
$^{1}/_{2}$ to $^{3}/_{4}$ cup cooked pasta (macaroni, spaghetti, noodles)
5 saltines
2 squares graham crackers

Foods Found in the Group
All breads and products made with flour
Breakfast cereals
Rice
Pasta
Grits
Bulgur (granulated wheat)
Oats
Barley
Buckwheat
Rye

Fig. 30–6. The bread and cereals group

nonessential group. Refined sugars, in all forms, are carbohydrates that provide no nutrients; these are empty calories. Carbohydrate needs can be best met from foods that provide other nutritional benefits.

Fats are needed in the diet. However, this nutritional need should not be met by selecting foods that provide mostly fat calories (such as butter and lard). Many of the available foods have fat in them; these fill the need for dietary fats. Consequently, foods that contain primarily fat calories are included in the nonessential group.

READING FOOD LABELS

The Food and Drug Administration (FDA) regulates the information on food labels. Nutrition labeling is mandatory only if a manufacturer adds nutrients to a food, or if a nutritional claim is made for a particular product. Some food manufacturers include information on a voluntary basis. A sample label is shown in Appendix A.

Information per Serving

The package must be labeled to include

- number of servings
- serving size
- calories per serving
- weight in grams per serving of protein, carbohydrate, and fat

Some labels include information on cholesterol, sodium, and potassium content.

Percentage of U.S. RDA

The United States Recommended Daily Allowance (U.S. RDA) is the measurement used in nutritional labeling on food packages. The label must show the percentage per serving of the U.S. RDA for

- protein
- vitamins A and C, thiamin, riboflavin, and niacin
- minerals—calcium, iron
- sodium content if not included in per serving data

Some food manufacturers include information on additional vitamins and minerals. It should be remembered that this listed information is in terms of U.S. RDAs, not RDAs. There is an important difference.

Carbohydrate Information

Some manufacturers of cereal may include a breakdown of carbohydrate information. This helps in estimating the amount of sugar or sweeteners in the product. Carbohydrate information, expressed in grams per serving, may include

- starch and related carbohydrates
- sugars (maltose, other sweeteners)
- dietary fiber
- total carbohydrates

Fat Information

Some labels on meat products, as well as peanut butter, contain a breakdown of fat per serving. This information may include

- fat—total grams
- percentage of calories from fat
- polyunsaturated fat
- saturated fat
- cholesterol

Sugars and Sweeteners

Most food ingredients are listed on the label in order of decreasing amounts present. Sugar can be judged by its position in the order of its listing.

Canned fruits, traditionally packed in heavy sugars, now are available packed in natural juices. These are labeled "no sugar added" or "packaged in natural juices." Some foods, once made with large amounts of sugar, are presently sweetened with artificial sweeteners. This change reduces sugar intake and the tendency of the food to promote tooth caries (decay). Tooth decay seems to be a disease of civilization, possibly associated with refined foods.

Low-Calorie Foods

A *low-calorie food* cannot contain more than 40 calories per serving or 0.4 calories per gram. A *reduced-calorie food* must be reduced in calories by one-third.

Sodium Content of Foods

Sodium, also called salt, is a necessary constituent of the body fluids and of the diet. When reading food labels, current terms may be helpful in determining the sodium content of a packaged food:

- low sodium—140 mg or less per serving
- very low sodium—25 mg or less per serving
- sodium-free—less than 5 mg per serving
- reduced sodium—product has at least 75 percent less sodium than before the reduction
- unsalted (no salt added)—no salt was used in processing the food

Misleading Terms on Labels

The FDA has yet to define the use of natural, organic, or health foods. These terms are misleading. Light, or lite, does not necessarily mean fewer calories. Perhaps the product still contains the same number of calories per ounce, but each serving weighs less. High-energy foods are usually high-calorie foods. Products whose content is higher in sugar and carbohydrates may be high-energy, but high in calories as well.

PROTEIN

A group of organic compounds containing carbon, hydrogen, oxygen, and nitrogen form proteins. *Protein* substances in the body are essential to its structure and function. None of the cells of the body can survive without an adequate supply of protein.

The end products of protein digestion are *amino acids*. Amino acids constitute about 20 percent of the cell mass and are the chief constituent of protein. Amino acids occur naturally in plant and animal tissues. More than twenty different amino acids are commonly found in proteins. Some of them can be produced in the body, but the human organism cannot manufacture others. These essential amino acids must be provided by protein foods in the diet.

Food proteins are of great nutritional importance, because they are necessary for the building and repair of all kinds of body tissues, especially of muscles and organs, heart, liver, and kidneys.

Functions of Proteins

The main function of protein is *tissue synthesis*, or tissue regeneration. *Synthesis* is a reaction, or series of reactions, in which a complex compound is created from elements and simple compounds.

Structural Protein (synthesized by body)

- Structures such as cell walls, various membranes, connective tissue, and muscles are mainly protein.
- Hormones, so important in the regulation of metabolism, are proteins.
- Enzymes that act as catalysts in the chemical reactions of metabolisms are proteins.
- One molecule of protein is composed of twenty-two different amino acids. To make body protein, the cell must have twenty-two of the amino acids simultaneously.

- Protein is the only nutrient that can *make new cells* and *repair tissues.*

Dietary Protein (supplied to the body from food)

- Builds new body tissues for growth during pregnancy, infancy, childhood, and for repair after injury or illness
- Maintains body structure
- Produces compounds essential for normal body functions, such as enzymes, hormones, hemoglobin
- Regulates body water balance
- Supplies an alternate energy source of protein (4 calories per gram)

Types of Amino Acids

Essential. Eight must be supplied by the diet.

- Used for growth and repair of tissues
- Cannot be stored for reserve, must be available simultaneously for tissue synthesis and maintenance

Source of Essential (high-quality or complete) Amino Acids

- Animal—lean meat, fish, poultry, dried beans, eggs and cheese. Egg is designated as the perfect protein against which other proteins are measured as a good source in human nutrition.

Nonessential. Twelve to fourteen are synthesized by the body.

- Can supply some essential amino acids, BUT are not used for tissue synthesis; are oxidized and nitrogen content excreted.

Source of Nonessential (low-quality or incomplete) Amino Acids

- Natural—grains (bread and cereal products), vegetable (peas, beans), small amounts of fruits

Nonessential amino acids are lacking in one or more essential amino acids and cannot perform the function of synthesis. *Complementary* amino acids are proteins that complement (work together) with other incomplete amino acids to supply missing or incomplete amino acids. For instance, gelatin taken from an animal source is not a complete protein. Pairing with vegetables or fruit enables the protein to function as effectively as complete proteins. Examples: bread complements milk, corn complements beans, and macaroni complements cheese. Such combinations enable the vegetarian to obtain a more adequate supply of dietary protein.

Protein Quality. The quality of dietary protein depends on whether

- it supplies all eight essential amino acids.
- the amount supplied will provide each amino acid in the amount needed for protein synthesis.

Amino Acid Balance. Dietary protein needs to supply each amino acid in the amount needed for protein synthesis in the body. When amino acids are supplied in amounts smaller than those needed, the total amount of protein that can be synthesized or used by other amino acids will be limited.

Although a daily supply of protein is essential to good nutrition, excess protein tends to put a strain on the liver and kidneys, as they process the excess. Protein intake greater than the RDA increases the urinary excretion of calcium and reduces the amount of calcium available for use by the body.

CARBOHYDRATES

Carbohydrates are a chemical compound of carbon, hydrogen, and oxygen. Carbohydrates are present, at least in small amounts, in most foods. Chief sources are sugars and starches.

Functions of Carbohydrates

Carbohydrates provide the major source of energy for the body.

- They convert carbohydrates into glucose, for tissues, cells, nerves, blood sugar, and muscular energy.
- They aid in oxidation of fats by combining with oxygen and removing hydrogen.
- They help to maintain body temperature.
- They store excess glycogen in the liver.

Types of Carbohydrates

Carbohydrates are chemically classified as

- monosaccharides (simple sugar)
- disaccharides (each molecule yields two molecules of monosaccharide—double sugar)
- polysaccharides (may yield ten or more molecules of monosaccharides—complex sugar)

Carbohydrate Conversion

- Sugar—yields simple carbohydrates (monosaccharides and disaccharides)
- Starches—yield complex sugar (polysaccharides) in digestible form for humans
- Dietary fiber—cellulose (polysaccharides) no enzyme can break it down, is not digestible

Digestive Process of Carbohydrates

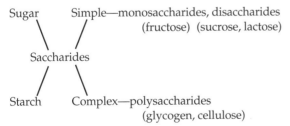

Carbohydrate Sources

- *Sugar* sources include refined table sugar (**sucrose**), syrups, honey, molasses, bread,

cookies, cakes. Naturally occurring sugars are found in fruits, vegetables, milk. Milk and dairy products contain carbohydrates in the form of milk sugar (lactose). Sugar is the only food that is nearly 100 percent carbohydrate.
- Starch sources include grains, grain products, starchy vegetables (such as potatoes and root vegetables).

Body Requirements

The body needs about 100 grams of carbohydrate, estimating 4 calories per gram, or 400 calories of carbohydrate, each day for energy and to ensure body maintenance and growth. Of all the major nutrients, carbohydrate is consumed in the greatest amount in the human diet.

Metabolism of Carbohydrates

Energy is needed for specific processes of metabolism: glucose for tissue cells, mainly the nervous system, depends solely on sugar for energy and must be in continuous supply.

- Brain cells are continually active whether a person is awake or asleep and need a continuous supply of glucose (sugar) in the fluid surrounding the cells.
- The brain and other nerves cannot make use of another energy source and are vulnerable to temporary deficiency in blood sugar.
- As mental processes originate in the brain, attitudes toward life are affected by the amount of glucose present in brain cells.
- The brain controls muscle reflexes.

Physical Conditions and Sugar Balance

- *Hypoglycemia*—abnormally low level of blood sugar
- *Hyperglycemia*—abnormally high blood glucose level

- *Diabetes mellitus*—a disorder of carbohydrate metabolism in which the ability to oxidize and utilize carbohydrates is lost, as a result of disturbances in the normal *insulin* mechanism (protein hormone, secreted by pancreas)

  Diabetic coma—insulin insufficiency (administer insulin to victim)

  Insulin shock—insulin insufficiency (provide victim with orange juice, sugar)

FATS

Fats (lipids) are a group of oily organic substances, insoluble in water but soluble in alcohol. The two basic units of fats in the human mechanism are fatty acids and glycerol (a sugar alcohol). Fats are a normal component of every living cell wall and membrane within the cell.

Function of Fats

Fats are a source of body fuel and provide efficient energy in a relatively small amount of food. Man cannot synthesize fat; therefore, it must be supplied by the diet.

Dietary fat is the most concentrated source of energy, 9 calories per gram. Normal tissue function is dependent on an adequate supply of fatty acids. Fat carries the fat-soluble vitamins A, D, E, and K.

Fats also help to maintain body temperature. They act as a cushion mechanism to protect vital organs and to pad various areas such as the buttocks, palm of the hands, and soles of the feet.

Types of Fats

The greatest portion of body and dietary fats are composed of complex molecules, called *triglycerides*. These fatty acids are of two types: *saturated* and *unsaturated*. Saturation is based on the number of hydrogen atoms a certain fatty acid contains.

Saturated Fatty Acids. *Saturated fatty acids* contain a greater number of hydrogen atoms and are often naturally solid at room temperature.

- Saturated fats are not an essential part of the diet.
- Saturated triglycerides tend to increase the amount of serum cholesterol in the blood.

Source of Saturated Fatty Acids

- Animal—fatty meats, whole milk (cream), egg yolk, animal organs (liver, kidney), butter, yellow (hard) cheese
- Plant—palm oil, coconut oil

Unsaturated Fatty Acids. Unsaturated fatty acids contain fewer hydrogen atoms and are often liquid at room temperature.

- Unsaturated fats provide essential fatty acids required by the body.
- Unsaturated triglycerides tend to lower the serum cholesterol when used to replace part of the saturated fat in the diet.

Source of Unsaturated Fatty Acids

- Vegetable—oils of safflower, sunflower, corn, soybean, cottonseed, peanut

Unsaturated fats are further divided into *monounsaturated* and *polyunsaturated* fats, depending on the hydrogen atoms present.

- *Mononusaturated* fats are those of olive oil and peanut oil. They neither raise nor lower serum cholesterol.

- *Polyunsaturated* fats include the common vegetable oils. Safflower and sunflower are the least saturated (10 percent). Corn and soybean are a bit more saturated (14 percent). Peanut oil is the most saturated (20 percent).

Hydrogenated oils are higher in saturated fat because of the process of adding hydrogen atoms to the oil. *Hydrogenation* is a process whereby polyunsaturated oils are changed into solid fats. Example: chemical change from vegetable oil (liquid) to margarine (solid).

Cholesterol. Cholesterol (sterols) is an essential body element that is present in nerve tissue, body fluids, blood, and bile. Cholesterol is important in body chemistry. The body's own production of cholesterol is necessary in the functioning of certain systems. For example: the nervous system.

- The greatest portion of cholesterol is converted into bile salts by the liver.
- It serves as the main building block of male and female sex hormones in the body.
- It is involved with vitamin D in calcium metabolism.
- There is a likely relationship between tension and cholesterol in blood.
- Reduced saturated fats in the diet may help to control blood cholesterol.

VITAMINS

The term *vitamin* comes from the Latin word *vita* that means *life* and is used to name a group of chemically unrelated compounds that are necessary for proper metabolism. Vitamins consist of various relatively complex substances occurring in plant and animal tissues and are smaller than the energy nutrients.

Vitamins cannot be made in sufficient quantities by the body and must be consumed through the diet. Very small amounts (milligrams) of vitamins fill the need for this essential nutrient.

Function of Vitamins

Vitamins are organic substances necessary for proper growth, development, and good health.

- They assist enzymes in the digestion, absorption, and metabolism of proteins, carbohydrates, fats, and minerals; they are termed *coenzymes.*

- They help enzymes to convert fuel food into energy needed for life-sustaining body functions.
- They participate in the formation of blood cells, genetic material, hormones, and chemicals of the nervous system.

Types of Vitamins

Vitamins are identified according to their solubility. There are thirteen vitamins, divided into two types: *fat-soluble* and *water-soluble vitamins,* table 30–1.

Fat-Soluble Vitamins. *Fat-soluble vitamins* can be dissolved in fat rather than water.

- They include vitamins A, D, E, and K.
- They are not destroyed by cooking and are stored in body fat and fatty tissue.
- It is not essential that they be consumed daily.
- Excessive amounts may build up to toxic (poisonous) levels.

Water-Soluble Vitamins. *Water-soluble vitamins* will dissolve in water.

- They include vitamin C and eight B vitamins.
- They cannot be stored in the body and must be consumed in the daily diet.
- They are naturally present in foods, are fragile, and may be washed away or destroyed during food preparation.

MINERALS

Minerals are inorganic (do not occur in the plant or animal worlds) substances. Various minerals are distributed throughout the body tissues.

Minerals must be supplied in the diet and generally can be obtained by a varied or mixed diet of animal and vegetable products that meet the energy and protein needs of the body. Minerals work together to maintain the health and well-being of the individual.

TABLE 30—1
VITAMINS

Vitamins	Sources	Important Functions	Deficiency Symptoms
Vitamin A	Fish liver oils. Liver. Vegetables (green and yellow). Fruits (yellow). Butter, margarine. Whole milk, cream. Cheese. Egg yolk.	Needed for growth. Health of the eyes, night vision. Structure and functioning of the cells of the skin and mucous membranes. Clear smooth skin.	Retarded growth. Night blindness. Increased susceptibility to infections. Changes in skin and mucous membranes.
Vitamin D	Vitamin D-enriched milk. Sunshine. Fish liver oil.	Absorption of calcium from digestive tract. Responsible for the body's assimilation of calcium and phosphorous.	Soft bones. Poor tooth development. Rickets. Osteoporosis and osteomalacia (softening of bones).
Vitamin E	Wheat germ oil. Vegetable oil. Vegetable greens. Egg yolk, milk fat, butter. Meat.	An antioxidant that helps to protect other nutrients from destruction by oxidation. Unites with oxygen to build the resistance of blood cells to ruptures.	Severe deficiency would result in the degeneration of body's skeletal muscles, paralysis of legs, and reproductive failure.
Vitamin K	Vegetable greens. Cabbage. Cauliflower. Soybean oil.	Normal clotting of blood. Normal liver function.	Delay in blood clotting (hemorrhages).
Vitamin B_1 (thiamin)	Yeast. Pork, organ meats. Wheat germ. Meat. Dried beans and peas. Whole-grain or enriched products.	Important in glucose metabolism. Normal function of nervous system. Promotion of normal appetite and digestion. Functioning of the heart, nerves, and muscles.	Retarded growth. Loss of appetite. Nerve disorder. Less resistance to fatigue. Impairment of digestion. Disease (beriberi).
Vitamin B_2 (Riboflavin)	Liver. Meat. Milk. Vegetable greens. Yeast. Fish, poultry, eggs. Enriched or whole-grain bread and cereals.	Needed for growth. Health of skin and mouth. Well-being and vigor. Functioning of the eyes. Important in energy and protein metabolism.	Retarded growth. Lesions at corners of mouth (cheilosis). Dimness of vision. Cataractlike symptoms. Intolerance to light. Premature aging. Dermatitis.
Niacin (nicotinic acid)	Meat, fish, poultry. Milk. Whole-grain or enriched products. Peanut butter.	Component of two enzymes. Helps cells to use other nutrients. Health of skin. Functioning of digestive and nervous systems.	Smoothness of tongue (glossitis). Skin eruptions. Digestive disturbances. Mental disorders. Disease (**pellagra**).
Vitamin B_{12}	Organ meat. Eggs. Saltwater fish.	Blood-regeneration cells in bone marrow and gastrointestinal tract.	Pernicious **anemia**.
Folic acid (folacin)	Yeast. Spinach.	Antianemic factor. Component of certain enzymes active in formation of red blood cells. Found in liver.	Megaloblastic anemia.

TABLE 30—1 [continued]

Vitamins	Sources	Important Functions	Deficiency Symptoms
Vitamin B$_6$	Liver. Pork. Muscle meat. Whole-grain cereals. Vegetables.	Functioning coenzyme in metabolism of all energy yielding nutrients. Requirement dependent on protein intake.	Rare.
Pantothenic acid	Yeast. Liver. Kidney. Eggs. Nuts. Whole-grain products.	Metabolism of protein.	Rare.
Biotin	Eggs yolk. Organ meat, muscle. Milk. Whole grains. Many vegetables. Some fruits.	Function for several enzymes systems. Involved in metabolism of protein, carbohydrates, and fats. Synthesized by intestinal bacteria.	Unlikely.
Vitamin C (ascorbic acid)	Citrus fruits. Melons. Berries. Other fruits. Tomatoes. Vegetables (especially raw).	Important role in formation and maintenance of collagen. Helps resist infection. Aids in healing. Cell activity. Maintaining strength of the blood vessels. Health of gingival tissue (gums).	Sore gingivae (gums). **Hemorrhage** around bones. Tendency to bruise easily. Disease (**scurvy**).

Functions of Minerals

When minerals are taken into the body as nutrients, they are absorbed through the gastrointestinal tract and excreted via the kidneys, bile, and other intestinal secretions as waste products.

- Minerals are component of the teeth and bones and give rigidity to their structure.
- They form compounds essential for normal metabolism.
- They activate cellular enzyme systems and hormones found in the body.
- They maintain the pH (acid-base balance) of body fluids and osmotic cell balance. _Note_: _osmosis_ is the process whereby molecules in two different solutions are separated by a semipermeable (allows passage) membrane. Molecules are capable of passing through the membrane inside the cell (intracellular) and outside the cell (extracellular).
- Minerals regulate the transmission of nerve impulses and the contraction of muscles.

Types of Minerals

Minerals may be classified into two groups: _macrominerals_ and _microminerals_ or _trace minerals_, table 30–2. Minerals that occur in large amounts in nature are needed in greater quantities by the body. Some authorities advocate the need for 100 milligrams (mg) or more of the macrominerals daily for optimum health. Microminerals (trace minerals) are those needed in only small amounts or a few milligrams per day.

Characteristics of Mineral. Minerals retain their chemical identity throughout the entire digestive process.

- Minerals will work together as long as a balance is maintained.

TABLE 30—2
MINERALS

Minerals	Sources	Important Functions	Deficiency Symptoms
Macrominerals			
Calcium (Ca)	Milk, cheese, sardines, and other whole canned fish. Vegetable greens. Some fruits.	Normal development and maintenance of bones and teeth. Clotting of the blood. Normal heart action. Iron assimilation. Nerve and muscle action.	Retarded growth. Poor tooth formation. **Rickets.** Slow clotting of blood. Osteoporosis. Osteomalacia.
Phosphorus (P)	Meat, poultry, fish. Milk. Cheese. Dried beans and peas. Whole-grain products.	Formation of normal bones and teeth. Maintenance of normal blood reaction. Maintenance of healthy nerve tissue. Normal muscle activity.	Retarded growth. Poor tooth formation. Rickets. Osteoporosis. Osteomalacia.
Magnesium (Mg)	Whole-grain cereals. Nuts. Small amounts in milk, meat, fish, eggs, and green vegetables.	Found in large amounts in bones. Major extracellular electrolyte. Controls body fluid concentration and volume.	Heavy perspiration or excessive water ingestion. Severe vomiting and diarrhea.
Potassium (K)	Fruit. Vegetables. Meat. Milk.	Major intracellular electrolyte. Controls normal pH of body.	Loss from large doses of certain drugs. Dehydration. Muscular weakness, paralysis, rapid heart beat. Low blood pressure, diarrhea, and intestinal distention.
Chlorine (Cl)	Salt, salty foods. Seafood and other animal foods.	Major extracellular electrolyte. Formation of hydrochloric acid found in digestive tract. Control blood pH. Activator for enzymes necessary for carbohydrate metabolism.	Occurs with dehydration.
Sulfur (S)	Eggs. Protein-rich foods.	Present in every cell in body. Present in hair, skin, and nails. Associated with protein, is a constituent of two amino acids. Active in energy metabolism.	Unlikely.
Microminerals			
Iron (Fe)	Liver, organ meat. Oysters. Vegetable greens. Dried beans and peas. Egg yolk. Whole-grain or enriched products.	Formation of hemoglobin in the red blood cells. Carrying oxygen to body tissues.	Anemia, characterized by weakness, dizziness, loss of weight, gastric disturbances, pallor.

TABLE 30—2 [continued]

Vitamins	Sources	Important Functions	Deficiency Symptoms
Copper (Cu)	Liver. Dried beans and peas. Meat. Nuts. Cereals.	Essential, occurs in all body tissues. Concentrated in brain, liver, heart, and kidneys. Necessary for normal absorption and utilization of iron.	Rare—severe malnutrition.
Iodine (I)	Seafoods. Iodized salt.	Formation of thyroxine, a hormone that controls metabolic rate.	Anemia. Enlargement of thyroid gland (goiter).
Fluorine (F)	Fluoridated water (1 ppm— one million parts of water). Plants and animals.	Formation of teeth. Resistance to dental caries.	Heightened tooth decay. _Excess amounts will result in mottled enamel._
Zinc (Zn)	Meat. Liver. Eggs. Seafood.	Found in most body tissues, particularly liver, voluntary muscles and bones. Needed for several body enzymes.	Retards sexual development. Severely stunts growth.
Chrominum (Cr)	Animal protein. Whole-grain products. Brewers' yeasts.	Needed for normal glucose metabolism and a cofactor for insulin.	Disturbances of glucose metabolism associated with old age and/or pregnancy.
Manganese (Mn)	Nuts. Whole grains. Fruits. Vegetables.	Large concentration in bones. Present in pituitary gland, liver, pancreas, gastrointestinal tissues. Essential for normal bone structure, reproduction, normal function of central nervous system and enzymes action.	Unknown.
Cobalt (Co)	Liver. Kidney. Oysters, clams. Lean meat. Salt water fish. Milk.	Integral component of vitamin B_{12}. Needed for the function of all cells, particularly those of the bone marrow, nervous system, and gastrointestinal tract.	Rare.

- One mineral, as a rule, cannot be administered without affecting the absorption and metabolism of other minerals.
- Increasing excess amounts of minerals beyond the RDA may in some cases be harmful.
- Serious risks are associated with megadose (excessively large) of minerals.

WATER

Water is the most abundant nutrient in the body. In fact, 65 to 70 percent body weight is water. Water is found in the plasma and lymph and surrounds each cell. Bone is one-third water; muscle is two-thirds water; and whole blood is four-fifths water.

Water is a critical and often forgotten nutrient, second only to oxygen as being essential for life. Humans can live longer without food than without water.

Functions of Water

In the circulatory system, water acts as a solvent (capable of dissolving other substances) for nutrients and hormones.

- Serves to transport waste products away from various parts of the body.
- Maintains blood volume.
- Serves as a catalyst in metabolic reactions.
- Acts as a lubricant.
- Regulates body temperature (perspiration helps to release excessive body heat and assists in the even distribution of heat in the body).

Water Sources for the Body

- drinking water and beverages consumed
- metabolic end-products of carbohydrates, protein, and fats
- water formed through oxidation of foods

Water Balance

The distribution of water inside and outside the cells depends on adequate protein and balanced mineral intake. Sodium (salt) and potassium are minerals largely responsible for water balance.

- Body maintains water balance through respiration, evaporation at the skin surface, and urinary excretion.

Conditions Arising from Water Imbalance

- Excessive water loss, which leads to severe alteration in body function.
- Reduction of 10 percent in volume of body fluids, which results in dehydration, fatal if left untreated.

- Heat exhaustion as a result of water depletion occurs when replacement of water is inadequate, coupled with prolonged sweating.
- Liquid intake of coffee, tea, and alcohol are diuretics and cause water to be excreted by the kidneys.

Symptoms of Water Imbalance

- Thirst, fatigue, infrequent urination, and fever occur.
- Severe cases lead to delirium, coma, and possible death.

Excessive Intake of Water

- May occur during exposure to heat.
- Adequate replacement of salt is lost through perspiration—essential to avoid salt depletion heat exhaustion.

Symptoms of Salt Depletion

- fatigue, nausea, vomiting, exhaustion, weakness

During periods of heavy labor or exercise, intake of adequate water and salt is recommended. One and one-half to two quarts of water should be consumed on the daily diet. The sodium content in prepared foods is generally adequate for sodium replacement.

DIETARY ANALYSIS

Dietary analysis is the primary tool used to determine the nutritional adequacy of a person's diet.

Limitations of Dietary Analysis

It is important to recognize the limitations of dietary analysis. There may be

- difficulty in getting an accurate recording of food intake

- variability in food stuffs and nutrient contents
- individual variations in the absorption of nutrients

The Diet Diary

A diet diary is used to gather information necessary to diet analysis. A person records everything consumed by himself or herself throughout the day. The entry should list all foods, both solid and liquid, as well as snacks. The entry should be specific as to what food was eaten, how it was prepared, the size of portion, and when it was eaten, figure 30–7.

Water, black coffee, tea without sugar, and diet soft drinks (nonessential foods) should be included, but not extended into any food group. Coffee with cream and sugar is still considered a nonessential.

The Diet Analysis

Use a prepared dietary analysis form, figure 30–8, and do the following:

- List each food, and determine the food group in which it belongs.
- Compare the amount eaten with the amount allowed for a serving of that food. For example, one apple is considered one serving. If only half an apple is consumed, it would be listed as a half serving. If two apples were eaten, the amount would be listed as two servings.
- Total the number of foods eaten in each group during the day. Compare this with the number that should have been eaten. This will help evaluate how well the person did in meeting the needs of all food groups.
- Review the nonessential foods eaten.
- Look for excesses, frequency of intake, and amount of cariogenic foods consumed.

SUGGESTED ACTIVITIES

- Apply your knowledge of the four food groups. Determine the food group in which each food recorded on your diet diary belongs.
- Prepare a written plan for a well-balanced diet for one day.
- Determine the nutritional needs for one day (making an entry each time a food is consumed). Use a prepared Diet Diary form for the entries.
- Record all information on a prepared Dietary Analysis form. Evaluate the nutritional adequacy of the one-day diet.

DIET DIARY

Name _____ Date_____ Day _____

Instructions

Details are important! Be certain to list everything you ate, how much you ate of each item, how it was prepared and when you ate it.

Start each day with a new page. Use as many pages as necessary per day.

TIME	FOOD (Note quantity and how it was prepared)

Fig. 30–7. A diet diary form (Courtesy Ehrlich, A. *Nutrition and Dental Health*, Delmar, Albany, NY, 1987)

DIET ANALYSIS FORM						
Name _____ Date_____ Day _____						
FOOD EATEN	**FOOD GROUP**					**CARIOGENICITY**
	MILK	MEAT	F&V	B&C	OTHER	High/Low
TOTAL SERVINGS						
FREQUENCY OF EATING (times per day) _____						
CARIOGENIC FOODS SCORE _____						
BASIC NUTRITION SCORE _____						

Fig. 30–8. A dietary analysis form (F&V, fruits and vegetables; B&C, breads and cereals) (Courtesy Ehrlich, A. *Nutrition and Dental Health*, **Delmar, Albany, NY, 1987)**

REVIEW

1. The two processes involved in digestion are

   a. _____ b. _____

2. The specific action of an enzyme is that _____

   _____.

3. The area of the digestive system where nutrients are absorbed into the body
   system is _____.

4. The first internal organ through which blood passes after leaving the small
   intestine is _____

5. The six key nutrients of a well-balanced diet are

   a. _____ b. _____ c. _____

   d. _____ e. _____ f. _____

6. Key nutrients are necessary for

   a. _____

   b. _____

   c. _____

   d. _____

7. Diet is defined as _____

   _____.

8. Give the caloric (calories per gram) value for protein, carbohydrate, fat, and
   alcohol.

   1 g protein = _____ calories   1 g carbohydrates = _____ calories

   1 g fat = _____ calories   1 g alcohol = _____ calories (no nutritional value)

9. List the four food groups

    a. _____   b. _____

    c. _____   d. _____

10. Information on food labels is regulated by the _____.

11. Nutritional labels on food packages show the percentage per serving, according to the U.S. RDA measurement, for

    a. _____   b. _____

    c. _____   d. _____

12. Carbohydrate information on food labels, expressed in grams per serving, includes

    a. _____   b. _____

    c. _____   d. _____

13. Fat information on food labels, expressed in grams per serving, may include

    a. _____   b. _____

    c. _____   d. _____

    e. _____

14. Sugar content on a food label can usually be judged in the _____.

15. Sodium information on a packaged food, expressed in grams per serving, may include the terms

    a. _____   b. _____

    c. _____   d. _____

16. Proteins are organic compounds of _____, _____,

    _____, _____.

17. The main function of protein is _____.

18. Protein is composed of at least _____ of amino acids.

19. The quality of dietary protein depends on whether

   a. _____

   b. _____

20. State the difference between essential and nonessential amino acids.

   a. _____

   _____

   _____

   b. _____

   _____

   _____

21. Sources of essential amino acids are_____, _____,

   _____, _____, _____, _____.

22. Sources of nonessential amino acids include_____, _____,

   _____.

23. The chief sources of carbohydrates are_____ and

   _____.

24. Carbohydrates provide the major source of _____ for the body.

25. Four functions of carbohydrates are to

   a. _____

   b. _____

   c. _____

   d. _____

26. Name the three types of carbohydrates.

    a. _____   b. _____   c. _____

27. Dietary fat cannot be synthesized by man; it must be supplied in the _____

    _____.

28. Dietary fats carry the fat-soluble vitamins_____, _____,

    _____, _____.

29. The two types of fatty acids (triglycerides) are _____ and

    _____.

30. Saturation of a fat is dependent on _____.

31. Polyunsaturated fats may be changed from an oil to a solid by the process of

    _____.

32. Vitamins cannot be stored in the body and must be supplied in the _____

    _____.

33. Thirteen vitamins, identified by their solubility, can be divided into two
    groups:

    _____ and _____.

34. The water-soluble vitamins include vitamins _____ and

    _____.

35. Minerals may be classified into two groups: _____ and

    _____ (_____).

36. Three minerals having a direct relationship with the formation of teeth are:

    _____, _____, and _____.

37. The most abundant nutrient in the body is _____.

38. Function of the water nutrient:

   a. _____

   b. _____

   c. _____

   d. _____

39. State the cause for the following systematic conditions:

Condition	Cause
a. goiter	_____
b. night blindness	_____
c. scurvy	_____
d. rickets	_____
e. osteoporosis	_____
f. cheilosis	_____
g. beriberi	_____
h. pellagra	_____
i. mottled enamel	_____
j. anemia	_____

Chapter 31: Basics in Dental Charting

INTRODUCTION

One of the many duties delegated to the dental assistant is the charting of the teeth. This is an exact recording of the dental conditions present, the dental services to be rendered, and serves as a legal record of the patient. It includes the types of dental restorations, treatment of periodontal tissues, extractions, the replacement of missing teeth, and other information regarding the oral condition of the patient.

GENERAL ANATOMY OF MOUTH

- A full complement of deciduous, or primary, teeth numbers twenty; a full set of permanent teeth includes thirty-two teeth.
- Teeth are classified as either those of the maxillary arch or mandibular arch.
- Each arch is divided by an imaginary line between the two central incisors, creating a right half and a left half.
- Each half arch constitutes one-fourth of the teeth, and each half-arch is referred to as a quadrant. Thus, there are four quadrants of teeth in the mouth.

- In referring to position, the teeth on the *patient's* right are indicated as right; those on the *patient's* left are indicated as left.
- If an adult has all thirty-two teeth, there are eight teeth in each quadrant. A child would have five deciduous teeth in each quadrant.

IDENTIFICATION OF TEETH

Identification of teeth may be made through the use of numbers and letters. Several systems have been developed that are used by dentists; the specific system used is, of course, a matter of preference.

Universal System

The American Dental Association (ADA) officially adopted the **Universal System** for charting teeth in 1968. In this system each tooth has its own number (permanent teeth) or letter (primary teeth), and this particular number or letter refers only to that one specific tooth.

The permanent teeth are numbered from 1 to 32, and the letters A–T are used for primary teeth.

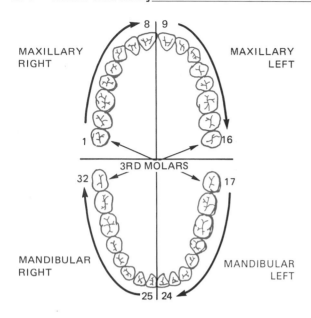

Fig. 31–1. Permanent teeth—Universal system

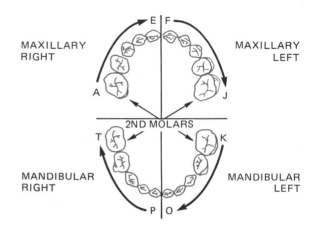

Fig. 31–2. Primary teeth—Universal system

MAXILLARY RIGHT	MAXILLARY LEFT
MANDIBULAR RIGHT	MANDIBULAR LEFT

Fig. 31–3. Arch and quadrant guide for Palmer system

Permanent Teeth, figure 31–1

1. Begin with tooth number 1, maxillary right 3rd molar, and work around the arch to number 16, maxillary left 3rd molar.
2. On the mandibular arch, start with tooth number 17, mandibular left 3rd molar, and work around to number 32, mandibular right 3rd molar.

Primary Teeth, figure 31–2

1. Begin with the letter A, maxillary right 2nd molar, and work around the arch to the letter J, maxillary left 2nd molar.
2. On the mandibular arch, start with the letter K, mandibular left 2nd molar, and work around the arch to the letter T, mandibular right 2nd molar.

Palmer System

In the Palmer System the teeth are numbered the same for each quadrant, 1–8 for permanent teeth and letters A–E for primary teeth. To distinguish which quadrant and tooth is to be recorded, a symbol or "bracket" is used to denote the maxillary and mandibular arch, as well as the right and left side of the patient.

To determine the correct arch and quadrant, figure 31–3, may be used as a guide.

Permanent Teeth, figure 31–4

1. In each quadrant the teeth are numbered from 1–8, beginning with the central incisors as 1 and working toward the 3rd molar, 8.
2. Use the quadrant bracket to denote the maxillary and mandibular arch and right or left side.
3. *Caution:* The correct bracket must be used with the tooth number for proper identification of tooth and quadrant.

   Examples: Maxillary right second molar $\underline{7|}$

   Mandibular left lateral $\overline{|2}$

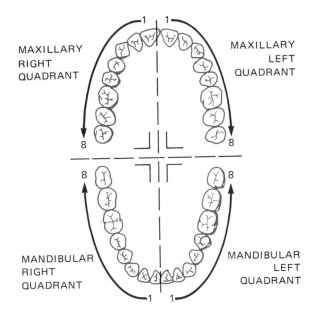

Fig. 31–4. Permanent teeth—Palmer system

Primary Teeth, figure 31–5

1. In each quadrant, the teeth are lettered A–E, beginning with the central incisors as A and working toward the 2nd molar, E.
2. Use the quadrant bracket to denote the maxillary or mandibular arch and right or left side.
3. *Caution:* The correct bracket must be used with the tooth letter for proper identification of tooth and quadrant.

   Examples: Maxillary left central |A̲
            Mandibular right second
            molar   D̄|

Fédération Dentaire International System

The Fédération Dentaire International System was designed to be used with the computer. The system uses a two-digit number to identify each tooth. The first number denotes the quadrant and the second number identifies the specific tooth in that quadrant. The quadrant numbers are 1–4 for the permanent teeth and 5–8 for the primary teeth, figure 31–6.

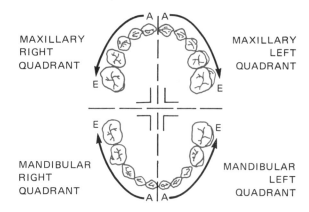

Fig. 31–5. Primary teeth—Palmer system

PERMANENT TEETH		PRIMARY TEETH	
MAXILLARY RIGHT		MAXILLARY RIGHT	
QUADRANT	1	QUADRANT	5
MAXILLARY LEFT		MAXILLARY LEFT	
QUADRANT	2	QUADRANT	6
MANDIBULAR LEFT		MANDIBULAR LEFT	
QUADRANT	3	QUADRANT	7
MANDIBULAR RIGHT		MANDIBULAR RIGHT	
QUADRANT	4	QUADRANT	8

Fig. 31–6. Quadrant numbering for International system

Permanent Teeth, figure 31–7

1. Teeth are numbered 1–8, beginning with the central incisors as 1 and 3rd molars as 8.
2. The quadrants are numbered 1–4 beginning with the maxillary right as #1, maxillary left as #2, mandibular left as #3, and mandibular right as #4.
3. Teeth in the maxillary right quadrant are recorded as: 11–18; the maxillary left quadrant, 21–28; mandibular left quadrant, 31–38; and mandibular right quadrant, 41–48.

   Examples: Maxillary right lateral: 12
            Mandibular left cuspid: 33

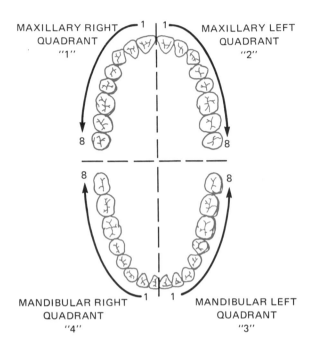

Fig. 31–7. Permanent teeth—International system

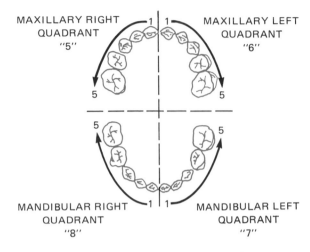

Fig. 31–8. Primary teeth—International system

Primary Teeth, figure 31–8

1. Teeth are numbered 1–5, beginning with the central incisors as 1 and 2nd molars as 5.
2. The quadrants are numbered 5–8, beginning with the maxillary right quadrant as #5, maxillary left quadrant as #6, mandibular left quadrant as #7, and mandibular right quadrant as #8.
3. Teeth in the maxillary right quadrant are recorded as 51–55; maxillary left quadrant, 61–65; mandibular left quadrant, 71–75; and mandibular right as 81–85.
   Examples: Maxillary right 1st molar: 54
   Mandibular left central incisor: 71

CAVITY CLASSIFICATIONS

A system for identifying tooth surfaces and teeth is used when recording dental conditions on a patient's dental chart.

G. V. Black (father of modern dentistry) developed the Stardard Classification of Cavities. There are five Classes, I, II, III, IV, and V. Each Class represents a particular type of **caries** (dental **cavity**) or restoration.

Class I, Anterior and Posterior Teeth

Class I caries occur in the developmental areas of the teeth, grooves, and **fossae**. When a developmental groove becomes faulty because of decay, it is called a fissure, and a defective fossa is called a pit. Pit and fissure caries are found on the following teeth.

1. On the occlusal surfaces of premolars and molars, figure 31–9.
2. On the facial (buccal) or lingual surfaces of molars, figure 31–10.
3. On the lingual surface of maxillary incisors, figure 31–11.

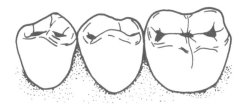

Fig. 31–9. Caries—occlusal surfaces of premolars and molars

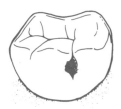

Fig. 31–10. Caries—facial and lingual surfaces of molars

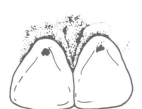

Fig. 31–11. Caries—lingual surface of maxillary incisors

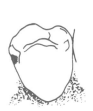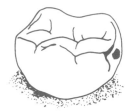

Fig. 31–12. Caries—proximal surfaces of premolars and molars

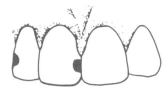

Fig. 31–13. Caries—proximal surfaces of incisors and cuspids

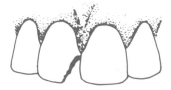

Fig. 31–14. Caries—proximal surfaces of incisors and cuspids involving incisal edge or angle

Class II, Posterior Teeth

In that class are caries that begin on the proximal surfaces (mesial or distal) of premolars and molars and involve two or more surfaces, figure 31–12.

Class III, Anterior Teeth

In that class are caries that begin on the proximal surfaces (mesial or distal) of incisors and cuspids, figure 31–13.

Class IV, Anterior Teeth

In that class are caries that begin on the proximal surfaces (mesial or distal) of incisors and cuspids and involve the incisal edge/angle, figure 31–14.

Class V, Anterior and Posterior Teeth

Class V caries occur on the gingival or cervical third of a tooth, facial or lingual surfaces, figure 31–15.

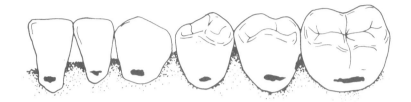

Fig. 31–15. Caries—gingival or cervical third of teeth

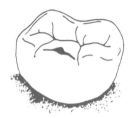

Fig. 31–16. Caries—defect on incisal edge or cusp tip of teeth

MO   MOD

MI

Fig. 31–17. Completed restorations

Class VI, Not a Part of the Standard Classification of Cavities

Class VI caries or defects that occur on the incisal edge or cusp tips of teeth, figure 31–16.

ABBREVIATION OF TOOTH SURFACES

In the charting of teeth and dental condition the surfaces of the teeth are abbreviated in order to aid in the recording of information.

The abbreviations for single tooth surfaces are:

- Mesial = **M**
- Distal = **D**
- Labial = **La**
- Lingual = **L** or **Li**
- Buccal = **B** or **Bu**
- Incisal = **I**
- Occlusal = **O** or **Occ**
- Facial (buccal and labial surfaces) = **F**

When two or more surface names are combined, such as mesial and occlusal, the combined two surfaces are referred to as mesio-occlusal or **MO**. In combining surfaces names the "**-al**" ending of the first surface is dropped and the letter *o* is substituted. If three surfaces are combined, the same rule applies to the second surface, and it is referred to as mesio-occluso-distal or **MOD**.

Common abbreviations for combining surface names include the following, figure 31–17:

- Mesio-occlusal = **MO**
- Disto-occlusal = **DO**
- Mesio-occluso-distal = **MOD**
- Mesio-incisal = **MI**
- Disto-incisal = **DI**
- Disto-lingual = **DL**
- Bucco-occlusal = **BO**
- Linguo-occlusal = **LO**

REVIEW

1. Universal System: Identify the following teeth by placing the correct tooth number or letter beside the tooth.

Permanent Teeth

a. Maxillary right 1st molar

b. Maxillary right lateral

c. Maxillary left central

d. Maxillary left cuspid

e. Maxillary left 3rd molar

f. Mandibular left 2nd molar

g. Mandibular left central incisor

h. Mandibular right central incisor

i. Mandibular right 1st molar

j. Mandibular right 3rd molar

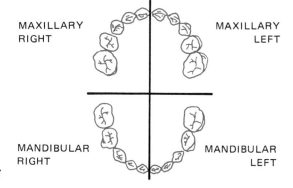

Primary Teeth

a. Maxillary right 1st molar

b. Maxillary right central incisor

c. Maxillary left lateral

d. Maxillary left 2nd molar

e. Mandibular left 1st molar

f. Mandibular left central incisor

g. Mandibular right central incisor

h. Mandibular right 2nd molar

2. Chart the following teeth in the Palmer System for both permanent and primary teeth.

	Permanent Teeth	Primary Teeth
a. Maxillary right 1st molar	_____	_____
b. Maxillary right lateral	_____	_____
c. Maxillary left central incisor	_____	_____
d. Maxillary left 2nd molar	_____	_____
e. Mandibular left cuspid	_____	_____
f. Mandibular left 2nd molar	_____	_____
g. Mandibular right central incisor	_____	_____
h. Mandibular right 1st molar	_____	_____

3. Chart the following teeth in the Fédération Dentaire International System for both permanent and primary teeth.

	Permanent Teeth	Primary Teeth
a. Maxillary right 1st molar	_____	_____
b. Maxillary right lateral	_____	_____
c. Maxillary left central incisor	_____	_____
d. Maxillary left 2nd molar	_____	_____
e. Mandibular left cuspid	_____	_____
f. Mandibular left 2nd molar	_____	_____
g. Mandibular right central incisor	_____	_____
h. Mandibular right 1st molar	_____	_____

4. Name the five standard classification of cavities and the tooth surface(s) involved.

   a. _____

   _____

   b. _____

   _____

   c. _____

   _____

   d. _____

   _____

   e. _____

   _____

5. Give the correct abbreviations for the following tooth surfaces:

   a. Mesial   _____

   b. Distal   _____

   c. Facial   _____

   d. Incisal   _____

   e. Occlusal   _____

   f. Lingual   _____

   g. Buccal   _____

   h. Labial   _____

6. Write the correct combining form for the abbreviated tooth surfaces:

   a. MO   _____

   b. DO   _____

   c. MOD   _____

   d. MI   _____

   e. DI   _____

Chapter 32: Interpretive Charting

After studying this chapter, the student will be able to:
- Identify the tooth surfaces on an anatomic and geometric diagram.
- Chart conditions present using appropriate charting symbols, abbreviations and code.
- Interpret the charted dental conditions from an anatomic and geometric diagram.
- Record Services Rendered in proper sequence on a dental chart.

INTRODUCTION

A patient's dental chart is a legal record of dental services. As with all legal records, any information must be current, accurate, complete, and concise. Care must be taken to ensure that they are properly filed and stored to prevent loss or damage.

There are many designs and types of dental charts; selection of a particular dental chart is based on the dentist's preference.

DENTAL CHARTS

Dental charts are used for recording clinical data obtained from the patient during an oral examination and radiographic diagnosis, figures 32–1 and 32–2.

The dental chart includes conditions present and dental treatment rendered while under the care of a particular dentist.

A system for recording this information must be one that is consistently practiced and can be completed in a minimal amount of time.

A dental chart may have several specific sections where patient information is recorded, indicated by letters in the list below and shown in figure 32–3.

A. *Patient personal information.* Full name of patient, age, home address and telephone number, billing address, employment, personal physician's name and address, and financial information.

B. *Charting area.* Representation of the maxillary and mandibular teeth.

C. *Medical precautions.* Patient's medical conditions of specific concerns must be noted and updated on subsequent visits.

D. *Anesthesia.* Consent, other pertinent remarks.

E. *Radiographic history.* Patient's radiographic history record.

F. *Remarks.* Reserved for the dentist's personal notations.

G. *Fee estimate.* Date, treatment plan, and fee.

Detailed description of services rendered, charges, payment received, and balance due are shown in figure 32–4, page 282.

ANTERIOR/POSTERIOR RELATIONSHIP OF TEETH

To accurately record dental conditions on a patient's chart, one must understand the anterior/posterior relationship of the teeth as they relate to the maxillary and mandibular arches. View of the maxillary and mandibular teeth with the mouth open is shown in figure 32–5, page 283. *Note:* Anterior/posterior relationship of the teeth remain the same whether viewed in the arches or on a straight line. For a view of the same teeth in a straight line, see figure 32–6, page 283.

Fig. 32–1. Dental chart (Courtesy Professional Publishers, Cupertino, CA. Reproduction prohibited by law)

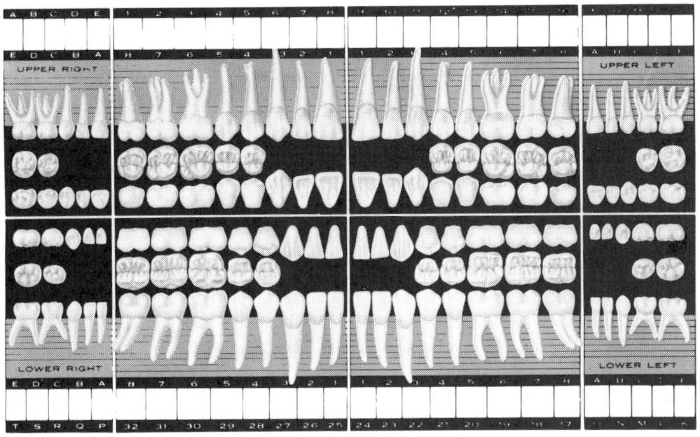

PATIENTS NAME _____   FINANCIAL ARRANGEMENT _____

BILLING NAME _____   _____

ADDRESS _____   _____

_____   _____

_____   _____

_____   _____

1 · 2 · 3 · 4 · 5

DATE	SERVICES	CHARGES	PAID	BALANCE

FORM C · 103 · C

Fig. 32–2. Reverse side of dental chart (Courtesy Professional Publishers, Cupertino, CA. Reproduction prohibited by law)

A. PATIENT PERSONAL INFORMATION

Name White   Ryan   J.   Home Phone (818) 123-0000 Business Phone (818) 541-0000   Date May 14, 1994
    Last   First   Middle
Home Address 1000 E. Green Street   City Pasadena   Date of Birth July 4, 1952   Age 41   Referred By M. Lamb

Occupation Engineer   Employer City Engineering   Employer Address 000 E. Walnut   City Pasadena, CA 91101

Marital Status Single   Spouse's Name ——   Spouse's Occupation ——

Employer ——   Employer's Address ——   City ——   Credit Rating Good

Person Financially Responsible Self   Relationship to You ——   Recall

Billing Address 1000 E. Green Street   City Pasadena   Zip 91101   Dental Insurance Delta Plan

Physician John V. Martin, M.D.   Phone (818) 300-0000 Former Dentist Deceased   Address ——

B. CHARTING AREA

C. MEDICAL PRECAUTIONS
MEDICAL PRECAUTIONS:

D. ANESTHESIA
ANESTHESIA: YES [ ]   NO [ ]
    REMARKS _____

E. RADIOGRAPHIC HISTORY
RADIOGRAPHIC HISTORY:

Date	Survey	Date	Survey

F. REMARKS

REMARKS: _____

G. FEE ESTIMATES
FEE ESTIMATES

DATE	TREATMENT	FEE

FORM C · 103 · B

Fig. 32–3. Parts of a dental chart (Form provided by Professional Publishers)

PATIENTS NAME	Ryan J. White		FINANCIAL ARRANGEMENT		
BILLING NAME	same		Delta Plan		
ADDRESS	1000 E. Green Street				
	Pasadena CA 91101				

1 • 2 • 3 • 4 • 5

DATE	SERVICES	CHARGES		PAID		BALANCE	
5-14-94	FM X-rays	65	00			65	00
5-14-94	FM Prophy	60	00			125	00
5-26-94	Radiogr Diag and Est	—	—			125	00
	CK 90-0012			125	00		
6-10-94	14 MOD Dycal, ZOE base Amal Anes Lido plain						
	1 cart	80	00			80	00
6-17-94	8 M Dycal, Copalite Adaptic Anes Lido Plain					80	00
	1 cart	75	00			155	00
6-24-94	19 FGCr prep and Imp Temp Cr seat ZOE Anes					155	00
	Lido plain 1 cart	—	—			155	00
7-01-94	19 FGCr seat ZnP	350	00			505	00

FORM C • 103 • C

Fig. 32–4. Area for recording services rendered (Form provided by Professional Publishers)

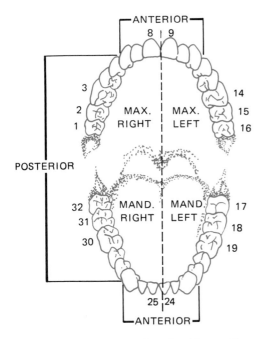

Fig. 32–5. View of teeth with mouth open

TOOTH DIAGRAMS

The most commonly used tooth diagrams on dental charts are anatomic and geometric representation.

Anatomic Diagram

The *anatomic diagram* may show only the crowns of the teeth, figure 32–7, crown and a small portion of the root, or crowns, and all of the root(s), figure 32–8. Tooth surfaces on the anatomic diagram may be difficult to identify. Figure 32–9 represents the facial, occlusal, and lingual tooth surfaces.

Rows 1 and 5 represent facial surfaces, posterior, and anterior teeth.
Rows 2 and 4 represent occlusal surfaces, posterior teeth.
Row 3 represents lingual surfaces, posterior, and anterior teeth.

Figure 32–10 represents the mesial and distal interproximal surfaces (anterior and posterior) as indicated by vertical lines on the chart.

Geometric Diagram

The *geometric diagram* represents teeth using the circle or circles. The coronal or crown surfaces of the teeth are shown in figures 32–11 and 32–12.

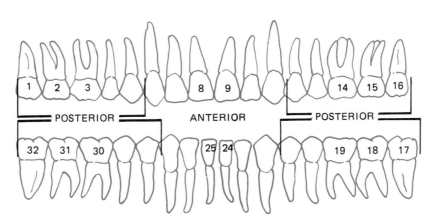

Fig. 32–6. View of teeth in a straight line

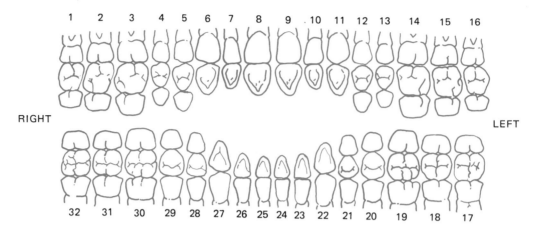

Fig. 32–7. Tooth crowns and small portion of root(s)

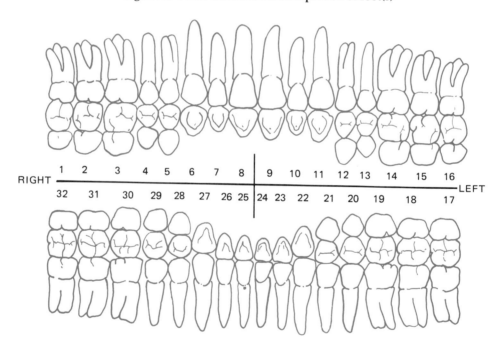

Fig. 32–8. Tooth crowns and roots

The geometric diagram shows only the crowns of the teeth of permanent dentition numbered 1–32, figure 32–13. The middle two rows represent primary dentition and are lettered A–T.

Tooth surfaces on the geometric diagram are less difficult to identify, because all five surfaces are represented within the circle. Figures 32–14 through 32–18 represent the different tooth surfaces with the geometric diagram method.

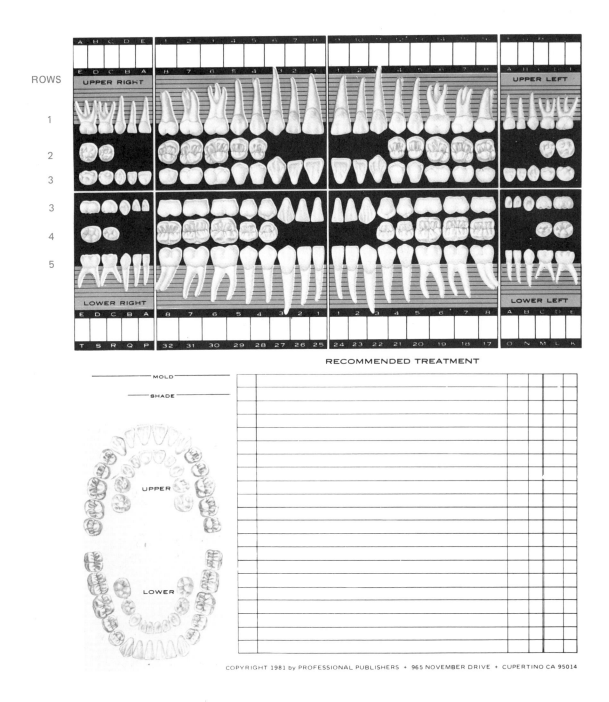

Fig. 32–9. A chart showing the facial, occlusal, and lingual surfaces (Courtesy Professional Publishers, Cupertino, CA. Reproduction prohibited by law)

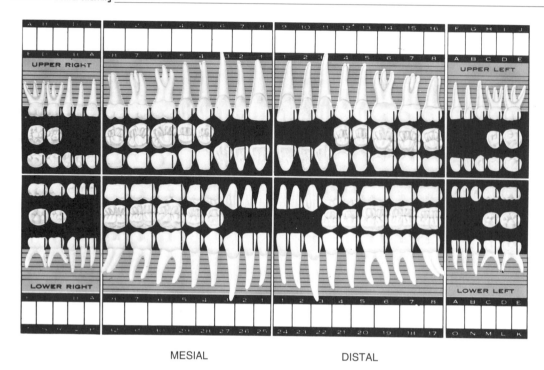

MESIAL   DISTAL

Fig. 32–10. Mesial and distal surfaces of teeth (Form provided by Professional Publishers)

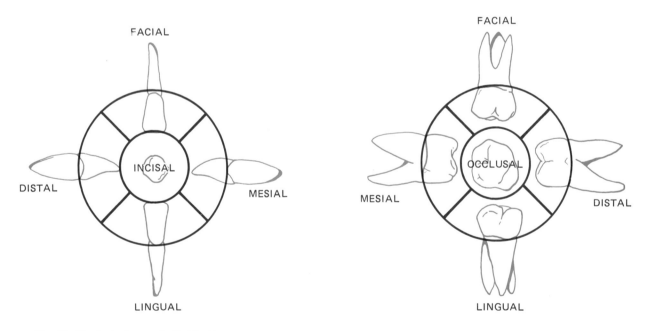

Fig. 32–11. Anterior tooth divided into five surfaces

Fig. 32–12. Posterior tooth divided into five surfaces

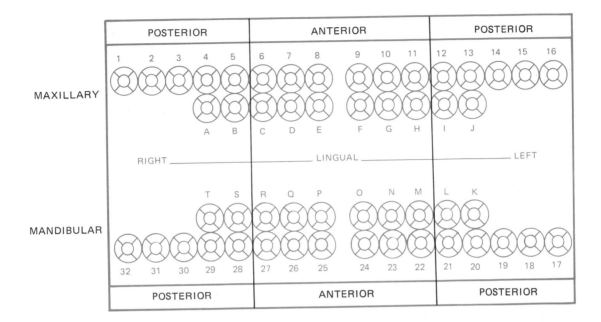

Fig. 32–13. Geometric representation of teeth

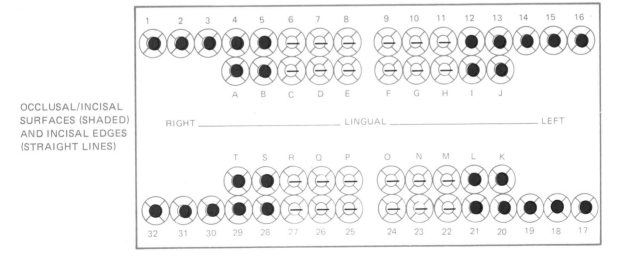

OCCLUSAL/INCISAL
SURFACES (SHADED)
AND INCISAL EDGES
(STRAIGHT LINES)

Fig. 32–14. Occlusal or incisal surfaces

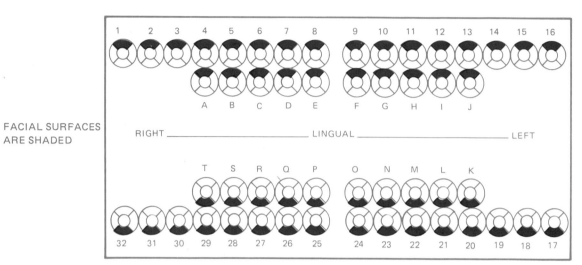

FACIAL SURFACES
ARE SHADED

Fig. 32–15. Facial surface

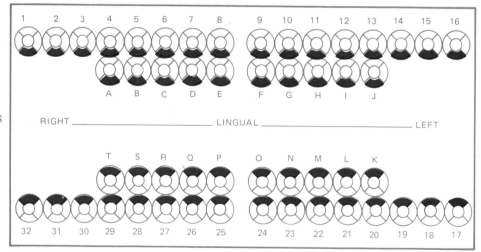

LINGUAL SURFACES
ARE SHADED

Fig. 32–16. Lingual surface

MESIAL SURFACES ARE SHADED, SHOWN AS "RIGHT"

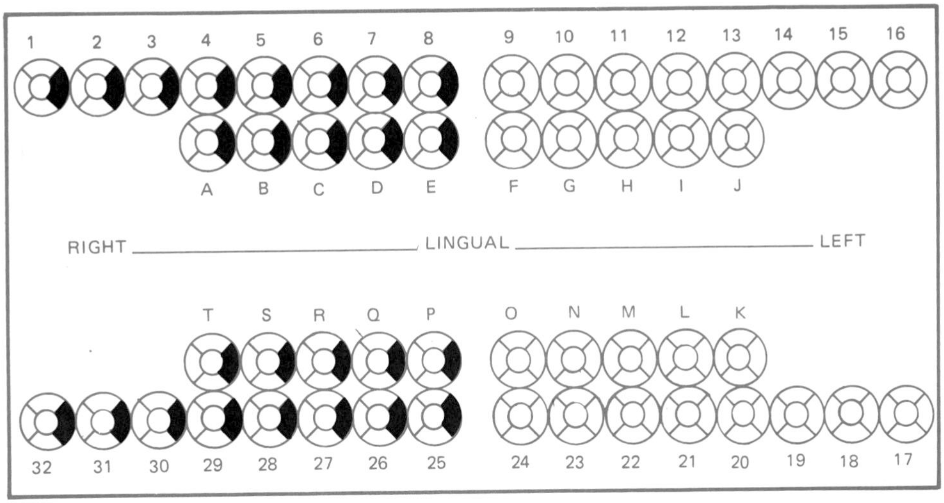

Fig. 32–17. Mesial surface

DISTAL SURFACES ARE SHADED, SHOWN AS "LEFT"

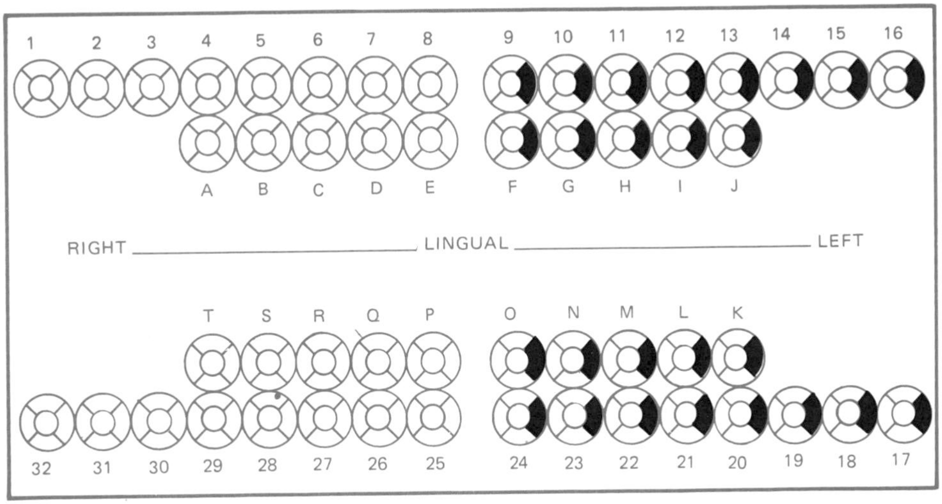

Fig. 32–18. Distal surface

CHARTING SYMBOLS

Missing Teeth—Refers to a tooth that has been surgically removed or to a tooth that has never formed. An *X* is drawn through the tooth.

MISSING

To Be Extracted—A tooth that is to be surgically removed. A diagonal line is drawn through the tooth.

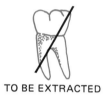

TO BE EXTRACTED

Unerupted or Impacted Tooth—Tooth that has not erupted and is encased in tissue or bone. Circle the tooth. An arrow is used to indicate the direction of an **impaction**.

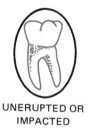

UNERUPTED OR
IMPACTED

Drifting Teeth—After teeth are removed and not replaced, opposing and surrounding teeth often drift into space created by the extraction. A

maxillary tooth will drift townward, and a mandibular tooth will move upward. This is indicated with vertical arrows.

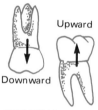

Upward

Downward

DRIFTING TEETH

Mesial or Distal Drift—A tooth may drift from mesial to distal or visa versa, and horizontal arrows are used to indicate direction.

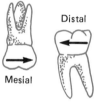

Distal

Mesial

MESIAL/DISTAL DRIFT

Three-quarter Crown—Covers the mesial, distal, lingual, and incisal or occlusal surfaces of a tooth. The facial surface of the tooth is *not* involved. This type of restoration is used on anterior teeth or maxillary premolars. The clinical crown is outlined and diagonal lines drawn on the lingual surface and around the edges of the facial surface.

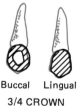

Buccal   Lingual
3/4 CROWN

Full Crown—The clinical crown is outlined and diagonal lines drawn through the crown.

FULL CROWN

Porcelain Crown Fused to Metal—Outline facial and lingual surface of crown. On lingual surface a moon shaped line with slash marks is drawn at cervical third of tooth.

PORCELAIN CROWN
FUSED TO METAL

Fixed Bridge—Indicate abutment teeth by outlining surface of restoration whether full or three-quarter crown(s). Draw an X through missing teeth. Draw horizontal lines through the crowns of abutments (anchor teeth for the **bridge**). Extend the lines through the pontinc (suspended portion).

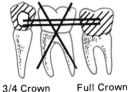

3/4 Crown   Full Crown
FIXED BRIDGE

Fractured Tooth—Draw a jagged line in area of fracture.

FRACTURE

Abscessed Tooth—To indicate an **abscess** (localized collection of pus) at apex of the root(s), draw a small circle over the end of the root(s) involved.

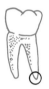

ABSCESS

Root Canal—Record endodontic (endo-, within; donto-, tooth) treatment by drawing a vertical line through the root canal(s).

ROOT CANAL(S)

Periodontal Pocket(s)—The pocket depth is recorded by using one or more diagonal lines in pocket area(s). The depth of pocket is recorded in millimeters (mm).

4 mm   4 mm
PERIODONTAL POCKET(S)

Periodontal Abscess—Draw a circle in area of the abscess.

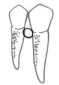

PERIODONTAL ABSCESS

Amalgam Restoration—Outline restoration and shade in surfaces involved, such as MO, DO, DLG, occ. or buccal pit.

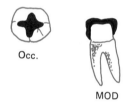

Occ.

MOD

AMALGAM RESTORATION

Composite Restoration—Outline tooth colored restoration. For Class III restoration, outline with a half-moon in the area of involvement. For a Class IV, include the incisal edge.

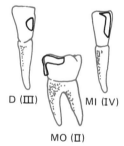

D (III)   MI (IV)

MO (II)

COMPOSITE RESTORATION

Overhanging Margin on Restoration—An overhanging margin on a restoration is indicated by placing a shaded triangle in the area of involvement, mesial or distal surface.

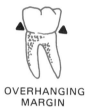

OVERHANGING
MARGIN

Brackets—Brackets are used to indicate a partial or full **denture**.

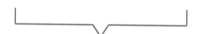

Partial Denture—Draw an *X* through the missing teeth and a bracket along the lingual surface of the arch, see page 293.

Full Denture—Draw an *X* through the entire arch and a bracket along the lingual surface, see page 293.

Suggested Abbreviations for Dental Terms

Abscess	Abs
Adjustment	Adj
Amalgam	Amal
Anesthetic	Anes
Bitewing	BW
Composite	Com
Crown	Cr
Denture	Dent
Diagnosis	Diag
Examination	Exam
Extraction	Ext
Estimate	Est
Fixed Bridge	Fix Br
Full Gold Crown	FGCr
Full Mouth	FM

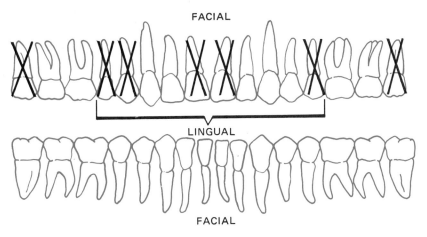

FACIAL

LINGUAL

FACIAL

PARTIAL DENTURE

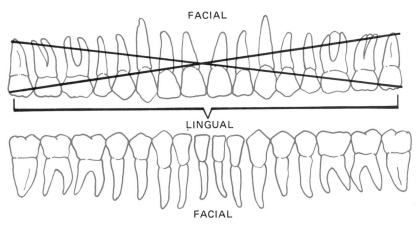

FACIAL

LINGUAL

FACIAL

FULL DENTURE

Full Upper	FU	Root Canal	RC
Gold **Inlay**	GI	Study Models	SM
Gold **Onlay**	GO	Temporary	Temp
Impression	Imp	Zing-oxide-eugenol	ZOE
Partial Upper	PU	Zinc Phosphate	ZnP
Porcelain Fused to Metal	PFM		
Preparation	Prep		
Prophylaxis	Prophy	*Anesthetics*	
Radiographs	Radiogr	Lidocaine	Lido
Removable	Rem	Xylocaine	Xylo

CHARTING CONDITIONS PRESENT

Chart conditions present using the appropriate charting symbols, abbreviations, and the following code.

Blue represents work completed or conditions not requiring treatment.

1. Outline, then shade in *blue* amalgam restorations in good condition.
2. Outline in *blue* tooth colored restorations.
3. Outline and place diagonal lines in *blue* gold restorations.
4. Indicate in *blue* missing teeth, root canal(s).

Red indicates that treatment is required.

1. Outline in *red* dental caries, fractures.
2. Indicate in *red* impactions, extractions, abscesses, periodontal pockets, overhanging margins.
3. *Solid blue, outlined in red* restoration present to be replaced.

Note: Because this text is only two color, it has only the red charting color; blue charting symbols are rendered in black. Your charting exercises, however, should be done correctly in red and blue.

Charting Anatomic Diagram

Posterior Teeth. Chart dental caries by outlining the occlusal and proximal (mesial and or distal) surfaces. *Outline* occlusal (A), facial (B), and lingual (C) surfaces in *red*, figures 32–19 and 32–20.

Anterior Teeth. Chart dental caries by drawing a half-moon on the proximal surface (mesial or distal) in the area of involvement (contact area), figures 32–21 and 32–22.

Restorations in *good condition* are *outlined* (tooth colored) or *shaded* (amalgam) in *blue*, figures 32–23 and 32–24. Indicate type of restorative material, using appropriate abbreviations.

Charting Geometric Diagram

Posterior Teeth. Chart dental caries by *outlining* occlusal and proximal (mesial and/or distal) surfaces in *red*, figures 32–25 and 32–26.

Anterior Teeth. *Outline* proximal (mesial or distal) surface in *red*, figures 32–27 and 32–28.

Restorations in *good condition* are *outlined* (tooth colored) or *shaded* (amalgam) in *blue*, figures 32–29 and 32–30. Indicate type of restorative material using appropriate abbreviations.

Charted anatomic and geometric diagram are shown in figures 32–31 and 32–32, respectively.

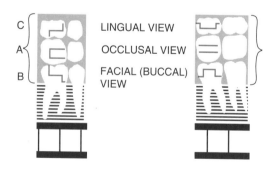

Fig. 32–19. Mesial caries

Fig. 32–20. Mesial and distal caries

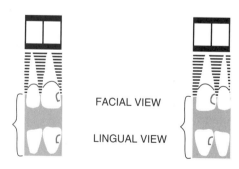

Fig. 32–21. Mesial caries

Fig. 32–22. Distal caries

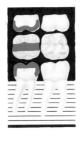

Fig. 32–23. MOD amalgam

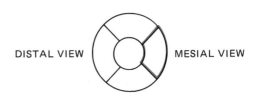

Fig. 32–27. Mesial caries

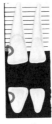

Fig. 32–24. M composite

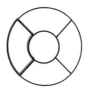

Fig. 32–28. Distal caries

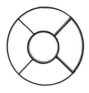

Fig. 32–25. Mesial caries

Fig. 32–29. Mesial composite

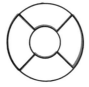

Fig. 32–26. Mesial and distal caries

Fig. 32–30. MOD amalgam

Dental charts, figures 32–31 and 32–32, represent charted conditions present.

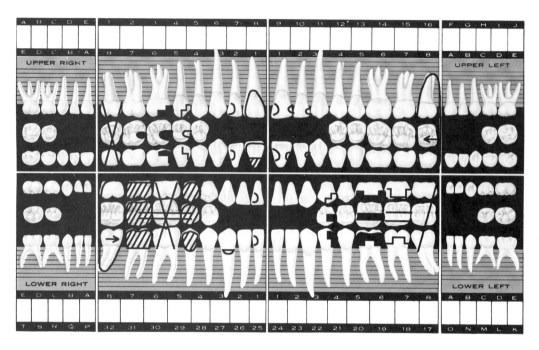

Tooth No.

1	Missing
2	Occlusal (mesial pit) amalgam
3	MO Amal
4	Mesial Caries
7	Distal Com
8	PFM
9	Mesial and Distal Caries
10	Distal Com
16	Impacted (mesially)
17	To Be Extracted

Tooth No.

18	Mesial and Distal Caries
19	MOD Amal
21	DO Amal
25	Distal Com
27	Facial V Com
29	FGCr – Pontic
30	Missing
31	FGCr – Pontic
32	Impacted (mesially)

Fig. 32–31. Anatomic chart (Form provided by Professional Publishers)

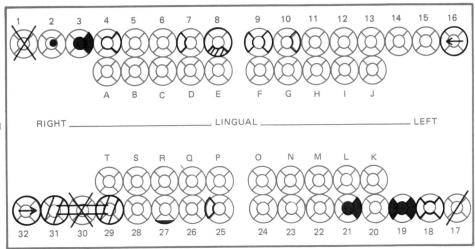

IAL SURFACES
SHADED, SHOWN
"RIGHT"

Tooth No.

1	Missing
2	Occlusal (mesial pit) amalgam
3	MO Amal
4	Mesial Caries
7	Distal Com
8	PFM
9	Mesial and Distal Caries
10	Distal Com
16	Impacted (mesially)
17	To Be Extracted

Tooth No.

18	Mesial and Distal Caries
19	MOD Amal
21	DO Amal
25	Distal Com
27	Facial V Com
29	FGCr – Pontic
30	Missing
31	FGCr – Pontic
32	Impacted (mesially)

Fig. 32–32. Geometric chart

RECORDING SERVICES RENDERED

Whenever a patient receives dental treatment, information regarding the treatment must be entered on the patient's chart under "services rendered." Other pertinent information, such as instructions to the patient, must also be recorded on the patient's chart. *Remember:* This information must be in ink or typewritten, accurate, complete, and concise.

A shorthand for recording dental treatment has been established that identifies the tooth by number or letter, the tooth surfaces by abbreviations, and other charting symbols.

Recording Services

1. All entries are to be printed or typed.
2. Record only one transaction per line.
3. Date each entry. Use numbers for date (2-17-94).
4. Use abbreviations to save time and space.
5. List entries in a given sequence.

Sequence in Recording Entries

Entries to be recorded must follow a particular sequence, figure 32–33.

1. Date treatment was rendered
2. Tooth/teeth, to be identified by a specific tooth number or letter and surface(s) involved
3. Dental procedure that involves the entire mouth, such as a prophylaxis and examination
4. Protective and restorative materials. List the type or protective material (Dycal, ZOE, Copalite) and restorative (composite, amalgam, gold) material.
5. Anesthetic: type used: indicate generic (Lidocaine) or brand name (Xylocaine) without vasoconstrictor (plain), number of cartridges (1.8 ml). With vasoconstrictor (epinephrine), record ratio (1:100,000) and number of cartridges.
6. Fee, cost of restoration or dental treatment
7. Payment, amount received
8. Balance, after payment

SUGGESTED ACTIVITIES

- Practice the following charting exercises, with the instructor's guidance.
- Practice making entries on the dental chart, with the instructor's guidance.

PATIENTS NAME __Ryan J. White__

BILLING NAME ___same___

ADDRESS ___1000 E. Green Street___

___Pasadena CA 91101___

FINANCIAL ARRANGEMENT

Delta Plan

1 • 2 • 3 • 4 • 5

DATE	SERVICES	CHARGES		PAID		BALANCE	
5-14-94	FM X-rays	65	00			65	00
5-14-94	FM Prophy	60	00			125	00
5-26-94	Radiogr Diag and Est	—	—			125	00
	CK 90-0012			125	00		
6-10-94	14 MOD Dycal, ZOE base Amal Anes Lido plain						
	1 cart	80	00			80	00
6-17-94	8 M Dycal, Copalite Adaptic Anes Lido Plain					80	00
	1 cart	75	00			155	00
6-24-94	19 FGCr prep and Imp Temp Cr seat ZOE Anes					155	00
	Lido plain 1 cart	—	—			155	00
7-01-94	19 FGCr seat ZnP	350	00			505	00

FORM C • 103 • C

Fig. 32–33. Recorded services rendered (Form provided by Professional Publishers)

REVIEW

1. Draw the correct charting symbol on the following teeth:

   a. Missing Tooth
   b. To Be Extracted
   c. D III Composite Restoration
   d. Unerupted or Impacted Tooth
   e. Drifting Teeth—Mesial

   f. Full Crown
   g. Fractured Tooth—mesio-incisal edge
   h. Abscessed Tooth
   i. Root Canal
   j. MOD amalgam restoration

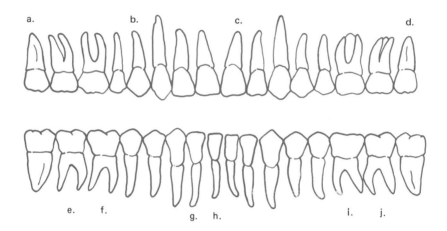

2. Chart teeth by using the Universal System. Indicate the condition present for each tooth on the following anatomic chart:

a. To Be Extracted
b. Full Gold Crown
c. Missing
d. Mesial Composite
e. Distal Caries
f. Missing
g. Mesial Caries
h. To Be Extracted

i. MOD Amalgam
j. Occlusal Amalgam
k. Distal Caries
l. Facial V Composite
m. DO Amalgam
n. Mesial and Distal Caries
o. Impacted—Mesially

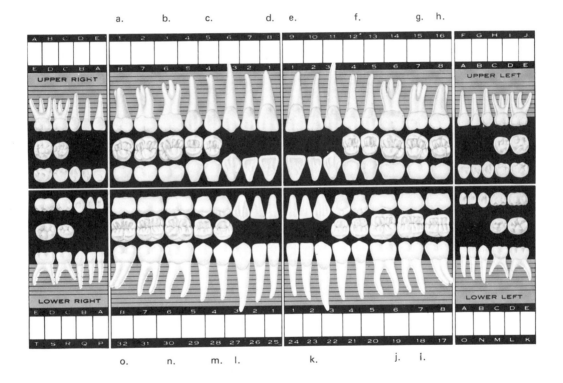

3. Identify by number the charted teeth and indicate the conditions present for each tooth. Use the Universal System and the following geometric chart:

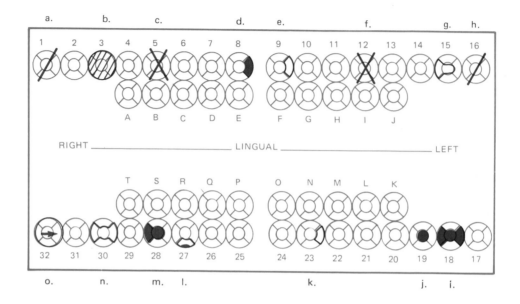

4. Chart the following dental caries by using the Universal System and anatomic diagram:

Teeth to Be Charted	Surfaces Involved
a. Maxillary Right 1st molar	Mesial Caries
b. Maxillary Right 2nd molar	Mesial and Distal Caries
c. Maxillary Right Lateral	Mesial Caries
d. Maxillary Left Lateral	Distal Caries
e. Maxillary Left 2nd premolar	Mesial and Distal Caries
f. Maxillary Left 1st molar	Mesial Caries
g. Mandibular Left 2nd molar	Occlusal Caries
h. Mandibular Left 1st molar	Distal Caries
i. Mandibular Left Cuspid	Mesial Caries
j. Mandibular Right Central	Mesial and Distal Caries
k. Mandibular Right 1st molar	Mesial Caries
l. Mandibular Right 2nd molar	Mesial and Distal Caries

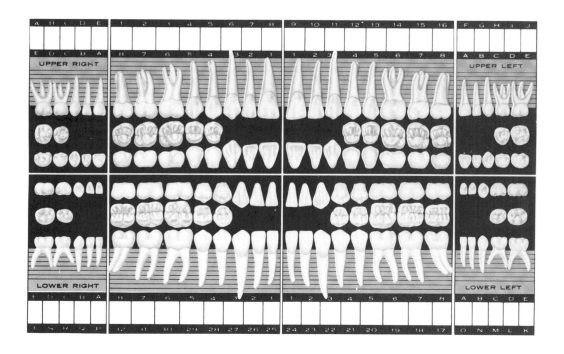

5. Chart the following dental caries by using the Universal System and geometric diagram:

Teeth to Be Charted	Surfaces Involved
a. Maxillary Right 1st molar	Mesial Caries
b. Maxillary Right 2nd molar	Mesial and Distal Caries
c. Maxillary Right Lateral	Mesial Caries
d. Maxillary Left Lateral	Distal Caries
e. Maxillary Left 2nd premolar	Mesial and Distal Caries
f. Maxillary Left 1st molar	Mesial Caries
g. Mandibular Left 2nd molar	Occlusal Caries
h. Mandibular Left 1st molar	Distal Caries
i. Mandibular Left Cuspid	Mesial Caries
j. Mandibular Right Central	Mesial and Distal Caries
k. Mandibular Right 1st molar	Mesial Caries
l. Mandibular Right 2nd molar	Mesial and Distal Caries

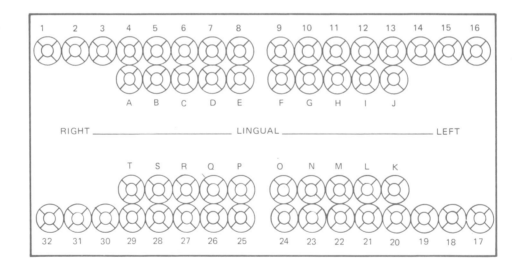

6. Chart the following dental conditions on the anatomic diagram. Use the Universal System for tooth identification with appropriate abbreviations for tooth surfaces and dental terms.

Teeth to Be Charted	Conditions Present
a. Maxillary Right 3rd Molar	Impacted—mesially
b. Maxillary Right 2nd Molar	Full Gold Crown
c. Maxillary Right 1st Molar	Mesio-occlusal amalgam
d. Maxillary Right Cuspid	Distal Composite
e. Maxillary Right Central	Porcelain Crown fused to metal
f. Maxillary Left Central	Mesial caries
g. Maxillary Left 1st Molar	Downward drift
h. Maxillary Left 3rd Molar	To be extracted
i. Mandibular Left 3rd Molar	To be extracted
j. Mandibular Left 2nd Molar	Full Gold Crown
k. Mandibular Left 1st Molar	Missing—Part of 3 Unit Fixed Bridge
l. Mandibular Left 2nd Premolar	Full Gold Crown
m. Mandibular Left Cuspid	Facial Class V Composite
n. Mandibular Right Central	Mesial Composite
o. Mandibular Right 1st Molar	Occlusal Amalgam
p. Mandibular Right 2nd Molar	Mesio-occluso-distal Amalgam
q. Mandibular Right 3rd Molar	Missing

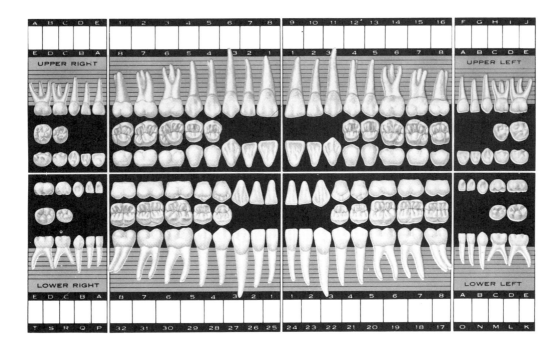

7. Chart the following dental conditions on the geometric diagram. Use the Universal System for tooth identification with appropriate abbreviations for tooth surfaces and dental terms.

Teeth to Be Charted	Conditions Present
a. Maxillary Right 3rd Molar	Impacted—mesially
b. Maxillary Right 2nd Molar	Full Gold Crown
c. Maxillary Right 1st Molar	Mesio-occlusal amalgam
d. Maxillary Right Cuspid	Distal Composite
e. Maxillary Right Central	Porcelain Crown fused to metal
f. Maxillary Left Central	Mesial caries
g. Maxillary Left 1st Molar	Downward drift
h. Maxillary Left 3rd Molar	To be extracted
i. Mandibular Left 3rd Molar	To be extracted
j. Mandibular Left 2nd Molar	Full Gold Crown
k. Mandibular Left 1st Molar	Missing—Part of 3 Unit Fixed Bridge
l. Mandibular Left 2nd Premolar	Full Gold Crown
m. Mandibular Left Cuspid	Facial Class V Composite
n. Mandibular Right Central	Mesial Composite
o. Mandibular Right 1st Molar	Occlusal Amalgam
p. Mandibular Right 2nd Molar	Mesio-occluso-distal Amalgam
q. Mandibular Right 3rd Molar	Missing

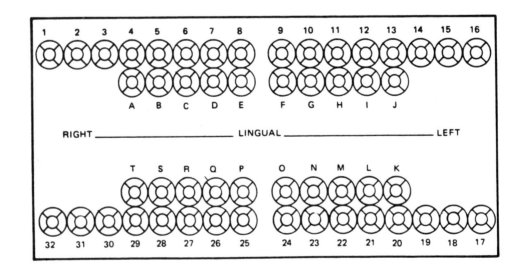

8. Record the following services rendered on a dental chart. Use the Universal System for tooth identification with appropriate abbreviations for tooth surfaces and dental terms.

<u>Services Rendered:</u>

a. Date - May 14, 1994

b. Full Mouth X-rays and Prophylaxis

c. Date - May 26, 1994

d. Diagnosis of radiographs and estimate

e. Upper and lower study models were taken—alginate

f. Date - June 10, 1994

g. Mandibular right 2nd premolar prepared for a full gold crown

h. Mandibular right 2nd molar prepared for a full gold crown

i. Impressions were taken

j. Temporary crowns were seated with zinc-oxide-eugenol

k. Anesthetic - Lidocaine plain, 1 cartridge

l. Date - June 10, 1994

m. Fixed bridge was seated for mandibular right 2nd premolar and 2nd molar

n. Fixed bridge was cemented with zinc phosphate

o. Maxillary left central, mesial composite was placed

p. Anesthetic for fixed bridge was Lidocaine plain 1 cartridge

No anesthetic was used with composite

Fees:	Full Mouth x-rays	$65.00
	Full Mouth Prophylaxis	$60.00
	Diagnosis and estimate	—
	Upper and lower study models	$55.00
	Fixed Bridge	$1500.00
	Mesial Composite	$75.00

Chapter 33: Dental Handpieces

OBJECTIVES:

After studying this chapter, the student will be able to:
- Identify the three basic parts of a dental handpiece.
- Identify dental handpieces according to design, mode of operation, and method by which the rotary instrument is held in the handpiece.
- Discuss the purpose of the dental chuck.
- Discuss the use of a fiberoptic system.
- Explain the importance of sterilizing handpieces.

INTRODUCTION

Dental **handpieces** are specifically designed to be used with various types of rotary instruments, such as burs, stones, and finishings discs. Most dental handpieces are used in the oral cavity. However, some are specifically designed for use in the dental laboratory.

The dental handpiece is used in operative and restorative dentistry (1) to cut tooth structure for various types of preparations; (2) to remove old metal restorations; and (3) to polish teeth and finish various types of restorative materials. The handpiece may also be used in oral surgery and for implant procedures.

Dental handpieces are classified according to the design, speed, mode of operation, and method by which the rotary instrument is held in the handpiece.

PARTS OF THE DENTAL HANDPIECE

The basic parts of a dental handpiece include the following, figure 33–1.

- *Head.* The head is the end of the handpiece that holds the rotary instruments, such as burs, mandrels, polishing stones, and the like.
- *Shank.* The **shank** is the handle portion of the handpiece.

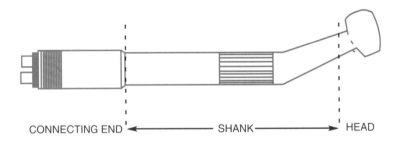

CONNECTING END ←————— SHANK —————→ HEAD

Fig. 33–1. Parts of a dental handpiece

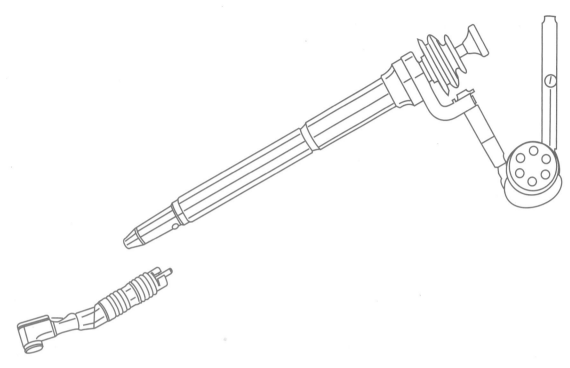

Fig. 33–2. Contra-angle and belt-driven straight handpiece

• *Connecting end.* The connecting end is where the handpiece attaches to the power source of the motor or unit.

BASIC HANDPIECE DESIGN

There are three basic handpiece designs: (1) the **straight handpiece**; (2) the **contra-angle handpiece**; and (3) the **right-angle handpiece**.

The Straight Handpiece

The *straight handpiece* is straight shanked and therefore can be used to hold a *contra-angle* or *right-angle* handpiece, figure 33–2. The straight handpiece may also be used with a straight-shanked rotary instrument on anterior teeth or where a direct approach to the teeth is possible.

A straight handpiece may be a low-speed, belt-driven type that is attached to an arm assembly made up of a series of pulleys and a belt that is mounted on an electric motor. One end of the belt is mounted over the pulley end of the handpiece and carried over the arm assembly pulleys to the dental motor pulley.

The straight handpiece may also be operated by compressed air or by electric power, figure 33–3. Handpieces that are operated by compressed air are attached to the dental unit by means of a flexible tubing with a "quick" connect-disconnect or threaded adaptor, figure 33–4. The connecting end of the handpiece is attached to the tubing adaptor, figure 33–5. The tubing adaptor may have 2 to 4 holes or input-output openings. The number of input-output holes is dependent on the handpiece. The connecting end of the handpiece is designed with the same number of tubes as there are input-output holes. The input-output holes provide the handpiece with air and water from the dental unit.

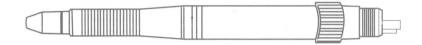

Fig. 33–3. Air-driven straight handpiece

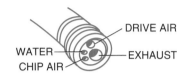

Fig. 33–4. Adaptor end of tubing

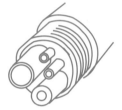

Fig. 33–5. The connecting end of the handpiece

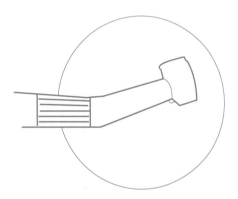

Fig. 33–6. Contra-angle handpiece

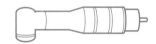

Fig. 33–7. A prophy-angle handpiece

angle to the shank. The most popular *right-angle handpiece* is the prophy-angle, figure 33–7. The right-angle handpiece is attached to the straight handpiece and is used for polishing teeth.

The Contra-Angle Handpiece

The *contra-angle handpiece* is designed to provide the operator with greater accessibility to the oral cavity during operative dentistry.

The head of the contra-angle handpiece is offset from the shank portion of the handpiece, figure 33–6. The contra-angle handpiece is available for use with the straight handpiece or as a single-unit handpiece. Refer to figure 33–1.

The Right-Angle Handpiece

The term *right-angle* refers to the way in which the head of the handpiece forms a 90° degree

DENTAL HANDPIECE SPEEDS

Handpieces may be classified as **low-speed**, slow-speed, or **high-speed** and are also referred to as *air-turbine* handpieces. Speed may be defined as the number of *revolutions per minutes* (rpm) or the number of times a rotating instrument, such as a bur, will make a full turn during a minute. The higher the rpm, the faster the speed of the handpiece.

Low-speed handpieces operate at a very low rpm, below 10,000, and are generally used with the dental laboratory engine. The slow-speed handpieces may operate at speeds up to 150,000 rpm. The slow-speed handpiece generally produces less friction heat (the rubbing or touching of one object against another). Frictional heat is the result of the rotary instrument coming in contact with the tooth structure or restorative material during the dental procedure. Frictional heat is generated regardless of the operating speed of the handpiece or the tooth structure or dental material the rotary instrument comes in contact with.

The high-speed, or air-turbine, handpieces operate at speeds of 500,000 rpm or more. Because high-speed or air-turbine handpieces operate at such high speeds, they produce a great deal of frictional heat. However, they are more efficient in cutting hard tooth structures. To minimize frictional heat, a coolant, such as air, water, or an air-water spray, must be used. If frictional heat is not controlled, the pulp may be seriously traumatized, resulting in permanent injury or damage to the tooth.

POWER SOURCE FOR THE DENTAL HANDPIECE

A source of energy (power) is needed to operate all dental handpieces. The flow of power may be activated by the use of a *foot control* or a *rheostat* (a device used to regulate an electric current without interrupting the circuit of flow). A rheostat is used with the belt-driven handpiece and is operated by electricity. A foot control is used with the air-turbine handpiece and is operated by compressed air.

METHODS FOR HOLDING ROTARY INSTRUMENTS IN HANDPIECES

The rotary instrument (**bur**) may be held in place by tightening a bur-rod knob at the end of the handpiece (straight handpiece), or by using a special bur tool provided by the manufacturer. Newer handpieces may have either a button or release lever that is used to secure and release the rotary instrument.

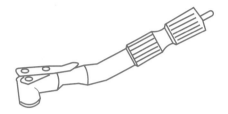

Fig. 33–8. Latch-type contra-angle handpiece

Inside the head of the handpiece is a small metal cylinder called a *chuck*. The chuck is designed to hold the shank portion of the rotary instrument in the handpiece.

Rotary instruments, such as burs, stone, and mandrels, are inserted into the chuck and are held in position by either a *latch-type* or *friction-grip* system. Refer to Chapter 34, *Rotary Instruments*.

A latch-type handpiece uses a special notched-shank rotary instrument. The rotary instrument is inserted into the chuck and is held in the handpiece by a moveable latch, figure 33–8.

Friction-grip rotary instruments are used with the air-turbine handpiece. The rotary instrument (bur) is inserted into a special metal chuck in the head of the handpiece and may be secured by a wrench-tightening system, figure 33–9. To secure the rotary instrument, either a control knob on the handpiece or a special tool is provided by the manufacturer for use with their handpiece.

The newer friction-grip/air-turbine handpiece may have an automatic button or release lever that allows the operator to secure and remove the rotary instrument instantly.

The head of a friction-grip or air-turbine handpiece is designed to hold a short, round-shanked, small-diameter, friction-grip rotary instrument.

FIBEROPTIC SYSTEM FOR HANDPIECES

Fiberoptic refers to a light system that uses special glass fibers called optical (vision) bundles (bound together) to carry a source of

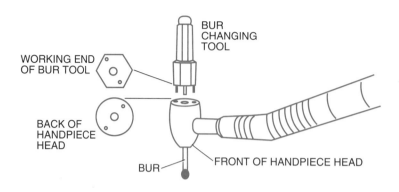

Fig. 33–9. Illustration of a bur changing tool

light to the dental handpiece. Fiberoptics may also be used with other diagnostic accessories or tools for use within the mouth. Fiberoptic systems can be used with both slow-speed and high-speed handpieces to provide an additional source of light to the oral cavity in addition to the dental light from the unit.

Two fiberoptic systems are available: one system carries the light via the optical bundles to the handpiece from a remote source, such as a control box. The second system, a bulb, is attached to the rear of the handpiece and the light is carried through the optical bundles within the tubing of the handpiece and from the dental unit.

An advantage of using the fiberoptic system is the improved visibility for the operator during tooth preparation.

STERILIZATION OF DENTAL HANDPIECES

It is no longer acceptable to merely wipe the handpiece with a disinfectant. Dental handpieces are exposed to and contaminated with many microorganisms during use. Because of the variety of dental handpieces available today, a single specific procedure for the sterilization, care, and maintenance of a handpiece is impossible.

According to the Centers for Disease Control recommendations, "handpieces should be steril-

ized after use with each patient, since blood, saliva or gingival fluid of patients may be aspirated into the handpieces or waterline. Handpieces that cannot be sterilized should at least be flushed, the outside surface cleaned and wiped with a suitable chemical germicide, and then rinsed. Handpieces should be flushed at the beginning of the day and after the use with each patient. Manufacturers' recommendations should be followed for use and maintenance of waterlines and check valves and for flushing of handpieces. The same precautions should be used for ultrasonic scalers and air/water syringes."

Precautions

Maximum effectiveness with minimum damage to the handpieces can be accomplished by using the following precautions:

1. Carefully follow the manufacturer's printed instructions, and do not vary from these instructions. If there is a doubt about any step, call the manufacturer.
2. After dismissing the patient, put on utility gloves.
3. Depress the foot control for at least fifteen seconds to remove as many contaminants

(saliva, blood, other debris) as possible from the internal tubings of the handpiece.

4. Stretch the tubing on the handpiece to the sink, and hand scrub the handpiece and tubing with soap and water. It is preferable to leave the bur in the handpiece to prevent any soap from entering the chuck.
5. Rinse and dry the handpiece. Remove the bur, and set aside for future sterilization.
6. Remove the handpiece from the tubing, and place in appropriate pouch or bag for sterilization.
7. Spray the handpiece tubing with a recommended surface disinfectant, and allow to dry for the prescribed time.
8. Wash, dry, and remove utility gloves.
9. Sterilize the handpiece in either a steam autoclave or a chemical vapor sterilizer. DO NOT USE DRY HEAT. *Note:* Various manufacturers furnish instructions on the care and maintenance of their handpieces, such as lubricating or oiling. These instructions must be followed in each individual case.

REVIEW

1. Name the three basic parts of a dental handpiece.

   a. _____   b. _____   c. _____

2. List the three basic designs for dental handpieces.

   a. _____   b. _____   c. _____

3. Give the advantage of using the contra-angle handpiece over the straight handpiece. _____

   _____

4. Define the term *revolutions per minute* (rpm). _____

   _____

   _____

5. When is frictional heat created? How may it be controlled? _____

   _____

   _____

6. Name the two ways in which a rotary instrument may be held in the head/chuck of a dental handpiece.

a. _____

b. _____

7. Why is it necessary to have a chuck in a dental handpiece? _____

_____

_____

8. What is the purpose for using a fiberoptic system in dentistry? _____

_____

_____

Chapter 34: Rotary Instruments

After studying this chapter, the student will be able to:
- Identify the parts of a cutting bur.
- Discuss the advantages of using tungsten carbide burs.
- Discuss the uses of the basic cutting burs.
- Discuss the advantages of using diamond rotary instruments.
- Recognize the various stones and discs used in dentistry.
- Discuss the procedure for sterilizing the various rotary instruments.

INTRODUCTION

Rotary instruments, such as *burs*, **stones**, and **discs**, are used with the dental handpiece. The different types of rotary instruments are classified according to how they are used within the oral cavity.

BURS

Cutting Burs

The most common rotary instruments are the *cutting burs*. The cutting burs are small rotary instruments that are inserted and held in the head/chuck of the dental handpiece. Cutting burs are used to cut and shape tooth structure for various types of restorations and for removing old restorations from the teeth.

Parts of a Cutting Bur

- *Head*, the cutting portion of the bur
- *Neck*, the portion of the bur that joins the head to the shank
- *Shank*, that part of the bur that is inserted and held in the head of the handpiece, figure 34–1

The head of the dental handpiece will determine the type of bur shank that can be used, straight, **latch-type**, or **friction-grip**. The straight handpiece will require a straight long-shanked bur. The contra-angle or the right-angle handpiece will use a latch-type or friction-grip bur depending on the handpiece, figure 34–2.

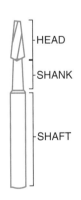

Fig. 34–1. Parts of the cutting bur

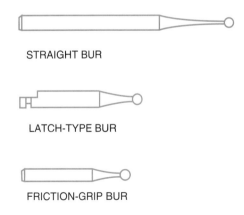

Fig. 34–2. Shank types of burs

Short-shanked burs ordinarily used in pediatric (childrens') dentistry are available in both latch-type and friction-grip.

Types of Cutting Burs. Cutting burs are made of either steel or tungsten carbide. *Tungsten carbide burs* are extremely hard and can be used many times for cutting hard tooth structures. Tungsten carbide burs are manufactured for use with the high-speed, or air-turbine, handpieces. The use of *steel burs* in operative dentistry is limited. Steel burs are not as hard as tungsten carbide and may become dull after one use when cutting hard tooth tissue such as enamel. Under this situation, the bur must then be discarded.

Cutting burs are named according to the shape of the bur head and the angle of the cutting blades. The name of the bur denotes the shape of the bur head, and the bur number indicates the size of the bur head. The lower the bur number in a series, the smaller the head of the bur. The numbers that are assigned to the individual bur groups may vary according to the manufacturer. The letter *L* following a number indicates a longer length cutting head.

The basic bur shapes include the following: round, inverted cone, straight and tapered fissure plain cut, straight and tapered crosscut, end-cutting, and wheel. The pear-shape and rounded-head straight and taper fissure burs are new additions to the list of cutting burs.

The *round bur* (Nos. 1/4, 1/2, 1–10) is used for opening pit and fissure cavities and for removing other dental caries. The round bur is ideal for opening pulpal chamber(s) in endodontic treatment, figure 34–3.

The *inverted cone* (Nos. 33 1/2-39, 36L, 37L) is designed for making undercuts of the pulpal wall of the tooth, to help retain the restorative material, figure 34–4.

The *plain fissure straight* (Nos. 56–60, 57L, 58L), figure 34–5, and the *crosscut fissure straight* (Nos. 556–560, 557L, 558L), figure 34–6, are used to form parallel walls and flat floors in preparations.

The *plain fissure taper* (Nos. 169–172, 168L, 170L, 171L), figure 34–7, and *crosscut fissure taper* (Nos. 699–703, 699L, 700L, 701L), figure 34–8, are used to create divergent (slightly narrowed at the pulpal floor) walls of the preparation and to avoid undercuts.

The *end cutting bur* (Nos. 957, 958) is used to prepare the shoulder for crown preparations, figure 34–9.

The *wheel bur* (No. 14) is used for cutting slots in preparations for crowns and inlays retention, figure 34–10.

The burs used for opening, shaping, and extending the internal line angles of occlusal restorations include the *pear-shape burs* (Nos. 329–332, 331L), figure 34–11; *plain fissure straight-rounded* head (Nos. 56R–59R), figure 34–12; *plain fissure taper-rounded* head (Nos. 1170, 1171), figure 34–13; crosscut fissure straight-rounded head (Nos. 1157–1159), figure 34–14.

Special burs include No. 245, figure 34–15, and Nos. 1931, 1958, figure 34–16; they are used for preparation and bulk removal of gold, amalgam, and other metals.

Surgical Burs

Surgical burs are available in various sizes and shapes and may be made of either steel or tungsten carbide. They are designed for use with varied shank lengths, figure 34–17. Surgical burs are used to cut through the bone of an impacted tooth or to split the crown or root(s) during an extraction. Surgical burs are also used for implant procedures, figure 34–18.

Finishing Burs

All *finishing burs* are available in various sizes, shapes, and lengths, figure 34–19. Finishing burs are made of either steel or carbide. The head of the bur may have as few as six or as many as forty cutting blades. The number of

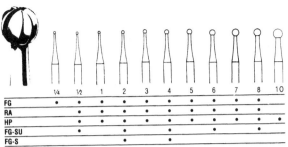

	1/4	1/2	1	2	3	4	5	6	7	8	10
FG	•	•	•	•	•	•	•	•	•	•	
RA		•	•	•	•	•	•	•	•	•	
HP		•	•	•	•	•	•	•	•	•	•
FG-SU		•		•			•		•		
FG-S			•		•						

Fig. 34–3. Round

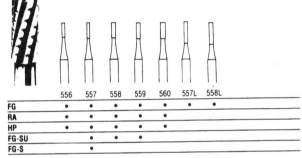

	33½	34	35	36	37	38	39	36L	37L
FG	•	•	•	•	•	•	•	•	•
RA		•	•	•	•	•	•		
HP	•	•	•	•	•	•	•		
FG-SU					•				
FG-S		•							

Fig. 34–4. Inverted cone

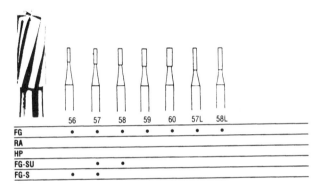

	56	57	58	59	60	57L	58L
FG	•	•	•	•	•	•	•
RA							
HP							
FG-SU						•	•
FG-S	•	•					

Fig. 34–5. Plain fissure straight

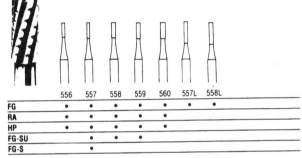

	556	557	558	559	560	557L	558L
FG	•	•	•	•	•	•	•
RA	•	•	•	•			
HP	•	•	•	•	•		
FG-SU		•	•	•			
FG-S	•						

Fig. 34–6. Crosscut fissure straight

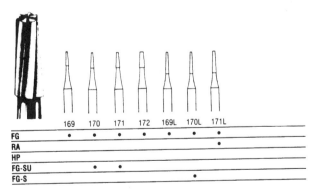

	169	170	171	172	169L	170L	171L
FG	•	•	•	•	•	•	
RA							•
HP							
FG-SU		•	•				
FG-S						•	

Fig. 34–7. Plain fissure taper

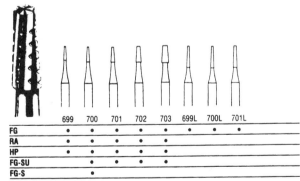

	699	700	701	702	703	699L	700L	701L
FG	•	•	•	•	•	•	•	•
RA	•	•	•	•				
HP	•	•	•	•	•			
FG-SU		•	•	•	•			
FG-S	•							

Fig. 34–8. Crosscut fissure taper

Figs. 34–3 – 34–8 (Courtesy Miltex Instruments Co., Lake Success, NY) FG, friction grip; RA, right angle; HP, handpiece; FG-SU, surgical; FG-S, short shank; •, available.

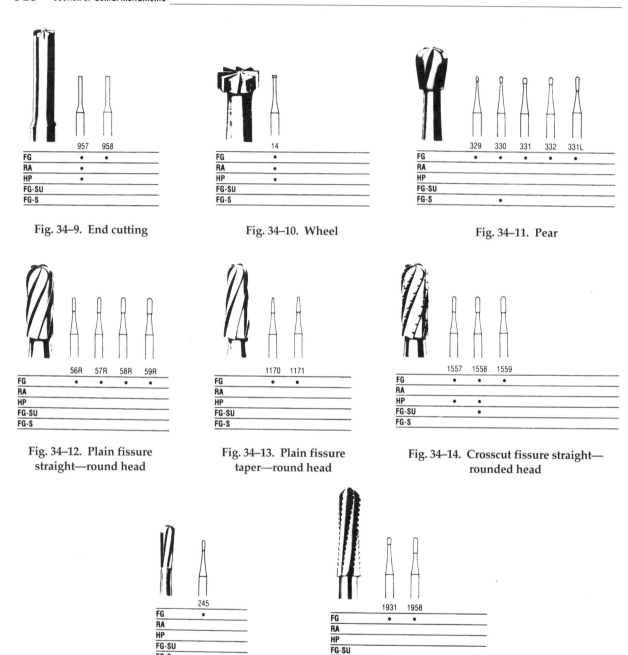

Fig. 34–9. End cutting

Fig. 34–10. Wheel

Fig. 34–11. Pear

Fig. 34–12. Plain fissure
straight—round head

Fig. 34–13. Plain fissure
taper—round head

Fig. 34–14. Crosscut fissure straight—
rounded head

Fig. 34–15. Special bur for
amalgam preparation

Fig. 34–16. Special bur used
for removal of metals

Figs. 34–9 – 34–16 (Courtesy Miltex Instruments Co., Lake Success, NY) FG, friction grip; RA, right angle; HP, hand-piece; FG-SU, surgical; FG-S, short shank; •, available.

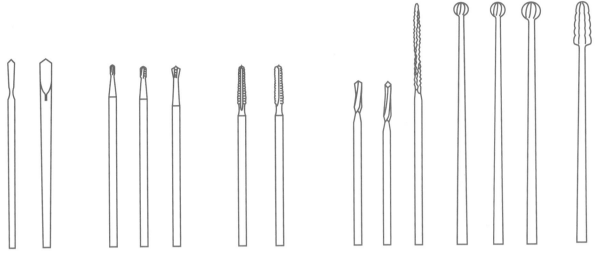

Fig. 34–17. Surgical burs

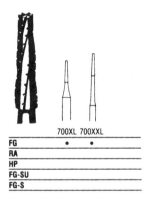

Fig. 34–18. Specialty burs for implants (Courtesy Miltex Instruments Co., Lake Success, NY)

cutting blades will determine the final smoothness or finish. The burs with the higher number of blades are used for ultrafine finishing of a restorative materials, such as composites and glass ionomers.

Vulcanite/Acrylic Burs

Burs that are used for quick removal of marginal excess or occlusal adjustments of partial and full dentures are the *vulcanite* or *acrylic burs*, figure 34–20.

MANDRELS

A **mandrel** is a metal-shanked rotary instrument that is designed to hold (mount) stones, discs, and wheels. The mandrel has a bur-type shank. The head of the mandrel may have a notched center or a screw to hold the disc of wheel on the mandrel. Mandrels are used with straight, contra- or right-angle and friction-grip handpieces, figure 34–21.

STONES

Stones used in dentistry are available in a full range of sizes, shapes, and grits. The *grit* (particle size of the abrasive that controls the cutting action) of a stone depends on the type of abrasive material that is used. Examples of abrasive materials include diamond, silicon carbide, and aluminum oxide.

The abrasive particles may be glued onto a backing material, or the abrasive particles may be mixed with a binding agent (matrix) that bonds the particles to one another. Some stones are molded onto a mandrel before the binder is

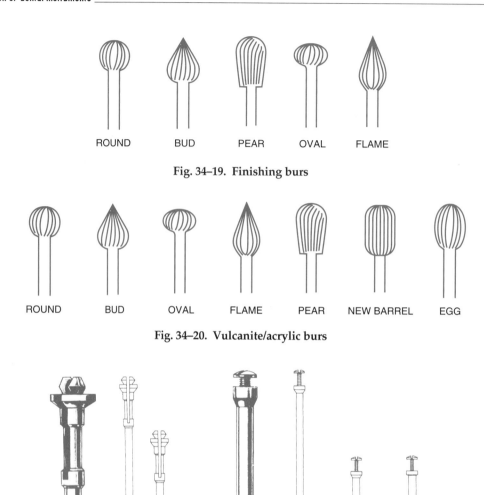

Fig. 34–19. Finishing burs

Fig. 34–20. Vulcanite/acrylic burs

Fig. 34–21. Mandrels (Courtesy Miltex Instrument Co., Lake Success, NY)

allowed to harden; these stones are referred to as *mounted stones*.

Diamond Instruments/Stones

The cutting portion of a diamond stone is composed of minute crystals of natural or man-made diamonds. The diamond crystals are either electroplated or bonded directly to a one-piece hardened stainless steel shank. Diamond stones are used because of their excellent abrasive or cutting action and are available in various grits from ultrafine to coarse. The grit determines the size and number of diamond crystals; the smaller the crystal, the finer the grit. Diamond stones vary in sizes, shapes, length, and function, figure 34–22. To help identify the various grits of a diamond stone, the manufacturer may notch or color-code the shank of the diamond stones.

Although carbide burs have basically six to eight cutting surfaces, diamonds stones have thousands of cutting edges.

Larger-size heads of diamond stones are used for gross reduction of tooth structure; other diamonds are used for cutting and shaping the tooth preparation. Diamond stones with an ultrafine grit may be used to finish and polish the surfaces of composite and glass ionomer restorative materials.

Abrasive Stones

Abrasive stones may be used within the oral cavity or in the dental laboratory. Although some abrasive stones are mounted directly on a mandrel, other stones are unmounted and require a mandrel.

Stones are available in a variety of colors and shapes. The color of the stone denotes the type of abrasive material and the grit.

One of the abrasives used for stones is *silicon carbide* and is generally recommended for working on ceramics, tooth structure, and plastics, figure 34–23. Additional stones made of either *garnet* or *aluminum oxide* may also be used for polishing metals. These stones are used in the laboratory.

Some abrasive stones are said to be *heatless* (creating less heat) and are composed of silicon carbide and rubber. During the finishing process the matrix material is weakened, causing the abrasive to be worn away as the stone comes in contact with the tooth structure or the restoration.

DISCS

Discs form a group of abrasive rotary instruments and are used for various operative and laboratory procedures. Discs may be rigid or flexible, paper, or with water-resistant plastic backing. The discs are available in a large variety

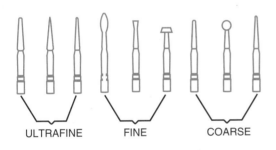

ULTRAFINE   FINE   COARSE

Fig. 34–22. Diamond stones

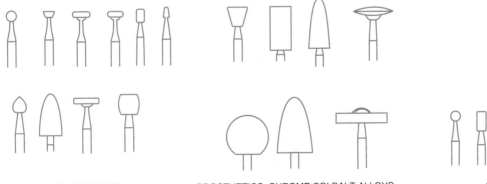

GENERAL ABRASIVES   PROSTHETICS, CHROME COLBALT ALLOYS   COMPOSITES

Fig. 34–23. Mounted abrasive stones

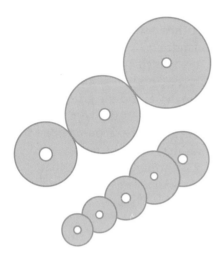

Fig. 34–24. Sandpaper discs vary in size.

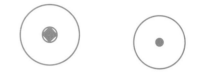

Fig. 34–25. Snap-on and pinhole discs

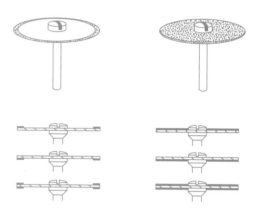

Fig. 34–26. Diamond discs

of grits and sizes, figure 34–24. The abrasive coating can be one of several materials, such as *diamond*, *garnet*, *quartz*, *sand*, and *aluminum oxide*. The shape of a disc may be flat, concave or convex and must be mounted on a suitable mandrel.

Discs are classified according to their grit, coarse to extra fine. When ordering discs, the size, shape, abrasive material, grit, and type of mandrel to be used must be specified.

Sandpaper Discs

The abrasive materials that are used for sandpaper discs may include sand, garnet, emery, and cuttlefish bone. The grit of the material will vary according to the abrasive material. Sandpaper discs must be mounted on a mandrel, and may be snap-on discs with either a metal or plastic centered notch or a pinhole to accommodate the screw-head mandrel, figure 34–25. Sandpaper discs are not reusable and should be removed from the mandrel before the mandrel is sterilized.

Diamond Discs

Diamond crystals or particles are bonded to a metal disc, some to the outer edge of the disc,

and others to the entire surface of the disc on one or both sides, figure 34–26. Diamond disc shapes vary from flat to concave to convex and are used for contouring and shaping tooth preparations.

Silicon Carbide (Carborundum) Discs

Silicon carbide discs are thin and very brittle and are used primarily in the laboratory; however, they can be used in the oral cavity in selective procedures. The disc may be used several times, but once damaged, it should be discarded.

Rubber Discs

Rubber discs are molded in the shape of wheels. These abrasive rotary instruments may be soft or hard with the abrasive particles embedded in the rubber. Two types of abrasives found in the rubber are silicon carbide and

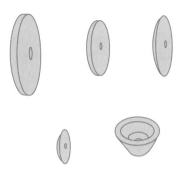

Fig. 34–27. Unmounted rubber discs

aluminum oxide. Rubber wheels are available in various grits, fine, medium, coarse, and may be mounted or unmounted, figure 34–27. They are used for finishing and polishing metal restorations.

STERILIZATION OF ROTARY INSTRUMENTS

Because rotary instruments are used within the oral cavity, they must be cleaned and sterilized or disposed of after each patient use.

Carbide and Steel Burs

The following methods are recommended for the care of carbide and steel burs. _Caution:_ Always wear heavy utility gloves when handling contaminated instruments.

1. Wearing utility gloves, place burs in a container with a solution of water and a neutral pH detergent or a recommended cleaner to loosen dried debris. _Note:_ An ultrasonic unit may be used to clean the burs. To prevent damage to the cutting blades of the bur, place burs in a heat-resistant bur block. This will keep the burs from touching one another during the cleaning (vibrating) process, because corrosion can occur when two different metals in a solution come in contact with each other during the cleaning cycle.
2. Remove burs from solution with appropriate instrument.
3. With a nylon or stainless wire bur brush, remove any remaining debris from the burs. Rinse burs under running water.
4. Thoroughly dry burs by placing them on an absorbent towel.
5. Place burs in a bur block, and prepare for sterilization. _Always_ follow the manufacturer's instructions regarding sterilization procedures.

Recommended methods for sterilizing carbide and steel burs include the following:

1. Dry heat, 170°C (340°F) for one hour
2. Chemiclave, (unsaturated) chemical vapor 132°C (270°F) 20 minutes at 20 psi (pounds per square inch)
3. Steam autoclave, 121°C (250°F) for 20 minutes at 15 psi. DO NOT USE COLD sterilizing solutions for the sterilization of carbide burs. The agents used in these solutions often contain strong oxidizing chemicals that may dull and weaken the carbide burs.

Diamond Instruments

The cleaning and sterilization of diamond instruments, stones, and discs are accomplished in the same manner as for the burs. Diamond stones and discs become clogged with hard and soft debris during use. This debris must be removed in order to clean and sterilize the diamond stones.

One may use disposable or nondisposable chips of aluminum oxide for cleaning clogged diamond stones and discs, figure 34–28. The use of disposable chips is recommended to prevent cross-contamination. Disposable chips should be discarded after use. Aluminum oxide chips can extend the life of diamond stones.

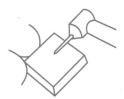

Fig. 34–28. Clean-a-diamond square

Stones

The various stones used within the oral cavity must be cleaned and sterilized according to the manufacturer's instructions.

Discs

The type of abrasive material used for the discs will determine whether they are to be discarded or sterilized. Sandpaper discs are always discarded. Rubber discs are cleaned and sterilized according to the manufacturer's instructions.

SUGGESTED ACTIVITIES

- Identify the various cutting burs and give uses of each.
- Identify the other rotary instruments and give uses of each.

REVIEW

1. List two uses of cutting burs.

   a. _____

   b. _____

2. Name the parts of a cutting bur.

   a. _____ b. _____ c. _____

3. What are the advantages of using a tungsten carbide bur?_____

   _____

   _____

4. What is the function of the bur number? _____

   _____

   _____

5. Name the eight basic cutting burs, and give the bur numbers of each.

a. _____   b. _____

c. _____   d. _____

e. _____   f. _____

g. _____   h. _____

6. Name the bur most commonly used for excavating caries from teeth. _____

_____

7. Name the bur used for making undercuts of the pulpal wall and for retention
   in cavity preparations. _____

8. Name the burs used to form parallel walls and flat floors in preparations. _____

_____

9. Finishing burs that have many cutting blades are best used for _____

_____.

10. What is the function of a mandrel? _____

_____

11. Define the terms *grit* and *abrasive.* _____

_____

12. Give the advantage of using diamond stones. _____

_____

13. Why are stones available in different colors? _____

14. What is the advantage of using a heatless stone? _____

_____

15. Why should carbide burs be sterilized in a heat-resistant bur block when you use an ultrasonic unit? _____

_____

Chapter 35: Hand Instruments for Operative Dentistry

OBJECTIVES:

After studying this chapter, the student will be able to:
- Select the basic examining instruments.
- Discuss the uses of the basic examining instruments.
- Name the parts of a cutting instrument.
- Identify the various cutting instruments.
- Discuss the uses of the various cutting instruments.
- Discuss the formula numbers of the cutting instruments.
- Identify the other hand instruments.

INTRODUCTION

Some **hand instruments** may be used for selected operative procedures within the oral cavity. Others may be used in a variety of procedures.

Hand instruments are classified into several groups. They include the basic examining instruments: *mouth mirror*, **explorer**, *periodontal probe*, and **cotton pliers (forcep)**. In addition, there are *cutting instruments*, *amalgam instruments*, *plastic instruments*, and *scalers*.

BASIC EXAMINING INSTRUMENTS

Explorers

The *explorer* is a slender, pointed instrument that is used primarily to examine the various tooth surfaces. The working portion or tip (point) of the explorer is very sharp and allows the operator to check the nautral surface(s) of a tooth/teeth, the grooves, and fossae for any defects and for other unusual conditions.

There are several styles of explorers with a variety of tips and angles; some, generally made of steel, are single- or double-ended, figure 35–1. Selection is determined by a specific need.

Uses of Explorers

- To examine the tooth for any developmental defects or faulty groove or fossa
- To check for faulty margins of a restoration
- To remove excess cement from around the margins of restoration during cementation

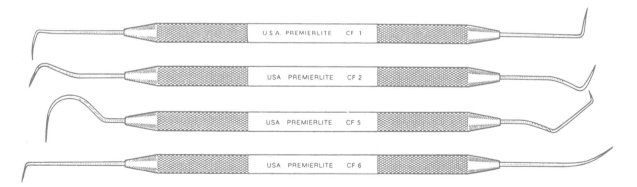

Fig. 35–1. Explorers (Courtesy Premier Dental/ESPE-Premier Sales Co.)

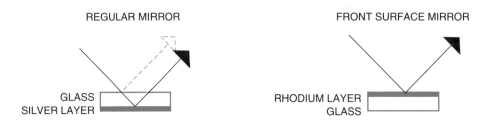

Fig. 35–2. Regular and front-surface mirrors (Courtesy Miltex Instrument Co., Lake Success, NY)

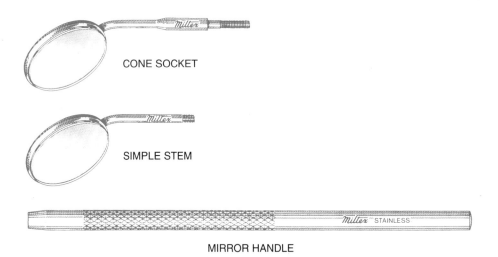

Fig. 35–3. Mirror stem styles (Courtesy Miltex Instrument Co., Lake Success, NY)

- To remove excess restorative material from around the matrix band before the band is removed
- To place gingival retraction cord prior to taking an impression

Mouth Mirror

The primary function of the *mouth mirror* is to allow the operator to see the various areas of the mouth that are impossible to see with direct vision. *Indirect vision* is a term used when the operator uses the mouth mirror to view an area within the mouth. This allows the operator to view the area as it is reflected in the mirror.

Dental mirrors are available with plane (regular) or magnifying surfaces. Regular mirrors are made with a silver coating on the back of the glass. This results in light being reflected from the surface of the glass as well as from the silver layer. This creates a "ghost image" and may cause considerable eye strain. The reflecting layer of a front-surface mirror is made with rhodium (a reflective metal) on the surface of the glass. The rhodium surface reflects a clear vision, free from all distortion, thereby eliminating the so-called ghost image, figure 35–2.

The stem portion of a mouth mirror may have either a simple- or a cone-socket stem, figure

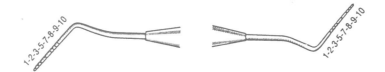

Fig. 35–4. Periodontal probe (Courtesy Premier Dental/ESPE-Premier Sales Co.)

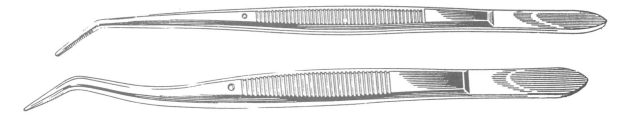

Fig. 35–5. Cotton pliers (forceps) (Courtesy Premier Dental/ESPE-Premier Sales Co.)

35–3. This type of stem allows the mirror to be replaced without having to purchase a new mirror handle when its surface becomes scratched or damaged.

Uses of Mouth Mirrors

- To view various areas within the oral cavity
- To retract the cheek and/or tongue for better access and visibility
- To reflect light into an area that is being examined or treated

Periodontal Probe

Periodontal probe has a round, tapered blade with a blunt tip. The blade is marked in millimeters (mm) and is used to measure the depth of the gingival sulcus, figure 35–4.

Cotton Pliers (Forcep)

Cotton pliers are a standard instrument used in most operative and restorative procedures. They allow the operator more flexibility in the manipulation of various materials that are used within the oral cavity.

The cotton plier is a two-bladed or beaked instrument and is available with either a locking or nonlocking handle. The beak may be straight or at an angle, figure 35–5.

Uses of Cotton Pliers

- To grasp or transfer materials from within or out of the mouth
- To retrieve other instruments or materials from sterile storage areas and to avoid contamination with the fingers
- To place and remove wedges from matrix bands
- To place and remove cotton rolls from the oral cavity

CUTTING INSTRUMENTS

Cutting instruments are used primarily to refine the walls and margins of cavity preparation. They are available in single-ended or double-ended styles. Double-ended instruments are more practical, because they reduce the number of instruments required for a given procedure.

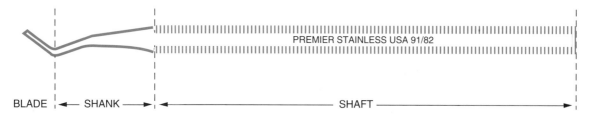

Fig. 35–6. Parts of a cutting instrument (Courtesy Premier Dental/ESPE-Premier Sales Co.)

Some cutting instruments are referred to as right and left and come in pairs (spoons, enamel **hatchets**). Other cutting instruments may be classified according to their use on the mesial or distal surfaces of a tooth (**bin-angle chisels**, special **hoes**, and **gingival margin trimmers**).

Parts of the Cutting Instrument

Blade, cutting portion
Shank, turned portion connecting shaft with blade; may be either straight or angled.
Shaft, the handle of the instrument, figure 35–6

Description of Cutting Instruments

Straight Chisel. A instrument with a straight blade, beveled on one side, figure 35–7.

- The longest side of the beveled blade is always toward the bulk of the tooth.
- Used on maxillary or mandibular anterior teeth in Class III or IV preparations.
- Can be used for planing down the enamel surface in cavity preparations.

Wedelstaedt. The **Wedelstaedt** chisel is an instrument with a curved blade beveled on one side. Similar to the straight chisel. Used in the same manner as the straight chisel, figure 35–8.

Bin-Angle Chisel. An instrument with a chisel blade placed at an angle to the shaft in the form of a hoe; i.e., two angles, figure 35–9.

- The longest side of the beveled blade is always toward the bulk of the tooth.
- Used on the maxillary posterior teeth in Class II.
- Used for smoothing or forming line angles of the buccal and lingual axial wall, either mesial or distal.

Enamel Hatchet. An instrument with a chisel blade placed at an angle to the shaft in the form of a hatchet, figure 35–10.

- The longest side of the beveled blade is always toward the bulk of the tooth.
- Used on the mandibular posterior teeth in Class II preparations.
- Used for smoothing or forming line angles of the buccal or lingual axial wall of the mesial or distal surfaces of the tooth.
- In pairs, right and left. (When right and left are indicated, this refers to the *patient's* right and left.)

Spoon. An instrument similar to a gingival margin trimmer in its angles and curve of blade but with the convex side of the blade beveled to form a cutting edge entirely around the periphery of the blade. This is a true lateral cutting instrument, figure 35–11.

- Used on all maxillary and mandibular teeth.
- Used to excavate decay; should be used instead of burs to remove decayed dentin, especially when close to the pulp.
- May also be used as an amalgam carver.
- Double-ended, in pairs, right and left.

Gingival Margin Trimmer. An instrument with a chisel blade placed at an angle to the shaft in the form of a hatchet, with the blade curved to buccal or lingual. The cutting edge is at a definite angle to the shaft of the instrument, figure 35–12.

- The beveled blade with the longest point toward, or away from, the shaft of the instrument will determine mesial or distal cutting.
- The short pointed end of the bevel is placed toward the floor of the gingival margin wall.
- Used on the maxillary and mandibular posterior teeth in Class II.
- A mesial and distal cutting, double-ended instrument.
- Used for placing the bevel on the gingival margin wall. Place one end of the instrument (short pointed end of the bevel) on the buccal wall, and, in a lateral motion, start planing the gingival margin floor from buccal to lingual wall; then reverse the instrument, and do the same operation, only from the lingual to buccal wall.
- Sometimes used in reverse position to form line angles and point angles in Class II preparations.

Special Hoe. An instrument with a bin-angle blade placed at an angle to the shaft, figure 35–13.

- Used on the maxillary posterior teeth.
- Used to plane the mesial and distal axial walls.

Angle Former. The **angle former** is similar to a hoe with the cutting edge placed at a definite angle to the long axis of the instrument, figure 35–14.

- The definite angle of the beveled blade (the longest point) is placed towards the mesial or distal surface of the tooth.

- Used on the maxillary and mandibular teeth in Class III and V.
- To make definite point angles and to sharpen line angles.
- May be used to establish cavo-surface bevels.

Cleoid-Discoid. The cleoid-discoid is an instrument with a disk-shaped blade placed at an angle to the shaft with a cutting edge around the entire periphery, figure 35–15.

- Used on the maxillary and mandibular teeth, usually in Class I, II, and V (posterior) preparations.
- Used primarily as a carver.
- Usually a double-ended instrument (the combination of both the cleoid and discoid).

Formula Numbers of Instruments

Formula numbers on the handle are descriptive of the size of the blade and the angle at which it is set to the shaft. Some consist of three numbers and others four.

1. Three numbers in the formula, figure 35–16.
   - The first number represents the width of the blade in tenths of a millimeter (A).
   - The second number designates the length of the blade in millimeters (B).
   - The third number shows in degrees the angle that the blade forms with the shaft (C).
2. Four numbers in the formula, figure 35–17.
   - The first number represents the width of the blade in tenths of a millimeter (A).
   - The second number represents in degrees the angle that the cutting edge of the blade makes with the shaft (B).
   - The third number designates the length of the blade in millimeters (C).
   - The fourth number shows in degrees the angle that the blade forms with the shaft (D).

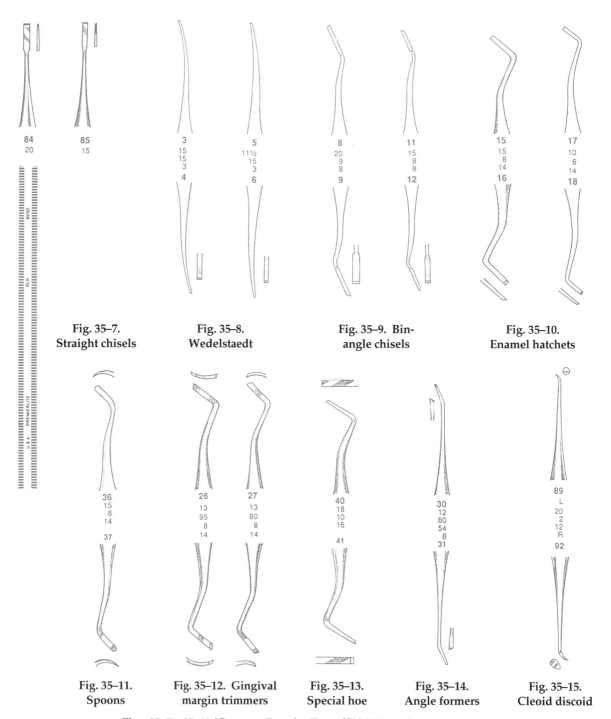

Fig. 35–7.
Straight chisels

Fig. 35–8.
Wedelstaedt

Fig. 35–9. Bin-
angle chisels

Fig. 35–10.
Enamel hatchets

Fig. 35–11.
Spoons

Fig. 35–12. Gingival
margin trimmers

Fig. 35–13.
Special hoe

Fig. 35–14.
Angle formers

Fig. 35–15.
Cleoid discoid

Figs. 35–7 – 35–15 (Courtesy Premier Dental/ESPE-Premier Sales Co.)

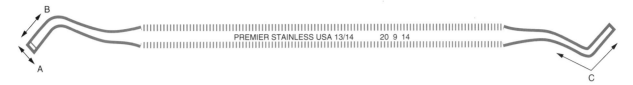

Fig. 35–16. Three-unit instrument formula. (A) Width of blade in tenths of mm. (B) Length of blade in mm. (C) Angle blade forms with shaft. (Courtesy Premier Dental/ESPE-Premier Sales Co.)

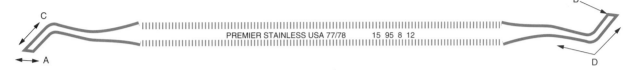

Fig. 35–17. Four-unit instrument formula. (A) Width of blade in tenths of mm. (B) Angle of cutting edge of blade with shaft. (C) Length of blade in mm. (D) Angle blade forms with shaft. (Courtesy Premier Dental/ESPE-Premier Sales Co.)

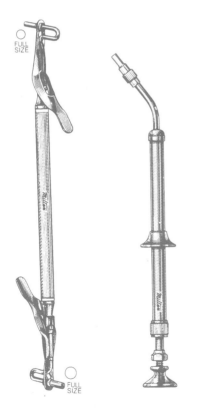

Fig. 35–18. Amalgam carriers (Courtesy Miltex Instrument Co., Lake Success, NY)

AMALGAM INSTRUMENTS

Amalgam instruments include the **amalgam carrier**, **condensors**, **carvers**, and **burnishers**.

Amalgam Carrier

The *amalgam carrier* is used to carry and dispense a pliable mix of silver amalgam into the tooth preparation.

The carrier may be single-ended or double-ended with both a large and small end and is made of metal or plastic. The carrier may have either a lever-action or plunger-type release, figure 35–18.

Amalgam Well

The **amalgam well** is made of stainless steel and is used to hold the triturated amalgam while loading the amalgam carrier, figure 35–19.

Amalgam Condensors

Amalgam condensors (pluggers) are used to condense (pack) restorative material into the cavity preparation.

Fig. 35–19. Amalgam well (Courtesy Miltex Instrument Co., Lake Success, NY)

The working end (nib) of the condensors is available in a variety of sizes and shapes, round, oval, rectangular, and diamond, and may be single- or double-ended.

The face of the nib may be smooth or serrated. The angle of the shaft of a condensor may vary. The variation in the angle of the shaft and the shape of the nib allows the operator access to specific areas within the tooth preparation, figure 35–20.

CARVERS AND BURNISHING INSTRUMENTS

Carvers

Carvers are used to recreate anatomy of the tooth before the amalgam restorative material has hardened. The working end of a carver may vary in design and size, from a pointed working end to an oval (disc) or rounded one. The angle of the blade may be shaped like a hoe or hatchet blade, figure 35–21.

Burnishers

Burnishers are used to smooth the surface and margins of an amalgam restoration while the

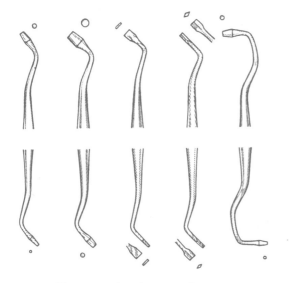

Fig. 35–20. Amalgam condensors

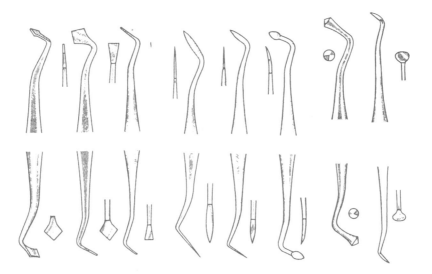

Fig. 35–21. Carvers

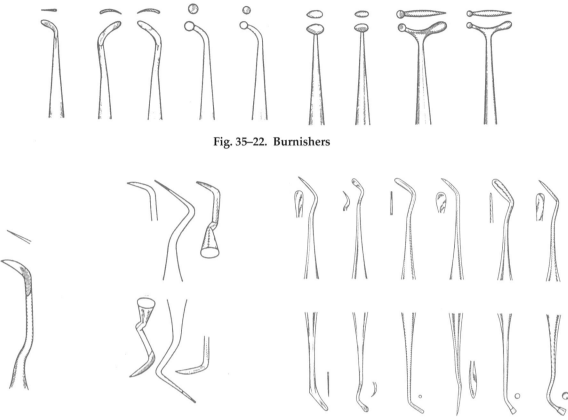

Fig. 35–22. Burnishers

Fig. 35–23. Gold knife

Fig. 35–24. Plastic instruments (Courtesy Premier Dental/ESPE-Premier Sales Co.)

material is still workable. A burnisher may have a working end that is smooth in the shape of a ball, egg, or combination of a ball and blade, figure 35–22.

Gold Knives

Gold knives are specific types of carvers that are used to remove excess restorative material. The cutting edge is a thin, sharp, double-ended, knife-type blade. It can be used on the interproximal surfaces of a tooth to eliminate improperly contoured or overhanging amalgam restorations extending from the occlusal to the gingival margins, figure 35–23.

PLASTIC INSTRUMENTS

Plastic instruments are a group of instruments used to place and condense restorative materials. They may be either of metal or plastic and single- or double-ended. The working end can vary, figure 35–24.

Plastic instruments should be used when placing tooth colored restorations; otherwise, the material may become discolored if a metal instrument is used. Plastic instruments are available in several designs.

Recently developed plastic carriers may be used in conjunction with the plastic instruments

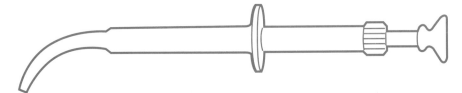

Fig. 35–25. Plastic syringe used for placing tooth restorative materials

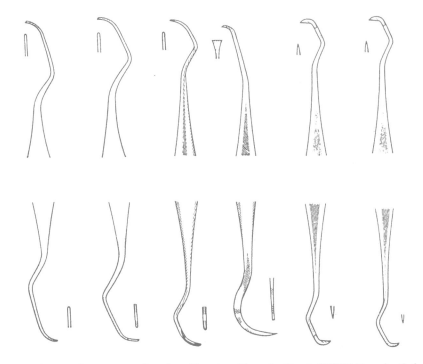

Fig. 35–26. Assorted curettes and scalers (Courtesy Premier Dental/ESPE-Premier Sales Co.)

to place composite and glass ionomer restorative material, figure 35–25.

CURETTES AND SCALERS

Curettes and *scalers* are designed to remove calculus deposits from tooth surfaces above and below the gingival attachment. The blades have cutting edges on the inner surface (face) of the blade. Curettes and scalers are paired instruments with various angled shanks and blades to allow access to all tooth surfaces of teeth. They may be purchased in a variety of blade sizes and shanks, figure 35–26.

CROWN AND BRIDGE SCISSORS

Crown and *bridge scissors* have small cutting blades designed to shape and trim temporary crowns (metal or plastic). The blades may be either curved or straight, figure 35–27. The handles may vary in length and size.

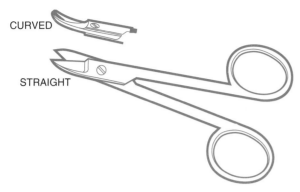

Fig. 35–27. Crown and bridge scissors (Courtesy Premier Dental/ESPE-Premier Sales Co.)

CEMENT SPATULAS

Cement spatulas are designed with a variety of blade lengths and widths. Cement spatulas are usually single-ended, metal instruments with a flat blade and a rounded end. They are used primarily for mixing dental cements, figure 35–28.

STERILIZATION OF HAND INSTRUMENTS

Refer to Chapter 26, _Infection Control in the Dental Setting._

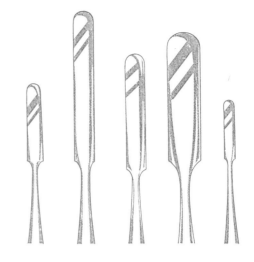

Fig. 35–28. Cement spatulas (Courtesy Premier Dental/ESPE-Premier Sales Co.)

SUGGESTED ACTIVITIES

- Identify the cutting instruments, and give the uses of each.
- Identify amalgam condensors, carvers, and burnishers.
- Recognize other hand instruments used in dentistry, and explain the use of each.

REVIEW

1. Name the basic four examining instruments used in dentistry.

   a. _____ b. _____

   c. _____ d. _____

2. The function of the periodontal probe is to measure the depth of the_____

   _____.

3. The primary function of the cutting instruments is _____

   _____.

4. Name the parts of the cutting instrument.

   a. _____

   b. _____

   c. _____

5. Which of the cutting instruments may be used for a maxillary Class II cavity preparation?

   a. _____   b. _____

   c. _____   d. _____

6. Which of the cutting instruments may be used for a mandibular Class II cavity preparation?

   a. _____   b. _____

   c. _____

7. The working end of a condensor is called_____.

8. The function of a carver is _____

_____.

9. The function of a burnisher is _____

_____.

10. A gold knife is used on _____

_____.

11. When placing tooth colored restorative material,_____

_____.

12. Curettes and scalers are used to _____

_____.

Chapter 36: Surgical Instruments

OBJECTIVES: After studying this chapter, the student will be able to:
- Identify various surgical forceps.
- Identify the other surgical instruments used in oral surgery.
- Select the surgical instruments needed for a specific oral surgery procedure.
- Select the correct armamentarium for extraction of a specific tooth.
- Discuss the procedure for sterilizing surgical instruments.

INTRODUCTION

Exodontics (ex, out; odont-, tooth) is the term used to describe the extraction of teeth. The term *oral surgeon* is given to the dentist, who is recognized as having the required skills, knowledge, and training in the speciality of oral surgery. The extraction of teeth is one of many procedures in oral surgery.

The indication for a tooth extraction may vary from the removal of a diseased primary tooth to the removal of a retained tooth (unerupted, embedded, impacted, malpositioned) or the retained roots of a tooth. In some orthodontic cases (ortho, to align or to straighten; donto-, tooth) teeth may be removed to allow space in a dental arch.

FORCEPS

The term *universal*, when associated with a forcep means that the forcep is designed for extracting teeth from either the right or left side of the same arch, but not for extracting teeth in the opposing arch. Forceps may also be identified by the angles and the notches on the beaks.

Maxillary Forceps

Maxillary and Mandibular Incisor Forcep (No. 69). This thin-beaked forcep is used on overlapping centrals and laterals. It is used, when

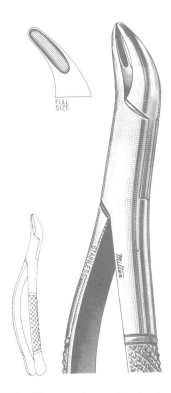

Fig. 36–1. Maxillary and mandibular incisor forcep (No. 69) (Courtesy Miltex Instrument Co., Lake Success, NY)

indicated, to avoid interference with the adjacent teeth or to remove root fragments, figure 36-1.

Maxillary Universal Incisors Cuspids, Bicuspids (Premolars) and Root Forcep (No. 150). A forcep

339

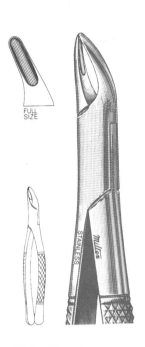

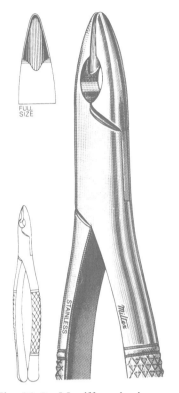

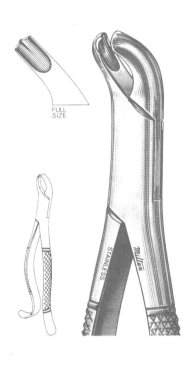

Fig. 36–2. Maxillary universal incisors, cuspids, bicuspids (premolars), and root forcep (No. 150) (Courtesy Miltex Instrument Co., Lake Success, NY)

Fig. 36–3. Maxillary incisors, cuspids, and bicuspids (premolars) forcep (No. 99C) (Courtesy Miltex Instrument Co., Lake Success, NY)

Fig. 36–4. Maxillary right first and second molar forcep (18R) (Courtesy Miltex Instrument Co., Lake Success, NY)

used in extracting centrals, laterals, bicuspids (premolars), and roots, figure 36-2.

Maxillary Incisors, Cuspids, and Bicuspids (Premolars) Forcep (No. 99C). The beaks of the forcep are parallel when employed on the tooth. The design of the forcep allows the beaks to grasp the entire periphery of the tooth at or above the gingival margin. The forcep is constructed in such a manner that the true force is placed along the axis, with the proper adaptation of the beaks to the root facilitating a rotary movement. This pressure on the forcep forces the tooth into the beak, where it is automatically locked, figure 36-3.

Maxillary Right First and Second Molar Forcep (No. 18R). The right-side beak is pointed and should be applied to the bifurcation of the two buccal roots; the left-side beak, which is rounded, should be applied to the lingual (palatal) root above the gingival margin, figure 36-4.

Maxillary Left First and Second Molar Forcep (No. 18L). The left-side beak is pointed and should be applied to the bifurcation of the two buccal roots; the right-side beak, which is rounded, should be applied to the lingual (palatal) root above the gingival margin, figure 36-5.

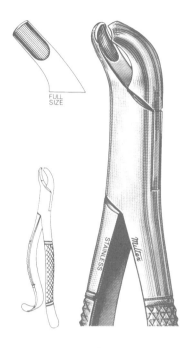

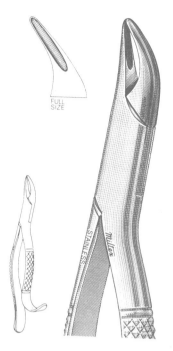

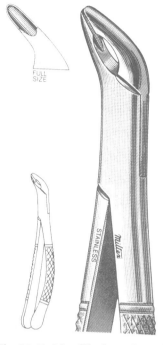

Fig. 36–5. Maxillary left first and second molar forcep (18L) (Courtesy Miltex Instrument Co., Lake Success, NY)

Fig. 36–6. Mandibular universal incisors, cuspids, bicuspids (premolars), and root forcep (No. 103) (Courtesy Miltex Instrument Co., Lake Success, NY)

Fig. 36–7. Mandibular universal incisors, cuspids, and bicuspids (premolars) forcep (No. 151A) (Courtesy Miltex Instrument Co., Lake Success, NY)

Mandibular Forceps

Mandibular Universal Incisors, Bicuspids (Premolars) and Root Forcep (No. 103). The forcep is constructed in such a manner that the thin, narrow beaks are at a angle and will allow proper application to all the anterior and crowded teeth, figure 36-6.

Mandibular Universal Incisors, Cuspids and Bicuspids (Premolars) Forcep (No. 151A). The edges of the beaks are sharp and can be used for breaking down the lingual and buccal alveolar bone plate to establish good subgingival root contact. This forcep is used for access to large cuspids and bicuspids (premolars), figure 36-7.

Mandibular Universal First and Second Molar Forcep (No. 17). The beaks of the forceps are sharp and pointed and deflect the soft tissue without injury. The beaks engage the bifurcation of the mesial and distal roots and form an extensive coverage of the crown, figure 36-8.

Mandibular Universal First and Second Molar Forcep (No. 16). This forcep is known as the "cow-horn" and is used on molars when the roots are not fused. The best application of the forcep is with full crowns or molars with badly broken-down crowns, figure 36-9.

Mandibular Universal Cuspids, Bicuspids (Premolars), and Molar Forcep (No. 85A). The forcep is designed so the beaks are parallel and

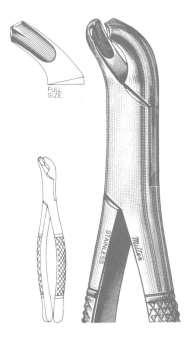

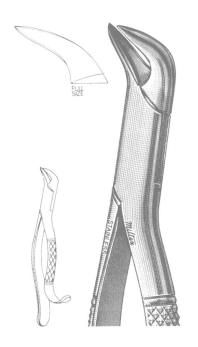

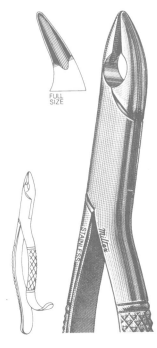

Fig. 36–8. Mandibular universal first and second molar forcep (No. 17) (Courtesy Miltex Instrument Co., Lake Success, NY)

Fig. 36–9. Mandibular universal first and second molar forcep (No. 16) (Courtesy Miltex Instrument Co., Lake Success, NY)

Fig. 36–10. Mandibular universal cuspids, bicuspids (premolars), and molar forcep (No. 85A) (Courtesy Miltex Instrument Co., Lake Success, NY)

their ends afford more than a two-point contact at the gingival margin. The raised portion (raised areas along the horizontal plane forming a curved incline) of the beaks grip almost the entire lingual and buccal surfaces of the tooth. The pressure on the handles pulls the crown into the opening between the forcep beaks and holds the tooth securely, figure 36-10.

ELEVATORS

Periosteal Elevator

A double-ended instrument with a blade at each end for lifting or raising the mucous membrane and underlying tissue covering the bone.

The angle and shape of the blades give access to all areas of the mouth. This elevator is used before the root elevator, figure 36-11.

Root Elevators

Root elevators are used on the maxillary or mandibular arch, and the concave blade is inserted between the root and the alveolar wall, figure 36-12.

Maxillary and Mandibular Root Elevators

A pair of root elevators, right and left, with the blades at a 90° angle to the shank. Maxillary and mandibular molar roots that are not fused can be easily removed with the right or left

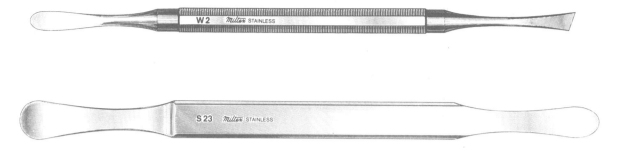

Fig. 36–11. Periosteal elevators (Courtesy Miltex Instrument Co., Lake Success, NY)

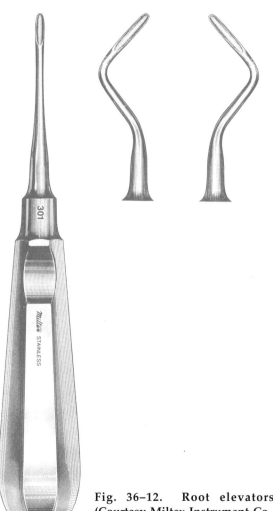

Fig. 36–12. Root elevators (Courtesy Miltex Instrument Co., Lake Success, NY)

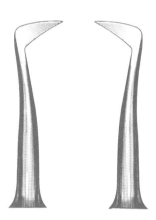

Fig. 36–13. Maxillary and mandibular root elevators (Courtesy Miltex Instrument Co., Lake Success, NY)

elevator by applying the point of the blade buccally at the bifurcation of the roots, forcing the point as far into the bifurcation of the roots as possible, figure 36-13.

SURGICAL INSTRUMENTS

Rongeur Forcep

A *rongeur* is a special type of forcep used to "trim" bone. The beaks may be round-nosed or square-nosed, with a hard, tough sharp blade extending along one side of the beak and curving around the extreme tip of the beak and along the opposite side. The rongeur may be used on the maxillary or mandibular arch, figure 36-14.

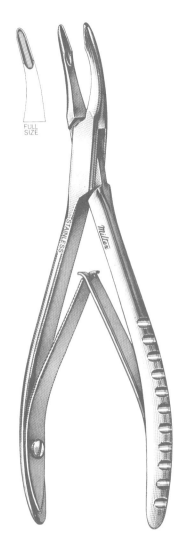

FULL
SIZE

STAINLESS

Miltex

Fig. 36–14. Rongeur forcep (Courtesy Miltex Instrument Co., Lake Success, NY)

Bone Files

Bone files are used after the rongeur forcep, chisel(s), and extractions for smoothing the alveolar process. The file blade is inserted and the tissue elevated. Pressure on the file causes it to engage the bone, and a pull toward the point of insertion removes rough, sharp fragments of bone, figure 36-15.

Root Tip Picks

Root tip picks may be straight or contra-angled and are used on the maxillary and mandibular arch. The straight pick is used in the anterior portion of the mouth, and the contra-angled pick is used in the posterior. Their purpose is to remove small root tips and bone fragments, figure 36-16.

Double-End Curettes

Double-end curettes are double-ended instruments used for removing soft diseased tissue and for establishing a flow of blood in the tooth socket. They are designed for application in all parts of the mouth. Double-end curettes are used after all extraction, figure 36-17.

Dressing Pliers

Dressing pliers are tweezer-type pliers with a serrated grip and slender pointed beaks for placing needed medication into the tooth socket, figure 36-18.

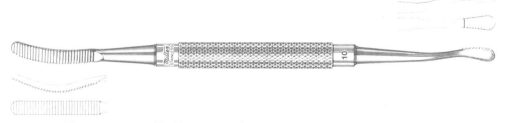

Fig. 36–15. Bone file (Courtesy Miltex Instrument Co., Lake Success, NY)

Scalpels/Surgical Blades

The *scalpel* is used in the mouth for making an incision in soft tissue, figure 36-19.

Surgical Mallet

The *surgical mallet* is used with bone chisels in reducing bone in selected oral surgery procedures, figure 36-20.

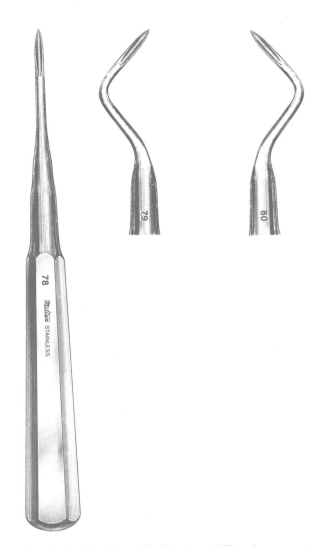

Fig. 36–16. Root tip pick (Courtesy Miltex Instrument Co., Lake Success, NY)

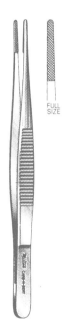

Fig. 36–18. Dressing pliers (Courtesy Miltex Instrument Co., Lake Success, NY)

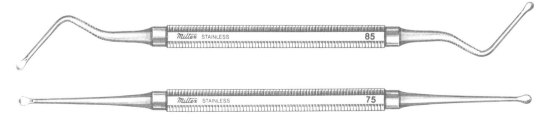

Fig. 36–17. Double-end curettes (Courtesy Miltex Instrument Co., Lake Success, NY)

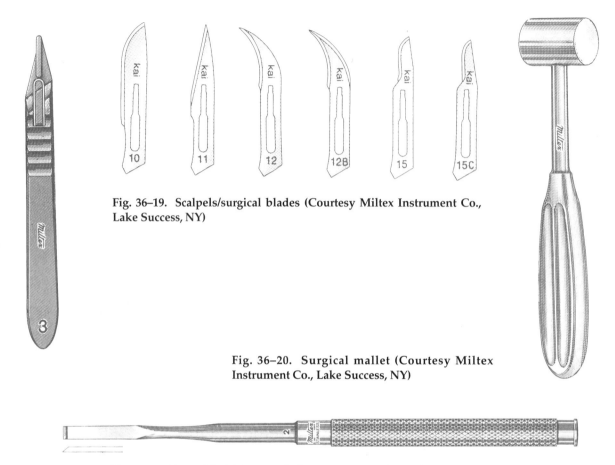

Fig. 36–19. Scalpels/surgical blades (Courtesy Miltex Instrument Co., Lake Success, NY)

Fig. 36–20. Surgical mallet (Courtesy Miltex Instrument Co., Lake Success, NY)

Fig. 36–21. Bone chisel (Courtesy Miltex Instrument Co., Lake Success, NY)

Bone Chisels

Bone chisels are designed for reducing bone structure in the maxillary or mandibular arch. Most bone chisels are used with a surgical mallet, figure 36-21.

Scissors

Scissors are used to trim soft tissue or for cutting suture material depending on whether the cutting ends are sharp or blunt. The cutting portion (blades) are available in plain (smooth) or serrated (horizontal, sharp, raised toothlike ridges) patterns. Surgical or tissue scissors with sharp delicate blades are used mainly for trimming soft tissue, and suture scissors with less delicate blades are used for cutting suture material. The shape of the blades may be straight, curved, or angled and of various lengths. Handles may be of varied lengths, figure 36-22.

Hemostat

A **hemostat** is a scissor-like instrument that is primarily used to clamp blood vessels. However, it can be used in dentistry to grasp tissue, root, or bone fragments. It is designed with serrated beaks that are either straight or curved.

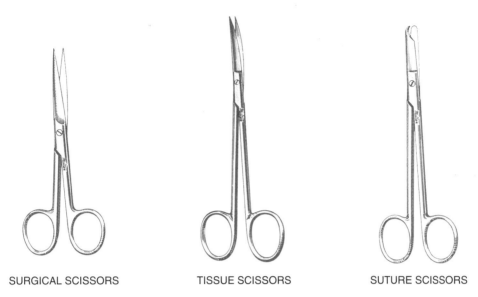

SURGICAL SCISSORS   TISSUE SCISSORS   SUTURE SCISSORS

Fig. 36–22. Scissors (Courtesy Miltex Instrument Co., Lake Success, NY)

The handles are designed to lock in position. The hemostat may be used in oral surgery to direct the suture needle throught soft tissue. In endodontic treatment it is often used to position a radiographic film, figure 36-23.

Needle Holder

A *needle holder* is similar in appearance to a hemostat. Unlike a hemostat's serrated beaks, the inner surfaces of the beaks have a crisscross pattern, allowing a firmer grasp of the suture needle. It is primarily used to grasp and manipulate a suture needle during suturing procedures, figure 36-24.

RECOMMENDED STEPS IN CLEANING, STERILIZATION, AND MAINTENANCE OF SURGICAL INSTRUMENTS

Instruments*

1. *Rinsing.* Immediately after surgery, rinse instruments under warm (not hot) running water. Rinsing should remove all blood, body fluids, and tissue.

2. *Cleaning.* (If cleaning is not done immediately after rinsing, instruments should be submerged in a solution of water and neutral pH (7) detergent.)
   A. *Ultrasonic cleaning*
   - For micro and delicate instruments, use manual cleaning (step C).
   - Instruments should be processed in the cleaner for the full recommended cycle time—usually five to ten minutes.
   - Place instruments in open position into the ultrasonic cleaner. Make sure that "sharps" (scissors, knives, osteotomes, etc.) blades do not touch other instruments.
   - All instruments have to be fully submerged.
   - Do not place dissimilar metals (stainless, copper, chrome plated, etc.) in the same cleaning cycle.

*List reproduced from the Miltex Instrument Catalog, 1989, pp. vi–vii. Courtesy Miltex Instruments Co., Lake Success, NY.

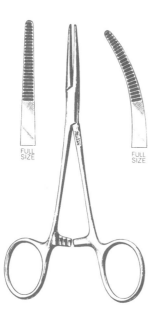

Fig. 36–23. Hemostat (Courtesy Miltex Instrument Co., Lake Success, NY)

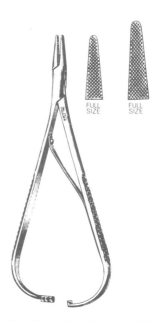

Fig. 36–24. Needle holder (Courtesy Miltex Instrument Co., Lake Success, NY)

- Change solution frequently—at least as often as manufacturer recommends.
- Rinse instruments after ultrasonic cleaning with water to remove ultrasonic cleaning solution.

B. *Automatic washer sterilizers.* Follow manufacturer's recommendations, but make sure instruments are lubricated after the last rinse cycle and before the sterilization cycle.

C. *Manual cleaning.* Most instrument manufacturers recommend ultrasonic cleaning as the best and most effective way to clean surgical instruments, particularly those with hinges, locks, and other moving parts. If ultrasonic cleaning is not available, observe the following steps:

  I. Use stiff plastic cleaning brushes (nylon, etc.). Do not use steel wool or wire brushes except specially recommended stainless steel wire brushes for instruments such as bone files or on stained areas in knurled handles.

  II. Use only neutral pH (7) detergents, because, if not rinsed off properly, low pH detergents will cause breakdown of stainless protective surface and black staining. High-pH detergent will cause surface deposit of brown stain, which will also interfere with smooth operation of the instrument.

  III. Brush delicate instruments carefully, and, if possible, handle them totally separately from general instruments.

  IV. Make sure all instrument surfaces are visibly clean and free from stains and tissue. This is a good time to inspect each instrument for proper function and condition. Check, and make sure that

- Scissors blades glide smoothly all the way (they must not be loose when in closed position). Test scissors by cutting into thin gauze. Three-quarters of length of blade should cut all the way to the scissors tips and not hang up.

- Forceps (pickups) have properly aligned tips. Hemostats and needle-holders do not show light between the jaws, lock and unlock easily, and joints are not too loose. Check needle-holders for wear on jaw surfaces.
- Suction tubes are clean inside.
- Retractors function properly.
- Cutting instruments and knives have sharp undamaged blades.
  V. After scrubbing, rinse instruments thoroughly under running water. While rinsing, open and close scissors, hemostats, needleholders, and other hinged instruments to make sure the hinge areas are rinsed out, as well as the outside of the instruments.

3. *After cleaning.* If instruments are to be stored, let them air dry and store them in a clean and dry environment.

4. *Autoclaving.* If instruments are to be reused or autoclaved:
   A. Lubricate all instruments that have any "metal-to-metal" action such as scissors, hemostats, needleholders, self-retaining retractors, etc. Recommended surgical lubricants such as instrument milk are best. Do not use WD-40 oil or other industrial lubricants.
   B. Put instruments up for autoclaving either individually or in sets.
      I. *Individual instruments.* Disposable paper or plastic pouches are ideal. Make sure you use a wide enough pouch (4" or wider) for instruments with ratchet locks such as needle holders and hemostats so the instrument can be sterilized in an open (unlocked) position.

II. *Instrument sets*
- Unlock all instruments, and sterilize them in an open position. Place heavy instruments on bottom of set (when two layers are required).
- Never lock an instrument during autoclaving. It will not be sterile, as steam cannot reach the metal-to-metal surfaces. The instrument will develop cracks in hinge areas because of heat expansion during autoclave cycle.
- Do not overload autoclave chamber, as pockets may form that do not permit steam penetration.
- Place towel on bottom of pan to absorb excess moisture during autoclaving. This will reduce the chances of getting "wet packs." Make sure the towels used in sterilization of instruments have no detergent residue and are neutral pH (7) if immersed in water. This can be a real problem as laundries frequently use inexpensive but high-pH (9–13) detergents and do not properly rinse out or neutralize those detergents in the final wash/rinse cycle. Also, sometimes bleaches such as Clorox are added and are not neutralized.
- *Caution.* At the end of the autoclave cycle, before the drying cycle, unlock autoclave door, and open it no more than a crack (about 3/4"). Then run dry cycle for the period recommended by the autoclave manufacturer. If the autoclave door is opened fully before the drying cycle, cold room air will rush into the chamber, causing condensation on the instruments. This will result in water stains on instruments and also cause "wet packs."

- If you have any unusual staining on your instruments during sterilization, contact your local instrument representative.

5. *Cold sterilization.* Most cold sterilization solutions render instruments sterile only after a 10-hour immersion. This prolonged chemical action can be more detrimental to surgical instruments than the usual 20-minute autoclave cycle. If the instruments need to be "disinfected" only, cold sterilization is okay as disinfection will take place in only 10 minutes, but keep in mind the difference between *sterile*—an absolute term (no living organism suvives)—and *disinfected*—basically clean.

- Always use the proper sterilization/cleaning technique to render the instrument in the required condition for use.

SUGGESTED ACTIVITIES

- Select and identify the various surgical instruments.
- Explain the use of each selected instrument.

REVIEW

1. Define the terms *exodontics, orthodontics,* and *universal* as they pertain to oral surgery.

    a. _____

    b. _____

    c. _____

2. List three reasons for tooth extractions.

    a. _____

    b. _____

    c. _____

3. Name the three forceps that may be used to extract a maxillary anterior tooth.

    a. _____

    b. _____

    c. _____

4. Name the forcep used to extract mandibular anterior teeth and bicuspid (pre-molars) and roots. _____

_____

5. Give the function of the periosteal elevator. _____

_____

6. Give the function of the rongeur._____

_____

7. Give the function of the bone file. _____

_____

8. Give the functions of the double-end curette. _____

_____

9. Give the main use of the surgical scissor._____

_____

10. Give three uses of the hemostat in dentistry.

a. _____

b. _____

c. _____

Chapter 37: Dental Equipment in the Operatory

OBJECTIVES:

After studying this chapter, the student will be able to:
- Identify the parts of the dental chair.
- Identify the parts of the dental unit.
- Expain the function of the dental lamp.
- Discuss the function of the oral vacuum system.
- State the requirements for a properly designed assistant's stool.
- State the requirements for a properly designed dentist's operating stool.

INTRODUCTION

The *dental operatory* (treatment room) is the primary work area of the dentist and of the chairside assistant. The size of the operatory and the floor plan and equipment should be designed and organized to offer comfort and convenience for the operator and assistant, figure 37-1.

The major equipment in a dental operatory includes the *dental chair*, *dental unit*, *dental operating light*, *operating stools*, and *mobile cart(s)* or cabinet.

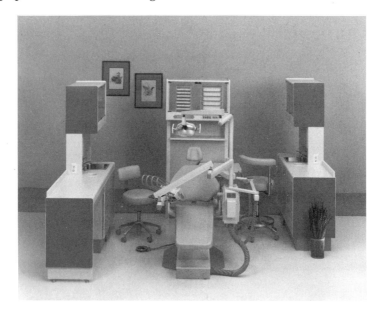

Fig. 37–1. Equipment in the dental operatory (Courtesy A-dec, Inc., P.O. Box 111, Newberg, OR)

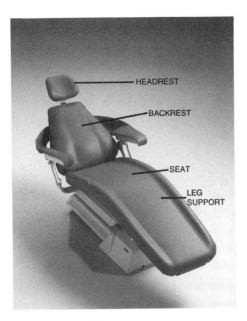

Fig. 37–2. The dental chair (Courtesy A-dec, Inc., P.O. Box 111, Newberg, OR)

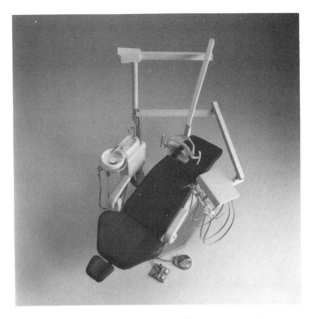

Fig. 37–3. Floor-mounted unit (Courtesy A-dec, Inc., P.O. Box 111, Newberg, OR)

THE DENTAL CHAIR

Most *dental chairs* used today are a lounge-type and are designed for use in four-handed sit-down dentistry. The dental chair supports the patient's head and body.

Part of the Dental Chair

- *Body of chair*. This includes the backrest, seat, and leg supports, figure 37-2.
- *Armrest*. Usually movable by lifting or sliding backward to allow easy access when seating patient, the armrest may have a sling to support and secure the patient's elbows.
- *Headrest*. Supports the patient head, figure 37-2.
- *Control panel*. Has controls that allow the body of the chair to be moved from the upright to the supine position and to raise and lower the height of the chair. Controls

may be located either on the side or on the back of the backrest.
- *Swiveled lever*. Allows the base of the chair to be rotated from side to side.

THE DENTAL UNIT

The *dental unit* is controlled by master on/off switches. The function of the dental unit is to supply water, air, electricity, and a system for oral evacuation.

Dental units are available in several designs. Some are mounted to the floor, figure 37-3, others are mobile, figure 37-4. The basic features of a dental unit include the dental handpieces, air-water syringe, oral evacuation system, and the unit may or may not have a *cuspidor* (a bowl with circulating water, used by the patient for spitting or emptying the mouth).

Today, with four-handed, sit-down dentistry the operator has greater flexibility with the use of either a mobile unit or cart.

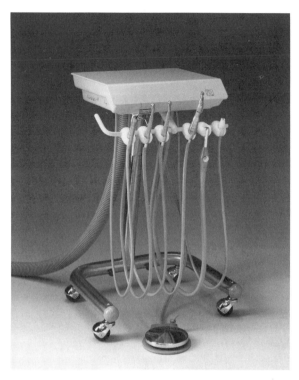

Fig. 37–4. Mobile dental unit (Courtesy A-dec, Inc., P.O. Box 111, Newberg, OR)

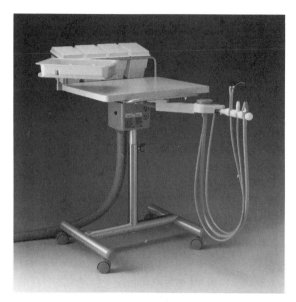

Fig. 37–5. Assistant's cart (Courtesy A-dec, Inc., P.O. Box 111, Newberg, OR)

The same features are available on the floor-mounted unit. However, the oral evacuation system may be a part of the assistant's cart, figure 37-5.

Parts of the Dental Unit

- *Dental Handpiece(s).* These are a part of the dental unit. The type of unit employed in the operatory will determine the dental handpiece arrangement.
- *Foot control.* The foot control is positioned on the floor close to the chair and activates the dental handpiece(s). The disc-shaped foot control is attached to the unit with flexible tubing, figure 37-6.
- *Air-water syringe.* Air is used to dry the surfaces of the teeth. Water is used to rinse the

oral cavity. Most air-water syringes will deliver (1) a stream of water; (2) a stream of air; and (3) a combination spray of air and water, figure 37-7.
- *Oral vacuum.* An oral vacuum is used to suction water and debris from the patient's oral cavity. With the used of the modern oral vacuum (evacuation) system, the unit cuspidor has virtually been eliminated. The placement of the oral vacuum tip during selected operative procedures aids in the retraction of the tongue and cheek, thereby keeping the field of operation free of water and debris while providing optimum visibility for the operator. In the washed field technique, the dental handpiece provides a fine jet of air/water spray during the preparation of a tooth. The oral vacuum system has proven to be the most efficient method to control and remove the water from the patient's oral cavity.
- *Saliva Ejector.* The function of the saliva ejector is to remove and control the saliva level and to hold the tongue away from the field

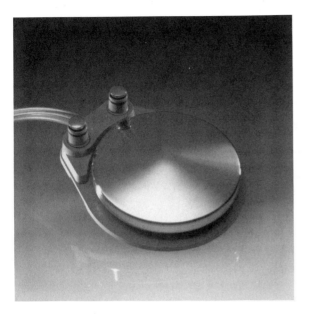

Fig. 37–6. Foot control (Courtesy A-dec, Inc., P.O. Box 111, Newberg, OR)

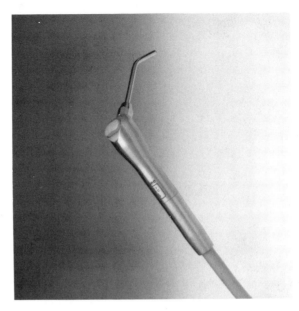

Fig. 37–7. Air-water syringe (Courtesy A-dec, Inc., P.O. Box 111, Newberg, OR)

of operation. A saliva ejector may also be used to maintain a dry environment during placement of restorative materials.

- *Cuspidor.* A cuspidor is used by the patient to empty the mouth of oral debris. A dental unit may or may not have a cuspidor. Cuspidors may be fixed to the dental unit or be a part of the oral evacuation system of a portable unit, figure 37-3.

THE OPERATING LIGHT

The dental operating light provides the bright light necessary for viewing the oral cavity.

The dental operating light may be attached to the dental unit, figure 37-8, or be ceiling-mounted, figure 37-9. The dental light is designed with two handles, one on either side. The handles allow the dental light to be adjusted according to the procedure.

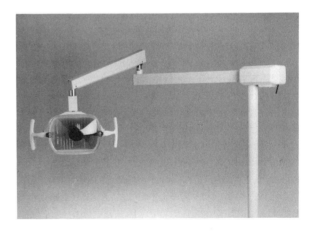

Fig. 37–8. Dental operating light attached to dental unit (Courtesy A-dec, Inc., P.O. Box 111, Newberg, OR)

Care and cleaning of the dental light should be conducted according to manufacturer's recommendations.

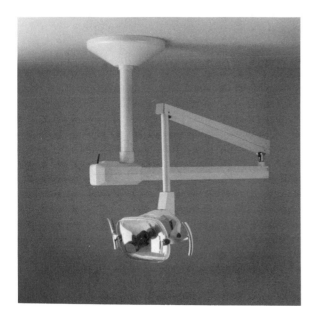

Fig. 37–9. Ceiling-mounted dental operating light (Courtesy A-dec, Inc., P.O. Box 111, Newberg, OR)

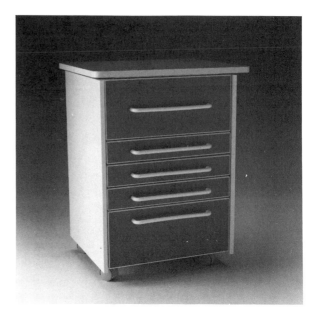

Fig. 37–10. Assistant's mobile cabinet (Courtesy A-dec, Inc., P.O. Box 111, Newberg, OR)

THE DENTAL CABINET

Dental cabinets may be fixed to the wall or free-standing and provide storage space for sterile instrument, tray setups, and any other supplies needed for the various dental procedures, figure 37-1. When a mobile cabinet is part of the operatory furnishings, it provides additional storage space as well as a working surface for the chairside assistant, figure 37-10. Generally, storage space in a mobile cabinet is limited to those materials and supplies needed immediately at the chair.

OPERATING STOOLS

Operating stools are used in four-handed, sit-down dentistry and allow the operator and chairside assistant to be seated. The stools used by the operator and assistant will vary in design. Features of a well-designed operator and assistant stools should include the following.

Operator's Stool, figure 37-11, left.

1. The seat of stool should be padded and may be flat-surfaced or contoured.
2. The stool base should have four to five casters to prevent tipping.
3. The stool must have an adjustable lever, beneath the seat, to adjust the height of the seat from the floor.
4. The stool must have an adjustable back support.

Assistant's Stool, figure 37-11, right.

1. The seat of the stool should be padded for the comfort of the assistant.
2. The stool should have five casters and be broad enough to prevent tipping.
3. The stool should have a foot ring to support the feet.
4. The stool must have a lever that can adjust leg length and for correct height.

5. The stool must have an adjustable support arm. The purpose of the arm is to provide the assistant with needed support to the upper body (torso).

X-RAY MACHINE

The x-ray machine may be a part of the operating or treatment room or housed in a separate area of the dental office. Refer to Chapter 79, *Radiation Protection*.

DISINFECTION OF DENTAL EQUIPMENT IN THE OPERATORY

It is advisable to always follow the manufacturer's recommendation when disinfecting dental equipment.

However, because of the variation in design, materials used, and technical aspects of the dental equipment, any procedure of disinfection must be systematic and thorough. Also it is imperative that barriers be used whenever possible. Refer to Chapter 39, *Preparation of the Operatory and Seating the Dental Patient*.

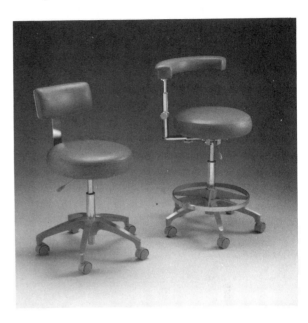

Fig. 37–11. (L) Operator's stool. (R) Assistant's stool. (Courtesy A-dec, Inc., P.O. Box 111, Newberg, OR)

REVIEW

1. Name the parts of the dental chair.

   a. _____ b. _____ c. _____

   d. _____ e. _____

2. List the parts of a floor-mounted dental unit.

   a. _____ b. _____ c. _____

   d. _____ e. _____ f. _____

3. State the main purpose of the oral vacuum system._____

   _____

4. Features of the operator's stool include the following:

a. _____

b. _____

c. _____

d. _____

5. Features of the assistant's stool include the following:

a. _____

b. _____

c. _____

d. _____

e. _____

Chapter 38: Positioning the Dental Team for Operative Dentistry

OBJECTIVES:

After studying this chapter, the student will be able to:
- Discuss the four operating zones as they relate to the dental team.
- Identify the three basic systems for instrument delivery.
- Explain the optimum seating position of the operator during operative dentistry.
- Explain the optimum seating position of the chairside assistant during operative dentistry.
- Explain the correct seating and head position of the patient for operative dentistry.

INTRODUCTION

The proper positioning of the patient and dental team may improve the delivery of dental care. The manner in which the operator and chairside assistant are positioned in relationship to the patient is important for efficiency and increased productivity.

Four-handed, sit-down dentistry provides the dental team with the opportunity to function as a coordinated and organized unit.

The system of four-handed, sit-down dentistry allows the operator and chairside assistant to work seated. The chairside assistant provides a second pair of hands for the operator.

The patient is placed in the **supine** (lying on back with face up) position in the dental chair, while the operator and chairside assistant are seated on either side of the chair.

OPERATING ZONES FOR DENTAL TEAM

The working zones in which the dental team must operate can best be described by the hours on the face of a clock. With the patient seated and placed into a supine position, the patient's oral cavity represents the center of the clock, figure 38–1.

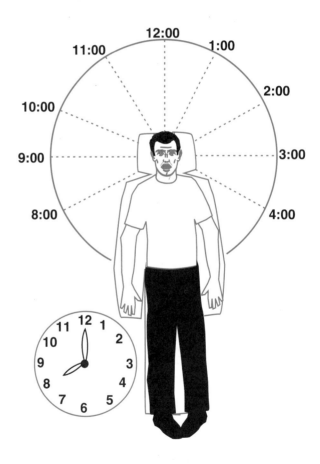

Fig. 38–1. Patient's oral cavity represented as the center of clock

359

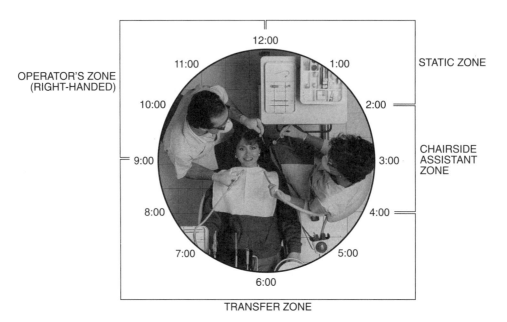

Fig. 38–2. Working zones (Photo courtesy A-dec, Inc., P.O. Box 111, Newberg, OR)

The operator and chairside assistant are positioned according to the hours on the face of a clock.

The clock may be divided into four working zones:

1. *The operator's zone—8 to 12 o'clock*, if the operator is right-handed, or *12 to 4 o'clock*, if left-handed. The operator's zone is the working area in which the operator is positioned to have access to all areas of the patient's oral cavity, figure 38–2.
2. *Assistant's zone—2 to 4 o'clock*, or *8 to 10 o'clock* if the operator is right- or left-handed, respectively. The assistant's working zone is generally limited to either the *3 o'clock* or *9 o'clock* position (left-handed operator) throughout the dental procedure, regardless of the operator's position, figure 38–2.
3. *Transfer zone—4 to 8 o'clock* position. The transfer zone is the area where the -operator and assistant will exchange

instruments and materials for delivery to and from the oral cavity during the dental procedure. This is also referred to as trans-thorax delivery (across the chest), figure 38–2.
4. *Static zone*—The *12 to 2 o'clock* or *10 to 12 o'clock* position is regarded as a nonactive zone. Equipment such as a mobile cabinet or cart may be placed in this zone, figure 38–2.

BASIC SYSTEMS FOR INSTRUMENT DELIVERY

Over-the-Patient Delivery

The majority of dentists use the over-the-patient delivery system. In this delivery system, the so-called dental unit is mounted on a post with an arm system that brings the controls to the operator, figure 38–3.

The *over-the-patient delivery system* is highly flexible in terms of positioning equipment and exchange of instruments. Instruments may be presented from across the patient's chest (trans-thorax) delivery or from either side of the patient. This system is ideal for either two or four-handed dentistry and may be used by the operator while in the seated or standing position. Instruments will be in full view of the patient at all times with this delivery system.

Advantages of the Over-the-Patient System

- Offers suitable instrumentation in the location and exchange of dental instruments.
- Allows for two- or four-handed, stand-up or sit-down dentistry.
- Allows the operator direct access to the lower quadrants.
- Requires minimal movement by operator and chairside assistant during operative dentistry.
- Minimizes eye fatigue, because the operator does not need to constantly adjust his or her eyes to oral cavity distance.
- Minimal operatory floor space is required for equipment.

Disadvantages of Over-the-Patient Delivery

- Reduces assistant's access to chair controls positioned on the operator's side of chair.
- Tubing from the unit to the handpiece(s) may drag over the patient's chest during operative procedure.

Side Delivery

The *side-delivery system* is developed specifically for four-handed sit-down dentistry. Instrument exchange is best achieved through the use of separate cart(s) for the operator and chairside assistant. In addition, the operator may use a wall- or cabinet-mounted unit along with the assistant's cart. With the side-delivery system, operative instruments are exchanged peripheral to the patient's view, i.e., outside his or her normal center of vision.

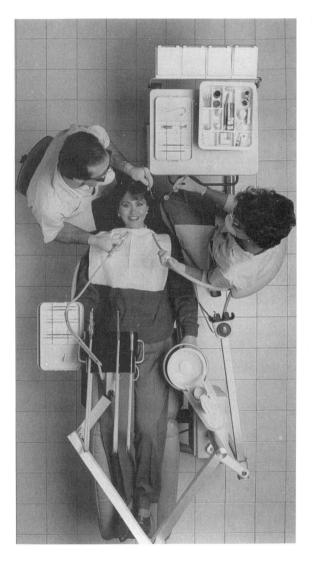

Fig. 38–3. Over-the-patient delivery system for instrumentation (Courtesy A-dec, Inc., P.O. Box 111, Newberg, OR)

Advantages of the Side-Delivery System

- Offers the operator and chairside assistant increased ability to view the oral cavity during all sit-down dental procedures.
- Offers flexible seating and instrument location.

- Offers the dental team mobility with the use of cart or mobile cabinets. Operator and chairside assistant are able to move more freely at the chair with the use of a cart or mobile cabinet.
- Tubing from the unit to handpiece(s) may be straight or coiled. Coiled tubing has less chance to drag across the patient.
- Provides operator and chairside assistant a better access to the patient and chair.
- Instruments are kept out of view of the patient.
- If wall-mounted units are used, minimal floor space is required.

Disadvantages of Side-Delivery System

- Requires more operatory floor space when split cart systems are used.
- A poorly located umbilical tubing arrangement may interfere with the ability of operator and chairside assistant to move freely within the working zone(s).
- Reduces assistant's access to operator's instruments.

Rear-Delivery System

In the *rear-delivery system*, the instruments are located behind the chair. A single cart or a cabinet- or wall-mounted unit can be used. The instruments are always at the rear of the chair and are generally out of the view of the patient, figure 38–4. Rear delivery is most effective in sit-down, four-handed dentistry.

Advantages of the Rear-Delivery System

- Operative instruments are out of the patient view.
- Provides excellent assistant access to operative instruments.
- Provides the assistant with a stable work surface when a dual-purpose cart or cabinet is used.

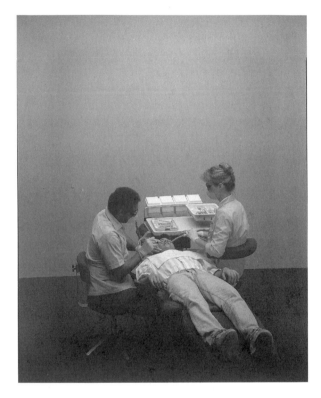

Fig. 38–4. Rear delivery system for instrumentation (Courtesy A-dec, Inc., P.O. Box 111, Newberg, OR)

- Allows the patient easy access to chair and efficient movement within the working zone(s) of the operator and chairside assistant.
- Requires minimal operator space.

Disadvantages of the Rear-Delivery System

- Limited to sit-down dentistry.

POSITIONING OF OPERATOR AND CHAIRSIDE ASSISTANT

Position of Operator

The position of the operator is critical to the fixed environment of the dental team. The entire system is based on the operator's position during the dental procedure. The operator must assume a desirable seated position. The patient, chairside assistant, and equipment are arranged according to this position.

The objectives for proper positioning of the operator should include the following criteria:

1. The operator must be seated so that the entire surface of the operator's stool is supporting his or her weight.
2. The height of the stool should be adjusted so that the operator's thighs are parallel to the floor.
3. The operator's elbows should be close to the body.
4. The operator is seated in a relaxed and unstrained position with the back and neck upright and with the top of the shoulders parallel to the floor.
5. The distance from the operator's eyes to the patient's oral cavity should be approximately 14 to 18 inches.

Position of the Chairside Assistant

The assistant must have easy access and visibility to the oral cavity during the treatment procedure. This can be accomplished when the dental team is seated and properly positioned.

For the assistant to function in an efficient manner the following criteria should be followed:

1. The assistant should be seated in the 3 o'clock position, for a right-handed operator or the 9 o'clock position for a left-handed operator.
2. The assistant's stool should be 4 to 6 inches higher than the operator's. This will allow the assistant greater visibility for most areas of the oral cavity.
3. The assistant should be seated as close to the dental chair as possible.
4. The assistant should be seated well back onto the seat of the stool. The stool back support must be properly adjusted in order to provide needed back support.
5. The assistant's back should be straight (erect) with the body-support arm adjusted to support the upper body just under the rib cage.
6. The assistant's legs should be directed toward the patient's head, with the assistant's thighs parallel to the seat of the chair.
7. The assistant's feet should rest on the foot support at the base of the stool.

REVIEW

1. Define the term supine._____

_____

2. What is the meaning of "four-handed, sit-down dentistry"? _____

_____

3. Name the four working zones in positioning the operator and the chairside assistant.

    a. _____   b. _____

    c. _____   d. _____

4. Briefly explain the operator's zone. _____

    _____

5. Give the working time zones for the chairside assistant when working with a right-handed operator. _____

    _____

6. Briefly explain the transfer zone. _____

    _____

7. What is the purpose of the over-the-patient delivery system? _____

    _____

8. What is the purpose of the side-delivery system? _____

    _____

9. What is the purpose of the rear-delivery system? _____

    _____

10. What criteria should be followed when positioning the chairside assistant?

    a. _____

    _____

    b. _____

    _____

c. _____

_____

d. _____

_____

e. _____

_____

f. _____

_____

g. _____

_____

After studying this chapter, the student will be able to:

- Discuss the correct procedure for using the spray-wipe-spray method for disinfecting the dental operatory.
- Prepare the dental operatory using the appropriate barriers.
- Discuss the proper position of the patient's oral cavity in relationship to the operator.
- Discuss the role of the chairside assistant in seating the patient for operative dentistry.
- Discuss the supine position as it pertains to the dental patient.

PREPARING THE OPERATORY

Materials Needed

- antimicrobial soap
- disposable towels
- utility gloves
- surface disinfectant
- sponge
- barrier materials

Preparing the dental operatory or treatment room requires that all work surfaces and equipment be either disinfected or protected with appropriate barriers.

Surfaces that cannot be barriered must be disinfected with an appropriate surface disinfectant, such as iodophors or other EPA-approved disinfectants.

The daily routine requires that the operatory be cleaned, disinfected, and ready for the placement of the barriers. It is recommended that at the beginning and the end of each day, the surfaces of the dental chair, unit, and countertop/cabinet(s) be sprayed with the surface disinfectant. However, only those surfaces that can withstand the application of a surface disinfectant should be sprayed. The technique of spray-wipe-spray is recommended. *Note:* Extreme care must be taken during the spray-wipe-spray procedure to avoid directing the spray onto the control panel of the chair, unit, and face of dental light. Should the spray accidentally come in contact with the electrical system, it may permanently damage the dental equipment.

To prepare for the spray-wipe-spray procedure the assistant should

1. Wash hands with antimicrobial soap in cool water for fifteen seconds, rinse, and dry.
2. Put on utility gloves.
3. Apply appropriate surface disinfectant to all working surfaces that can safely withstand the surface disinfectant. First spray, then wipe surfaces with sponge or disposable towel using a frictional wiping action. Spray a second time, and allow surfaces to dry for ten minutes.
4. Wash and dry utility gloves once equipment and working surfaces have been disinfected.
5. Spray outer surface of gloves with disinfectant and hang to dry.
6. Wash hands in cool water and dry.

PLACING BARRIERS

The routine spray-wipe-spray procedure between patients will depend on the extent to which *barriers* are used. The placement of barriers will save time between patients in disinfecting the operatory.

Many barriers are available for use and include disposable plastic covers, baggies, plastic perforated sheet wrap, and aluminum foil. For barriers to be effective they must be impervious (resists passage) to moisture and the penetration of microorganisms.

Dental Chair

- Cover headrest and body of chair with a disposable plastic full-chair drape, figure 39–1.

Dental Unit

Dental handpieces—autoclave.
- Handpiece hoses/tubing—cover with disposable plastic sleeve, figure 39–2.

Air-water syringe
- Handle and tubing—cover with disposable plastic sleeve, figure 39–3.
- Syringe tip—autoclave, or if disposable, discard.

Oral vacuum
- Suction hose or tubing—cover with disposable plastic sleeve, figure 39–3.
- Vacuum tip—autoclave, or if disposable, discard.

Saliva ejector
- Hose/tubing—cover with disposable plastic sleeve.
- Ejector tip—disposable, discard.

Dental Operating Light

- Handles—use plastic bags or perforated plastic sheet wrap, figure 39–4.
- Light switch—use perforated plastic sheet wrap.

X-ray Machine

- Tubehead/arms—use disposable plastic bag or perforated plastic sheet wraps.
- Exposure button/handle—cover with disposable tube-shaped plastic bag.

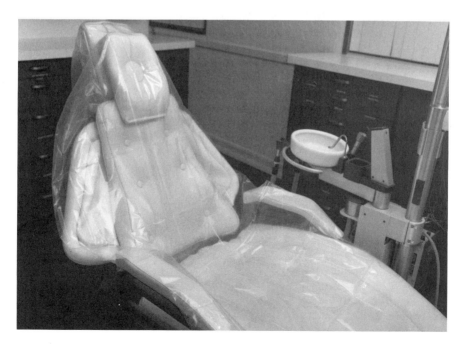

Fig. 39–1. Full chair drape (Courtesy Perio Support Products, East Irvine, CA)

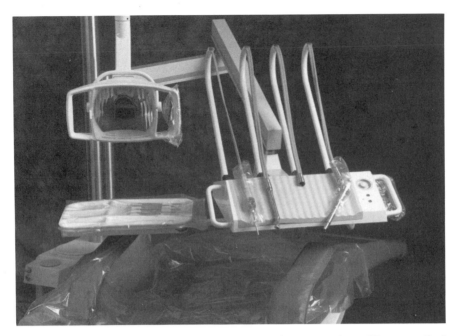

Fig. 39–2. Disposable sleeves for handpiece and water syringe (Courtesy Perio Support Products, East Irvine, CA)

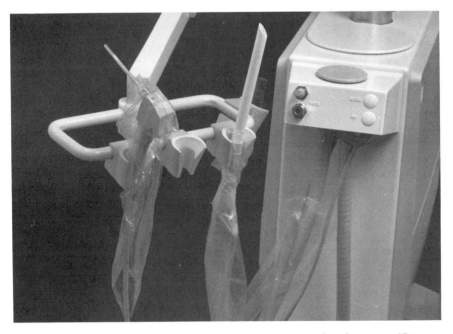

Fig. 39–3. Disposable tubing cover for air-water syringe and oral vacuum (Courtesy Perio Support Products, East Irvine, CA)

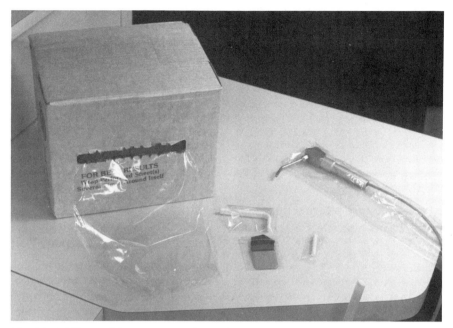

Fig. 39–4. Disposable wrap or perforated sheets for various applications (Courtesy Perio Support Products, East Irvine, CA)

- Cone/cylinder—cover with disposable tube-shaped plastic bag. *Note:* Use facial tissue to adjust exposure dial when exposing x-ray films.

Bracket and Instrument Trays

- Use disposable tray covers or liners on unit bracket tray and instrument tray(s). All metal and/or plastic instruments trays should be sterilized after each patient.

SEATING THE DENTAL PATIENT FOR OPERATIVE DENTISTRY

Materials Needed

- antimicrobial soap
- disposable towel(s)
- patient chart
- pen
- drape/neckchain/bib
- disposable oral vacuum tip

- disposable saliva ejector
- sterile handpiece(s) in pouch
- sterile basic instrument setup in pouch
- stethoscope/aneroid, mercury-type manometer
- appropriate tray setup
- protective eyewear
- face mask
- disposable gloves/gowns

The assistant's and operator's protective eyewear, face mask, gloves, and disposable gowns should be available for immediate use.

Once the operatory has been disinfected and the appropriate barriers placed, the patient is escorted from the reception/waiting room to the operatory by the assistant. Once the patient is in the operatory, the assistant will:

1. Adjust the height of the chair so that the patient can easily be seated.

2. Invite the patient to be seated. *Note:* It is suggested that an area be set aside for the patient's coat or wrap. Do not allow the patient to leave personal articles in the reception or waiting room. There should be a designated area/place in the operatory, in view of the patient, for his or her handbag or other valuables.

3. The patient is in an upright position for placement of drape and/or bib and should remain in this position until the operator is seated. If the patient is wearing lipstick, offer a tissue, and ask the patient to remove lipstick.

4. At this time, the patient's health history is reviewed, and any changes should be recorded on the patient's chart. Refer to Chapter 28, *Dental and Medical Emergencies.*

5. Vital signs are taken and recorded on the patient's chart.

6. Next, the assistant will wash hands for fifteen seconds using an antimicrobial soap and cool water. Then rinse hands in cold water, dry with disposable paper towel.

7. Don gloves and slightly rinse in cool water. Dry.

8. With gloved hands, sterile items such as the saliva ejector, air/water syringe and oral vacuum tip are placed. The dental handpiece(s) are removed from the sterilizing pouch and attached to the appropriate hose(s)/tubing.

9. Sterile instruments or tray setup are selected and placed according to the system used for instrumentation.

10. Should the basic setup of the mouth mirror, explorer, periodontal probe, and cotton pliers be sterilized in a separate pouch, they may be removed and placed on the tray at this time.

Positioning the Patient

Generally, it will be the operator who will place the patient in the supine position.

Dental chairs that are automatically programmed for positioning the chair, tend to place the patient into the supine position too quickly. This could frighten the patient. Therefore, the patient should be slowly lowered into the supine position.

In the supine position, the patient's legs and head should be at the same level. The patient should be positioned in the chair with little bending at the waist. Patients who are placed with their legs higher than their head are not considered to be in a supine position. Placing a patient for a long time in such a position is not recommended, causing a numbness of the feet and legs.

Once the patient is seated and the instruments are in place, the operator is notified.

1. Upon entering the room the operator greets the patient.
2. Reviews the patient's chart, and checks any notation made on the chart by the assistant.
3. Discusses the procedure to be done.
4. Washes and dries hands.
5. Dons protective eyewear, face mask, disposable gown/jacket, and gloves.
6. Positions him or herself on the operator's stool.
7. Places patient in supine position. It is important that the dental patient be in proper position with the patient's oral cavity centered in the vicinity of the operator's lap and at the height of the operator's elbows. The operator must have access and visibility in order to work in all areas within the oral cavity.
8. Once the patient and dental team are properly seated, the dental operating light

is brought into position. *Note:* When turning the dental light on, the beam of light is first directed toward the patient's chest, then directed toward the patient's oral cavity. Care must be taken to avoid directing the light beam into the patient's eyes.

9. The dental team starts the dental treatment.

COMPLETION OF DENTAL TREATMENT

When the dental procedure has been completed, services rendered must be entered on the patient's chart. The operator will direct the assistant to record these, then, the assistant will

1. Wash gloved hands with antimicrobial soap and water, rinse, and dry. Remove gloves. Refer to Chapter 25, *Principles of Personal Protection in Dentistry.*
2. With pen, enter on patient's chart services rendered.
3. Record all instructions given the patient on the patient's chart.

The operator will

1. Return patient to upright position.
2. Excuse him/herself and proceed to wash gloved hands with antimicrobial soap and water, rinse, and dry. Remove gloves and gown, and place in appropriate waste receptacle.
3. Thank the patient and leave the operatory.

DISMISSING THE PATIENT

The assistant will

1. Remove drape or bib. Set aside.
2. Lower the chair to height that will enable the patient to comfortably leave the chair.

3. Raise arm of chair, and assist the patient out of the chair. Check to make certain the patient has gathered any personal items.
4. Escort patient to the reception desk.

CLEANING UP THE OPERATORY

After each patient the assistant will remove barriers, disinfect needed surfaces, then replace barriers. Surfaces that are not barriered must be disinfected.

The assistant will

1. Put on utility gloves.
2. Remove all barriers, and place in appropriate waste receptacle. Blood- and/or saliva-contaminated items must be placed in a suitably labeled BIOHAZARD receptacle.
3. Remove dental instruments from operatory to the sterilization area for further care. Refer to Chapter 26, *Infection Control in the Dental Setting.*
4. Spray surface disinfectant on those surfaces that were not barriered, and wipe with sponge or disposable paper towel, using a frictional wiping action to remove debris.
5. Once the disinfection process is completed, with utility gloves on, wash, rinse, and dry your hands. Spray gloves with an approved disinfectant. Hang to dry.
6. Replace barriers. Operatory is now prepared for the next patient.

SUGGESTED ACTIVITIES

- Practice preparing dental operatory and/or dental chair and unit using appropriate spray-wipe-spray procedures.
- Practice placing appropriate barriers on dental chair and unit.

REVIEW

1. Discuss the daily routine required in preparing the dental operatory. _____

   _____

   _____

2. What is the advantage of using barriers?_____

   _____

3. Barriers to be effective must be impervious to _____

   _____

4. What is the correct position of the patient's head and legs in the supine position? _____

   _____

5. What is the proper position of the patient's oral cavity in relationship to the operator?

   a. _____

   b. _____

6. What procedure should be followed when turning on the dental operating light? _____

   _____

7. What is the procedure the assistant should follow when recording services rendered on the patient's chart?

   a. _____

   b. _____

   c. _____

8. Give the procedure the assistant should follow when cleaning the operatory after each patient.

a. _____

b. _____

c. _____

d. _____

e. _____

f. _____

Chapter 40: Principles and Application of Oral Evacuation

OBJECTIVES:

After studying this chapter, the student will be able to:
- Discuss the washed-field technique.
- State the advantages for using oral vacuum/high-velocity suction.
- List the parts of the oral vacuum system.
- Demonstrate the correct thumb-to-nose and modified pen grasp hand positions.
- Discuss the basic rules for oral vacuum tip placement.
- Demonstrate the correct oral vacuum tip placement for maxillary and mandibular posterior teeth.
- Demonstrate the correct oral vacuum tip placement for maxillary and mandibular anterior teeth.

INTRODUCTION

Today, most dental handpieces operate at speeds higher than 150,000 rpm and require the use of a water coolant to reduce the frictional heat that is produced during the cutting and shaping of tooth tissues. The use of water as a coolant in operative dentistry is called the *washed-field technique*.

Because a considerable amount of water is released from the handpiece during this procedure, a *high-velocity suction* or *oral vacuum system* is needed. This system provides a quick and efficient method for the removal of water and debris from the oral cavity.

THE ORAL VACUUM SYSTEM

Parts of the Oral Vacuum System

- *Removable oral vacuum tip*—plastic or metal, open-ended cylinder, figure 40–1.
- *Handle*—where tip is inserted and the on/off control dial or button is located, figure 40–2.
- *Hose*—flexible tubing that connects the handle to the suction or vacuum source of the unit, figure 40–3.

The universal oral vacuum tip is slightly curved in the middle, and the tip ends are beveled. One end of the beveled tip is for use on the anterior maxillary and mandibular teeth,

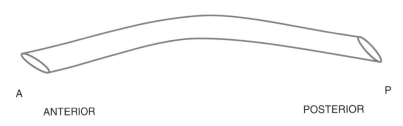

A   P

ANTERIOR   POSTERIOR

Fig. 40–1. Oral vacuum tip

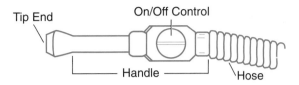

Fig. 40–2. Parts of the oral vacuum system

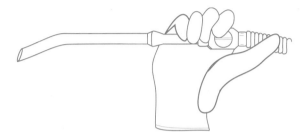

Fig. 40–3. Thumb-to-nose grasp for holding oral vacuum with tip in place

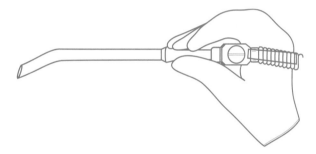

Fig. 40–4. Modified pen grasp for holding oral vacuum with tip in place

whereas the opposite end is used for the maxillary and mandibular posterior teeth.

To identify which end of the oral vacuum tip is anterior or posterior, the bend in the tip may be used as a guide. If the beveled end of the tip faces toward the floor, the tip is used for the maxillary and mandibular anterior teeth, designated as *A*, figure 40–1. For the maxillary and mandibular posterior teeth, the bevel will be directed upward, designated as *P*, figure 40–1.

The hose/tubing must be flexible and long enough to allow access to each quadrant or area within the oral cavity.

Hand Grasp for Oral Vacuum Tip

The two methods for holding the oral vacuum tip/handle/hose include the *thumb-to-nose grasp*, figure 40–3, and the *modified pen grasp*, figure 40–4. The thumb-to-nose grasp is used for the maxillary and mandibular posterior teeth. The thumb-to-nose grasp is very effective in controlling the oral vacuum tip when used for retracting the patient's cheek and tongue. The modified pen grasp is used when working on the anterior maxillary and mandibular teeth.

Advantages of the Oral Vacuum System

1. Allows for rapid removal of oral fluids, water, and debris from oral cavity.
2. Oral vacuum tip may be used in the retraction of tongue or cheek.
3. Allows the operator greater visibility with proper placement of oral vacuum tip.
4. Reduces chair time, because patient can remain in the supine position without having to be placed in an upright position for rinsing and emptying mouth.

Disadvantages of the Oral Vacuum System

1. The oral vacuum may be noisy when on.
2. If oral vacuum tip is too close to oral tissues, it may accidentally grab them and cause serious damage.
3. May trigger gag reflex should the tip touch the soft palate.
4. Improper placement of tip may interfere with operator's access and visibility.

BASIC RULES FOR ORAL VACUUM TIP PLACEMENT

An assistant working with a right-handed operator will hold the oral vacuum tip/handle with the right hand, while the left hand is free to hold the air/water syringe or transfer instruments. (The procedure is reversed when working with a left-handed operator.)

1. The beveled portion of the oral vacuum tip should be parallel to either the buccal or lingual surfaces of the teeth.
2. The tip should be as close to the tooth as possible and slightly distal of the tooth being prepared.
3. The middle of the tip opening should be even with the occlusal surface, figure 40–5. Care must be taken not to draw the water coolant away from the bur or handpiece before it has a chance to cool the tooth.

4. The oral vacuum tip should be in position before the operator places the handpiece and mouth mirror in the oral cavity. The relationship between the mouth mirror and oral vacuum tip will depend on the quadrant or teeth being prepared.

The general operating zone for the operator is the 9 to 11 o'clock position and the 2 to 3 o'clock for the assistant. Refer to Chapter 38.

Quadrant	Oral Vacuum Tip Placement Chart
Maxillary right	Adjacent to the lingual surfaces of posterior tooth being prepared, figure 40–6.
Maxillary left	Adjacent to the buccal or facial surfaces of the posterior tooth being prepared, figure 40–7.
Mandibular right	Adjacent to the lingual surface and slightly posterior to the tooth being prepared, figure 40–8. Oral vacuum tip may aid in retraction of the tongue.
Mandibular left	Placed along the buccal or facial surfaces of the teeth. The tip will aid in the retraction of the cheek, figure 40–9.

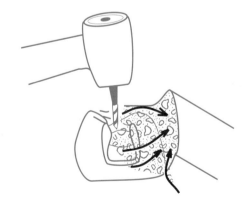

Fig. 40–5. Correct placement of oral vacuum tip

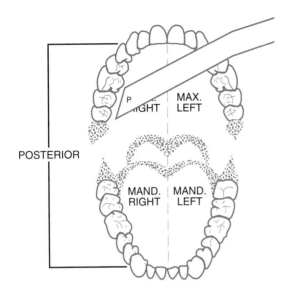

Fig. 40–6. Oral vacuum placement for maxillary right quadrant

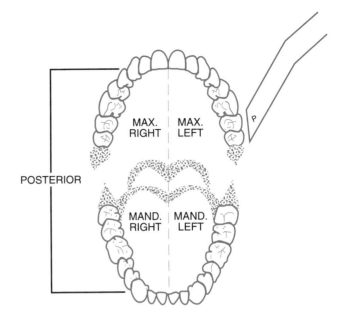

Fig. 40–7. Oral vacuum placement for maxillary left quadrant

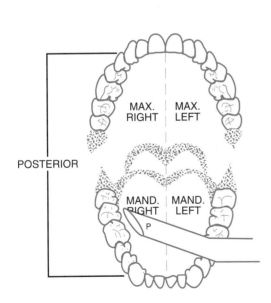

Fig. 40–8. Oral vacuum placement for mandibular right quadrant

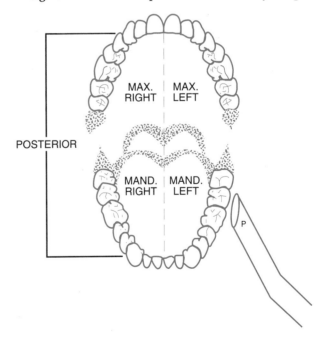

Fig. 40–9. Oral vacuum placement for mandibular left quadrant

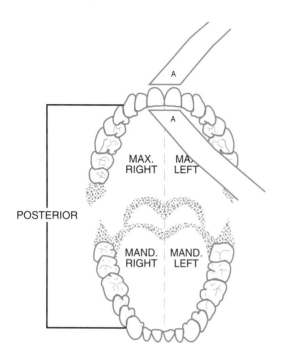

Fig. 40–10. Oral vacuum placement for maxillary anterior teeth, facial/labial and lingual approach

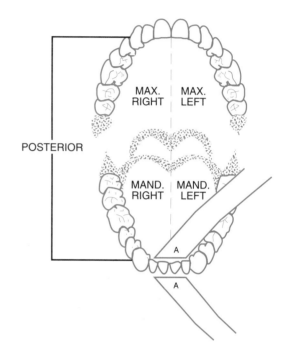

Fig. 40–11. Oral vacuum placement for mandibular anterior teeth, facial/labial and lingual approach

Maxillary Anterior

Facial/labial approach — Adjacent to the lingual surface near the incisal edge of tooth being prepared, figure 40–10.

Lingual approach — Same as for the facial/labial approach, figure 40–10.

Mandibular Anterior

Facial/labial approach — Adjacent to the lingual surface of the tooth being prepared, figure 40–11.

Lingual approach — Adjacent to lingual surface of the tooth being prepared, with tip resting in the vestibule by the lower lip and surfaces of the anterior teeth, figure 40–11.

SUGGESTED ACTIVITIES

• Practice oral evacuation while in groups of three. One serves as the patient, another as the operator and the third as the chairside assistant.

• Using the air-water syringe, the operator will spray water on a tooth of the patient. The chairside assistant will evacuate the patient's mouth following the basic rules for oral vacuum tip placement.

1. What is meant by the *washed-field* technique? _____

_____

2. Which hand grasp is used for the posterior maxillary and mandibular teeth?

_____

3. State the basic rules for oral vacuum tip placement.

   a. _____

   b. _____

   c. _____

   d. _____

4. State the position of the oral vacuum tip for the maxillary right quadrant.

_____

5. State the position of the oral vacuum tip for the maxillary left quadrant.

_____

6. State the position of the oral vacuum tip for the mandibular right quadrant.

_____

7. State the position of the oral vacuum tip for the mandibular left quadrant.

_____

8. State the position of the oral vacuum tip for the maxillary anterior teeth, facial and lingual approach.

_____

9. State the position of the oral vacuum tip for the mandibular anterior teeth, facial and lingual approach.

_____

OBJECTIVES:

After studying this chapter, the student will be able to:
- Discuss the chairside assistant's role in the retrieval and delivery of hand instruments.
- Cite the basic rules for instrument transfer.
- State the advantages for using a fulcrum when working in the oral cavity.
- Discuss the reasons for using the pen grasp, modified pen grasp, palm grasp and palm-thumb grasp.
- Demonstrate instrument transfer following the sequence; approach, retrieval and delivery.

INTRODUCTION

There are several ways in which instruments may be transferred between assistant and operator. In four-handed, sit-down dentistry, the most frequently used instrument transfer involves the retrieval and delivery of instrument(s) into and out of the operator's hand during a dental procedure.

The transfer of instruments between operator and assistant takes place in the transfer zone near the patient's chin. Effective instrument transfer should involve little movement of the operator's fingers or eyes. A smooth transfer of instruments occurs when the chairside assistant is able to anticipate the operator's needs.

To aid the assistant in the delivery of the instruments, it is best to identify the fingers and thumb of the hand. The *thumb* is referred to by the letter *T*, and the fingers are numbered; *index finger (1)*, *middle finger (2)*, the *ring finger (3)*, and *little finger (4)*, figure 41–1.

If the operator is right-handed, the assistant's left hand is used to transfer and retrieve instruments. This frees the assistant's right hand to use the oral vacuum or for retraction. For a left-handed operator the procedure is reversed.

In instrument transfer, the chairside assistant will select the correct instrument and hold it in his/her hand with the appropriate fingers until the operator signals the exchange. The assistant will remove the used instrument from the operator's hand, and place the new instrument.

To hold the instrument to be delivered, the thumb, index (1), and middle (2) fingers work together to deliver the instrument, while the little finger (4) is used in the retrieval of the

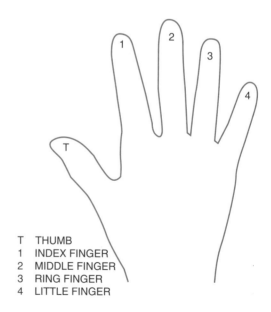

T	THUMB
1	INDEX FINGER
2	MIDDLE FINGER
3	RING FINGER
4	LITTLE FINGER

Fig. 41–1. Hand with fingers identified by numbers

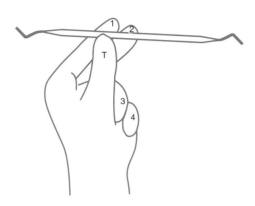

Fig. 41–2. Hand position for instrument transfer

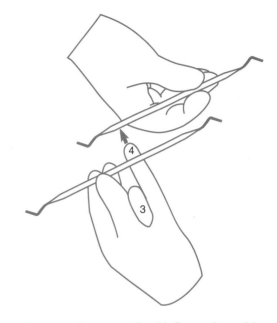

Fig. 41–3. The approach with fingers in position

instrument from the operator's right hand. For greater stability in retrieval and delivery of an instrument, fingers 3 and 4 may be used.

BASIC RULES FOR INSTRUMENT TRANSFER

1. Hold instrument with thumb (T) and fingers 1 and 2, figure 42-2.
2. Hold instrument close to the end opposite from the one that is to be used by the operator.
3. Hold instrument with working end in proper operating position for the tooth being treated.
4. Working end of hand instrument or bur in handpiece should be directed downward for mandibular arch and upward for maxillary arch.
5. Hold instrument to be passed in a position parallel to the instrument held by the operator. Instruments should be as close to one another as possible, but without becoming entangled during instrument exchange.

SEQUENCE FOR INSTRUMENT TRANSFER

A system for the passing and receiving of instruments may include the following movements: (1) the approach, (2) the retrieval, (3) and the delivery.

1. *Approach.* Finger 4 is extended, figure 41–3, and the instrument is grasped by the handle (shaft) at the end opposite to that held by the operator, figure 41–4.
2. *Retrieval.* Finger 4 is closed around the instrument handle and rests between fingers 3 and 4. As the unwanted instrument is lifted from the operator's hand, the assistant lifts the new instrument to a position slightly above the level of the operator's hand, figure 41–5.
3. *Delivery.* The assistant lowers the new instrument into the operator's fingers; the delivery is complete when the operator

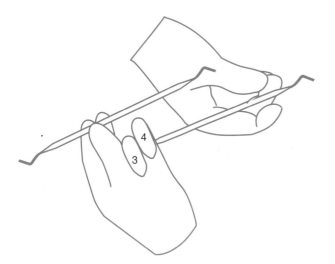

Fig. 41–4. Position of fingers for removal of instrument

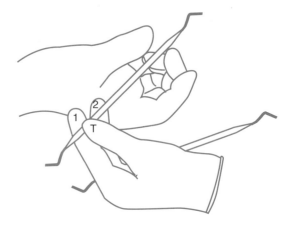

Fig. 41–5. Delivery of new instrument into operator's hand

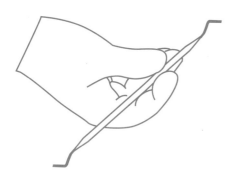

Fig. 41–6. Instrument retained, fingers closed

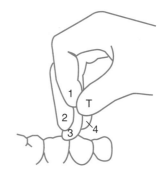

Fig. 41–7. Finger rest position

grasps the instrument, figure 41–6. *Note:* If the same two instruments are to be transferred a second time, immediately reposition the retrieved instrument from the little finger into the delivery finger position. One-handed instrument transfer is primarily used for hand instruments, the dental handpiece and the air-water syringe. In the transfer of the air-water syringe, the syringe is held by the nozzle tip, and the handle is delivered into the operator's hand.

INSTRUMENT GRASPS

The first requirement when working within the oral cavity is to establish control of the dental instrument or handpiece. This is accomplished by the use of a *finger rest* that provides support or a point of rest for the fingers on the tooth surface, figure 41–7.

The finger rest serves as a **fulcrum**, or base of support, for the fingers and allows the hand to move or rotate. The pad of the ring finger (3) is positioned on a given surface of a tooth, prefer-

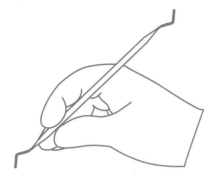

Fig. 41–8. Modified pen grasp

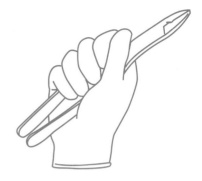

Fig. 41–9. Palm grasp

ably in the same arch and as close to the tooth being treated as possible, figure 41–7.

Finger rests and fulcrums, when used properly, will provide the needed stability to control the action of the instrument or dental handpiece, thereby preventing injury to the patient's oral tissues.

The most common instrument grasps used in operative dentistry are the modified pen grasp, palm grasp, and palm-thumb grasp.

Modified Pen Grasp. The conventional pen grasp is used as a foundation for the modified pen grasp. In the conventional pen grasp, the instrument is held with the thumb and index finger and the side of the middle finger.

With the modified pen grasp, the instrument is held with the same fingers, except that the pad of the middle finger (2) is held against the shank of the dental instrument. The ring finger acts as the finger rest and helps to hold and guide the movement of the instrument, figure 41–8.

Palm Grasp. The handle of the instrument is held in the palm of the hand, and fingers grasp the handle of the instrument, figure 41–9. The palm grasp is used with surgical and other types of forceps.

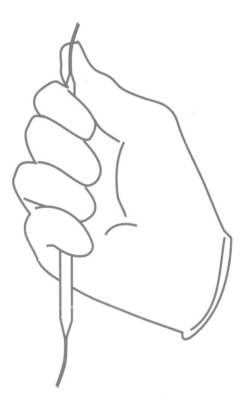

Fig. 41–10. Palm-thumb grasp

Palm-Thumb Grasp. The instrument is held firmly in the palm of the hand with the four fingers grasping the handle while the thumb is extended upward from the palm, figure 41–10. This grasp is used with instruments having a straight shank and blade, such as the straight chisel or wedelstaedt.

SUGGESTED ACTIVITIES

• Work in pairs; one will serve as the assistant, the other as the operator. Using the sequence of instrument transfer, each student will practice passing and receiving instruments.

REVIEW

1. How do the thumb and fingers function in the delivery of an instrument?

   _____

   _____

   _____

2. Name the three steps involved in the passing and receiving of instruments. Briefly explain each step.

   a. _____

   b. _____

   c. _____

3. Give the basic rules for instrument transfer.

   a. _____

   b. _____

   c. _____

   d. _____

   e. _____

4. Define the term *finger rest*. _____

_____

5. Define the term *fulcrum*. _____

_____

6. What are the three instrument grasps used to hold the various dental instruments.

a. _____

b. _____

c. _____

Chapter 42: Use and Care of the Aspirating Syringe

INTRODUCTION

Dental syringes used for intraoral injections (local **anesthesia**) are available in metal and plastic.

Two basic types of metal syringe are the conventional, or *nonaspirating syringe* and the *aspirating syringe*. The aspirating syringe is the one recommended for use in dentistry as part of the standard of care guidelines.

ASPIRATING SYRINGE

The aspirating syringe is designed to allow the operator to check the placement of the needle in order to determine whether or not the needle has entered or penetrated a blood vessel. If the needle has entered a blood vessel, a slight amount of blood may appear in the cartridge solution. Should this occur, the needle is withdrawn, repositioned, and tested again until there is evidence that the needle is no longer in the blood vessel. The injection is then completed. The use of an aspirating syringe is for the safety and comfort of the patient.

A plastic autoclavable aspirating syringe is available and is made like the metal syringe. There is a single-use disposable-reusable syringe. The ring mechanism is reusable, but the rest of the syringe is disposable.

Parts of the Aspirating Syringe

The parts of an aspirating syringe, include the following, figure 42–1.

- *Thumb ring*—for placement of thumb.
- *Finger grip/bar*—supports the index and middle fingers as the anesthetic solution is introduced into the oral tissues.
- *Syringe barrel*—holds the anesthetic cartridge.
- *Piston rod*—used to push down the silicone rubber plunger of the anesthetic cartridge.
- *Harpoon*—the barbed tip, positioned at the end of the piston rod that engages the silicone rubber plunger in the cartridge. The

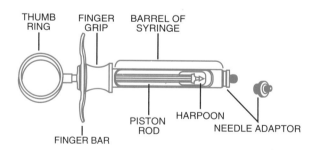

Fig. 42–1. Parts of an aspirating syringe (Courtesy Miltex Dental Instruments, Lake Success, NY)

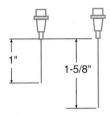

Fig. 42–2. Length of dental needles

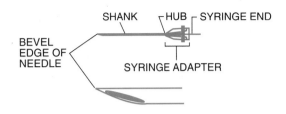

Fig. 42–3. Parts of a dental needle

harpoon allows the piston rod to be withdrawn as the anesthetic is injected (forced) through the needle into the tissues.
- *Needle adaptor*—where the needle is attached to the syringe.

NEEDLE

The needle is used to direct the local anesthetic solution from the anesthetic cartridge into the tissues surrounding the needle tip. Most dental needles used today are made of stainless steel and are presterilized and disposable.

The selection of a needle for use is based on the type of injection to be given. Two factors that must be considered are the diameter, or gauge, and the length of the needle. The internal opening of the needle, through which the anesthetic solution flows, is called the **lumen**.

The needles used in dentistry range from 25 gauge to 30 gauge. The smaller the gauge number, the larger the lumen of the needle; the larger the gauge number, the smaller the lumen. The 25 gauge needle is recommended for intraoral use.

Dental needles are available in two lengths; long (1-5/8") or short (1"), figure 42–2. The long needle is indicated when the injection requires the penetration of several thicknesses of soft tissue, such as with a nerve block. Short needles are used for injections that require the penetration of only the surface soft tissue (infiltration).

Parts of a Needle, figure 42–3

- *Bevel*—the slanted tip of the needle that will penetrate the soft tissues.
- *Shank*—the length of the needle from the hub to the tip of the bevel.
- *Syringe adaptor*—the part of the needle that screws onto the syringe and is either metal or plastic.
- *Hub*—the part of the needle that attaches to the syringe adaptor.
- *Syringe end of the needle*—the end of the needle that punctures the diaphragm of the glass cartridge.

Care of the Dental Needle

1. Never use a needle for more than one patient.
2. The needle should be changed after three injections for the same patient. Each time the needle penetrates the soft tissue, it becomes a little duller. Therefore, after the second or third injection with the same disposable needle, it is recommended that the needle be replaced. Failure to change the needle may result in injury to the patient's tissues and cause postoperative pain.
3. A needle must be covered with its protective cap whenever the needle is not in use. See *Procedure for Recapping Needle*, page 391.

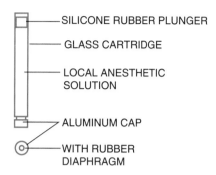

SILICONE RUBBER PLUNGER

GLASS CARTRIDGE

LOCAL ANESTHETIC SOLUTION

ALUMINUM CAP

WITH RUBBER DIAPHRAGM

Fig. 42–4. Parts of the anesthetic cartridge

ANESTHETIC CARTRIDGE

The *anesthetic cartridge* is a glass cylinder that contains the anesthetic solution.

Parts of an Anesthetic Cartridge, figure 42–4

- *Glass cartridge*—that contains the anesthetic solution.
- *Silicone rubber plunger*—located at the harpoon end of the cartridge. An acceptable silicone rubber plunger in the cartridge is slightly indented.
- *Aluminum cap*—located on the opposite end of the cartridge from the silicone plunger. It fits tightly around the neck of the glass cartridge and holds the thin rubber diaphragm in position.
- *Rubber diaphragm*—the rubber diaphragm located under the aluminum cap at the end of the cartridge and that will be penetrated by the syringe end of the needle.

Color-coding (different colors) of the cartridge plunger is no longer used to identify the drug content of the cartridge. The selection of a cartridge should be based on the information printed on the side of each cartridge.

Recognizing a Damaged Anesthetic Cartridge

Bubbles in the Cartridge. Small bubbles in the solution are bubbles of nitrogen gas and are considered harmless to the patient. A large bubble present may cause the plunger to extend beyond the end of the cartridge. Such cartridges should be discarded.

Extruded Plunger. An *extruded plunger* means that something has happened to the cartridge. The cartridge may have been frozen, causing the solution inside to expand, and forcing the plunger past its normal position.

Also, a cartridge with an extruded plunger and with no bubble(s) indicates that cartridge has been stored too long in a chemical disinfectant and that some of the solution has entered the cartridge. Such cartridges should be discarded.

Burning Sensation upon Injection. A burning sensation during the injection may be the result of the cartridge becoming contaminated with disinfecting solution.

Corroded Aluminum Cap. A corroded aluminum cap indicates that the anesthetic cartridge has been immersed too long in a disinfecting solution. Aluminum-sealed cartridges should be disinfected with either 91% isopropyl alcohol or 70% ethyl alcohol. A corroded aluminum cap will leave a white deposit on the aluminum cap. Such cartridges must be discarded.

Rust on Aluminum Cap. Rust on the aluminum cap indicates that at least one cartridge has broken in the tin container. This will cause the tin in the container to rust, leaving a red deposit on the cartridge. These cartridges must be discarded.

COMMON PROBLEMS RELATED TO HANDLING SYRINGES

Leakage of Anesthetic Solution

Leakage of the solution during injection indicates that the needle did not penetrate the center

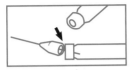

Fig. 42–5. Off-centered needle (Courtesy Astra Pharmaceutical Products, Westborough, MA)

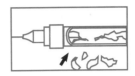

Fig. 42–6. Broken cartridge (Courtesy Astra Pharmaceutical Products, Westborough, MA)

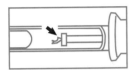

Fig. 42–7. Bent harpoon (Courtesy Astra Pharmaceutical Products, Westborough, MA)

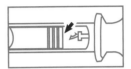

Fig. 42–8. Disengagement of harpoon from plunger during aspiration (Courtesy Astra Pharmaceutical Products, Westborough, MA)

of the rubber diaphragm. An off-centered needle will prevent the diaphragm from sealing itself around the needle. Therefore, some solution may leak from the cartridge between the needle and diaphragm into the patient's mouth, figure 42–5.

Broken Cartridges

A cartridge that is cracked, chipped, or damaged in any way should not be used. The pressure exerted on the cartridge during the injection may cause the cartridge to shatter inside the patient's mouth, figure 42–6.

Bent Harpoon

The harpoon should be sharp and straight. A bent harpoon will puncture the rubber plunger off-center, causing it to rotate as it travels down the cartridge. This could cause the cartridge to break, figure 42–7.

Disengagement of Harpoon from Plunger during Aspiration

Aspiration should be completed by gently pulling the plunger in a backward motion. A

forceful action is not necessary and may cause the harpoon to become disengaged from the plunger, figure 42–8.

Taking Care of the Anesthetic Cartridge

1. The anesthetic cartridge must NEVER be used on more than one patient.
2. Do not use cartridges beyond the expiration date indicated by the manufacturer.
3. Cartridges should be stored at room temperature.
4. Cartridges should not be warmed before use.

Disinfecting the Anesthetic Cartridge

Materials Needed

- aspirating syringe
- disposable needle
- disinfectant solution (91% isopropyl or 70% ethyl alcohol)
- 2" × 2" dental sponge

Anesthetic cartridges can be stored in their original containers. When the cartridge is

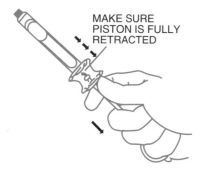

Fig. 42–9. Retraction of piston for placement of cartridge (Courtesy Astra Pharmaceutical Products, Westborough, MA)

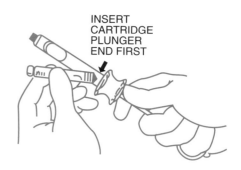

Fig. 42–10. Inserting cartridge (Courtesy Astra Pharmaceutical Products, Westborough, MA)

removed for use, the rubber diaphragm should be wiped with a 2″ × 2″ sponge moistened with 91% isopropyl alcohol or 70% ethyl alcohol. Prior to loading the syringe, the cap end of the cartridge must be wiped with a 2″ × 2″ alcohol moistened sponge.

LOADING THE ASPIRATING SYRINGE

The procedure is for a right-handed individual. (Use opposite hand if left-handed.)

Preparing the Aspirating Syringe

1. With washed, gloved hands, select the appropriate needle for the type of injection to be administered.
2. Select correct disinfected anesthetic cartridge to be used for the given dental procedure.
3. Remove the sterile syringe from the autoclave pouch/bag.
4. Hold syringe with left hand, and use the thumb ring to retract the piston rod to its full position, figure 42–9.
5. With the piston fully retracted, place the cartridge into the barrel of the syringe, plunger end first, figure 42–10.

6. With moderate pressure, gently push the piston rod forward until the harpoon is firmly engaged in the plunger, figure 42–11. *Do not* hit the piston rod in an effort to engage the harpoon, as this may cause the glass cartridge to crack or shatter.
7. Place needle on the syringe. Remove protective cap from the end of needle. Screw the needle onto the syringe. *Note:* A metal-hubbed needle has a threaded hub and can be screwed onto the end of the syringe. If a plastic-hubbed needle is used, the needle is pushed onto the threaded tip of the syringe while constantly turning the needle. Do not screw the needle tightly against the end of the syringe. Leave at least the thickness of a fingernail between the two. This allows the operator to adjust the bevel of the needle as needed.
8. Carefully remove the protection cap from the needle. Next, test the syringe by expelling a few drops of solution to test for proper flow of solution, figure 42–12.
9. If a second cartridge is required for the dental procedure on the same patient, the cartridge is removed. See *Disassembling the Syringe*, steps 1–3. Because the needle

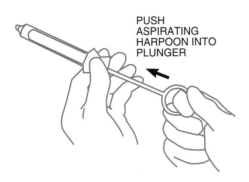

Fig. 42–11. Engaging harpoon (Courtesy Astra Pharmaceutical Products, Westborough, MA)

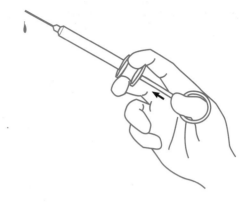

Fig. 42–12. Testing flow of anesthetic (Courtesy Astra Pharmaceutical Products, Westborough, MA)

is already on the syringe, the second disinfected cartridge is placed directly into the barrel of the syringe.

10. While holding the syringe firmly with the left hand, the operator will give a quick, sharp blow to the end of the thumb ring with the right hand. This will engage the harpoon into the plunger. If the operator simply pushes the cartridge into position as for loading the cartridge the first time, the harpoon will not penetrate the plunger. This will allow the anesthetic solution to be injected through the needle but will not allow the operator to retract the plunger and aspirate.

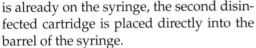

RECAPPING THE NEEDLE

After the injection, the syringe is removed from the patient's mouth. The needle should be capped immediately. The procedure recommended by most state safety and health agencies is termed the *scoop* technique.

The operator should not hold the protective cap while recapping the needle. The cap should be placed on a table or counter.

1. Immediately after removal of syringe from the patient's mouth, replace protective cap on needle.

2. Using the scoop technique, slide the uncapped needle into the needle cap that has been placed on the table/counter, figure 42–13.

3. The needle must be safe within the cap before you attempt to pick up the capped needle.

4. Never place an uncapped needle on a table or countertop. An uncapped needle must never be allowed to touch *anything* before or after the injection.

UNLOADING THE ASPIRATING SYRINGE

1. Pull the cartridge away from the needle with the thumb and forefinger as the piston is retracted. This will disengage the harpoon from the plunger, figure 42–14.

2. Invert syringe, and allow the cartridge to fall freely from the barrel. Discard cartridge in the appropriate container, figure 42–15.

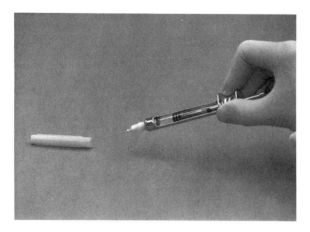

Fig. 42–13. Scooping technique for recapping needle after injection

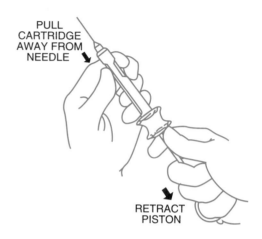

Fig. 42–14. Retraction of piston for cartridge removal (Courtesy Astra Pharmaceutical Products, Westborough, MA)

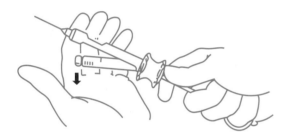

Fig. 42–15. Removal of cartridge from syringe (Courtesy Astra Pharmaceutical Products, Westborough, MA)

3. Carefully remove the capped needle. Should a syringe have its own needle adaptor, care must be taken not to remove the adaptor with the needle.
4. After removing the capped needle from the syringe, the needle is placed in a Sharps container for proper disposal.

TAKING CARE OF THE ASPIRATING SYRINGE

1. After each use, the syringe must be thoroughly washed, rinsed, and dried. The syringe must be free of any anesthetic solution, saliva, or other foreign matter.
2. Place the clean syringe in a labeled autoclavable pouch or bag. The syringe is now ready to be autoclaved. *Note:* It is recommended that after a syringe has been used and autoclaved five times, it should be disassembled and all threaded parts lightly lubricated. Reassemble the syringe, place in a labeled pouch and autoclave for future use.

SUGGESTED ACTIVITIES

- Practice loading the aspirating syringe following the step-by-step procedure.
- Practice unloading the anesthetic syringe following the step-by-step procedure.

REVIEW

1. What is the advantage of using an aspirating syringe over a nonaspirating syringe? _____

    _____

2. Give the two factors that must be considered when selecting a needle.

    a. _____

    b. _____

3. What does the gauge number of a dental needle indicate? _____

    _____

4. When would a long needle be considered for an injection? _____

    _____

5. What procedure should be followed if a needle has been used for three injections for the same patient? Explain why. _____

    _____

    _____

6. What does an extruded plunger indicate? _____

    _____

    _____

7. What would cause an anesthetic solution to leak into the patient's mouth during an injection? _____

    _____

    _____

8. Give the suggested procedure for recapping a needle.

a. _____

_____

b. _____

_____

c. _____

_____

d. _____

_____

Chapter 43: Punching a Rubber Dam

OBJECTIVES:

After studying this chapter, the student will be able to:

- Select the armamentarium for both punching a rubber dam and clamp placement.
- Prepare a precut square of rubber dam for punching, using a ruler and pencil to mark the general guidelines.
- Punch a rubber dam for the maxillary and mandibular arch, following the detailed instructions.

INTRODUCTION

A *rubber dam* is a thin, flexible piece of rubber used to isolate one or more teeth during various dental procedures. The purpose for using a rubber dam is to provide an optimum working environment for the dentist and the assistant, while protecting the patient during operative procedures.

The advantages of using a rubber dam are: maintaining a clean, dry operative field, protecting the patient from inhaling debris during the dental procedure, and allowing the placement of various dental materials without the fear of moisture contamination.

There are also contraindications, such as partially erupted teeth, malaligned teeth, fixed bridge work, and patients who strongly resist the use of the rubber dam as might asthmatics or claustrophobics.

MATERIALS NEEDED

- ruler
- ballpoint pen
- rubber dam—precut
- rubber dam punch
- rubber dam clamps
- rubber dam forceps

INSTRUCTIONS

Selection of Rubber Dam Materials

Rubber Dam. Rubber dam material may be purchased in rolls or precut sheets. The roll of rubber dam is 6 inches wide and 18 feet long. It must be cut into the desired size. Precut dam is available in 5" × 5" sheets for children or 6" × 6" sheets for adults.

Rubber dam may be purchased in different weights (thicknesses): (1) light; (2) medium; (3) heavy; (4) extra heavy; and (5) special heavy.

The heavier rubber dam is more functional in that it is less likely to tear or be damaged by rotary instruments. It is also more effective in tissue retraction, but it is more difficult to place.

Rubber dam is available in various shades. Dark gray or green dam is used because of the color contrast between the dam and tooth structure, and because it reflects less light.

Rubber Dam Clamps. A *rubber dam clamp* is used to anchor or secure the rubber dam to a tooth. Clamps are available in various shapes and sizes and are classified according to their shape:

- *Winged clamp*—a clamp with engaging projections, figure 43–1
- *Wingless clamp*—a clamp without engaging projections, figure 43–2
- *Cervical clamp*—for Class V, facial restoration, figure 43–3

395

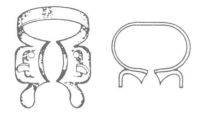

Fig. 43–1. Winged clamp

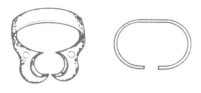

Fig. 43–2. Wingless clamp

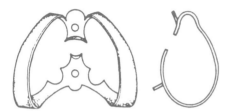

Fig. 43–3. Cervical clamp

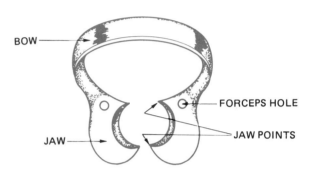

Fig. 43–4. Wingless rubber dam clamp

Parts of a wingless rubber dam clamp as seen in figure 43–4: (1) bow; (2) jaw(s); (3) forceps hole(s); and (4) jaw points.

Classification of clamps is also done according to the manufacturer, number, and use, figure 43–5. For example, classification of anterior and premolar (bicuspid) clamps would be as follows (an asterisk denotes the most commonly used clamp):

Manufacturer: S.S. White

- Number: 212; use: cervical clamp for Class V
- Number: 27; use: premolars and small third molars

Manufacturer: Ivory

- Number: 00*; use: lower incisors
- Number: 0; use: small premolars
- Number: 2*; use: general purpose—premolars
- Numbers: 51, 52, 53; use: cervical clamp

And for molar clamps, the classification would be as follows:

Manufacturer: S.S. White

- Numbers: 1A*, 2A*; use: deciduous molars
- Number: 26; use: general purpose—premolars
- Numbers: 30*, 31*; use: cervical clamp for gingival restorations

Manufacturer: Ivory

- Number: 3*; use: small molars
- Number: 4; use: cervical clamp for upper molars
- Number: 7*; use: lower molars
- Number: 8*; use: upper molars
- Number: 8A; use: partially erupted molars
- Numbers: 14, 14A*; use: partially erupted molars, larger than 8A

Rubber Dam Guide. The rubber dam must be punched properly. Therefore, it is recommended that some type of guide be used as an aid in

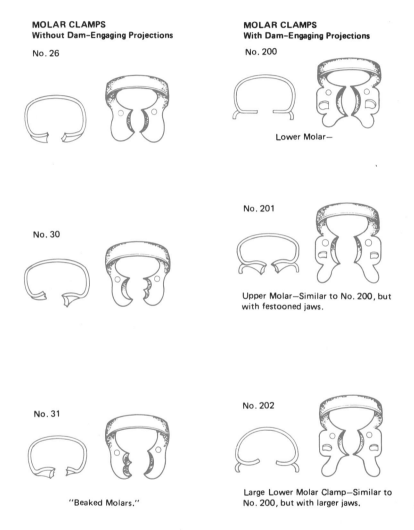

MOLAR CLAMPS
Without Dam-Engaging Projections

No. 26

No. 30

No. 31

"Beaked Molars."

MOLAR CLAMPS
With Dam-Engaging Projections

No. 200

Lower Molar—

No. 201

Upper Molar—Similar to No. 200, but with festooned jaws.

No. 202

Large Lower Molar Clamp—Similar to No. 200, but with larger jaws.

Fig. 43–5. Molar clamps and bicuspid clamps (Courtesy S.S. White Company, a division of the Pennwalt Corporation, Philadelphia, PA)

BICUSPID CLAMPS
With Dam-Engaging Projections

No. 206
(20793)

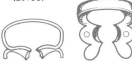

No. 27 provided with dam-engaging projections. For upper and lower bicuspids.

No. 207

Same as No. 206, but with flat jaws-

BICUSPID CLAMPS
Without Dam-Engaging Projections

No. 27

No. 29

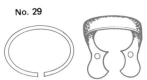

CERVICAL CLAMPS

No. 212
(20811)

 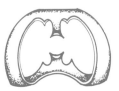

Dr. W. I. Ferrier's design of cervical clamp for labial cavities on anterior teeth.

LABIAL CLAMPS
With Dam–Engaging Projections

No. 210

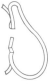 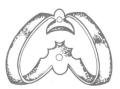

Useful on centrals and cuspids and also in some cases on bicuspids.

No. 211

 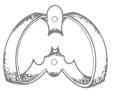

Universal for labial cavities on the twenty anterior teeth.

Fig. 43–5. (Continued)

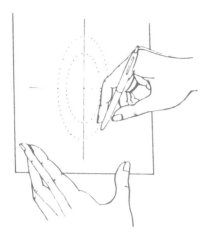

Fig. 43–6. Marking holes on the dam

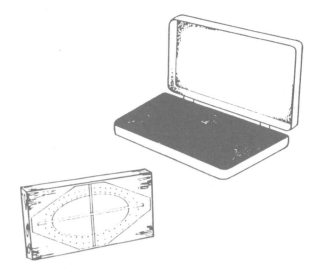

Fig. 43–7. Rubber dam stamp and inked pad

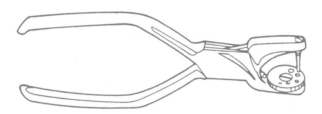

Fig. 43–8. Rubber dam punch

punching the dam. A plastic stencil or template with holes punched for the primary and permanent dentition can be used. The stencil is placed over the dam, and a pencil or pen is used for marking the holes on the dam, figure 43–6.

In the case of a patient with malposed teeth, it is suggested that a wax bite or study model be used as a guide.

The rubber dam stamp has holes for the teeth embossed (raised) on the surface of the stamp and requires the use of an inked pad to transfer the pattern to the rubber dam, figure 43–7.

The rubber dam punch is designed with an adjustable wheel or disc with five or six hole sizes. The punch must be adjusted to the proper hole size before the dam is punched. Care must be taken to align the punch point directly over the hole on the wheel table to be punched to prevent breaking or dulling the punch point, figure 43–8.

Rubber Dam Forceps. Rubber dam forceps, figure 43–9, carry the rubber dam clamp to and from the tooth. The forceps beaks will spread the jaws of the rubber dam clamp allowing the clamp to be positioned on the tooth. When in proper position, the handle lock is released and the forcep removed. In placing the clamp on the tooth, hold the forceps with a palm grasp, figures 43–10 and 43–11.

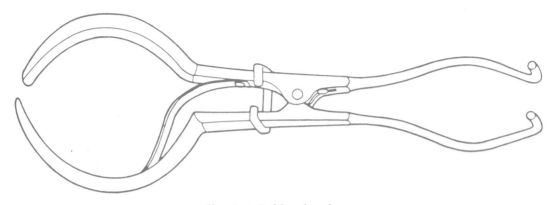

Fig. 43–9. Rubber dam forcep

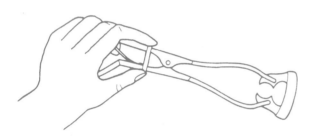

Fig. 43–10. Position of forcep for mandibular arch (*Note:* **The clamp is being placed with the left hand.**)

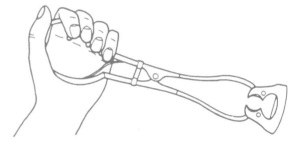

Fig. 43–11. Position of forcep for maxillary arch

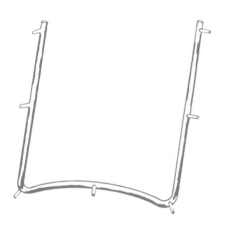

Fig. 43–12. Young frame

Rubber Dam Holders. The function of the *rubber dam holder* is to maintain the position of the dam on the patient's face while holding the dam in place. There are basically three types of holders used to hold the rubber dam in position—the Young Frame, the Woodbury, and the Ostby. The Ostby is used primarily for endodontics. The Young Frame is a metal frame that holds the rubber dam in place with projections that extend from the frame, figure 43–12. Woodbury uses two straps attached to two clip arms. One clip arm secures the rubber dam on one side of the face, while the straps are placed behind the patient's head, to the opposite side, where the other clip arm is fastened to the dam and length adjusted, figure 43–13.

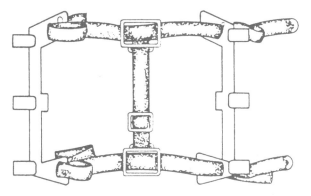

Fig. 43–13. Woodbury frame

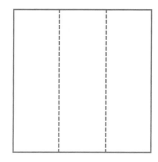

Fig. 43–14. Dam is divided into thirds.

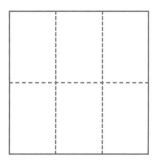

Fig. 43–15. Dam is divided in half.

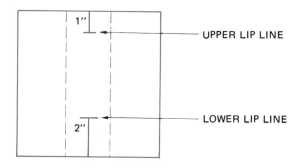

Fig. 43–16. The center of the dam is marked.

Rubber Dam Napkin. The *rubber dam napkin* is made from an absorbable material—paper, gauze, or flannel. The napkin is used for patient comfort and is placed underneath the rubber dam to prevent the dam material from coming into contact with the patient's skin.

PREPARING THE RUBBER DAM

Prepare the rubber dam for punching; use 6″ × 6″ precut squares. Mark the rubber dam, using a stencil, a rubber stamp, or a pencil and ruler as a guide. To mark the rubber dam with a pencil and ruler, use the following guidelines as a reference:

1. Divide the dam into thirds vertically, figure 43–14.
2. Divide the dam in half, horizontally, figure 43–15.
3. Mark the center of the dam. Measure 1 inch from the upper edge of the dam; this represents the upper lip line. Next, measure 2 inches from lower center of the dam; this represents the lower lip line, figure 43–16.
4. Punch holes equidistant from one another, approximately 3.5 mm. The distance from one hole to the next is equal to the distance from the middle of one tooth to the middle of the adjacent tooth. Work to be done on the maxillary arch requires that the central incisors be punched first, figure 43–17.

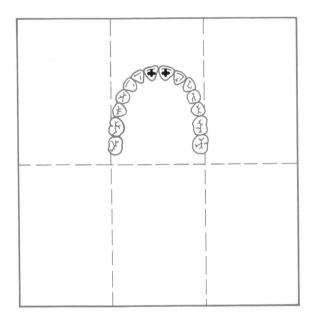

Fig. 43–17. The central incisors are first to be punched in the arch and are marked ++.

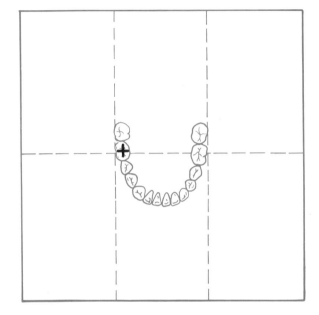

Fig. 43–18. Position of mandibular first molar

Maxillary Arch

1. Standard positions, punch 1 inch from center of top edge of the dam.
2. Variation in position:
   a. Distance from top edge of the dam should be increased for a patient with a moustache.
   b. Distance from top edge of the dam should be decreased for a patient with a very thin upper lip.
3. Punch remaining holes following arch form.
4. Punch to include cuspid on opposite side of arch.
5. For anterior tooth (teeth) being prepared, punch to maxillary first molar.

Mandibular Arch

1. The first tooth to be punched is the clamp tooth.

2. Position mandibular first molar on the line where vertical and horizontal lines cross, figure 43–18.
3. Punch hole for tooth to receive clamp. If tooth other than first molar is to be the clamp tooth, adjustments must be made for clamp hole.
4. Punch remaining holes to correspond to arch form.

Class V (Cervical Area) Restoration

1. Punch hole for Class V restoration 1 mm facially from normal alignment.
2. Allow 1 mm between the adjacent teeth in arch.
3. For work to be done on either arch, the clamp tooth is punched first.
4. To punch a dam for Class V, the hole is punched facially 1 mm, figure 43–19. This compensates for the dam having to be stretched to fit the clamp.

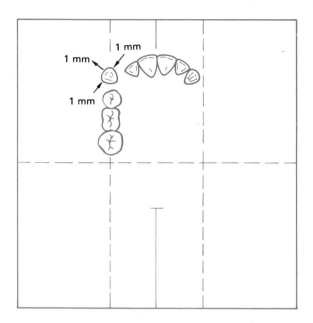

Fig. 43–19. Punching a dam for Class V

5. When punching the dam without the aid of a guide, care must be taken not to punch the width of the arch too shallow (flat) or too curved. In either case, the dam will not seat properly. The improper punching of the dam will result in puckering on the lingual or facial surface of the dam or in stretching the dam too taut, causing it to tear.

GUIDELINES FOR PUNCHING THE RUBBER DAM

The diameter of the hole increases with the number. (See figure 43–20.)

- hole number 1—lower incisors
- hole number 2—upper incisors
- hole number 3—cuspids and premolars
- hole number 4—molars
- hole number 5—molars, used for anchor tooth

Select the correct hole size on the punch plate for teeth to be isolated, figure 43–21. Mark adjustment for missing or malpositioned teeth. Care should be taken in selecting the hole size. Too large a hole will result in leakage around the tooth; too small a hole will tear the dam. Punch clean-cut holes in the dam. There should be no rubber tags or frayed edges that would prevent the dam from properly sealing the area around the tooth or cause the dam to tear during placement.

For better access and visibility, punch the dam two teeth distally from the tooth to be treated and across to the cuspid on the opposite side of the arch. A minimum of three teeth must be isolated, except in endodontic treatment, when one tooth is isolated.

SUGGESTED ACTIVITIES

- Prepare precut squares of rubber dam for punching. Use ruler and pencil to mark the general guidelines.
- Practice punching a rubber dam for maxillary and mandibular arch until you can punch a dam properly and with ease and confidence.

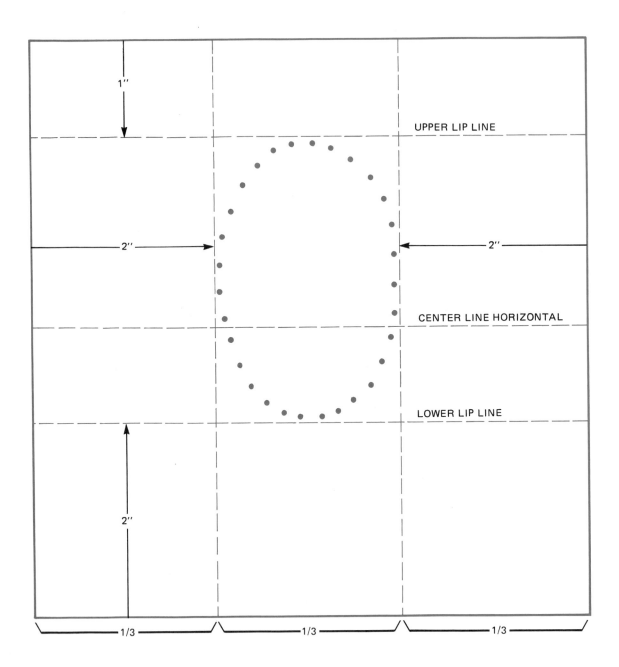

Fig. 43–20. Diagram to facilitate punching the rubber dam

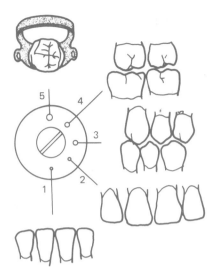

HOLE NUMBER 1 – LOWER INCISORS
HOLE NUMBER 2 – UPPER INCISORS
HOLE NUMBER 3 – CUSPIDS AND PREMOLARS
HOLE NUMBER 4 – MOLARS
HOLE NUMBER 5 – MOLARS, USED FOR ANCHOR TOOTH

Fig. 43–21. Wheel table

REVIEW

1. Give the advantages for using a heavier rubber dam material.

   a. _____

   b. _____

2. Which of the two shades of rubber dam would provide the best operative environment for the dentist? Why? _____

   _____

3. Name the three types of rubber dam clamps.

   a. _____

   b. _____

   c. _____

4. Give two reasons why the holes punched in the rubber dam must be clear-cut.

   a. _____

   b. _____

5. In preparing a rubber dam for the mandibular arch, which tooth is punched first?

   _____

6. It is advisable to punch a rubber dam to include the cuspid of the opposite side of the arch. Why? _____

   _____

7. Care should be used in selecting the hole size for teeth to be isolated for a dental procedure. Why?_____

   _____

8. In punching the rubber dam, what guideline is used to determine the distance from one hole to the next? _____

   _____

9. What diameter of hole is recommended for the anchor or clamp tooth?

   _____

10. Name the four parts of a rubber dam clamp.

    a. _____

    b. _____

    c. _____

    d. _____

11. Give the guidelines for marking a rubber dam when using a ruler and pencil.

a. _____

b. _____

c. _____

Chapter 44: Placing and Removing a Rubber Dam

OBJECTIVES:

After studying this chapter, the student will be able to:
- Select the armamentarium needed for rubber dam placement.
- Punch a rubber dam for the mandibular right quadrant, with the right second molar as the clamp anchor tooth.
- Place and remove the punched rubber dam on a mannequin, following the detailed instructions.

INTRODUCTION

A rubber dam is used in operative dentistry to maintain a clean, dry operating field while providing protection for the patient. A rubber dam aids in the retraction of the lips, tongue, and gingival tissues, allowing for better access to the field of operation during the preparation, placement, and finishing of a restoration. The use of a rubber dam can be a positive step toward providing the dental patient with quality dentistry.

MATERIALS NEEDED

- rubber dam
- rubber dam punch
- rubber dam forceps
- rubber dam clamp(s)
- rubber dam holder—Woodbury or Young
- rubber dam napkin
- dental floss (ligature) four 18-inch lengths of floss
- lubricant—water-soluble shaving cream or greaseless lubricant
- vaseline
- cotton roll
- inversion instrument
- crown and collar scissors
- stick compound
- matches
- Bunsen burner

- basic setup (mouth mirror, explorer, cotton pliers)

INSTRUCTIONS

Placement

1. Examine the patient's mouth. Check the position of the teeth, and note any deviation in alignment and size of teeth.
2. Check contact or interproximal areas with dental floss (ligature). Teeth and soft tissue should be free of debris and calculus.
3. Select and try-in clamp(s). The clamp jaws must rest securely on the tooth.
4. Tie a piece of dental floss around the bow of the clamp as a safety precaution. Should the clamp slip off the tooth accidentally, the floss provides a means for retrieving it.
5. Punch a rubber dam for teeth to be isolated. See Chapter 43.
6. Punch an identification hole in the upper right corner of the dam.
7. Lubricate the dam. Use a water-soluble shaving cream or a greaseless lubricant. The lubricant is applied to the undersurface of the dam. This aids in the placement of the dam.
8. Lubricate the patient's lips with vaseline.
9. Position clamp on anchor or clamp tooth with the bow of the clamp toward the distal surface of the tooth. When the clamp is

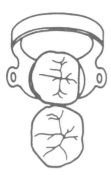

Fig. 44–1. Proper position for clamp

placed on the tooth, position the lingual jaw of the clamp at the cervical surface (neck of tooth), then seat facial jaw of clamp. This is done by rotating the clamp from the lingual surface to the facial surface of the tooth. Both points on each jaw must be in contact with the tooth to prevent the clamp from rocking, figure 44–1. Care should be taken not to impinge on the gingival tissue with the clamp.

10. Place the punched rubber dam with anchor hole over the bow of clamp, then the jaws, using forefingers of both hands.

11. Slip the dam over opposite cuspid, and secure with dental floss. Fashion a loose knot in a length of dental floss. Slip over cuspid. Tighten knot, making certain the floss remains on top of the rubber dam.

12. If the Woodbury holder is used, place the dam napkin as detailed in Chapter 43. Carefully pull dam material through opening of napkin. Arrange the napkin so it is flat against the patient's face.

13. Fasten two clips on one side of rubber dam. Pass straps of holder around back of patient's head and fasten the clips of the straps on the opposite side.

14. Complete dam placement.
    a. Stretch the remaining dam holes over the respective teeth to be isolated.
    b. Use a knifing action to pass the dam septums through the contact areas.
    c. With another piece of dental floss, pass the floss through the contact areas to help seat the dam. Note: If the Young frame is used, follow steps 1–3. Then, secure dam to the frame by the projections on the frame.

15. Invert the dam, lingually and facially. With a suitable inversion instrument, such as a beavertail burnisher or a Hartzell instrument, invert the dam. Take the air syringe, and direct a stream of air on each tooth while the instrument inverts the edges of the dam into the gingival sulcus.

16. Should the clamp require further stability, softened stick compound may be applied to the bow of the clamp and tooth.

17. Place saliva ejector. The saliva ejector may be placed under the rubber dam in the floor of the mouth, on the opposite side of the arch from the working area. An alternative is to cut a small hole in the dam just behind the mandibular incisors and place the saliva ejector tip through the hole in the dam. *Note:* Other techniques for placing a rubber dam may be used, such as placing the bow of the clamp through the anchor hole in the dam first, then positioning the dam and clamp on the tooth as a unit. Once the clamp is securely placed on the tooth, the dam is slipped over the jaws of the clamp.

Removal

1. Remove saliva ejector.

2. To remove the dam, use scissors to cut the dental floss tie. Proceed to cut each septum of the rubber dam. This is done by stretching the dam toward the facial surface and placing a finger under the dam by each septum as it is being cut. Tips of the scissors should be directed away from

the arch. Cut each septum of the rubber dam with one quick snip. This procedure is to protect the gingival tissue from being accidentally cut.

3. Remove the rubber dam holder.
4. Remove the rubber dam clamp with forceps.
5. Remove the rubber dam and the napkin. With napkin, wipe area around the patient's mouth.
6. Inspect the dam to determine if all of its parts are intact. No tags of rubber dam should be missing; no bits of rubber dam should remain between teeth or in sulcus; if so, check interproximal areas of teeth with dental floss. Remnants of a rubber dam often cause periodontal problems.
7. Gently massage gingival tissue.
8. Rinse patient's mouth with warm water.

Care of Rubber Dam Armamentarium

1. Remove dental floss tie from bow of clamp. Wash clamp, clamp holder, and Young frame with soap and water. Dry and prepare for autoclave.
2. Wipe the rubber dam punch with an antibacterial cleanser (gluteraldehydes).

SUGGESTED ACTIVITIES

- Practice placing and removing a rubber dam on a mannequin.
- Place and remove a rubber dam from the following teeth: maxillary right first premolar, mandibular left first molar, mandibular left central incisor, and maxillary left lateral incisor.
- If state law permits, practice placing and removing a rubber dam on classmate or patients.

REVIEW

1. Why should dental floss be tied to the bow of the clamp? _____

_____

2. In seating a rubber dam clamp, the bow of the clamp is directed toward

_____

3. In positioning the rubber dam clamp on a tooth, which jaw of the clamp is seated first? _____

4. Give the procedure for seating a rubber dam clamp._____

_____

_____

5. Give the procedure for inverting a rubber dam.

 a. _____

 b. _____

6. In removing a rubber dam, why should the finger be placed under each septum as the dam is being cut? _____

_____

7. What is the purpose of using stick compound during rubber dam placement?

_____

_____

> **OBJECTIVES:**
> After studying this chapter, the student will be able to:
> - Identify the parts of the Tofflemire matrix retainer.
> - Prepare and assemble a Tofflemire retainer and matrix band for a designated maxillary and mandibular tooth.
> - Apply the principles of wedging.

INTRODUCTION

The most common and generally accepted matrix retainer used today is the **Tofflemire**. The Tofflemire has two parts: the **retainer** and **matrix band**. The retainer is a device used to hold and stabilize the matrix band. The matrix band is a contoured, thin strip of stainless steel and is used to form the missing wall(s) of a prepared tooth (Class II). It helps establish proper anatomic contour and restores correct proximal contact.

PARTS OF THE TOFFLEMIRE RETAINER

The parts of a Tofflemire retainer are as follows, figure 45–1.

- *Frame*—the main body of the retainer to which the vise, spindle, and adjustment knobs are attached.

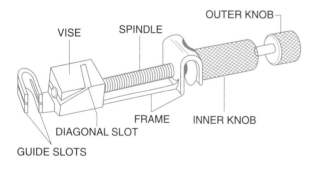

- *Vise*—holds the ends of the matrix band in the diagonal slot.
- *Guide slots*—slots that enable the matrix band loop to be positioned to the right or left of the retainer.
- *Spindle*—a screwlike rod with a pointed tip used to lock the ends of the matrix band in the vise.
- *Outer knob or set screw*—used to tighten or loosen the spindle against the matrix band in the vise.
- *Inner knob*—used to slide the vise along the frame to either increase or decrease the size of the matrix band loop.

Tofflemire Matrix Bands

Matrix bands are supplied in assorted sizes for use with the Tofflemire retainer.

- *universal band*, figure 45–2
- *medium band*, figure 45–3
- *medium MOD band*, figure 45–4

The universal matrix band is used for premolars and molars with moderate gingival MOD extensions, and the medium and wide bands are used for deep MOD gingival extensions. Observe figure 45–5 to determine the occlusal and gingival edge of the matrix band.

The highest curve of the matrix band is the occlusal edge and the inner curve is the gingival edge.

Fig. 45–1. Parts of the Tofflemire retainer

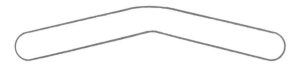

Fig. 45–2. Universal band

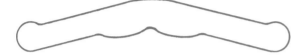

Fig. 45–3. Medium band

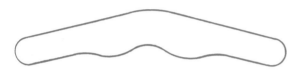

Fig. 45–4. Medium MOD band

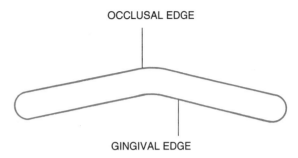

Fig. 45–5. Occlusal and gingival edges of band

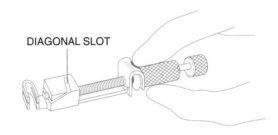

Fig. 45–6. Diagonal slot of vise

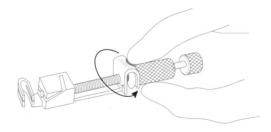

Fig. 45–7. Inner knob of retainer

MATERIALS NEEDED

- Tofflemire retainer
- matrix band(s)
- wedge(s) wood/plastic
- ball burnisher
- cotton or lab pliers
- mouth mirror

INSTRUCTIONS

Assembling the Tofflemire Retainer

1. Prepare the retainer to receive the matrix band. Hold the retainer so that the *diagonal slot* of vise is visible, figure 45–6.
2. Turn the *inner knob*, figure 45–7, counter-clockwise until the vise is positioned next to the guide slots. To accomplish this, the spindle tip must be inserted in the vise.
3. Turn the *outer knob*, figure 45–8, clockwise until the point of the spindle is barely visible in the diagonal slot.
4. With the opposite hand select the appropriate matrix band. The band should be determined according to the quadrant and before threading the band.

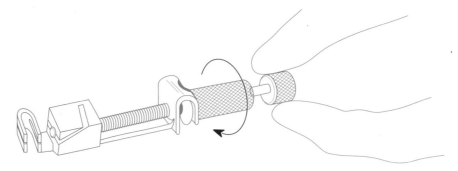

Fig. 45–8. Outer knob of retainer

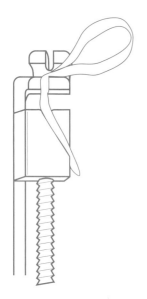

Fig. 45–9. Loop in place for maxillary right

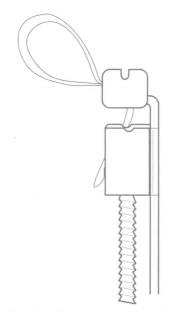

Fig. 45–10. Loop in place for mandibular left

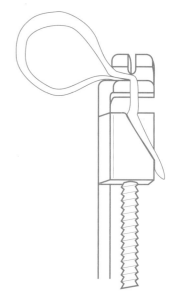

Fig. 45–11. Loop in place for maxillary left

In preparing the matrix, use the patient's maxillary arch and the operator's right and left hand as a reference guide. The retainer/band may be used interchangeably for the maxillary and mandibular quadrants. If the retainer/band is to be used for the maxillary right quadrant, figure 45–9, it may also be used for the mandibular left quadrant by merely inserting the retainer,

figure 45–10. To load the retainer for the maxillary right and mandibular left quadrant, the loop of the matrix band will be directed toward the operator's right hand. To load the retainer for the maxillary left and mandibular right quadrants, the loop of the matrix band will be directed toward the operator's left hand. The retainer/band for the maxillary left quadrant, figure

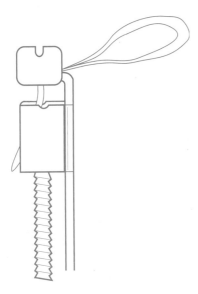

Fig. 45–12. Loop in place for mandibular right

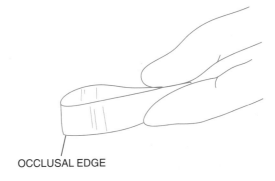

OCCLUSAL EDGE

Fig. 45–13. Occlusal edge of band directed toward floor

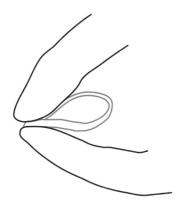

Fig. 45–14. Folding ends of band to form loop

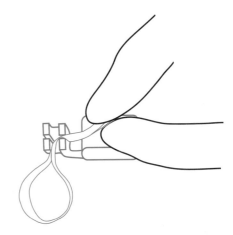

Fig. 45–15. Band positioned in diagonal slot

45–11, may be used for the mandibular right quadrant by inserting the retainer, figure 45–12.

5. With opposite hand, hold the matrix band with the occlusal edge pointed toward the floor, figure 45–13.

6. Loop the band end-to-end between thumb and forefinger. Hold joined ends together, allowing the band to remain in a tear-shaped loop and without a crease, figure 45–14.

7. Slide the joined ends of the band into the diagonal slot of the vise, figure 45–15. Continue threading the joined band so that it emerges from between the prongs of the guide slot according to Instructions.

8. Turn the *outer knob* clockwise until the tip of the spindle engages the matrix.

9. Use the handle of the mouth mirror to contour band, figure 45–16.

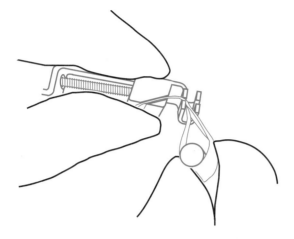

Fig. 45–16. Contouring matrix band

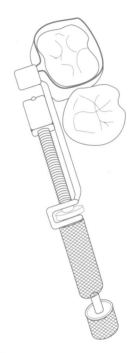

Fig. 45–17. Positioning the loop

Placing the Retainer

1. Place the loop around the prepared tooth (gingival edge first), with the retainer frame parallel to the buccal surfaces of the teeth and with the slotted portion of the retainer facing the gingiva. This will place the loop lingually around the tooth, figure 45–17.
2. Seat the loop into the interproximals, using one finger of one hand to stabilize the retainer. With the other hand, tighten the inner knob of the retainer by turning clockwise to close the band around the tooth, figure 45–18.
   a. Sometimes jiggling the retainer is necessary to carry the gingival edge of the band past the gingival margin of the preparation.
3. Check to see that the guide slot is centered on the buccal of the tooth.

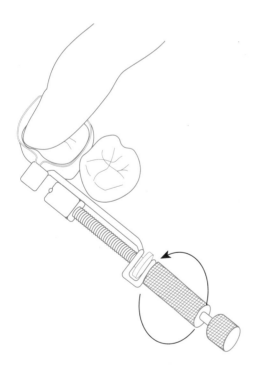

Fig. 45–18. Stabilizing the loop

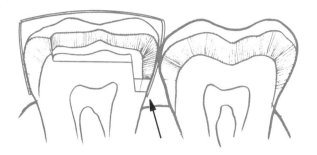

Fig. 45–19. Cross section of matrix band, gingival margin

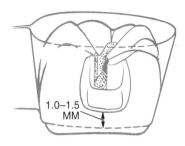

Fig. 45–20. Distance between gingival margin of band and gingival step, 1.0—1.5 mm

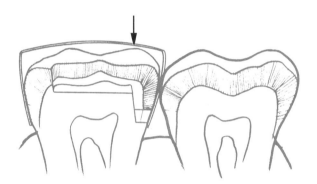

Fig. 45–21. Cross section showing height of matrix band

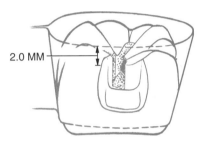

Fig. 45–22. Distance between highest cusp of tooth and occlusal border, 2.0 mm

4. The matrix band should extend no more than 1.0 to 1.5 mm below the gingival margin of the preparation, figures 45–19 and 45–20. The matrix band should extend no more than 2.0 mm above the highest cusp of the tooth, figures 45–21 and 45–22.
5. Adapting the band is necessary to ensure contact with adjacent teeth. To adapt the band, use the ball burnisher, and contour the inner surface of the band so it is slightly concave at the contact area of the prepared tooth.
6. Check the band for tightness. A band drawn too tightly will produce a flat contour lacking in correct proximal contact, figure 45–23. Too loose a band will cause an overcontoured restoration, figure 45–24. Either may result in a change in anatomic contour and/or incorrect proximal contact.

Problems of Improper Band Placement

1. Failure to seat band beyond the gingival step of the preparation, figure 45–25.
2. The band width is too narrow and does not extend beyond the gingival step of the preparation, figure 45–26.
3. The band is improperly seated because it impinges on the rubber dam, figure 45–27.
4. The band is improperly seated because it impinges on the gingival tissue, figure 45–28.

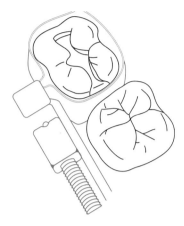

Fig. 45–23. Band too tight, lacking contour

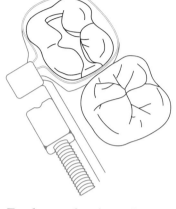

Fig. 45–24. Too loose a band, causing overcontoured band

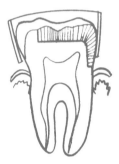

Fig. 45–25. Band does not extend beyond tooth preparation

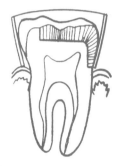

Fig. 45–26. Band extends only to step of preparation

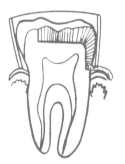

Fig. 45–27. Band impinges on rubber dam

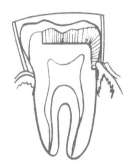

Fig. 45–28. Band impinges on gingival tissue

Wedging the Matrix Band

Once the matrix band has been placed on the tooth, a wedge is used to stabilize the matrix band. Wedges are wooden or plastic, are triangular in shape, and come in assorted sizes. Wedges are inserted between the teeth after the matrix band is placed around the tooth. Wedge(s) act as a brace to hold the matrix band against the tooth and prevent overhangs of restorative material. Wedge(s) separate the teeth slightly to compensate for the thickness of the matrix band.

1. Observe the size of the embrasure(s) involved, and select the proper wedge(s), figure 45–29.
2. A wedge is generally placed in the lingual embrasure. Wedges are placed mesially (M), distally (D), or both if the restoration is mesio-occluso-distal (MOD). Occasionally, buccal wedging is required.
3. With cotton pliers, choose the appropriate wedge. Use the beaks of the instrument to grasp the wedge at the base. Insert the wedge into the linguo-gingival embrasure next to the preparation and the band, figure 45–30.

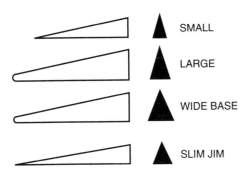

Fig. 45–29. Wedge sizes

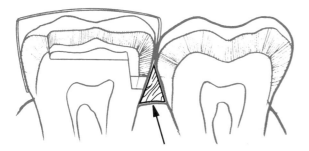

Fig. 45–31. **Cross section of tooth with band and wedge in proper position**

4. Base of the wedge should fit snugly on the gingival crest, figure 45–31, with the point of the wedge directed into the lingual embrasure.

Problems with Improper Wedging

1. Improper placement of the wedge results in an overhang of the finished restorative material.
2. If the matrix band is not wedged firmly enough to slightly separate the adjacent teeth, the restorative material will not provide a proper contact with the adjacent tooth.
3. When the matrix is not wedged properly, the restorative material will not provide the desired contact, contour, and protection of the interproximal gingiva.

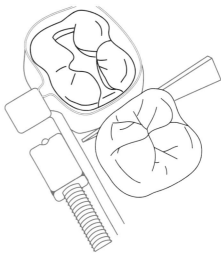

Fig. 45–30. **Wedge placed in lingual embrasure**

Removing the Wedge and Matrix

1. To remove the wedge, use cotton or lab pliers to grasp the wedge at the base, and remove from lingual embrasure, figure 45–32.
2. Holding the matrix firmly in place with the finger(s) of one hand, figure 45–33, slowly turn the *outer knob* of the retainer counterclockwise with the opposite hand.
3. Loosen the ends of matrix band from the retainer.
4. Carefully remove the retainer toward the occlusal and away from the gingiva. Thus, the holder is removed, while the band remains in place.
5. Using cotton or lab pliers, gently free the ends of the band from around the tooth, figure 45–34.
6. With fingers, grasp either the mesial or distal portion of the band.
7. Gently lift the matrix band from the proximal surface(s) of the restoration in an occluso-lingual direction, using a rocking motion. *Note:* If possible, remove the side of the matrix band that is away from the restored proximal surface first.

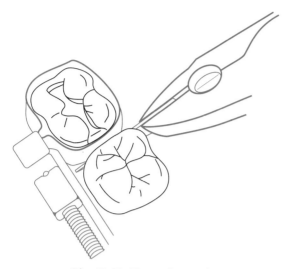

Fig. 45–32. Removing wedge

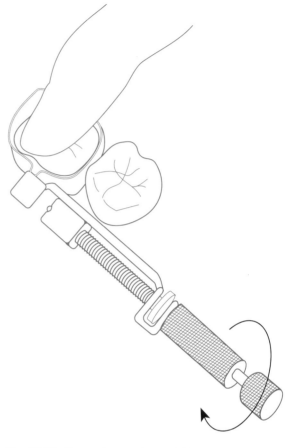

Fig. 45–33. Removing retainer while stabilizing band

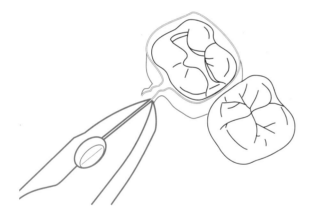

Fig. 45–34. Removing band from tooth

SUGGESTED ACTIVITIES

- Practice assembling the Tofflemire retainer and matrix band for maxillary and mandibular first molars.
- Use a typodont to practice placing a Tofflemire retainer/band on the following

teeth: maxillary right first molar, mandibular left first molar, maxillary left first molar, and mandibular right first molar.
- Practice wedge placement with the Tofflemire retainer in place.
- Practice removal of wedge, retainer, and matrix band.

REVIEW

1. What is the function of the Tofflemire matrix and retainer? _____

_____

_____

2. List the parts of the Tofflemire retainer, and give the function of each. _____

_____

_____

_____

_____

_____

3. The purpose of a matrix band is _____

_____.

4. What are the three types of stainless steel matrix bands? Give the use of each
   type. _____

_____

_____

_____

5. When placing the Tofflemire, what should be the position of the retainer
   frame? _____

_____

6. A properly placed matrix band will extend no more than _____ to _____
   mm below the gingival margin of the preparation and no more than _____
   mm above the highest cusp of the tooth.

7. The function of the ball burnisher is _____

_____.

8. How does the tightness of a matrix band affect the contour of a restoration? __

_____

_____

9. What is the function of wedges? _____

_____

_____

Chapter 46: Zinc Phosphate Cement

OBJECTIVES:

After studying this chapter, the student will be able to:
- Explain why water is the most critical ingredient in the liquid.
- List the steps that can be used to reduce the exothermic reaction when spatulating zinc phosphate cement.
- Discuss the reason for using a cool glass slab when mixing zinc phosphate cement.
- State the purpose for using a thin-consistency mix when seating a permanent restoration.

INTRODUCTION

Zinc phosphate is commonly referred to as a *crown* and *bridge cement*. Zinc phosphate can be used as an insulating base under restorations and for permanent cementation of crowns, inlays, onlays, fixed bridges, and orthodontic appliances.

COMPOSITION

The cement is supplied as powder and liquid that must be mixed together by hand on a cool glass slab. The principal constituent of zinc phosphate powder is zinc oxide, plus a small amount of magnesium oxide. Zinc phosphate powders are available based on particle size, *Type I* and *Type II*.

Type I is a fine-grain cement powder that when spatulated with the liquid forms a thin-film thickness. Film thickness is an important factor in the seating of gold or porcelain restorations. The reason for this is that the thin layer of cement will flow into the minute internal surface irregularities of the cast restoration and the retentive features of the tooth preparation, resulting in greater retention.

Type II is a medium-grain powder which may be used as a posterior temporary restoration.

The liquid is principally orthophosphoric acid and water. The water content of the liquid is carefully established by the manufacturer; this must be maintained. When dispensing the liquid, the cap should not be left off the bottle, nor should the liquid be placed on the mixing slab for any period of time. Water content of the liquid may either evaporate or gain water if the relative humidity (amount of water in the air) is high. In either case, the setting time and properties of the cement will be affected.

The liquid may or may not contain zinc salts that act as a buffering agent. A buffer will counteract the effects of the acid in the liquid and improve its storage behavior.

When the powder and liquid are mixed, a chemical reaction occurs, and heat is released. This reaction is called **exothermic** (exo-, outer; thermos, heat). As heat is produced, it speeds up the reaction even more. To reduce this reaction, and provide reasonable working time, any heat created must be dissipated (driven off) by spatulating over a large area.

To slow the exothermic reaction (to help dissipate the heat), the following steps may be taken during mixing: (1) use a cool glass slab; (2) spread the mix over a large area of the glass slab; and (3) add small increments (portions) of powder to the liquid. All of the above steps will affect to some degree the setting time.

Zinc phosphate cement must be mixed on a glass slab, never on a paper pad. The paper pad will not dissipate the heat of the mix. A thicker mix will set faster than a thin mix, with less powder.

The American Dental Association's (ADA) specifications for zinc phosphate cement state that the setting time be in the range of five to nine minutes. Of all the mixing of cements used in dentistry, mixing of zinc phosphate cement is more critical, and each procedural step must be followed.

MATERIALS NEEDED

- zinc phosphate powder
- zinc phosphate liquid
- spatula—metal
- **dappen dish**
- paper towels
- sodium bicarbonate solution

INSTRUCTIONS

1. Place clean spatula and cool glass slab on paper towel, along with the powder and liquid, figure 46–1. The temperature of the glass the slab should be approximately 65–75°F (18–24°C). In selecting the powder and liquid, check to see that the brand of cement is the same for each bottle.
2. Shake powder before removing cap.
3. Place appropriate amount of powder onto the right end of the slab (left side if you are left-handed), figure 46–2. The amount of powder to be used is determined by the liquid-powder ratio and the amount of cement required for the procedure.
4. Level powder with flat side of the spatula blade into a layer about 1 mm thick.

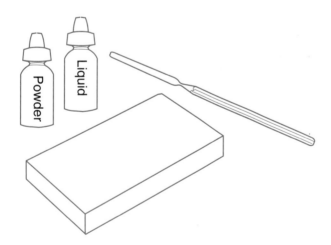

Fig. 46–1. Assembling of materials

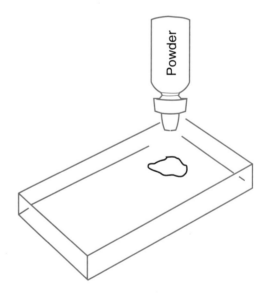

Fig. 46–2. Dispensing powder onto glass slab

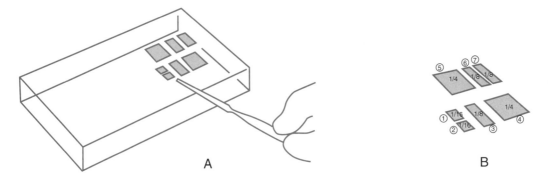

Fig. 46–3. (A) Powder divided into increments. (B) Powder in incremental portions.

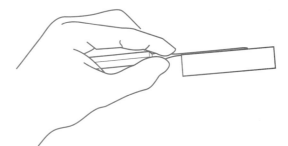

Fig. 46–5. Spatula blade flat against glass slab

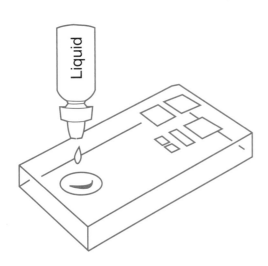

Fig. 46–4. Dispensing the liquid

5. Divide powder into two equal portions with the spatula; divide each of these into quarters, then the first eighth into six-teenths, and the last quarter into eighths, figure 46–3.
6. Shake liquid. Dispense liquid from drop-per bottle according to powder-liquid ratio required for mix, figure 46–4. To pro-duce uniform drops, hold bottle vertical while dispensing the required numbers of drops on to the glass slab.
7. Place the correct number of drops (two for base and eight for cementation) on to the slab, approximately $1^1/_2$ to 2 inches away from the powder.
8. Replace cap immediately after dispensing liquid.
9. Hold spatula with an overhand grasp, with index finger resting near the neck of the spatula blade and your thumb along the side of the spatula handle.
10. Incorporate the first one-sixteenth of pow-der into the liquid. Use the flat size of the spatula blade to wet the powder particles.
11. Hold the spatula blade flat against the glass slab, figure 46–5. Using a wide sweeping motion, spatulate the powder and liquid over a large area of the glass

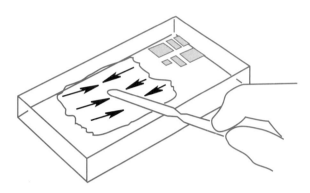

Fig. 46–6. Spatulate mix over large area of glass slab

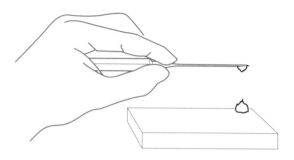

Fig. 46–7. Puttylike consistency for insulating base

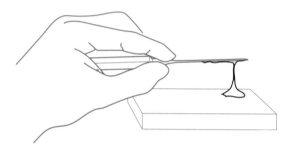

Fig. 46–8. Consistency for cementation

slab, figure 46–6. The first increment of powder will be spatulated for fifteen seconds. Adding small amounts of powder will help neutralize the acid and achieve a smooth consistency of the mix. Each increment of powder must be thoroughly incorporated into the mix. The mix must be smooth, with no unmixed particles of powder or liquid remaining on spatula or around the outer edge of mix.

12. Add the second increment; spatulate for fifteen seconds; add the third increment, and spatulate for fifteen seconds.

13. At this time, turn the spatula blade on edge, and gather the mass with two or three strokes to check the consistency.

14. Continue adding additional increments into the mix until desired consistency is reached and within the prescribed time. The approximate time for each increment is: 15, 15, 15, 20, 20, 15, and 20 seconds, for a total mixing time of 120 seconds (2 minutes).

15. Gather entire mass into one unit on the glass slab. The consistency for a base should be puttylike, figure 46–7, and can be rolled into a cylinder with the flat side of the spatula blade. The consistency for cementation is creamy and will follow the spatula for about 1 inch as it is lifted off the glass slab before breaking into a thin thread and flowing back into the mass, figure 46–8. *Remember:* Zinc phosphate cement must be spatulated over a large area of the cool glass slab to help the heat dissipate. This will allow the maximum amount of powder to be incorporated into the mix, which will result in a stronger cement.

16. Total spatulation time: 120 seconds (2 minutes).

Seating the Cast Restoration for Cementation

The tooth is prepared with certain retentive features that provide the mechanical retention needed to hold the cemented cast restoration on the tooth. Also, the internal surface of the casting must be roughened, which helps in the retention of the cemented restoration.

Prior to cementation, the casting or restoration must be tried on the tooth to check for fit, occlusion, and the margins of the casting.

The cement for cementation must be thin enough to allow it to flow over the tooth and the surface irregularities of the casting. The function of the dental cement is to seal the margins of the restoration. If the cement is too thick, it will interfere with the seating of the restoration. In this case, the exposed layer of cement, the cement line (the layer of cement formed around the margin of the restoration), will gradually dissolve and disintegrate permitting the development of a space between the tooth and the restoration (microleakage) that may lead to recurrent dental caries.

Preparing the Cast Restoration for Cementation

The assistant's responsibility during this procedure is to prepare the casting restoration for cementation. The preparation of the casting must be done prior to spatulating the zinc phosphate cement.

1. The cast restoration must be washed in water, using a brush to remove any debris. The cast restoration is dried and placed in a clean dappen dish and next to the glass slab.
2. When the operator is ready to seat the cast restoration, the assistant will spatulate

and apply the cement to the cast restoration, making sure the cement covers the entire internal surface of the casting.
3. The assistant will hold the glass slab, while the operator removes a small amount of cement on a instrument to coat the tooth preparation.
4. The assistant will hold the cast restoration in the palm of her or his hand for the operator to remove and place on the tooth. Note: The tooth or teeth to receive the restoration must be isolated from moisture. The vicinity immediately surrounding the area of cementation must be kept dry while the restoration is being placed and during hardening of the cement.

Cleaning the Slab and Spatula

1. Remove cement or excess powder from the glass slab with the spatula, and discard on a paper towel.
2. Wash spatula and glass slab in cool water.
3. Set particles may be removed with a solution of bicarbonate solution.
4. Thoroughly rinse glass slab and spatula. Dry.

SUGGESTED ACTIVITIES

- Practice spatulating zinc phosphate to the correct consistency for permanent cementation.
- Practice spatulating zinc phosphate to the correct consistency for an insulating base.

REVIEW

1. List the principal constituents of zinc phosphate powder. _____

2. List the principal ingredients of zinc phosphate liquid. _____

_____

3. What are the principal uses for zinc phosphate cement?_____

_____

_____

4. Give the advantages for using Type I powder. _____

_____

_____

_____

5. What effect does a buffer have in zinc phosphate liquid?_____

_____

6. How would an increase or decrease in the water content of the liquid affect the cement? _____

_____

7. What should the consistency of the cement be for cementation?_____

_____

_____

8. Spatulation of the liquid and powder should be done over a large area of the glass slab. Why? _____

_____

_____

9. List the three steps that can control the setting time of zinc phosphate cement?

a. _____

b. _____

c. _____

Chapter 47: Zinc Polyacrylate Cement

OBJECTIVES:

After studying this chapter, the student will be able to:
- Discuss the advantages for using zinc polyacrylate cement.
- Prepare a mix of zinc polyacrylate cement for cementation.
- Recognize the proper consistency of zinc polyacrylate for cementation.

INTRODUCTION

Zinc polyacrylate (carboxylate or polycarboxylate) is used for cementation of permanent restorations, orthodontic bands, and for bases under other types of restorations. The cement is manufactured with powder and liquid components.

COMPOSITION

The composition of the powder is zinc oxide with a small amount of magnesium oxide. However, some manufacturers substitute magnesium oxide with stannous fluoride, which is added to the powder to increase strength and to reduce the film thickness. The liquid is polyacrylic acid and water.

When the powder and liquid are mixed together, the result is a cement that is extremely acid at the time of placement, pH of 1.7. However, the acid is rapidly neutralized during the setting reaction. Despite the acidity of the cement, zinc polyacrylate is less irritating to the pulpal tissue and is comparable to zinc oxide eugenol cement in that it is a soothing agent.

Zinc polyacrylate cement has an advantage over other dental cements in that it has the ability to adhere directly to the tooth structure. Through a process called *chelation* (a chemical reaction between two substances that join together to form an adhesive bond), the polyacrylic acid combines with the calcium in the tooth structure to form a primary adhesive bond. Because of this bonding action, when properly prepared, zinc polyacrylate cement can be used to attach orthodontic brackets directly to tooth enamel. A procedure called **acid etching** is used to prepare the enamel, which will allow the chelation or bonding to occur between the tooth enamel and orthodontic bracket. The same procedure may also be used when cementing crowns or fixed bridges.

However, gold or porcelain restorations must be thoroughly cleansed prior to cementation. Contaminants, such as chemical residue left from the acid pickling solution, will prevent the cement from adhering to the restoration. The inside of the gold restoration may be cleaned with an air abrasive or an abrasive bur, then washed and dried.

MATERIALS NEEDED

- zinc polyacrylate powder
- zinc polyacrylate liquid or calibrated dispenser
- paper mixing pad—nonabsorbable—or glass slab
- measuring scoop
- spatula

INSTRUCTIONS

1. Dispense one scoop of powder onto mixing pad or glass slab. Press measuring scoop firmly into powder. Withdraw measuring scoop from bottle, and remove

430

excess powder with spatula. Powder should be flush with top of measuring scoop.

2. Place three drops of liquid on mixing pad near powder. Liquid should never be placed on the mixing pad or glass slab until just ready to be mixed. Exposure to air will cause loss of water and will result in the premature thickening of the mix. If liquid is dispensed from the plastic squeeze bottle, hold the bottle in a vertical position and squeeze. Release pressure when the drop separates from the nozzle tip. Should a calibrated liquid dispenser be used, push plunger rod to release three full calibrations, as marked on the plunger barrel.

3. Incorporate powder into the liquid in one increment. Begin spatulation. Spatulation should be rapid and be completed within thirty seconds. Do not overspatulate!

4. The consistency of polyacrylate cement for cementation is smooth and creamy, and the mass will flow from the spatula in a thin strand. The cement must be applied to the tooth and the object to be cemented while the mix is glossy. If the cement loses its sheen or becomes stringy, do not use it; it has started to set. For a base, the consistency should also be glossy. To facilitate the setting of the base, an instrument dipped in powder or in alcohol will cause the base to set faster.

5. The setting time for zinc polyacrylate is three to four minutes.

Cleaning the Spatula and Instrument

1. Immediately rinse spatula and instrument in cool water. If cement adheres to the spatula or instrument, it can be removed with a 10% solution of sodium hydroxide.

2. Dry and prepare instruments for sterilization.

SUGGESTED ACTIVITY

• Practice mixing zinc polyacrylate for cementation.

REVIEW

1. Why is the liquid placed on the mixing pad or glass slab just prior to spatulation? _____

_____

_____

2. What procedure should be followed when preparing a gold or porcelain restoration? _____

_____

_____

3. Why can zinc polyacrylate cement be used to cement orthodontic brackets directly to the tooth structure?_____

_____

_____

Chapter 48: Zinc Oxide Eugenol Cement

OBJECTIVES:

After studying this chapter, the student will be able to:
- State the advantages for using zinc oxide eugenol cement.
- State the advantage for using reinforced zinc-oxide cement over the conventional zinc oxide eugenol cement.
- Prepare zinc oxide eugenol cement for a base.
- Prepare zinc oxide eugenol cement for a temporary restoration.

INTRODUCTION

Zinc oxide eugenol (ZOE) cement is noted for its sedative or soothing effect on the dental pulp. It is used as an insulating base to protect the pulp against mechanical and thermal trauma, for cementation of treatment restorations (See Chapter 54, table 54–1), for temporary restorations before permanent restorations are placed, and for root canal fillings.

COMPOSITION

The powder for the conventional zinc oxide eugenol cement is zinc oxide, resin, zinc acetate, and an accelerator. The liquid, **eugenol**, is found in clove oil. The improved or reinforced zinc oxide powder includes the addition of alumina and polymers (resins), and ethoxybenzoic acid (EBA) is added to the eugenol. The new additives to the powder and liquid increase the strength of the cement.

MATERIALS NEEDED

- zinc oxide powder
- eugenol liquid
- parchment mixing pad
- metal spatula
- measuring device
- alcohol—91% isopropyl or 70% ethyl alcohol
- 2" × 2" sponge

INSTRUCTIONS

1. Place powder on mixing pad.
   a. Fluff powder before removing cap.
   b. Dispense one scoop of powder from large well with the measuring device, and place on mixing pad. A clean spatula may be used instead of the measuring device to dispense a portion of powder.
   c. Replace cap on powder bottle to avoid spilling and contamination.
   d. Divide powder into four equal portions.
2. Place liquid on slab.
   a. Shake liquid.
   b. With pipette in liquid bottle, draw liquid into pipette; remove and hold pipette perpendicular (vertical) to the mixing pad.
   c. Dispense one drop of liquid onto pad, near powder, but not touching powder, figure 48–1.
3. Spatulate cement.
   a. Draw first portion or quarter of powder into the liquid, and thoroughly spatulate.
   b. Draw next portion of powder into the mix, and continue to spatulate. Repeat procedure until desired consistency is reached.
   c. The spatulation time may vary with brand, generally between thirty seconds and one minute.

433

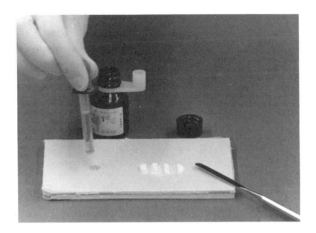

Fig. 48–1. Dispense liquid onto pad.

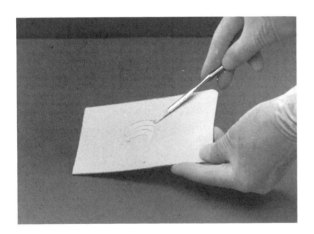

Fig. 48–2. Consistency for temporary cementation

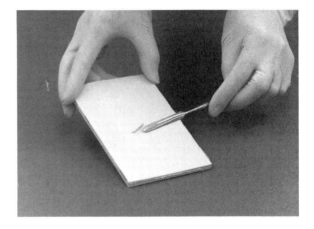

Fig. 48–3. Puttylike consistency for base

    d. The consistency for temporary cementation of a crown is creamlike frosting, figure 48–2.

    e. The consistency for an insulating base is puttylike. It can be rolled into a cylinder, using the blade of the spatula, figure 48–3.

  4. Clean spatula.

    a. Wipe spatula with a 2″ × 2″ sponge moistened with alcohol.

    b. Wash, rinse, and dry.

SUGGESTED ACTIVITY

- Practice spatulating zinc oxide eugenol cement for an insulating base.
- Practice spatulating zinc oxide eugenol cement for a temporary restoration.
- Practice spatulating zinc oxide eugenol cement for cementation of a temporary crown.

REVIEW

1. Give the main advantage for using zinc oxide eugenol cement. _____

   _____

2. List four uses for zinc oxide eugenol cement.

   a. _____

   b. _____

   c. _____

   d. _____

3. State the consistency of zinc oxide eugenol cement for temporary cementation. _____

Chapter 49: Applying a Cavity Varnish

OBJECTIVES:

After studying this chapter, the student will be able to:
- Define the composition of a cavity varnish.
- Explain the difference between a cavity varnish and a cavity liner.
- Describe the basic technique for applying a cavity varnish.

INTRODUCTION

A cavity **varnish** is a special liquid used in conjunction with dental cements and restorative materials.

COMPOSITION

The varnish is composed of either a natural gum or resin (e.g., copal) or of a synthetic resin dissolved in an organic solvent of acetone, chloroform, or ether.

After the varnish is applied to a cavity preparation, the solvent evaporates, leaving a thin film on the tooth surface that seals the exposed dentinal tubules against chemical irritants from certain cements and restorative materials. The varnish acts as a semipermeable membrane, preventing the passage of acids from the cements along the dentinal tubules to the pulp. A cavity varnish may also be applied when placing an amalgam restoration, because the varnish aids in reducing the number of metallic ions penetrating the tissues of the dentin and enamel, thus minimizing the discoloration of the tooth structure next to the restoration.

The use of a cavity varnish depends on the type of cement or restorative material to be used. It is suggested that the cavity varnish be applied prior to the placement of zinc phosphate cement, amalgams, and gold foil restorations. A cavity varnish is applied after calcium hydroxide preparation, zinc oxide, and carboxylate cements. See figure 54–1, page 451.

A cavity varnish may be used with certain composite restorations, but as specified by the manufacturer; otherwise, it may interfere with the setting reaction of the material.

A varnish to be effective must be thin, enabling it to flow over and seal the dentinal tubules. If the varnish becomes too thick to use, a thinner may be added to the solvent, since a thick layer will not seal the tubules as well.

Another type of cavity sealant, called a *cavity liner*, is available. It is different from a cavity varnish in that it contains either calcium hydroxide or zinc oxide suspended in a solvent of natural or synthetic resins. The liner is applied to the cavity preparation in the same manner as a cavity varnish. However, the liner must not go beyond the dentinoenamel junction of the preparation, because it will eventually dissolve and cause marginal leakage.

MATERIALS NEEDED

- cavity varnish
- cotton pellet
- cotton pliers or applicator
- cotton roll

INSTRUCTIONS

1. Clean and dry the cavity preparation.
2. Select cotton pellet for size of preparation.
3. Remove cap from varnish bottle. Quickly take cotton pliers with pellet and touch surface of varnish until pellet is moistened. Replace cap. Should pellet become

saturated with excess varnish, press pellet against cotton roll to remove excess. *Note: The cap of the bottle must be replaced immediately after each application; otherwise, the solvent will evaporate and the remaining solvent will become thick.*

4. Apply varnish to the cavity preparation. Coat the entire surface of the preparation, dentin and enamel. It is not necessary to remove the varnish from the cavo-surface margins of the tooth.

5. Dry with gentle stream of air, using air syringe, for fifteen to twenty seconds.

6. Apply second application of varnish. Two successive applications are necessary to provide a continuous layer without voids. A third application may be desired.

7. Dispose of cotton pellet in appropriate waste receptacle; clean and sterilize cotton pliers or applicator.

SUGGESTED ACTIVITY

• Practice the application of a cavity varnish on a prepared stone model.

REVIEW

1. What is the main purpose for applying a cavity varnish?_____

_____

2. Why are cavity varnishes not recommended for use with certain composite restorations? _____

_____

3. Why should the cap be replaced on the varnish bottle immediately after each use? _____

_____

Chapter 50: Preparing Calcium Hydroxide

OBJECTIVES:
After studying this chapter, the student will be able to:
- Select the materials needed to prepare calcium hydroxide for a base.
- Prepare calcium hydroxide for a base.

INTRODUCTION

Calcium hydroxide is a cement-type material used in deep cavities and for microscopic pulp exposures or near-exposures. The benefit of calcium hydroxide is in its therapeutic effect on the pulp, for it tends to stimulate the formation of secondary dentin—the most effective barrier to any further irritants.

As a rule, the thicker the dentin, whether primary or secondary, between the surface of the cavity and the pulp, the better the protection from chemical and physical trauma. However, when a cavity penetrates the dentinoenamel junction more than 0.5 mm, calcium hydroxide is the ideal choice for a base.

Calcium hydroxide is placed in the deepest portion of the preparation, figure 50–1, approximately 0.5–1.0 mm in thickness. With some calcium hydroxide–based cements (aqueous type), this layer does not provide sufficient hardness or strength to warrant its use alone as base in a deep cavity. For this reason, it is usually overlaid with a stronger cement in order to provide protection against the forces of condensation and mastication.

COMPOSITION

Suspensions of calcium hydroxide are of two types: aqueous or nonaqueous. Aqueous calcium hydroxide is formed when calcium hydroxide powder is mixed with distilled water. Nonaqueous calcium hydroxide contains calcium hydroxide and zinc oxide powder suspended in a chloroform solution of a natural or synthetic resin.

MATERIALS NEEDED

- calcium hydroxide base or catalyst pastes
- paper mixing pad
- ball-point instrument or small spatula

INSTRUCTIONS

1. Dispense an equal amount of both base and catalyst paste onto mixing pad.
2. With ball-point instrument or spatula, immediately incorporate base and catalyst together, using a circular motion, until a homogenous mix is achieved, usually within thirty seconds or less.

SUGGESTED ACTIVITY

- Practice mixing calcium hydroxide base material.

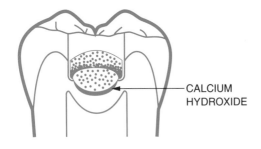

CALCIUM HYDROXIDE

Fig. 50–1. Application of calcium hydroxide

REVIEW

1. When would a calcium hydroxide base be indicated?_____

   _____

2. What is the main reason for using calcium hydroxide as a base material?_____ .

   _____

   _____

3. Name the two types of calcium hydroxide suspensions. How do they differ?

   _____

   _____

   _____

4. Explain why the thickness of dentin, whether primary or secondary, is important to the health of the tooth. _____

   _____

After studying this chapter, the student will be able to:
- Name the two inorganic fillers used in a composite restoration.
- Name the polymer matrix material used in a composite restoration.
- State the two methods used in the polymerization of a composite restoration.

INTRODUCTION

Composite restorations have a natural toothlike appearance and are used primarily in anterior teeth, Class III and V. However, newer composites are available for posterior teeth.

COMPOSITION

Composite restorative material is composed of a polymer matrix, dimethacrylate (BIS-GMA), and inorganic filler particles such as quartz and lithium aluminum silicate. The inorganic filler particles are treated with an organic silane coupling agent that provides a bond between the inorganic fillers and the resin matrix. To make the material more radiopaque (whiter or lighter in appearance), composites may contain one of several elements such as barium, strontium, zinc, or zirconium.

The composites are classified according to particle size and the distribution of the inorganic fillers. Composites may contain fine irregularly shaped particle fillers or microfine particle fillers. The composites that are used today are a combination of the two particle sizes.

Commercial composites are available as a *single-* or *two-paste system*. The *single-paste system* is supplied in disposable syringes and comes in various shades. The composite may be dispensed into a special composite syringe that is used to place the material into the cavity preparation. Once the composite material has been placed, polymerization of the composite is accomplished by shining a small beam of visible blue light onto the restoration for approximately twenty to thirty seconds. *Precaution:* The operator and chairside assistant should always wear light-filtering glasses or use a light-screening safety tip when using visible blue light.

In the *two-paste system*, one paste is the base material and the second paste is the catalyst. The base contains an initiator, peroxide, and the second paste contains an activator, amine (an organic compound containing nitrogen), that serves as the catalyst when they are combined. The two pastes are spatulated together and packed into the tooth preparation with a plastic instrument. The mix will begin to harden within one to two minutes. Polymerization is the result of a chemical reaction that has occured between the initiator, peroxide, and the activator, amine. This reaction is called the amine-peroxide polymerization system.

MATERIALS NEEDED

- composite base paste
- catalyst paste
- mixing pad
- disposable plastic spatula (supplied by manufacturer)

INSTRUCTIONS

Measure equal amounts of both base and catalyst paste on to mixing pad.

1. Use one end of the spatula to remove a small amount of base paste, and place on to the mixing pad.
2. With the other end of the spatula, remove an equal amount of catalyst paste, and place on to mixing pad. *Note:* Care must be taken not to cross-contaminate base paste with catalyst paste; otherwise, material will harden in jars.
3. With the same disposable spatula, spatulate base paste and catalyst together. Spatulation time is usually within thirty seconds. The mix will have a doughy consistency.
4. Throw used disposable spatula away after procedure.

REVIEW

1. Give the composition for a composite restoration. _____

_____

2. Why are the inorganic fillers treated with the silane coupling agent?

_____

_____

3. Name the two methods used in the polymerization of composite restorations.

    a. _____

    b. _____

4. Name the elements that are used to make a composite restoration radiopaque.

_____

_____

Chapter 52: Glass Ionomers

OBJECTIVES:

After studying this chapter, the student will be able to:
- State the advantages of using glass ionomer cement.
- State four uses of glass ionomer cement.
- Discuss the bonding reaction of glass ionomer cement to enamel and dentin.
- Discuss the importance of removing the "smear layer" from the tooth preparation prior to placing a glass ionomer restoration.
- Prepare a glass ionomer for cementation by following the prescribed instructions.

INTRODUCTION

Glass **ionomer** cements are used because of their high strength and low solubility and film thickness. They are relatively "kind" to the pulp. However, in the case of a deep cavity preparation or near-pulp exposure, a protective base such as calcium hydroxide is recommended. Glass ionomer cement also has the ability to release fluoride, which helps protect both the immediate and surrounding tooth structure from dental caries.

Glass ionomer cement has the ability to bond to tooth structure (enamel and dentin). The bonding reaction occurs between the polyacrylic acid and the calcium of the tooth. In order for bonding to occur, the tooth surface must be free of debris. After the tooth is prepared, a microscopic layer of mineralized tooth and bacterial debris (smear layer) remains on the tooth. This smear layer must be removed before bonding can taken place. To remove the smear layer, one must thoroughly cleanse the tooth structure with a conditioner composed of a 25% solution of polyacrylic acid. A blue coloring agent is added to the conditioner for visibility. The conditioner is applied directly over the dentin, including the dentoenamel junction, for a minimum of ten seconds. The tooth is rinsed with a steady flow of water for at least 30 seconds, then air-dried with a gentle stream of air. Care must be taken to avoid dehydrating the tooth, as this may cause postoperative tooth sensitivity. This is particularly true when cementing crowns and bridges.

The conditioner is applied prior to placing the glass ionomer base or restorative material. The conditioner may be placed directly onto the tooth, using the disposable applicator tip(s). The use of the conditioner is contraindicated when cementing crowns and bridges. In this case, the smear layer provides a protective layer for the tooth or abutment teeth.

Glass ionomer cement may be used as dentin replacement material (base), figure 52–1, and for the permanent cementation of crowns and bridges, orthodontic bands, cast posts, and core buildups, figure 52–2.

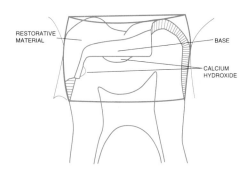

Fig. 52–1. Placement of calcium hydroxide, dentin replacement base and restoration (Courtesy Premier Dental/ESPE-Premier Sales Co.)

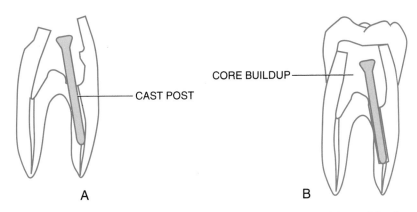

Fig. 52–2. (A) Cast post cemented in tooth. (B) Core buildup with glass ionomer cement (Courtesy Premier Dental/ESPE-Premier Sales Co.)

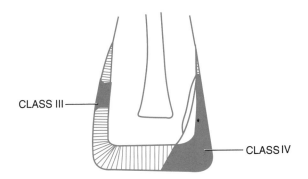

Fig. 52–3. Anterior restorations, Class III and IV (Courtesy Premier Dental/ESPE-Premier Sales Co.)

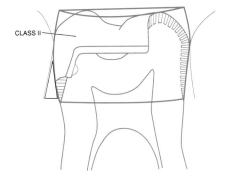

Fig. 52–4. Posterior restoration, Class II (Courtesy Premier Dental/ESPE-Premier Sales Co.)

As a restorative material, glass ionomers may be used for anterior and posterior teeth, figures 52–3 and 52–4, and are ideal for cervical or erosion lesions, root caries, and for repair of crown margins.

Glass ionomer restorations pass through two setting stages and must be protected against moisture contamination and dehydration. A light-cure surface sealant or glaze is recommended to protect the restoration(s) during setting.

Glass ionomer cement is available as a powder and liquid and in capsules, figure 52–5. The capsules require the use of a high-speed amalgamator to mix the cement, figure 52–7.

MATERIALS NEEDED

- amalgamator—high speed
- capsule(s)—glass ionomer
- capsule activator
- glass ionomer powder
- glass ionomer liquid
- scoop
- mixing pad
- spatula

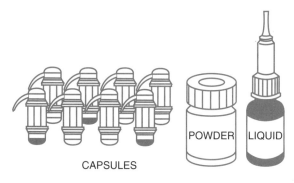

Fig. 52–5. Systems for dispensing glass ionomer cements (Courtesy Premier Dental/ESPE-Premier Sales Co.)

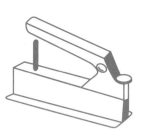

Fig. 52–6. Capsule activator (Courtesy Premier Dental/ESPE-Premier Sales Co.)

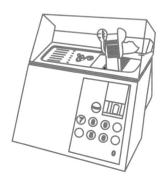

Fig. 52–7. Trituration of capsule with amalgamator (Courtesy Premier Dental/ESPE-Premier Sales Co.)

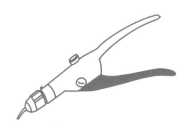

Fig. 52–8. Capsule in applier (Courtesy Premier Dental/ESPE-Premier Sales Co.)

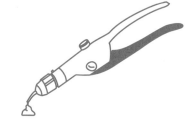

Fig. 52–9. Applier used to express cement (Courtesy Premier Dental/ESPE-Premier Sales Co.)

INSTRUCTIONS

Preparing Ionomer Cement Using an Amalgamator

1. Activate the capsule with the activator, figure 52–6.
2. Insert the activated capsule in the high-speed amalgamator.
3. Triturate for about ten seconds. *Note:* The amount of time may vary depending on the make of the amalgamator, figure 52–7.
4. Remove the capsule, insert it into applier, and immediately remove the sealing pin. The nozzle tip of the capsule should be positioned at a 90° degree for better access to the cavity preparation, figure 52–8.
5. Express the material directly into the tooth preparation by squeezing the applier, figure 52–9.
6. Working time will vary from one and one-half to two minutes depending on glass ionomer.

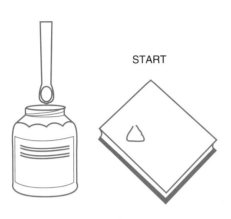

Fig. 52–10. Measuring powder with scoop (Courtesy Premier Dental/ESPE-Premier Sales Co.)

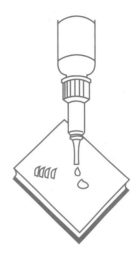

Fig. 52–11. Dispensing liquid onto pad (Courtesy Premier Dental/ESPE-Premier Sales Co.)

Preparing Glass Ionomer Cement (Powder and Liquid System)

Cementation

1. Shake powder to fluff material.
2. Dispense one level scoop of powder onto mixing pad, figure 52–10.
3. Divide each scoop of powder into small increments, figure 52–11.
4. Holding the liquid bottle vertical, dispense two drops of liquid onto mixing pad, figure 52–11. Liquid should be placed on mixing pad just prior to mixing. Exposure to air will cause loss of water to the atmosphere. Keep bottles tightly sealed when not in use.
5. Draw the first increment of powder into the liquid. Spatulate each increment thoroughly before adding the next increment, figure 52–12. Spatulation must be completed within sixty seconds, and the cement should have a glossy appearance. *Note:* Working time can be extended by mixing cement on a chilled, dry glass slab.

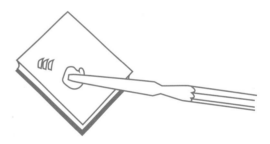

Fig. 52–12. Adding increments of powder into liquid (Courtesy Premier Dental/ESPE-Premier Sales Co.)

Dentin Replacement (Base)

1. Select the desired shade of powder to match or vary from the dentin shade.
2. Dispense one level scoop of powder on to the mixing pad, figure 52–10.
3. Divide each scoop of powder into small increments, figure 52–11.
4. Holding the liquid bottle vertical, dispense one drop of liquid on to the mixing pad, figure 52–11.

5. Draw the first increment of powder into the liquid. Spatulate each increment thoroughly before adding the next increment, figure 52–12. Spatulation must be completed within thirty seconds.

Placing Glass Ionomer Restoration

1. Place calcium hydroxide in deepest areas of preparation.
2. Apply conditioner to dentin for ten seconds to remove smear layer.
3. Rinse tooth with a steady flow of water for thirty seconds.
4. Dry tooth with a gentle stream of air. Do not dehydrate tooth.
5. Apply base to cover dentin, including dentoenamel junction. Allow base to set for two minutes.
6. Next, etch enamel with etching gel/liquid for thirty seconds.
7. Rinse tooth with water for sixty seconds.
8. Dry tooth with a gently stream of air. Do not dehydrate tooth.
9. Place glass ionomer restorative material. Place protective surface sealant when indicated.

SUGGESTED ACTIVITY

• Practice mixing glass ionomer cement for cementation, using the powder and liquid system.

REVIEW

1. State three uses for glass ionomer cement.

   a. _____

   b. _____

   c. _____

2. State four advantages for using glass ionomer cement.

   a. _____

   b. _____

   c. _____

   d. _____

3. Define the term *smear layer*. _____

_____

4. State the procedure used to remove the smear layer from the tooth preparation. _____

_____

_____

5. Explain the bonding reaction of glass ionomer cement with the tooth.

_____

_____

6. When is the use of the glass ionomer conditioner contraindicated?

_____

Chapter 53: Pit and Fissure Sealants

OBJECTIVES: After studying this chapter, the student will be able to:
- State the advantage for using pit and fissure sealants.
- Select the materials needed for the preparation and placement of a pit and fissure sealant.
- Explain the procedure for preparing the tooth surfaces for receiving a sealant.

INTRODUCTION

In preventive dentistry, the application of *pit* and *fissure sealants* are recommended for newly erupted teeth with defective fissures, both deciduous and permanent teeth. The purpose is to seal the surfaces against the possibility of dental caries.

The anatomy of a tooth is important in the prevention of dental caries. During normal tooth development, the occlusal surface of posterior teeth form smooth-based depressions called *grooves*. These grooves are easily cleansed by the usual excursion of food and the use of a toothbrush. However, if during the state of development the enamel fails to coalesce (grow together) properly, a faulty groove will result. This is called a *fissure*. The lack of enamel coalescence may only involve the enamel, or it may extend down to the dentinotenamel junction. The defective fissure becomes a potential trap for food debris, thereby increasing the chance of dental caries. The prevention of such caries may be controlled through the use of pit and fissure sealants.

COMPOSITION

Although various types of resins have been used, the currently used commercial pit and fissure sealants are the **bisphenol-A-glycidyl methacrylate (BIS-GMA)** resins. The polymer is an epoxy resin with an acrylic monomer, bisphenol A, and glycidyl methacrylate. The BIS-GMA sealant may be polymerized by the conventional amine-peroxide system or with the use of a visible "blue" light. With the light-cured system, the light, rather than a chemical, is the activator, the initiator is a light-sensitive chemical diketone that is actived by the visible light of a certain wavelength. By shining a small beam of visible blue light onto the resin surface, the light decomposes the initiator, causing polymerization to take place.

The success of the sealant technique depends on the ability of the resin to complete adaption with the tooth surface. Therefore, the sealant should be of low viscosity in order for it to flow easily into the prepared pit or fissures, allowing the material to come in contact with all the small surface irregularities of the tooth. This requires special treatment to the tooth surface(s) prior to the placement of the sealant. The enamel surfaces must be cleaned thoroughly then etched with an acid or conditioner—usually a concentrated solution of phosphoric acid (35–50%) is used. This procedure produces a selective dissolution (dissolving) of the enamel surface, thereby providing the mechanical retention needed to hold the sealant. The open pores of the enamel will allow the resin to flow into the surface irregularities to form what are referred to as resin *tags*. This mechanical interlocking of the resin to the enamel surfaces increases the bond strength of the resin to the tooth structure.

MATERIALS NEEDED

- basic setup (mouth mirror, explorer, and cotton pliers)
- prophy handpiece
- prophy brush/cup
- nonfluoride prophy paste
- rubber dam setup
- etching solution
- sealant
- cotton pellet
- applicator or syringe
- articulating paper
- small white or diamond stones
- light-cured system, depending on type of sealant

INSTRUCTIONS

1. Clean the teeth with a prophy brush and nonfluoride paste.
2. Rinse and dry the teeth.
3. Place a rubber dam to isolate the teeth to be treated.
4. Moisten a cotton pellet with the etching solution or conditioning agent, and apply to the occlusal surface(s) of the tooth or teeth.
5. Allow the etching solution to remain on the tooth surface(s) for approximately thirty to sixty seconds. Care must be taken not to apply the solution to other surfaces of the tooth or teeth.
6. Rinse the teeth thoroughly (ten to fifteen seconds) with water to remove the decalcified tooth debris from the etched surfaces.
7. Dry the tooth surfaces with a stream of air for at least fifteen to thirty seconds. This step is critical, because moisture contamination will interfere with the retention of the sealant. The prepared surface(s) should have a dull, slightly chalky appearance.
8. Apply the sealant with the applicator or syringe, depending on brand of sealant to be used. Avoid air voids when applying the sealant.
9. If the sealant is being set with the "blue" light, position the tip of the gun about 2 mm from the sealant, and expose to the light for approximately twenty seconds.
10. Once the sealant has set, examine the occlusal surface(s) with an explorer to determine whether the fissure or pit has been completely covered.
11. Check the occlusal surface(s) with articulating paper. White or diamond stones may be used to adjust the contour of the sealant.
12. Remove the rubber dam, and rinse the patient's mouth with warm water.

SUGGESTED ACTIVITY

- Prepare a procedure for the application of a sealant.

REVIEW

1. Explain the purpose for using a pit and fissure sealant. _____

2. Why is a low-viscosity resin used in pit and fissure sealants? _____

_____

3. Give the reason for etching the tooth surface prior to the placement of the sealant._____

_____

4. Why is it necessary for the tooth to be completely dry before you place the sealant? _____

_____

Chapter 54: Applying Dental Cements and Restorative Materials

OBJECTIVES:

After studying this chapter, the student will be able to:
- Describe the technique for applying a cavity varnish to a prepared tooth.
- Describe the technique for applying a liner to a prepared tooth.
- Demonstrate the application of a varnish, base, and temporary restoration on a prepared stone model.

APPLYING VARNISH AND LINER

Varnish

A *varnish* is applied to the enamel and dentin walls up to the cavo-surface margin, figure 54–1. The varnish should be applied *before* zinc phosphate, amalgam, and gold foil and *after* calcium hydroxide and zinc oxide eugenol.

Liner

A **liner** is applied *only* to the dentinal walls up the dentinoenamel junction, figure 54–2.

APPLYING BASE AND TEMPORARY RESTORATION

Base

A **base** is applied to the cavity preparation, followed by the varnish, figure 54–3.

A base may be one of the following: calcium hydroxide, zinc oxide eugenol, zinc phosphate, zinc polyacrylate, and glass ionomers cement.

Double Base and Temporary Restoration

A *double base* is used in deep cavity preparations for additional protection.

Calcium hydroxide is placed first, followed by another base material. Base material may serve as the temporary restoration or another type of temporary cement may be used, figure 54–4.

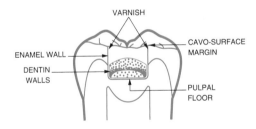

Fig. 54–1. Applying varnish

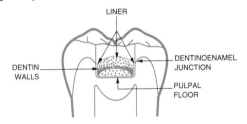

Fig. 54–2. Applying liner

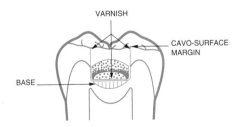

Fig. 54–3. The base is applied as shown.

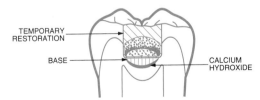

Fig. 54–4. Double base and temporary restoration

451

Table 54–1 lists the dental cements and restorative materials in columns according to their function and use. The column heading states the use of the cement or restorative material. In each column the names and brands of the various cements or restorative materials that may be used are listed.

TABLE 54–1
DENTAL CEMENTS AND RESTORATIVE MATERIALS

Cavity Varnishes and Liners	Bases for under Restorations	Temporary Restorations
Seals the dentinal tubules, protects pulp from chemical irritants in certain cements and restorative materials	Protects pulp from mechanical, thermal or electrical stimuli	Protects tooth until permanent restoration is placed
Cavity varnish —a solvent that, when applied to a cavity preparation, evaporates, leaving a resinous film on the surface. Applied to dentin and enamel walls. *Do not use with resins or composites.* • Copalite • Cavaseal • Caulk Varnish • S.S. White Cavity Varnish	**Calcium hydroxide** —stimulates the formation of secondary dentin. Used in deep cavities and for pulp capping • Dycal • Pulpdent Paste • Hydrex • Pro Cal • ESPE AlkaLiner	**Zinc oxide eugenol** —placed into prepared cavity preparation • Caulk ZOE B&T • S.S. White ZOE no. 2 with fibers • Wards Tem Pak • Wards Tem Pak or for temporary cementation of crowns
Cavity liner —a varnish-type material that contains calcium hydroxide or zinc oxide a solvent that, when applied to a cavity preparation, evaporates, leaving a film of calcium hydroxide or zinc oxide on the surface • Hydroxyline • Chembar	**Zinc oxide eugenol (ZOE)** —soothing effect on irritated pulp. Adds bulk to cavity preparation when needed • Cavitec • S.S. White ZOE • Caulk ZOE B&T	**Reinforced zinc oxide eugenol** —intermediate restoration, longer lasting temporary • Caulk IRM • Zinroc
• Pulpdent —a paste applied for a cavity preparation. Applied to the dentin walls *only* • Illypocal	**Reinforced zinc oxide eugenol** —stronger than regular ZOE but less soluble • Caulk IRM	**Zinc polyacrylate** —adheres to enamel and is stronger than zinc phosphate • Durelon • P.C.A. • Carboset • Poly-C
	Zinc phosphate —stronger than ZOE, but acid in cement is irritating to pulp when used in deep cavity preparations • S.S. White Zinc Improved • Modern Tenacin • Mizzy, Fleck	**Zinc phosphate** —may be used as a temporary restoration • S.S. White Zinc Improved • Modern Tenacin • Mizzy, Fleck
	Zinc Polyacrylate —mild effect on pulp comparable to zinc phosphate • Durelon • P.C.A.	
	Glass Ionomer —strong, kind to pulp, releases fluoride, anticarogenic property • ESPE-KETAC-BOND • GC Dentin Cement	

TABLE 54–1 [Continued]

Cementation	Direct Esthetic Restorative Material	Surgical Cements and Periodontal Dressings
To cement "lute" (to seal) gold inlays, onlays, crowns, bridges, and orthodontic band to permanent teeth	Restorations where esthetics are of primary importance	Applied to surgical wound to aid healing
Zinc phosphate —cement is applied to both the tooth/teeth and to the gold casting(s) or orthodontic bands • S.S. White Zinc Improved • Modern Tenacin • Mizzy, Fleck	**Composite resins**—Used in anterior teeth and posterior teeth in *limited areas only*. Class III, IV, and I and II in limited conditions • Adaptic • Concise • Prestige	**Surgical Cement** —placed over a surgical wound to aid in the retention of medication • Wards Wondr-Pak
Zinc polyacrylate • Durelon • P.C.A.	**Pit and fissure sealants** —used to prevent occlusal caries in newly erupted primary and permanent molars • Delton • Epoxylite • Prisma Shield	**Periodontal dressing** —placed over surgical wound following periodontal surgery or gingival curettage **(Eugenol)** • Wards Wondr-Pak • "PPC" • Kirkland (non-eugenol) • Coe-Perio Pak
Glass Ionomer —cementation of crowns and bridges, PJC; bonds to clean tooth structure enamel and dentin • Ketac-Cem • Fuji Type I	**Glass Ionomer** —used in small anterior restorations Class III, IV, posterior teeth Class I and II, Class V, and erosion or abrasion lesions • Ketac Fil • Fuji Type II	

Chapter 55: Dental Amalgam

OBJECTIVES:

After studying this chapter, the student will be able to:
- Define the terms lathe-cut and spherical alloy.
- State the advantages for using a high-copper alloy.
- Discuss the chemical composition of a dental alloy.

INTRODUCTION

The dental *amalgam* is one of the oldest restorative materials still in use today. A dental **alloy** is composed of two or more metals. A dental amalgam is the result of **amalgamation** of a dental alloy combined with mercury (a metal that is liquid at room temperature). A dental alloy and mercury are placed in a capsule, **triturated** (mixed) to form a pliable mass capable of being condensed (packed) into a cavity preparation. Dental amalgams do not adhere to the tooth structure. Therefore, adequate tooth structure must be present and the cavity preparation must offer sufficient retention.

TYPES OF AMALGAMS

Dental alloys available today consist of the conventional (traditional) low-copper and high-copper alloys. The conventional low-copper alloys are composed of *lathe-cut* (filings) or spherical particles. High-copper alloys are a combination of lathe-cut and spherical particles or a single composition of spherical particles.

Before 1961, lathe-cut (filings) alloy was the only type of alloy available. Lathe-cut alloy is produced by melting silver, tin, copper, and sometimes zinc together to form an ingot (metal cast into a bar). The ingot is then placed on either a lathe or a milling machine to produce alloy particles (filings) that are irregular in shape and have rough edges. This type of alloy requires more mercury to be used when triturated.

Spherical or spheroidal alloy particles are formed by atomization (to separate into atoms), a process in which the molten alloy is sprayed into a mist and the droplets are cooled with either air or water. As the droplets solidify, spherical (round) particles of different sizes are formed. This produces an alloy with a smoother surface that requires less mercury when triturated. Spherical alloys allow for improved carving and polishability of the amalgam restoration.

The American Dental Association's (ADA) specification No. 1 for dental alloys has been changed regarding the proportion of copper to other elements in the formula. Dental alloys that contain 6 percent or less copper are designated as low-copper, or conventional (traditional), alloys. Amalgam alloys that contain more than 6 percent copper are referred to as high-copper alloys.

High-copper alloys are classified according to particle shape, such as lathe-cut (filings), spherical, or a combination of particles (admixed). Admixed alloy is a combination of the low-copper lathe-cut alloy and high-copper spherical alloy particles. Alloys with smaller particle sizes will usually produce amalgams with a smoother surface when carved and will result in a stronger restoration.

SETTING REACTION

During trituration of the conventional low-copper alloy, the silver-tin alloy particles will react with the mercury (Hg). This reaction will result in the combination of silver with mercury referred to as (gamma phase-1) and tin with mercury referred to as (gamma phase-2). *Gamma* is a particular arrangement of atoms. *Phase* denotes a change in structure.

With the new high-copper alloy in gamma phase-2, copper will combine with tin, rather than tin with mercury. Both reactions form a matrix that holds the unreacted powder particles. The amalgam can be thought of as original alloy particles surrounded by a continuous matrix of silver-mercury and a little tin mercury in the conventional amalgam, or copper-tin in high-copper amalgams. The tin-mercury phase is the weakest phase in the conventional amalgam most likely to corrode. **Corrosion** is a chemical reaction of a nonmetallic substance with a metal. This phase is usually not present in the high-copper amalgams, which explains their superior properties.

Because high-copper alloys eliminate the weak tin-mercury phase, the result is an amalgam with improved strength, increased resistance to corrosion, and reduced marginal breakdown and failure. Over 90 percent of amalgams purchased today are high-copper alloys.

COMPOSITION

The chemical composition of a dental alloy may contain the following metals: silver (Ag), Tin (Sn), Copper (Cu), and Zinc (Zn). *Note:* Not all alloys contain zinc.

Each metal used in dental alloy has certain qualities that are needed in order to produce the desired restoration. The effects of each component are as follows:

Silver

- Used to form the metallic compound with mercury (Hg) that determines the dimensional changes that occur during hardening.
- Increases strength of restoration.
- Increases expansion.

- Is slow to amalgamate.
- Hardens rapidly.
- Tarnishes easily.
- Decreases setting time.

Tin

- Aids in the amalgamation (chemical combining) of the alloy with the mercury because of its strong affinity for mercury.
- Reduces expansion during setting.
- Reduces strength.
- Setting time is slower.
- More susceptible to corrosion (conventional alloy).
- Tends to weaken the amalgam.

Copper

- Increases strength and hardness.
- Increases expansion of amalgam during hardening.
- Reduces flow of finished restoration.
- Resists corrosion (high-copper).
- Reduces marginal failure (high-copper).

Zinc

- Used to minimize the oxidation of the other metals present in alloy during manufacturing. Zinc is a scavenger and reacts with oxygen, preventing it from combining with silver, tin, or copper. *Note:* Should moisture contamination occur during manipulation or condensation of the amalgam, delayed expansion may occur. Zinc-containing dental amalgams are particularly sensitive to moisture. Zinc reacts with water to form the zinc oxide and hydrogen gas that may cause the unwanted and excessive expansion of the set amalgam restoration.

ADVANTAGES OF DENTAL AMALGAMS

1. They can be triturated into a smooth plastic mass within seconds, remain this way

for approximately three minutes, allowing for proper placement and condensation.

2. They can be placed, condensed, and readily adapted to the cavity walls.
3. They can receive and retain a polish twenty-four hours after the restoration has been placed.
4. When correctly manipulated, the restoration will have limited dimensional changes (expansion and contraction).

DISADVANTAGES OF AMALGAMS

1. They lack edge-strength and will fracture if not supported by the presence of adequate tooth structure.
2. They lack esthetic appeal because of their silver color; therefore, they are used in posterior teeth for Class I, II, and V.
3. They have a tendency to tarnish (simple surface discoloration of a silver alloy).

REVIEW

1. Name the two dental alloys used in dentistry today. _____

_____

_____

2. What is the advantage for using a high-copper alloy over the conventional low-copper lathe-cut alloy? _____

_____

_____

3. Give the composition of an admixed high-copper alloy.

_____

_____

_____

4. What are the desirable and undesirable effects of each metal used in a dental alloy? _____

_____

_____

_____

_____

_____

_____

5. Why is it necessary to have adequate tooth structure when placing an amalgam restoration? _____

_____

6. Define the terms *dental alloy* and *dental amalgam.* _____

_____

_____

Chapter 56: Mercury

> **OBJECTIVES:**
> After studying this chapter, the student will be able to:
> - Discuss the hazards of mercury vapor.
> - Discuss the principles of mercury hygiene as they apply to dental office personnel.
> - Discuss the principles of mercury hygiene in the dental operatory.

INTRODUCTION

The properties of mercury for use in the production of dental amalgams must meet the specification listed by the Council on Dental Materials, Instruments and Equipment of the American Dental Association, Specification No. 6.

Dental mercury is one of the most commonly used metals in dentistry and it is highly toxic (poisonous). It is the only metal that is liquid and vaporizes (particles of matter scatter and freely float in the air) at a relatively low room temperature. Mercury vapor has no color, odor, or taste and cannot be readily detected. Mercury may be absorbed into the body through inhalation or through the pores of the skin. Mercury vapor inhalation may occur during trituration, dispensing the amalgam mass from the capsule, and when polishing new amalgam restorations. Also, during the cutting and removal of amalgam restorations, mercury vapor and amalgam dust are created. The frictional heat created by grinding the amalgam causes the surface mercury to separate from the alloy, resulting in mercury vapor and amalgam dust (minute particles of alloy and mercury).

Mercury will penetrate the pores of the skin when touched with bare hands. Therefore, squeezing of the amalgam mass to express excess mercury should be avoided and is no longer an accepted technique.

Mercury plays an important role in the clinical behavior of the individual amalgam restoration. The average well-condensed amalgam should contain approximately 50 percent or less mercury.

RECOMMENDATIONS FOR MERCURY HYGIENE

The American Dental Association (ADA) recommends that a program of mercury hygiene be established within each dental practice. The dentist has a dual responsibility to the dental staff and him or herself to control mercury vapor in the dental office.

In 1984, the Occupational Safety and Health Act (OSHA) mandated that the dentist provide a workplace that is free from any occupational hazards.

Potential office hazards involving mercury can be eliminated by practicing appropriate mercury hygiene. A great deal of concern has been directed toward the biological effects of mercury. To inform the dental profession of the potential dangers of mercury, the Council on Dental Materials, Instruments and Equipment of the American Dental Association, has established the following guidelines:

Dental Office Personnel Responsibilites

1. Wear disposable gloves, face mask, and glasses or shield when working with dental amalgam.
2. A no-touch technique should be used when handling mercury. Skin that is exposed to mercury should be cleansed

with soap and water. Rinse thoroughly under running water.

3. The use of premeasured capsules allows for exact ratio of alloy and mercury. This type of capsule eliminates the use of the mercury dispensers and any possibility of mercury spillage. The ideal premeasured capsule that is electronically welded presents no hazard.

4. Use an amalgamator that has a protective hood to reduce the chance of any mercury vapor being released into the atmosphere and to confine mercury that might be sprayed from a traditional capsule with an ill-fitting cap. Screw-type or frictional-fit capsules that must be pressed together may also leak during trituration. Both can be checked for leakage by wrapping adhesive tape around the point where the two parts of the capsule join. Leakage will show up as small drops of mercury on the adhesive tape. Leaking capsules should be discarded.

5. All used capsules should be reassembled immediately after dispensing the amalgam. The used dental amalgam capsule is highly contaminated with mercury vapor.

6. Office personnel should have periodic urinalyses to check for any mercury in the body. The ADA suggests that mercury testing be a part of all dental office personnel on a regular health evaluation basis. More information concerning a mercury testing service is offered by the ADA Council on Dental Therapeutics, 211 East Chicago Avenue, Chicago, IL 60611. Request pamphlet 3-005-3.

Dental Operatory

1. Unwanted mercury and amalgam scraps should be stored in a tightly sealed, unbreakable jar containing used x-ray fixer, glycerin, or mineral oil. Storing scrap amalgam under water is not an effective means of controlling mercury vapor.

2. Carpeted floors in dental operatories is not recommended. Mercury in carpeting is impossible to retrieve and significantly increases mercury hazard. Never use a household vacuum to clean up mercury spills, as it tends to vaporize the mercury rather than collect it.

3. Water spray and high-volume evacuation should be used when cutting old amalgams or finishing new restorations, because the heat created will release some mercury vapor. A face mask should be worn to reduce mercury vapor and amalgam dust inhalation.

4. Avoid working with mercury or amalgam near a heat source.

5. Perform all operations involving mercury over areas that have an impervious and suitable lipped surface. This will allow easier recovery of unwanted mercury or amalgam scraps.

6. Treatment rooms should have proper ventilation to reduce the possibility of mercury vapor inhalation. Frequent changes in the office air-filter system is of utmost importance.

7. Dispose of mercury-contaminated items such as gloves, mask, used capsules, squeeze cloths, and the like, by placing and sealing in a labeled polyethylene bag.

Suggestions for Controlling Mercury Spills

1. Clean up mercury spills immediately regardless of amount. Small droplets may be recovered by using a fresh mix of amalgam or lead foil from a x-ray film packet. Spills of mercury should be cleaned up, because small droplets of mercury have a high vapor potential as atmospheric temperature increases. That is to say, the

higher the room temperature, the more likely it is that mercury will vaporize.

2. Dental offices that use large quantities of mercury should be equipped with a mercury-spill kit. The kit should include disposable rubber gloves, a mercury-vapor respirator, a hypodermic needle with a large lumen, a syringe, adhesive tape for picking up droplets, polyethylene bags for disposal, and a sulfur solution for coating droplets prior to retrieval and disposal.

3. The Council on Dental Materials, Instruments and Equipments, specifically advises against the use of ultrasonic condensors when condensing amalgam, because mercury vapor is released from the amalgam.

REVIEW

1. How does mercury differ from other metals used in dentistry? _____

_____

2. By what two means may mercury enter the body system?_____

_____

3. The average well-condensed amalgam should contain approximately _____ percent or less mercury.

4. Why should an amalgamator with a protective hood be used? _____

_____

_____

5. How can leakages from a capsule be determined during trituration? _____

_____

_____

6. How should unwanted mercury and amalgam scraps be stored?_____

_____

7. Give the four precautionary measures that dental office personnel can take to reduce the potential hazards of mercury vapor.

a. _____

b. _____

c. _____

d. _____

8. What procedure should be followed when cutting or removing old amalgams?

_____

_____

9. How should mercury contaminated items be disposed of? _____

_____

Chapter 57: Use of the Dental Amalgamator

OBJECTIVES: After studying this chapter, the student will be able to:
- Compare the types of capsules that can be used with a dental amalgamator.
- Discuss the advantages of using a premeasured sealed capsule over the traditional screw or friction-fit capsule.
- Explain the proper procedure for preparing a dental amalgam.
- Demonstrate the correct procedure for loading an amalgam carrier.

INTRODUCTION

A dental **amalgamator,** or *triturator*, is a specially designed machine used to triturate (mix) a dental alloy with mercury to produce a silver amalgam restorative material, figure 57–1.

Today several types of amalgamators are available. Although some amalgamators may operate at a single speed, others have variable speeds (low, medium, or high) and frequency levels (rate of speed and path in which the capsule moves during trituration).

The manufacturers of amalgamators provide information about which speed or frequency and trituration time are required for their particular type of amalgamator. Each amalgamator must be set for the type of dental alloy used, slow, medium, or fast.

Medium- and high-speed frequency amalgamators are recommended for use with improved high-copper alloys.

Generally the higher the speed or frequency, the shorter the trituration time. However, less than six seconds is not recommended, as it is insufficient to remove the alloy's oxide layer, a necessary step so that the particles can combine with mercury. Usually, trituration of the alloy or mercury for ten to fifteen seconds will produce a homogeneous and uniform mix.

CAPSULE

Amalgamators may be used with the traditional **capsule** and pestle or the premeasured sealed capsules containing both the alloy particles and mercury.

The traditional capsules are plastic or metal, screw-type or friction-fit. This type of capsule must be loaded with the dental alloy and mercury before trituration. If the traditional capsule is to be used, the choice of a screw-type capsule over the friction-fit is better, because the friction-fit may release mercury vapor during the trituration process. Any type of capsule that releases mercury vapor is a health hazard to dental personnel.

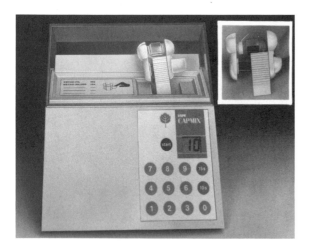

Fig. 57–1. Dental amalgamator (Courtesy Premier Dental/ESPE Premier Sales Co.)

462

Premeasured sealed capsules contain both dental alloy and mercury. The alloy powder particles and mercury are separated by a nonreactive thin foil that must be punctured by compressing or twisting the two parts of the capsule together. This releases the mercury into the alloy inside the capsule.

Another type of premeasured sealed capsule is electronically welded together. A plastic wafer inside the capsule contains the mercury and premeasured alloy. During the trituration cycle, the mercury is released from the plastic wafer, and the empty wafer is forced against the end of the capsule.

Some of the advantages of using premeasured sealed capsules are: (1) the portions of the alloy and mercury are consistent; (2) they prevent any chance of mercury spill; and (3) they prevent the possibility that mercury vapor will be released during trituration.

TRITURATION

Trituration is the mechanical means of combining the dental alloy with mercury. Amalgamation is the actual chemical reaction that occurs between the alloy and mercury to form the silver amalgam.

To attain the maximum properties and desirable working characteristics of a dental amalgam, the manufacturer's instructions for trituration time must be followed.

CONDENSING THE AMALGAM

An amalgam is placed into a cavity preparation by using an amalgam carrier and **condensing** instruments. The dental amalgam is carried to the preparation with the amalgam carrier, then packed with the **condensers**. The dental amalgam must be placed rapidly and with enough force to ensure proper adaptation of the amalgam to the cavity walls of the preparation. Failure to condense the amalgam immediately

after trituration can weaken the amalgam and may cause the amalgam to set before it is placed in the preparation. If the amalgam is not condensed within three to four minutes, a fresh mix should be prepared.

MATERIALS NEEDED

- gloves, mask, glasses, or face shield
- amalgamator
- premeasured sealed alloy or mercury capsule
- squeeze cloth, amalgam well, or dappen dish
- amalgam carrier
- scrap container for amalgam

INSTRUCTIONS

1. Assemble materials, figure 57–2. Select trituration time and speed for type of alloy and amalgamator used.
2. Prepare capsule according to type being used.
3. Insert capsule into prongs or clip of amalgamator, figure 57–3. The capsule must be properly inserted; otherwise, it may become dislodged during trituration.

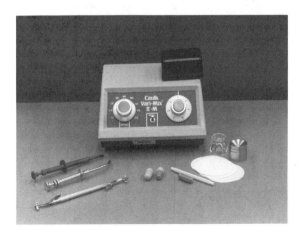

Fig. 57–2. **Assembled materials**

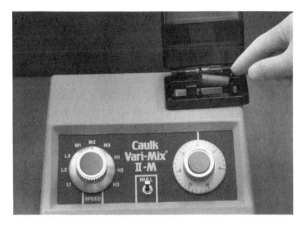

Fig. 57–3. Capsule inserted into prongs or clip of amalgamator

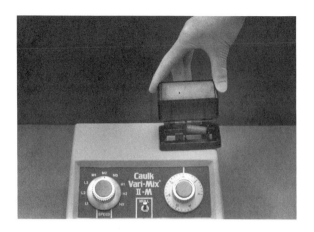

Fig. 57–4. Close cover over capsule.

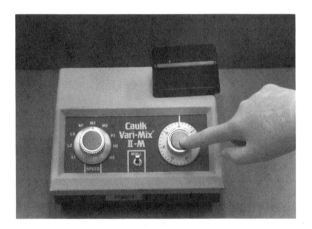

Fig. 57–5. Activate timer.

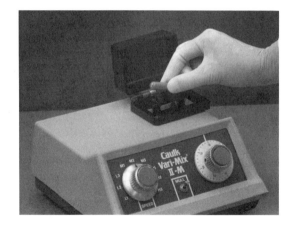

Fig. 57–6. Remove capsule from amalgamator.

4. Close cover of amalgamator, figure 57–4.
5. Triturate for prescribed time according to manufacturer's instructions (generally between ten to fifteen seconds depending on type of alloy used, and whether the machine is set on slow, medium, or fast).
6. Activate timer, figure 57–5. The timer will automatically switch off after the prescribed trituration time.

7. Lift cover, and remove capsule from prongs or clip, figure 57–6. If a traditional capsule or pestle is used, the pestle must be removed and the cap replaced on the capsule, then mulled for one or two seconds.
8. Separate capsule, and empty contents into a squeeze cloth, the amalgam well, or the dappen dish, figure 57–7. Avoid touching amalgam, even with gloved hands.

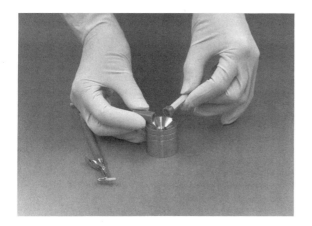

Fig. 57–7. Place amalgam in amalgam well.

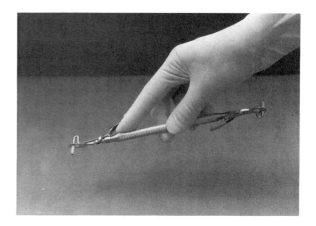

Fig. 57–8. Hand position for amalgam carrier

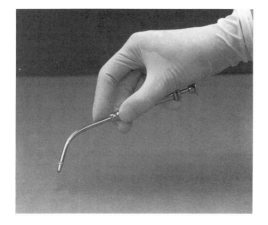

Fig. 57–9. Hand position for amalgam carrier

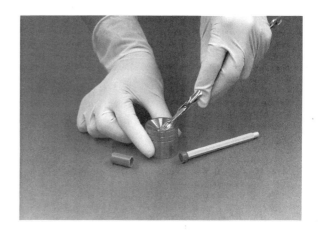

Fig. 57–10. Begin loading carrier.

Note: A well-mixed amalgam should have a glossy appearance with a smooth velvety consistency. An amalgam that crumbles when loading a carrier should be discarded, because it will be impossible to condense.

9. Immediately recap capsule to reduce mercury vapor released during trituration.

Loading the Carrier

1. Hold amalgam carrier with an overhand grasp, figures 57–8 and 57–9.

2. Begin loading carrier, figure 57–10.
3. Pack carrier to form a compact cylinder, figure 57–11. After carrier is packed, immediately pass to operator. Operator will dispense amalgam and return the carrier to the assistant. The assistant will exchange the carrier for a condenser. The operator now proceeds with condensing, while the assistant reloads the carrier. This procedure will be repeated until a sufficient amount of amalgam has been condensed into the tooth preparation.

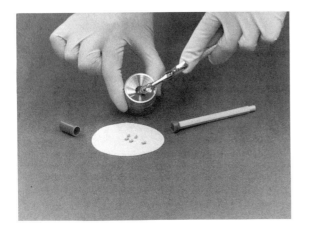

Fig. 57–11. Amalgam carrier dispenses compact amalgam cylinders.

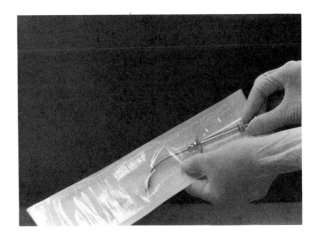

Fig. 57–12. Carrier placed in sterilizing pouch

Cleaning Up

1. Expel any excess amalgam into appropriate container. See Chapter 56, *Mercury*.
2. Disinfect carrier with surface disinfectant. Place in Chemiclave pouch for sterilization, figure 57–12.

SUGGESTED ACTIVITIES

- Practice using the amalgamator, and prepare a mix of amalgam.
- Practice loading the amalgam carrier from a squeeze cloth, an amalgam well, or dappen dish.

REVIEW

1. How long after trituration may amalgam be permitted to stand before it is condensed into the preparation? _____

   _____

2. Define the term *trituration*. _____

   _____

3. Define the term *amalgamation*. _____

   _____

4. The approximate working time for condensing an amalgam is_____

   _____.

Chapter 58: Alginate Impression Material (Irreversible Colloids) _____

OBJECTIVES: After studying this chapter, the student will be able to:
- Discuss the basic composition of an irreversible colloid.
- Discuss the physical and chemical properties of alginate.
- Discuss the factors that influence the stability of alginate.

INTRODUCTION

Alginate is used for making study models, for *primary impressions* of **edentulous** mouths, and for making impressions in areas in which partial dentures are to be fabricated.

COMPOSITION

Alginates are salts of alginic acid (crystalline compounds that are typically water-soluble) and are extracted from seaweed. However, alginate is insoluble until potassium or sodium salts are added to make it soluble. When alginate is mixed with water, it has the ability to set or gel.

Dental alginates are called **irreversible colloids**. A **colloid** is a gelatinous substance with large inorganic molecules that remain suspended and do not diffuse or spread once the chemical change occurs. The material is supplied as flour-like powder and consists essentially of soluble potassium alginate and calcium sulfate. The exact proportion of each chemical may vary with the manufacturer. A basic formula for alginate impression material follows (percentage of total weight):

potassium alginate	15%
calcium sulfate	16%
trisodium phosphate	1%
diatomaceous earth	60%
zinc oxide	4%
potassium titanium fluoride	3%

When mixed with calcium sulfate, a *reactor* (causes a chemical change), potassium alginate produces an insoluble calcium alginate. This chemical reaction must be delayed until the impression material has been mixed with water, placed on the impression tray, and carried to the mouth. A third soluble salt, trisodium phosphate, is added as a **retarder**.

Calcium sulfate will react first with the trisodium phosphate before reacting with the soluble potassium alginate. As long as trisodium phosphate is present, the gelation reaction between the potassium alginate and calcium sulfate will be prevented. Therefore, when the trisodium phosphate is exhausted, the calcium ions will begin to react with the potassium alginate.

The purpose of diatomaceous earth is to act as a filler. Proper amounts of filler can increase the strength and stiffness of the mix and ensure a firm surface that is not tacky. Fillers also help to form the sol by dispersing the alginate powder particle in the water. Zinc oxide is also added as a filler and has some influence on the setting time.

Potassium titanium fluoride is added to ensure a hard, dense stone cast surface.

Alginate powder contains about 60 percent finely ground silicate filler (diatomaceous earth). When fluffed, these particles can be inhaled and may prove to be a health hazard. (Recent studies have shown dental alginate to be a health hazard.) A new dustless alginate has been introduced to eliminate the presence of these fine airborne particles. Jeltrate Plus is coated with a glycol (an alcohol derived from a carbohydrate) to make it dustless. Jeltrate Plus has a strength 50 percent higher than standard Jeltrate. The powder is more easily wetted by the water when mixed.

Currently, a two-paste alginate system, Ultrafine, is available. Ultrafine is supplied as two pastes (base and catalyst) that contain water and a silicone oil. Ultrafine is similar to standard alginate in strength but is easier to mix because of the two-paste system.

GEL STRUCTURE

The gelation of a hydrocolloid is the changing of a **sol** to a **gel**. The *sol* is the colloidal solution, and the semi-solid state is termed colloidal *gel*. During this phase of changing from a sol to a gel, fibrils will branch and intermesh to form a brush heap structure. These fibrils are composed of chains, sometimes called *micelles*. The structure resembles the intermeshing of twigs in a brush pile. The final structure can be envisioned as a brush heap of calcium alginate fibrils in a network of filler particles and excess water.

GEL STRENGTH

Manipulation of alginate material will affect the wet strength. For example, if too much or too little water is used in mixing, the gel will be weakened. Proper water to powder ratio is specified by the manufacturer. When an insufficient amount of time is used for mixing, the strength of the final gel will be radically reduced. When there is insufficient spatulation (undermixing), the ingredients do not dissolve enough to permit the chemical reactions to proceed uniformly throughout the mass. Overmixing also produces poor results, because any calcium alginate gel formed during prolonged spatulation will be broken up. The strength of the mix depends on

exact measurements of powder and water, as well as correct spatulation to obtain a smooth, creamy mix within the specified time.

GELATION TIME

Manufacturers make dental alginates that have different properties. Some, for instance, are made to set faster than others (Type I, fast set); some set slower for additional working time (Type II, regular or normal set).

Type I, Fast Set

Working Time	*Setting Time*
68°F (20°C), 1 min., 45 sec.	1 min., 45 sec.
72°F (22°C), 1 min., 45 sec.	1 min., 45 sec.
75°F (24°C), 1 min., 30 sec.	1 min., 45 sec.

Type II, Regular Set

Working Time	*Setting Time*
68°F (20°C), 2 min., 15 sec.	2 min., 15 sec.
72°F (22°C), 2 min.	2 min., 15 sec.
75°F (24°C), 2 min.	2 min.

Cool water will delay gelation time, and warm water will hasten it. It is of the utmost importance to *read and carefully follow the manufacturer's directions.*

It is always wise to use alginate that has been certified by the Council on Dental Materials, Instruments and Devices.

DIMENSIONAL STABILITY

Alginate impressions should be poured as soon as possible, because the material undergoes dimensional changes as time elapses. Such changes in dimensions are termed **syneresis** or **imbibition**. *Syneresis* refers to a loss of water by evaporation due to exposure to the air; the result is a shrinkage in dimension. *Imbibition* may occur when a substance takes on additional water, causing a swelling of the material. Consequently, alginate impressions should not be stored in water. Either of these dimensional changes produce an inaccurate impression in the poured model or cast.

Alginate gels currently used in dentistry exhibit reasonably good dimensional stability in an atmosphere of 100% humidity. If the alginate impression has to be preserved for a short time, it should be placed in an airtight container with a moistened paper towel to produce an atmosphere of 100 percent humidity. However, for the most accurate and satisfactory results, impressions should be poured immediately after being taken. There is no adequate method for storage of any of the hydrocolloid impressions materials.

REVIEW

1. The correct term for the final set alginate is _____.

2. Three major uses for alginate impression material are

    a. _____

    b. _____

    c. _____

3. Give the composition of alginate impression material and the function of each compound in the basic formula.

    a. _____

    _____

    b. _____

    _____

    c. _____

    _____

    d. _____

    _____

    e. _____

    _____

    f. _____

    _____

4. The best the way to alter the gelation time for alginate is _____

_____.

5. Synereris is _____

_____.

6. Imbibition occurs when _____

_____.

Chapter 59: Mixing Alginate Impression Material

OBJECTIVES: After studying this chapter, the student will be able to:
- Select the armamentarium needed to mix alginate impression material.
- Measure correct water to powder ratio.
- Spatulate mix to a creamy, smooth homogeneous mass.

INTRODUCTION

The major physical and chemical properties of alginate have been described in Chapter 58. Alginate impressions are taken by (1) inserting impression trays loaded with alginate impression material onto one arch of the dental patient; (2) allowing the material to gel or set; (3) removing the impression from the mouth; and finally (4) pouring up the impression in plaster.

Mixing or spatulation of alginate impressions material requires practice in order to obtain the smooth, homogeneous mass needed to take an accurate impression of the dental arch.

MATERIALS NEEDED

- protective glasses
- face mask
- alginate impression material
- water measure
- powder scoop
- paper cup or paper towel
- room-temperature water
- plaster bowl
- spatula, plaster

INSTRUCTIONS

Assemble all materials needed for the procedure, figure 59–1.

1. Measure required amount of room-temperature (70 to 72°F) water. Carefully read **meniscus** (the concave surface of a column of liquid with its lowest point in the center) on measuring gauge, figure 59–2.
2. Pour water into mixing bowl, figure 59–3.

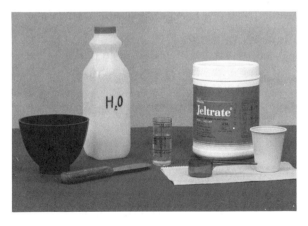

Fig. 59–1. Materials assembled

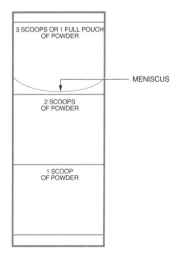

Fig. 59–2. Reading meniscus

471

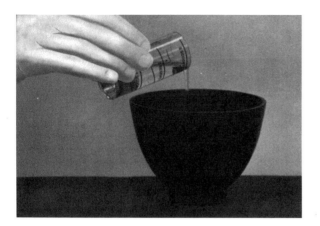

Fig. 59–3. Placing water into bowl

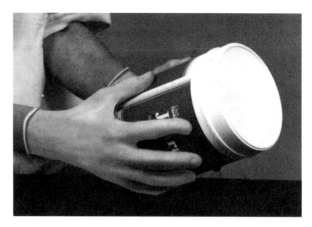

Fig. 59–4. Rotating alginate container

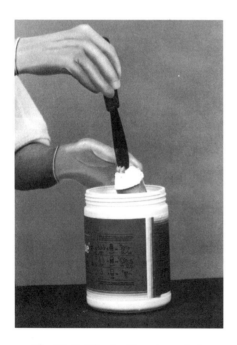

Fig. 59–5. Eliminating air pockets

side several times, figure 59–4. Otherwise, a hazardous aerosol cloud (aerosol, fine particles that float in the air) will form inside the container. Therefore, it is best to allow the container to be left unopened for about two minutes. After opening the container, disturb the contents as little as possible. If the alginate powder is inhaled, it can become a health hazard; wearing a face mask can reduce this risk.

4. Fill powder scoop. Gently tap handle of scoop against rim of container. Cut powder with spatula inside scoop to avoid air pockets, figure 59–5. Level powder with spatula, figure 59–6. Place powder in paper cup or on paper towel.

5. Replace alginate container cover immediately.

6. Carefully sift powder into water, figure 59–7. If using premeasured packets, open with scissors and gently tap entire contents into water.

7. Stir the mix to wet all powder particles, figure 59–8.

3. Fluff alginate powder when using powder from a vacuum-sealed container. *Do not shake*, but roll the container from side to

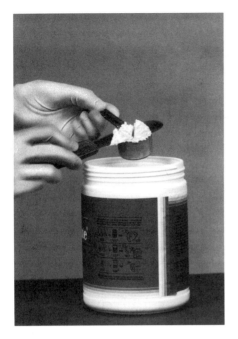

Fig. 59–6. Leveling powder with spatula

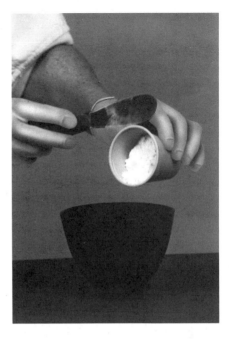

Fig. 59–7. Sifting powder into water

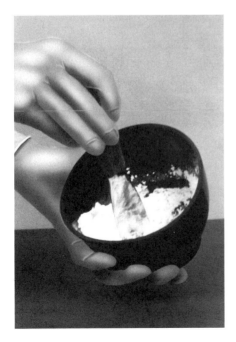

Fig. 59–8. Wetting powder particles

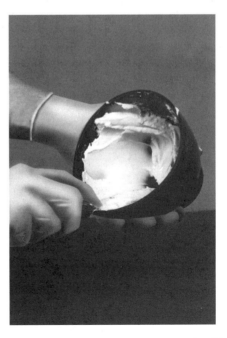

Fig. 59–9. Spatulating material against side of bowl

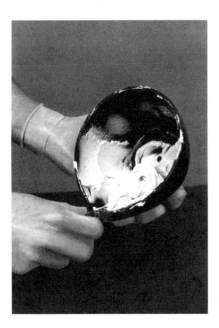

Fig. 59–10. Gathering material

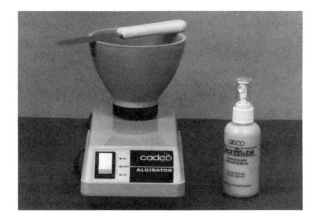

Fig. 59–11. Mechanical mixer

8. Begin spatulation in a stropping (back and forth) motion. Rotate bowl during spatulation, and, at the same time, spread the mix against the side of the bowl to dissolve all the granules and to eliminate air voids, figure 59–9. Do not allow alginate to spill out of the bowl.

9. Gather alginate mix with spatula after approximately twenty seconds; replace mix in bottom of bowl, figure 59–10. Continue spatulation until mix is creamy. Gather mass on spatula and load tray. Total mixing time of steps 6 to 9 is not to exceed one minute for regular set. *Note:* Alginate may be hand-mixed or mixed with a mechanical mixer (alginator), figure 59–11.

SUGGESTED ACTIVITIES

• Select materials needed for mixing alginate impression material.

• Spatulate alginate impression material within the prescribed time.

Chapter 60: Loading Alginate Trays

OBJECTIVES:
After studying this chapter, the student will be able to:
- Select a tray for a full-arch maxillary alginate impression.
- Select a tray for a full-arch mandibular alginate impression.
- Spatulate alginate material and load the trays.

INTRODUCTION

The first consideration when taking an impression is the proper selection of the tray(s). The purpose of the tray is to control, carry and confine the impression material in the patient's mouth. Trays may be made of disposable styrofoam, perforated or solid (rim lock) metal, or plastic. Trays may be full arch, anterior only or right or left quadrant.

MATERIALS NEEDED

- impression trays
- alginate impression material
- measuring devices
- plaster bowl
- small rubber bowl
- spatula, plaster (ovoid)
- paper cup
- room-temperature water
- paper towels

INSTRUCTIONS

Loading the Tray for a Mandibular Impression (2 scoops of powder)

Assemble all materials needed for the procedure.

1. Spatulate alginate according to instructions. Refer to Chapter 59.
2. Remove half the alginate mix from bowl and load one side of tray, figure 60–1.
3. With spatula, press alginate mix into tray, figure 60–2.
4. Repeat procedure for opposite side of tray.
5. Wet fingers, and smooth the surface of the tray mix while gently pressing material to obtain retention, figure 60–3.

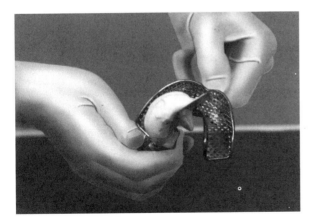

Fig. 60–1. Loading half of mandibular tray

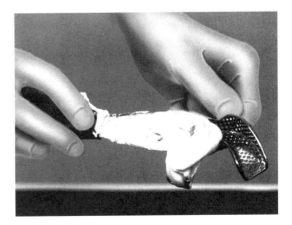

Fig. 60–2. Pressing alginate mix into tray

475

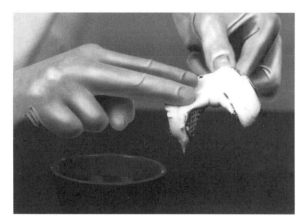

Fig. 60–3. Smoothing surface of alginate with wet fingers

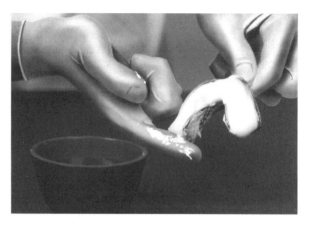

Fig. 60–4. Removing unwanted material from border of tray

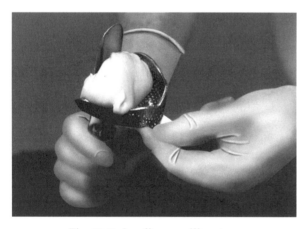

Fig. 60–5. Loading maxillary tray

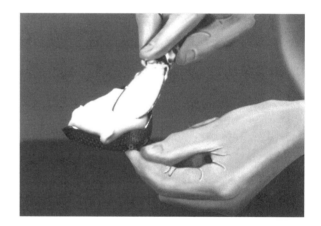

Fig. 60–6. Pressing alginate mix over entire tray

6. Remove any unwanted material from border of the tray, especially the tongue area, figure 60–4.
7. Loading time should approximate thirty seconds.

Loading the Tray for a Maxillary Impression (2–3 scoops of powder)

1. Have a small bowl of water ready for smoothing tray alginate.
2. Spatulate alginate according to instructions.

3. Remove alginate from bowl in one mass.
4. Place all of the alginate in the posterior area of the tray while holding spatula vertical to the plane of the tray, figure 60–5.
5. With spatula, spread alginate evenly over entire tray, making certain that no open voids are created, figure 60–6.
6. Wet fingers, and smooth the surface of the tray mix while gently pressing material to obtain retention.
7. Remove any unwanted material from border of the tray.

8. Loading time should approximate thirty seconds.

Cleaning Up

1. Remove impression material from tray(s), and place in ultrasonic unit with tray-cleaning solution. Rinse and dry tray(s).
2. Wash and dry bowls and spatula.
3. Return all items to proper place.
4. Clean work station.

SUGGESTED ACTIVITIES

- Measure the alginate and water for the maxillary arch.
- Practice spatulating alginate and loading the maxillary tray.
- Measure the alginate and water for the mandibular arch.
- Practice spatulating alginate and loading the mandibular tray.

Chapter 61: Taking Alginate Impressions for Study Models

OBJECTIVES:

After studying this chapter, the student will be able to:
- Select and prepare the appropriate maxillary and mandibular tray for an alginate impression.
- Take a maxillary and mandibular alginate impression, to include the accurate reproduction of all teeth, supporting tissues (soft tissue, muscle attachments, tuberosities, or retromolar pads).
- Prepare wax, and take a wax bite for centric occlusion.

INTRODUCTION

Through legislative measure, under their respective state Dental Practice Acts, some states have legally afforded additional duties and responsibilities to the dental assistant. Among these is taking alginate impressions for study **models**. For that reason, the object of this chapter will be to detail the essential steps in taking alginate impressions of the dental arches of patients.

The study models are taken for several reasons. They are used in diagnosis and treatment planning, patient education, comparison for "before" and "after" models, recording tooth size and position (in case of an accident), rotated and malaligned teeth, height of the soft tissue, and for occlusal relationship of maxillary and mandibular teeth.

MATERIALS NEEDED

- protective glasses
- face mask or shield
- disposable gloves
- maxillary and mandibular perforated trays
- beading wax
- lubricant
- cotton rolls
- mouthwash
- plastic drape or patient napkin
- spatula, plaster
- lab knife
- alginate scoop
- alginate powder
- water vial
- room-temperature water
- paper cup or paper towel
- mixing bowls, large and small

INSTRUCTIONS

Seating and Preparing the Patient for Impressions

1. Seat patient upright in chair.
2. Drape and place patient napkin. *Note:* At this time the operator should wash and glove hands and don a face mask or shield.
3. Examine patient's mouth with mouth mirror.
4. Apply lubricant to patient's lips.

Selecting Impression Trays

1. The trays should cover the most distal teeth or the tuberosity/retromolar pads, whichever is most posterior.
2. The trays should allow about 3 mm (1/8") of impression material on buccal, lingual, and facial surfaces of all teeth involved.
3. Incisors should set in the deepest anterior portion of the tray.
4. The tray should not impinge on the soft tissues.

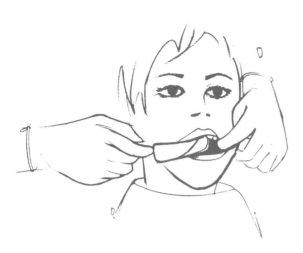

Fig. 61–1. **Trying in mandibular tray**

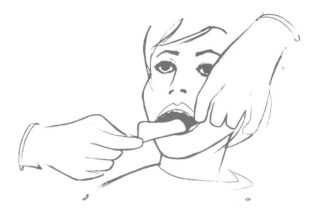

Fig. 61–2. **Trying in maxillary tray**

Preparing Impression Trays

1. Try maxillary and mandibular trays in patient's mouth.
2. Slide tray in sideways and center in mouth as shown, figures 61–1 and 61–2.
3. Observe trays, making certain that ample space is provided. Trays should *NEVER* impinge on soft tissues.
4. Adapt beading wax to peripheral edges of tray(s), figure 61–3 (figure 61–3 is illustrated on a typodont to show proper seating of tray filled with alginate). This adds to patient comfort and prevents impinging on the tissues. Beading wax may be added to the length and dimension of tray(s) and helps to retain impression material in tray. For a high vault, a wax strip may be placed over the palatal area.
5. Retry prepared trays in patient's mouth.
6. Explain procedure to patient. The mandibular impression is taken first to accustom the patient with the taste, feel, and consistency of the impression material. Patients are less likely to gag on the lower impression. Should the gag reflex become

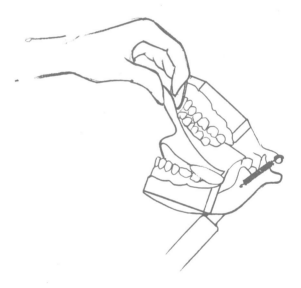

Fig. 61–3. **Depressing heel of tray**

a problem the following instructions may be given:
a. Ask the patient to relax, pant, or breathe rapidly through mouth and or nose.
b. Use "temple tapping." This involves having the operator firmly tapping both temples of the patient and at the same

time maintaining direct eye contact, while repeating the phrase "You will not gag" with each tap.

c. Direct the patient to extend one leg upward and concentrate on maintaining it in same position until the impression is completed.

d. Place a small amount of imitation table salt on distal portion of tongue and instruct the patient to swallow. *Note: NoSalt* has a potassium chloride base, rather than the commonly used sodium chloride table salt.

e. Children may be given a mental chore, such as counting backward beginning with 100.

Taking the Impression(s)

Mandibular Arch. The position of the operator for the mandibular impression is between 8 and 9 o'clock, and for the maxillary impression between 9 and 12 o'clock. The patient's shoulder should be positioned at about the same height as the elbow of the operator.

Instruct the patient to rinse with mouthwash just prior to taking impression(s).

1. Mix alginate, and load tray.
2. Insert tray.
3. Hold tray in one hand and, with the other hand, retract cheek.
4. Slide tray in sideways until one half of tray is inside the mouth, then rotate tray and seat. See figure 61–1. The handle of the tray should be centered (aligned with nose) and perpendicular to the anterior teeth. The anterior portion of the tray must be positioned over centrals or laterals in order to provide adequate impression material in the vestibular area. *Note:* Alginate impressions must provide detail of the facial surfaces of the anterior teeth and labial frenum and also of the muco-buccal attachment. The peripheral roll

should be accurately duplicated in impression(s). Examine the impression(s) for detail. Large voids and lack of detail or completeness are reasons enough for retaking the impression(s).

5. Ask the patient to close his or her mouth slightly; this will relax the facial muscles and help the operator to seat the tray.
6. Depress heels of tray (posterior teeth) first, figure 61–3.
7. Have the patient elevate tongue (toward roof of mouth), then depress tray downward, bringing it parallel to the occlusal plane, figure 61–4. (Figure 61–4 is illustrated on a typodont to show proper seating of tray filled with alginate.)
8. Assist the patient in lifting the lip and cheek areas to allow complete seating of tray.
9. Position tray by pressing firmly on the occlusal and incisal surfaces of the mandibular teeth, using the index and middle fingers of each hand on top of tray and resting thumbs under the mandible.
10. Instruct patient to breathe deeply and slowly through mouth or nose while tray is in place.
11. When the impression material has set, lift cheek on one side with index finger and

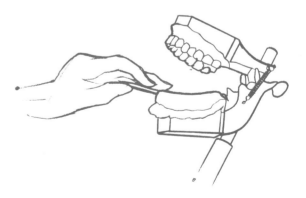

Fig. 61–4. Tray position, parallel to occlusal plane

then on the other side to break atmospheric seal. Insert fingers over the handle portion of the tray to protect the opposing teeth.

12. Separate the impression from the teeth in one continuous vertical motion (upward for the mandibular arch).

13. Rinse impression in room-temperature water following Centers of Disease Control (CDC) guidelines. The CDC and the American Dental Association (ADA) guidelines on the care of hydrocolloid impression materials specify that blood and saliva should be thoroughly cleaned from the impression material that has been used in the mouth. Therefore, the dental assistant or auxiliary should rinse the impression(s) in room-temperature water for thirty seconds, shake off excess water, then spray with one of three disinfectants: Regular iodophor diluted according to the manufacturer's instructions, an acid gluteraldehyde (diluted 4 parts water to 1 part gluteraldehyde), or sodium hypochlorite (household bleach) diluted 10 parts water to 1 part bleach. Place impressions(s) in a baggie for ten to thirty minutes and label baggie with patient's name. After impression(s) have been disinfected, rinse, and pour immediately. Place in airtight container for one hour while plaster hardens.

Maxillary Arch

1. Mix alginate, and load tray with bulk of material toward the anterior portion of the tray.

2. Insert tray.

3. Hold tray in one hand, and with the other hand retract cheek.

4. Slide tray in sideways until one half of tray is inside the mouth, then rotate tray and seat. The handle of the tray should be centered (aligned with nose) and perpendicular to the anterior teeth. The anterior portion of the tray must be positioned over centrals and laterals in order to provide adequate impression material in the vestibular area.

5. Seat posterior of tray first. This will expel material forward, instead of toward the throat.

6. Continue seating the anterior portion of the tray, figures 61–5 and 61–6. (Figures 61–5 and 61–6 are illustrated on a typodont to show proper seating of tray filled with alginate.)

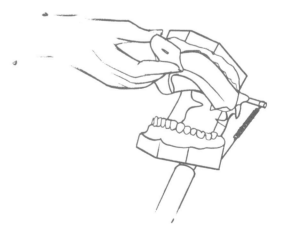

Fig. 61–6. Bringing anterior of maxillary tray into position

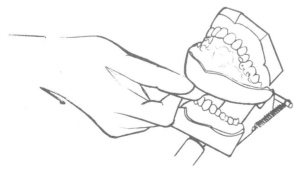

Fig. 61–5. Seating posterior of maxillary tray

7. Lift upper lip to free it from the tray. Have patient relax cheeks and lips. Direct patient to use a "sucking on straw" technique to help bring lip over tray and obtain impression of muscle attachments.
8. Patient's head should be tipped forward to prevent material from flowing into the throat, which could cause patient to gag.
9. Instruct patient to breathe deeply and slowly through mouth or nose while tray is in place.
10. When impression material has set, lift cheek on one side with index finger, then on the other side, to break atmospheric seal. Insert fingers under the handle portion of the tray to protect the opposing teeth.
11. Separate the impression from the teeth in one continuous vertical motion (downward for the maxillary arch).
12. Follow the same procedure as directed for handling mandibular impression, step 13.
13. Shake excess water from impression, and wrap in wet paper towel and place in humidor. *Note:* After wax bite is taken, immediately pour impression. Refer to Chapter 72.

Taking a Wax Bite

A wax **bite** provides occlusal relationship of the maxillary and mandibular teeth.

1. Place wax bite (horseshoe-shaped wax) in hot water to soften.
2. Take softened wax, and place over patient's mandibular teeth. Extend wax $1/4''$ beyond incisal edge of maxillary centrals.
3. Have patient close firmly on wax until it has hardened. Patient must be in his or her true **centric occlusion**.
4. An air syringe may be used to hasten the cooling of wax bite.
5. Carefully remove wax bite and chill under cold water.
6. Remove wax bite from water and spray with appropriate disinfectant.
7. Place patient's initials in upper right-hand corner of wax for identification purposes.
8. Retain wax bite. During model trimming, use to maintain centric occlusion.

Note: Before dismissing the patient, remove any excess impression material from his or her face.

REVIEW

1. Give the criteria for selecting a maxillary and mandibular tray for alginate impressions.

   a. _____

   _____

   b. _____

   _____

c. _____

_____

d. _____

_____

2. List the procedural steps to be followed when preparing the patient for alginate impressions.

a. _____

b. _____

c. _____

d. _____

e. _____

3. What procedure should be followed to reduce the mucous saliva prior to taking the alginate impressions? _____

_____

4. What procedure should be followed when removing an alginate impression from the patient's mouth?

a. _____

_____

b. _____

_____

c. _____

_____

5. Give the position of the operator when taking a maxillary and mandibular impression. _____

_____

6. Give three reasons why beading wax may be used in preparing tray(s).

a. _____

b. _____

c. _____

7. Give six reasons why study or diagnostic models may be used.

a. _____

b. _____

c. _____

d. _____

e. _____

f. _____

8. Explain how the "gag reflex" can be minimized when taking alginate impressions for adults and children.

a. _____

_____

b. _____

_____

c. _____

_____

d. _____

_____

e. _____

_____

f. _____

_____

9. What is the purpose of taking a wax bite? _____

_____

OBJECTIVES:

After studying this chapter, the student will be able to:
- Discuss the basic composition of a reversible hydrocolloid impression material.
- Discuss the need for borax and potassium sulfate in hydrocolloid impression material.
- Discuss the factors that influence the dimensional stability of hydrocolloid impression material.

INTRODUCTION

Hydrocolloid materials were the first of the elastic impression materials to be developed. However, other types of elastic impressions materials are currently available. Hydrocolloids are capable of producing extremely accurate **dies** with excellent reproduction of detail well-suited for the constructions of wax patterns for cast restorations.

Reversible hydrocolloid (series of particles suspended in water) can be used repeatedly simply by heating and cooling. The term *reversible* indicates the capacity of the hydrocolloid to change from a liquid (sol) state to a semi-solid (gel) state and vice versa under certain conditions. This physical effect is induced by a change in temperature. The temperature at which the change from the sol state to a semi-solid material occurs is known as the **gelation temperature**. The final gel is composed of a brush-heap arrangement of *fibrils* of agar-agar enmeshed in water and is no different than the original fluid sol.

Reversible hydrocolloid is used for construction of crown and bridge work and partial dentures. The principal use of this material is where accuracy and detail are demanded.

COMPOSITION

Agar-agar (seaweed)	8–15%
Water by weight	80–85%
Borax	(small amount)
Potassium sulfate	2%
Fillers	remaining %

Agar-agar, extracted from a certain type of seaweed, provides a suitable colloid as a base for hydrocolloid impression materials. A colloid is a suspension of particles, or small groups of molecules, in some type of dispersing (i.e., distributed more or less evenly throughout) medium, which, in this case, is water.

Borax, in small amounts, is added by the manufacturer to increase the strength of the gel. Borax is a retarder for the setting of gypsum products. Thus, the presence of borax and the gel itself are detrimental to the impression material in that it retards the set of the gypsum die material that is poured into the impression. Therefore, to overcome the presence of borax in the impression material, potassium sulfate (approximately 2 percent) is currently added to commercial dental hydrocolloid impression materials. However, the impression may be immersed in a 2% potassium sulfate (K_2SO_4) solution for a minimum of five minutes prior to pouring the impression. Care should be taken not to leave impressions in the solution for over twenty minutes. Potassium sulfate will harden the surface of the stone and will give a better model.

Fillers, preservatives, and flavorings comprise the remaining components.

GEL STRENGTH

Hydrocolloid gels are relatively weak **elastic** solids that are subject to tearing if the stress is applied rapidly and not maintained for a prolonged time. When a complete uniform gel is reached, the impression is removed with a quick "snap-out" action rather than a slow, teasing movement.

GELATION TIME

Gelation of the hydrocolloid occurs when circulating cool water is drawn through the tray at approximately 60 to 70°F (16 to 21°C) for no less than five minutes. As gelation begins near the base of the tray, ice water should not be used, because it will promote rapid gelation and a concentration of stress in the hydrocolloid material. The minimum five-minute gelling time is required in order to allow gelation to process until the gel is strong enough to resist distortion or fracture during removal.

DIMENSIONAL STABILITY

Because the large fraction of the volume of a hydrocolloid gel is occupied by water, the water content of such a gel has a considerable influence on the dimensional stability of the impression material. Loss of water results in shrinkage, and uptake of water produces swelling. Such changes in dimensions are termed *syneresis* or *imbibition*. Syneresis refers to the loss of water by evaporation due to the exposure to the air;

the result is a shrinkage in dimension. If a hydrocolloid gel is stored in contact with water, it will absorb additional water by the process of imbibition. Obviously, either circumstance will lead to a dimensionally unstable gel.

ADVANTAGES

- It is one of the most accurate of reproduction materials.
- It can be manipulated with comparative ease to get the impression.
- It allows the operator to take impressions of multiple preparations at one time.
- There is comparative ease in reproducing contour, anatomy, and detail.
- It is a relatively inexpensive material and convenient to use.
- The technique affords a clean and highly controlled procedure.

FAILURES

There are several common causes for failures in the use of reversible hydrocolloid materials. The numbered items are the imperfections. The bulleted items under each number are the probable causes.

1. Grainy material
   - inadequate boiling
   - conditioning temperature too low
   - conditioning time unduly long
2. Separation of tray and syringe material
   - water-soaked layer of tray material not removed
   - undue gelation of either syringe or tray material
3. Tearing
   - inadequate bulk
   - moisture contamination at gingiva
   - premature removal of impression tray from mouth

- syringe material partially gelled when tray seated
- improper removal of tray from the mouth

4. Irregularly shaped voids
   - moisture or debris on tissue
   - material too cool or grainy
5. Rough or chalky stone cast
   - inadequate cleansing of impression
   - excess water or potassium sulfate solution left in impression

- premature removal of stone cast from impression
- improper manipulation of stone; water-powder ratio

6. Distortion, inaccuracy
   - impression not poured immediately
   - movement of tray during gelation
   - premature removal of tray from mouth
   - improper removal of tray from mouth
   - use of ice water during initial stages of gelation

REVIEW

1. Give the composition of a reversible hydrocolloid.

   a. _____   b. _____   c. _____

   d. _____   e. _____

2. Explain why hydrocolloid impressions should be placed in a 2% solution of potassium sulfate. _____

   _____

3. What is meant by gelation time? _____

   _____

4. In which area of the tray does gelation first occur. Why?_____

   _____

5. What causes hydrocolloid material to become grainy?

   a. _____

   b. _____

   c. _____

6. What causes hydrocolloid material to tear?

   a. _____

   b. _____

   c. _____

   d. _____

   e. _____

7. List the six advantages for using reversible hydrocolloid impression material.

   a. _____

   b. _____

   c. _____

   d. _____

   e. _____

   f. _____

8. What causes a rough or chalky stone cast?

   a. _____

   b. _____

   c. _____

   d. _____

9. What would cause the tray and syringe material to separate?

   a. _____

   b. _____

10. Give five reasons for the cause of an inaccurate or distorted impression.

   a. _____

   b. _____

   c. _____

   d. _____

   e. _____

11. Describe the technique used when removing a hydrocolloid impression from the mouth._____

   _____

12. Define the term *reversible hydrocolloid.*_____

   _____

   _____

Chapter 63: Use of the Hydrocolloid Conditioner

OBJECTIVES:

After studying this chapter, the student will be able to:
- Identify the three compartments of a hydrocolloid conditioner, and give the appropriate function and temperature for each compartment.
- Describe the proper procedure for preparing the three types of hydrocolloid syringe material.
- Describe the tempering process for reversible hydrocolloid impression material.

INTRODUCTION

Hydrocolloid impression material is distributed by the manufacturer in a solid state and includes both tray and syringe material, figure 63–1.

The tray material is supplied in tubes and in five different **viscosities** (having a fluid consistency, but with a tendency to resist flow) and colors. The type used may vary according to dentist preference.

The syringe material is manufactured in various colors and three viscosities and forms (stick, backloading tubes, and prefilled vials). The color of the material denotes its viscosity. The difference of color between the tray and syringe material provides contrast and detail to the hydrocolloid impression.

It is essential that hydrocolloid be boiled and changed from a solid (gel) to a liquid (sol) state before it can be used. This may be accomplished by the use of a controlled temperature conditioner. Moving from left to right, the conditioner has one compartment for liquefying the material, one for storage after boiling, and one for conditioning (tempering) the hydrocolloid, figure 63–2.

When the material is being liquefied, the temperature of the boiling compartment must reach 212°F (100°C), the storage compartment 150 to 155°F (66 to 68°C), and that of the tempering compartment 110 to 120°F (43 to 49°C). On the hydrocolloid conditioner, the temperatures are thermostatically regulated.

PREPARATION OF HYDROCOLLOID IMPRESSION MATERIAL

Check the water level of each compartment. Care must be taken to avoid over- or underfilling the three compartments with water. Space in both boiling and storage compartments must be allowed to compensate for the displacement of water that occurs as the tubes of impression material and syringes are placed into the compartment. New electronic conditioners may require that an electrolyte solution be added to

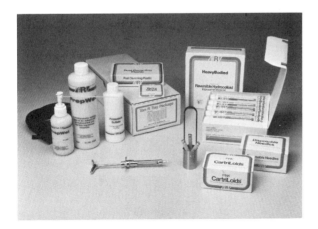

Fig. 63–1. Hydrocolloid products (Courtesy Van R Dental Products, Inc., Los Angeles, CA)

491

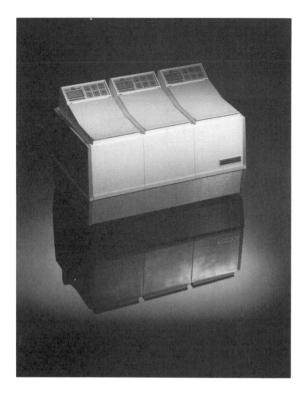

Fig. 63–2. Hydrocolloid conditioner and accessories (Courtesy Van R Dental Products, Inc., Los Angeles, CA)

the water prior to use. A beeping sound will warn the operator that it must be added to the water or that the water level is low in one of the compartments.

Boiling Compartment

1. Tighten caps on tray or syringe tubes, and place tubes cap down in the boiling compartment. This will prevent air pockets from forming at the tip of the nozzle.
2. Prepare syringe material according to form used. Polytube-type syringe material and the prefilled glass vials must be liquefied (metal cap up), then placed in appropriate syringe prior to being used. Stick syringe

material must be placed in syringe prior to being liquefied or boiled.
3. Allow impression material to boil at 212°F (boiling point) or 100°C for ten minutes. No hydrocolloid material should be reboiled more than four times before being discarded.

Storage Compartment

1. After boiling, place hydrocolloid material in the storage bath at 150°F (65°C) for a minimum of ten minutes before using; this will reduce the temperature of the hydrocolloid material to a point where it can be easily handled. *Note:* Prefilled glass vials must be stored with metal cap up.
2. Hydrocolloid material may be stored in the storage bath from one to five days, *providing the conditioning unit remains on.* If the material is not used or the conditioner is turned off, remove impression material from the storage bath and place back in boiling compartment to be reboiled.

Tempering Compartment

1. Hydrocolloid tray material must be tempered to reduce the temperature of the material to avoid burning the oral tissues of the patient. Tempering increases the viscosity of the material, thereby preventing the material from flowing out of the tray.
2. The tray must be filled and placed in the tempering compartment for the required tempering time, a minimum of five minutes. *Syringe material always remains in the storage bath until ready for use.*

Types of Hydrocolloid Impression Trays

Impression trays used for hydrocolloid impressions are of the water-cooled type and include full upper and lower arch, figure 63–3,

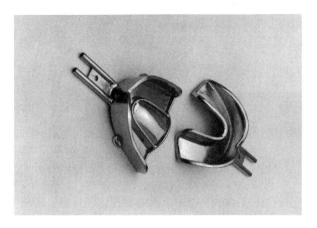

Fig. 63–3. Full upper and lower water-cooled trays (Courtesy Van R Dental Products, Inc., Los Angeles, CA)

full quadrant, and double-bite. All water-cooled trays require a tubing hose that is attached to the tray at one end; the water/vacuum source on the dental unit is attached at the opposite end. Refer to Chapter 64, figure 64–1.

Selection of the proper tray(s) for taking a hydrocolloid impression will depend on the type of impression to be taken; quadrant, full upper, or lower arch. The tray will be prepared according to the type being used. Full lower trays may require wax occlusal stops that help to anchor the material to tray and to prevent overseating. Some quadrant trays may be dammed with stick wax to help retain the material in the tray to prevent pushing the tray too far onto the teeth and to aid in maintaining stability during the critical period of gelation.

Preparation of Tray Material

1. Remove tray material from storage bath, and fill prepared tray. Remember to keep the nozzle tip of the tray material against the base of the tray as material is expelled. This will prevent air pockets from forming.
2. With a moistened finger, smooth the surface of the tray material.

3. Place tray in tempering bath. Water must cover entire tray material.
4. Set timer for the prescribed tempering time, a minimum of five minutes.

Preparing the Hydrocolloid Syringe

Hydrocolloid syringe materials are designed to be used with prefabricated sticks and backloading polytube material. However, manufacturers also supply syringe material in prefilled glass vials. Prefilled glass vials must be liquefied, then loaded in an anesthetic-type syringe prior to use. Stick hydrocolloid is used with a regular hydrocolloid syringe that requires the stick be placed directly in the syringe, then liquefied.

Once the hydrocolloid material has been boiled and transferred into the storage compartment (for a minimum of ten minutes), the hydrocolloid syringe is ready for use.

Backloading polytube syringe material can be loaded in the hydrocolloid syringe at this time. To fill the syringe from the backloading polytube, the following steps are recommended:

1. Remove clean syringe from storage compartment. Remove cap from needle and plunger from barrel of syringe.
2. Remove polytube syringe material from storage compartment, and dry off excess water from tube.
3. Unscrew cap and place the nozzle of the polytube against the barrel of the syringe.
4. Hold the end of the polytube against the syringe, and squeeze the tube, forcing the material into the barrel of the syringe. Care should be taken to avoid overfilling the syringe, as the plunger must be inserted into the syringe.
5. Next, guide the plunger into the barrel of the syringe (minimum of $1/4$ inch), forcing some syringe material through the needle.
6. Replace the protective cap on the needle. Return the syringe to the storage compartment until ready for use.

Taking a Hydrocolloid Impression

1. Once tempering time is completed, remove syringe from storage bath, and test the flow of the material by expelling a small amount on a 2″ × 2″ sponge.
2. Quickly pass the syringe to the operator.
3. While the operator is expelling the syringe material, the assistant removes tray from tempering bath and attaches tubing to tray. Surface water must be removed with a dry 2″ × 2″ sponge. *Note:* Removal of the surface water is necessary in order for bonding to occur between the tray and syringe material. Surface water acts as a separating medium between the tray and syringe material.
4. The assistant attaches the tubing hose to the dental unit. One tubing hose is inserted into the dental unit oral vacuum attachment, and the other tubing hose to the water source. If a "quick-connect" attachment is required, attach the quick-connect to the water source at this time.
5. Operator will pass the syringe to the assistant and, in return, receive the tray. See *Taking Care of the Hydrocolloid Syringe.*
6. While the operator seats and positions the tray, the assistant will immediately turn on the oral vacuum system and, at the operator's command, will establish water flow.
7. The assistant will set the timer for a minimum of five minutes.
8. After the hydrocolloid impression has gelled for a minimum of five minutes, the operator will remove the impression from the patient's mouth. As the operator is removing the impression, the assistant will turn off the water, then the oral vacuum. The assistant will disconnect the tubing hoses from the unit as the operator is inspecting the impression for accuracy.

Taking Care of the Impression

1. Take the impression and tubing to the sink, remove the tubing from the impression tray, and drain.
2. Next, rinse the impression with room-temperature water for thirty seconds to remove any debris. Run water into the gloved cupped palm of one hand while inverting the impression into the running water with the other hand. This method of rinsing the hydrocolloid impression will prevent the breaking of the fragile interseptal areas of the impression.
3. To disinfect the hydrocolloid impression, immerse in one of the following solutions: A regular iodophor diluted according to the manufacturer's instructions, an acid gluteraldehyde (diluted 4 parts water to 1 part gluteraldehyde), or sodium hypochlorite (household bleach) diluted 10 parts water to 1 part bleach.
4. Immerse impression for a minimum of ten minutes but no longer than thirty minutes.
5. Remove impression from the disinfecting solution after the prescribed time. Rinse the impression in room-temperature water, and prepare to pour in stone. If the hydrocolloid impression cannot be poured immediately, place in the humidor, *but not more than four hours.* Should the impression remain in the humidor for four hours, the impression must then be placed in a potassium sulfate solution for twenty minutes before pouring in stone. However, it is best to pour the impression in stone as soon as possible to prevent distortion.
6. After the impression has been poured in stone, it is placed in a humidor for one hour, while the stone hardens. The impression should now be removed from the stone model. Otherwise, the result will be a chalky surface.

Taking Care of the Hydrocolloid Syringe(s)

The syringe that is used in the patient's mouth should be disinfected or sterilized.

When the anesthetic-type syringe is used with the prefilled vials, the vial and needle tip are discarded, and the anesthetic-type syringe sterilized in the autoclave or Chemiclave.

If the regular hydrocolloid (plunger-type) syringe is used, expel the remaining syringe material from the syringe. Remove the plunger from the syringe barrel, and rinse the syringe under hot tap water to flush any remaining hydrocolloid material that may have hardened in the needle tip. Replace the plunger and the protective cap on the needle. Disinfect with an ADA-approved surface disinfectant.

Should impression material be left to harden in the syringe, disinfect the syringe first before reboiling to remove the hardened hydrocolloid.

SUGGESTED ACTIVITIES

- Prepare hydrocolloid tray and syringe material for taking an impression of a typodont.
- Work in pairs, one as the operator, the other as the assistant; take an impression of the typodont following the prescribed instructions.

REVIEW

1. Name the three parts of the hydrocolloid conditioner, and give the function and temperature of each.

   a. _____

   b. _____

   c. _____

2. Give the two reasons why reversible hydrocolloid should be tempered.

   a. _____

   b. _____

3. State two reasons why a hydrocolloid impression tray should be dammed.

   a. _____

   b. _____

4. Explain why the outer layer of hydrocolloid material is removed just prior to taking an impression. _____

_____

5. Why is the syringe material manufactured in a color different from the tube material's?_____

_____

6. Describe the care and cleaning of the regular hydrocolloid syringe.

a. _____

_____

b. _____

_____

c. _____

_____

d. _____

_____

Chapter 64: Preparing and Using the Double-Bite Hydrocolloid Tray

OBJECTIVES:

After studying this chapter, the student will be able to:
- Select and prepare the armamentarium for a double-bite reversible hydrocolloid impression.
- Prepare a double-bite tray for a reversible hydrocolloid impression.
- State the correct sequence for establishing a flow of water before taking the impression and then terminating that flow.

'INTRODUCTION

The *double-bite tray* is designed to be used for either the patient's right or left side of the mouth and to take both the maxillary and mandibular quadrant at the same time. The reason for this is that one side of the tray will be used to take the impression of the prepared teeth, while the other side will provide the opposing bite. A special cut paper, called an *occlusal insert*, is placed into the middle of the tray. This insert serves to separate the tray into an upper and lower quadrant. The occlusal insert paper is then secured with red stick wax. A small amount of stick wax is placed on each side of the tray and paper to secure the paper insert in place.

To take the impression, the operator must first determine the arch where the prepared tooth or teeth are, maxillary or mandibular, and whether they are on the patient's right or left side. Once that has been determined, the tubing is attached to the tray. The tubing is attached before the occlusal insert paper is inserted and secured to the tray. This procedure will prevent the double-bite tray from being bent and from causing a break in the tray rim that will leak when the water is circulated through the tray during the gelation process.

Loading the double-bite tray requires that the "bite side" of the tray be filled first, then the opposite, or preparation side, last.

MATERIALS NEEDED:

- hydrocolloid unit
- hydrocolloid tray material (tube)
- hydrocolloid syringe material (syringe)
- water cooled tray (double-bite)
- occlusal tray insert
- stick wax (red)
- 2″ × 2″ sponge
- tray tubing

INSTRUCTIONS

Loading the Double-Bite Tray

1. Attach tubing to tray, figure 64–1.
2. Place occlusal insert into tray, small end of insert placed from the large side of the

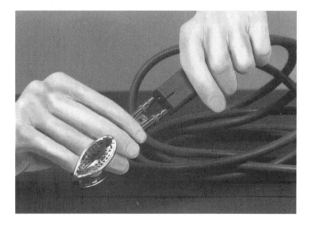

Fig. 64–1. Attaching tubing to double-bite tray

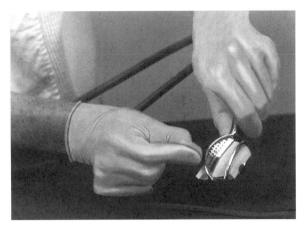

Fig. 64–2. Securing occlusal insert with stick wax

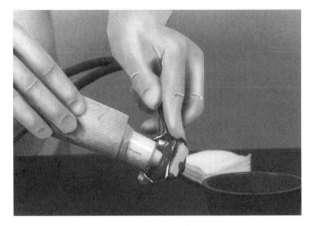

Fig. 64–3. Loading double-bite tray

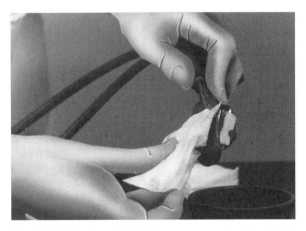

Fig. 64–4. Placing 2″ × 2″ sponge over hydrocolloid material, "bite side"

tray. Secure each side of insert with stick wax. One side of the occlusal insert must be attached facing up, and the opposite side must be facing down, figure 64–2.

3. Load *bite side of tray first* with hydrocolloid tray material. With nozzle of tray material against one side of tray, begin expelling material with a continuous motion, forcing material through the perforations of the tray, figure 64–3. If necessary, moisten

finger with water and press hydrocolloid through perforation of tray for retention.

4. Open a 2″ × 2″ sponge, and place half of the sponge over the surface of the impression material on the "bite" side of the tray, figure 64–4. With index and middle fingers supporting the bite side of the tray, turn the tray over and load the opposite "preparation" side of the tray in the same manner as for the bite side.

6. Bring remaining half of the 2″ × 2″ sponge, and cover the surface of the "preparation" side of the tray, figure 64–5.

7. Place the prepared tray in a tempering bath for approximately five minutes to temper the material from 150°F to approximately 110–115°F.

8. Immediately return unused hydrocolloid tray material to storage bath.

9. At this time, attach tubing hoses to dental unit. Insert one tubing hose into the dental unit oral vacuum attachment and the other tubing hose to the water source. If a "quick-connect" attachment is needed, attach the quick-connect to the water source at this time. Should the location of the hydrocolloid unit and the vacuum-

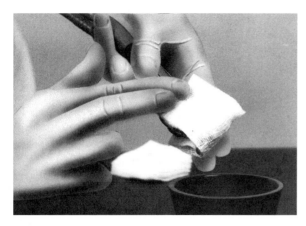

Fig. 64–5. Carrying 2" × 2" over "preparation side" of tray

water source make this impossible, the prepared tray and tubing must be attached at the time the operator receives the tray.

Taking Hydrocolloid Impression with a Double-Bite Tray

1. When the tempering process for the tray is completed, immediately remove syringe from storage bath, unscrew protection cap from nozzle, test, and pass to the operator. If prefilled glass vials are to be used, have an anesthetic syringe ready for loading.

2. While operator is injecting the syringe material onto the prepared tooth or teeth, remove the tray from the tempering bath. Carefully remove the 2" × 2" sponge in a "peeling," rather than "pulling" off, motion from the hydrocolloid tray. If surface water is present on preparation side of tray, use a dry 2" × 2" sponge to remove the water layer from the hydrocolloid material.

3. Exchange the double-bite tray for the syringe.

4. Immediately turn on the unit oral vacuum system, and, at the operator's command, establish water flow.

5. After hydrocolloid impression has gelled for a minimum of five minutes, the operator will remove the impression from the patient's mouth. As the operator is removing the impression, turn off the water and then the oral vacuum. Disconnect the tubing hoses from the unit as the operator is inspecting the impression.

6. Take the impression and tubing to the sink to drain any remaining water from the tubing. Carefully disconnect the tubing from the impression tray.

7. Rinse impression with room-temperature water for thirty seconds to remove any debris. This is done by running water into the gloved cupped palm of one hand, while inverting the impression into the running water with the other hand and gently raising and lowering the impression in the water flow.

8. Then disinfect the impression by placing it in an appropriate solution. Refer to Chapter 63, *Use of Hydrocolloid Conditioner, Taking Care of the Impression.*

9. Clean up operatory and equipment.

SUGGESTED ACTIVITIES

- Practice placing the occlusal insert into the tray.
- Practice loading the double-bite tray with the impression material.

Chapter 65: Elastomeric Impression Materials

OBJECTIVES: After studying this chapter, the student will be able to:
- Discuss the advantages of using elastomeric impression materials over hydrocolloid impression material.
- Identify the four types of elastomeric impression materials.
- State the advantage(s) for using each type of elastomeric material.
- Discuss the disinfecting procedure used for each type of elastomeric impression.

INTRODUCTION

The rubberlike *elastomeric impression* materials *polysulfide*, *silicones*, and *polyether* offer several advantages over hydrocolloid impression materials. The elastomer or rubberlike materials are stronger and more tear-resistant than hydrocolloid. In other words, when the impression is removed, the material will not tear. They also do not have the dimensional problems of syneresis or imbibition. With one exception, polyether is a hydrophilic (capable of taking up water) and, if placed in water, will swell.

The elastomeric impression materials use a base and **accelerator** system. The base material is supplied in paste form, and the accelerator (a substance that speeds up a reaction) or catalyst (a substance capable of promoting or altering the speed of a chemical reaction, but that does not take part in the reaction) may be a paste or a liquid. The materials are classified according to their viscosity (thickness). The four classes are identified as (1) very high viscosity with puttylike consistency, used for custom trays; (2) high viscosity or heavy-bodied tray material; (3) medium or regular viscosity, used for full-arch impressions; (4) low viscosity or light-bodied syringe material.

POLYSULFIDE IMPRESSION MATERIAL

The first rubber-base material introduced to dentistry was *polysulfide*, later changed to *mercaptan* for the chemical contained in the base paste. The term *mercaptan* or polysulfide may be used interchangeably; however, it is more acceptable to refer to the spatulated material as mercaptan and the set rubberlike impression material as polysulfide. It is during polymerization (process of changing two or more like molecules to form a more complex molecule) that mercaptan reacts with the accelerator, lead dioxide.

Composition

Polysulfide is supplied in a two-paste system. The base contains the mercaptan polymer (containing many parts), and the accelerator contains lead dioxide, sulfur, and fillers added to form a paste. Lead dioxide is the substance that gives the final impression material its brown color. However, if the reactor is an organic peroxide, dyes may be added, making it possible to have many other colors of impression materials.

Uses

Polysulfide is used for single- or multiple-tooth preparations, quadrant, and full-arch impression.

Advantages. Polysulfide material provides accuracy and a detailed impression of the margins of the tooth preparations. They offer excellent tear resistance as the impression is removed from the mouth.

Disadvantages. Polysulfide impressions should be poured within one hour to minimize polymerization shrinkage and to ensure accuracy of the impression. Polysulfide is difficult to mix and handle. Care must be taken to avoid contact with the skin and clothing, as it will permanently stain fabrics. Patients often find the odor and color of the material objectionable.

Disinfecting Polysulfide Impressions

The American Dental Association (ADA) states that an impression should be rinsed as soon as it is removed from the mouth to remove saliva, blood, and debris prior to disinfection.

Polysulfide impressions may be immersed in an ADA-approved disinfectant. The ADA's list includes chlorine compounds, iodophors, combination synthetic phenolics, and various glutaraldehyde formulations. It is advisable to follow the manufacturer's recommended disinfectant for care of a particular elastomeric impression material.

The impression should be rinsed after it has been exposed to the disinfectant to remove any remaining solution that could affect the surface of the poured stone model.

CONVENTIONAL SILICONE IMPRESSION MATERIAL

Conventional *silicone* rubber-base impression material was originally developed as a replacement for polysulfide because of the latter's objectionable odor, staining ability, and the difficulty encountered in spatulating it.

Composition

Conventional silicone paste is composed of dimethylsiloxane and the reinforcing agent silica. Silica is added to control the viscosity of the paste and helps to reduce polymerization shrinkage. The catalyst is tin octoate, and the reactor is alky silicate. The manufacturer may supply the catalyst as either a liquid or a paste.

As with polysulfide, it is spatulated with the accelerator to form the silicone rubber.

Uses

The conventional silicone impression materials are used for crown, bridge, and full-arch impressions.

Advantages

Silicone is easy to spatulate and to handle. It is odorless and more pleasing in appearance.

Disadvantages

Conventional silicone material should be poured within the first hour after removal from the patient's mouth. The set silicone impression has poor tear strength and tends to rip when it is removed from the patient's mouth. It is expensive to purchase and generally is said to have a shorter shelf life (the stability of a dental material when it is stored). To extend the shelf life of a conventional silicone, it is recommended that it be stored in the refrigerator.

Disinfecting Silicone Impressions

As with polysulfide, the silicone impression should be rinsed immediately after removal from the mouth and prior to disinfection. Silicones can be disinfected in the same manner as polysulfide impressions using the immersion technique.

POLYETHER IMPRESSION MATERIAL

Polyether rubber impression material is a fast-setting and more accurate impression material than either polysulfide or conventional silicone.

Composition

Polyether impression material is supplied in a two-paste system. The base material is a polyether polymer, and the catalyst is alky aromatic sulfonate.

Uses

Polyether impression material is used for quadrant and full-arch impressions.

Advantages

Polyether is like silicone in that it is easy to manipulate and care for. Polyether also has less dimensional change during polymerization and storing than polysulfide or conventional silicone. Because polyether is very stable, the finished impression retains its accuracy for extended periods of time; it is unnecessary to pour the impression within the first hour as with polysulfide and the conventional silicone materials.

Disadvantages

Because polyether is a hydrophilic impression material, it should not be exposed to high humidity or stored in water. Also, the overall stiffness of the set material makes removing the impression from the mouth more difficult. Care should be taken when working with the catalyst to avoid skin contact, as it may cause skin irritation.

Disinfecting Polyether Impressions

Rinse polyether in the same manner as for the other elastomeric impressions. However, the ADA recommends that the spray disinfection method be used to disinfect the polyether impression because of its hydrophilic nature. Immersion disinfection could adversely affect the dimensions (shape) and the stability of the material.

POLYSILOXANE OR POLYVINYLSILOXANE IMPRESSION MATERIAL

Polysiloxane or *polyvinylsiloxane* impression material, an improved silicone, is more accurate than the conventional condensation silicone. It is available in a range of viscosities for various uses, including the two-phase or "wash" tech-

nique. With the wash technique, the puttylike material is used to make a custom tray prior to the tooth being prepared. It is then set aside while the dentist prepares the tooth or teeth. The custom tray is used for the final impression.

A more recent hydrophilic polyvinylsiloxane impression material has been introduced. The stated advantage over the nonhydrophilic silicone is the improved marginal detail and the fact that it is not adversely affected by contact with the oral fluids. This allows the material to spread evenly over moist surfaces (tooth) without developing voids in the final impression.

Composition

Polysiloxane is supplied as a two-paste system. The base contains two polymers, polysiloxane and poly (vinyl) siloxane. The catalyst is a platinum salt.

Uses

Polysiloxane impression material is used for crowns and edentulous (without teeth) impressions.

Advantages

Polyvinylsiloxane materials are highly accurate and exhibit long-term dimensional stability (the ability to retain their shape and size). The material has a shorter working and spatulation time. Polyvinylsiloxane is easy to spatulate, odor-free, and clean to handle.

Disadvantages

Because polyvinylsiloxane has a shorter working and spatulation time, it tends to produce hydrogen gas (bubbles) on setting. For this reason, a waiting period is usually recommended before pouring the stone cast. However, newer hydrophilic polyvinyl siloxane materials have an added additive that absorbs the hydrogen bubbles. It should be noted that certain latex gloves may inhibit the setting of the puttylike impression material. Therefore, vinyl gloves must be worn when working with the material.

Disinfecting Polyvinylsiloxane Impressions

Care and disinfection of polysiloxane impression is the same as for other silicone impression material.

Most elastomeric impression materials are spatulated on a paper mixing pad and with a stiff spatula. However, with the newer polyvinylsilioxane materials an automix hand gun may be used. Refer to Chapter 68 for assembling the gun.

REVIEW

1. Elastomeric impression materials are classified according to their viscosity and class. List and give the uses of each.

   a. _____

   b. _____

   c. _____

   d. _____

2. State the advantages of using polysulfide impression material.

   a. _____

   b. _____

3. What are the disadvantages of using polysulfide material?

   a. _____

   b. _____

   c. _____

   d. _____

4. State the advantages of using conventional silicone impression material.

   a. _____

   b. _____

5. What are the disadvantages of the conventional silicone materials?

   a. _____

   b. _____

   c. _____

6. State the advantages of using polyether impression material.

   a. _____

   b. _____

   c. _____

7. What are the disadvantages of the polyether material?

   a. _____

   b. _____

8. State the advantages of using polyvinylsiloxane.

   a. _____

   b. _____

   c. _____

   d. _____

9. Which of the elastomeric impression materials may be immersed in an approved disinfected solution?

   a. _____

   b. _____

Chapter 66: Making Quadrant Custom Acrylic Trays

OBJECTIVES: After studying this chapter, the student will be able to:
- Discuss the two types of custom-made trays used for elastomeric impression material.
- Explain the function of a wax spacer.
- Make an acrylic custom-made tray using a plaster model.

INTRODUCTION

Two types of *custom-made trays* may be fabricated for use with rubber-base impression materials. One type is a silicon putty (Chapter 68), a second, a self-cured acrylic resin tray for polysulfide impression material.

The recommended procedure for constructing an acrylic custom-made tray requires that an alginate impression of the individual's mouth be taken. The impression is poured in plaster and allowed to dry. The acrylic custom-made tray is then fabricated on this model.

MATERIALS NEEDED

- plaster model
- base plate wax
- bowl of hot water
- acrylic powder
- acrylic liquid
- small spatula
- paper cup
- vaseline
- lab knife
- pencil
- measurers for resin
- glass square or slab
- acrylic bur or dental instrument with straight handpiece

INSTRUCTIONS

1. Outline with a pencil where the peripheral edge of the tray will be.
2. Prepare selected quadrant of plaster model with a thin layer of vaseline.
3. Cut base plate wax to the width and length of the selected quadrant. One or two thicknesses of base plate wax may be used. The wax provides the necessary space needed for the impression material. This wax is called a spacer.
4. Place wax in bowl of hot water to soften.
5. Remove softened wax from water and adapt to prepared quadrant. If necessary, trim excess wax with lab knife. Wax should cover crown portions of the teeth and extend approximately 4 mm beyond the gingival margin and the buccal and lingual surfaces, figure 66–1. Cut out holes to serve as "stops." This will prevent overseating of tray. Do not place holes in the tray over a prepared tooth.
6. Coat the top surface of the wax spacer with vaseline. Set aside.
7. Measure liquid, and place in paper cup.

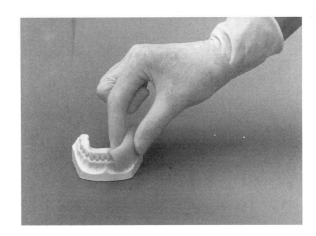

Fig. 66–1. Place wax spacer.

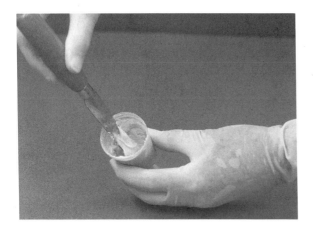

Fig. 66–2. Spatulate monomer and polymer.

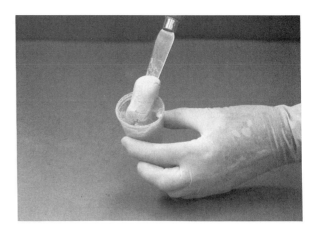

Fig. 66–3. Resin set to doughy consistency

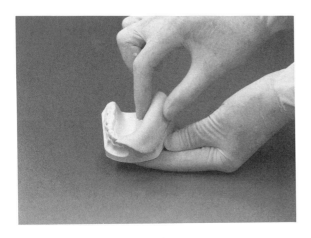

Fig. 66–4. Adapt resin over wax spacer.

8. Measure powder, and carry into liquid. *Note:* Follow manufacturer's instructions for proportions.

9. Spatulate for thirty seconds, figure 66–2.

10. Allow acrylic to set for two to three minutes to doughy stage, when gloss has disappeared and is nonsticky, figure 66–3.

11. Lightly lubricate glass slab and hands with vaseline.

12. Remove acrylic mix from paper cup with spatula. With finger tips, form into a ball.

13. Place dough on glass slab, and flatten with hands to a uniform thickness, $1/8$ inch.

14. Carefully remove from glass slab, and adapt over wax spacer, figure 66–4. Do not extend acrylic beyond wax spacer.

15. While material is pliable, form handle over anterior teeth. Handle should be parallel to the occlusal surfaces of the teeth. Should a separate handle be fashioned, place a drop of liquid where it will attach.

16. Remove acrylic tray from model before final curing has completed, figure 66–5.

17. Remove wax spacer before wax melts. Reposition tray on the model for final curing, about seven to ten minutes (from initial mix to final set), figure 66–6. *Note:* As acrylic begins to cure, an exothermic reaction occurs (heat is given off).

18. Trim tray. Remove excess or rough areas on the tray with acrylic bur. The completed tray should be smooth in appearance, without undercuts, and uniform in thickness, figure 66–7. The bur may also be used on the inside of the tray to remove excess tray

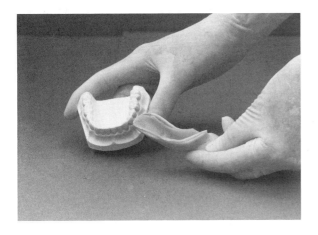

Fig. 66–5. Remove tray and liner from model.

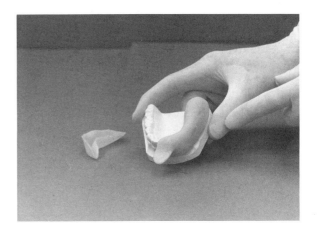

Fig. 66–6. Reposition tray on model for final curing.

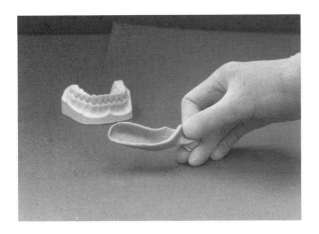

Fig. 66–7. Completed acrylic quadrant tray

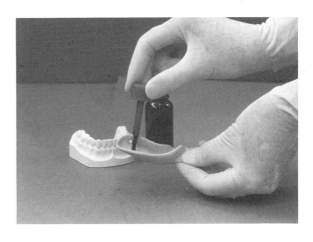

Fig. 66–8. Apply tray adhesive.

material. This will provide the necessary depth for the impression material.

19. Prepare tray with tray adhesive. The adhesive must be applied to the tray so that the impression material will adhere to the acrylic tray. Two to three applications of the tray adhesive are required well in advance of the impression procedure, figure 66–8.

SUGGESTED ACTIVITY

• Make an acrylic quadrant custom-made tray on a plaster model.

REVIEW

1. Why is base plate wax used when constructing a custom-made tray? _____

_____

2. Why must a tray adhesive be used with the acrylic tray? _____

_____

3. At which stage may the self-cured acrylic resin mix be molded? _____

_____

Chapter 67: Preparing and Using Polysulfide Impression Material

OBJECTIVES:

After studying this chapter, the student will be able to:
- Select the materials needed to prepare polysulfide impression material.
- Prepare polysulfide rubber-base impression material for both the syringe and tray.
- Take an impression using a typodont.

INTRODUCTION

Polysulfide products are dispensed as a two-paste impression system. The two pastes are spatulated together to form a rubber-like impression material.

To take an impression with polysulfide, a custom-made tray should be used. The custom-made tray permits only enough space between the tray and teeth (or the part to be duplicated) for the impression material. As with all rubber-base impression materials, the less distance there is between the tray and the teeth, the more accurate the final impression. The thickness of the material between the teeth and sides of the tray should be approximately 2 to 4 mm.

Generally, a multiple mix of syringe and the tray material is used. In this procedure, the syringe material is mixed first. This enables the dentist to inject small amounts of the syringe material directly into the cavity preparation(s) and other areas where precise detail is needed. While the syringe material is being injected, the tray material is mixed and placed into the prepared tray.

Retention of the impression material in the tray is critical to the achievement of an accurate impression. Considerable force is generated when removing the impression from the patient's teeth. This force tends to pull it out of the tray. Therefore, tray adhesive is applied to prevent this from occurring.

MATERIALS NEEDED

- steel spatulas, tapered (2)
- mixing pads (2)
- polysulfide impression material, base and accelerator
- acrylic tray (prepared with tray adhesive)
- typodont with prepared teeth
- paper towels
- brush (to clean barrel of syringe)

INSTRUCTIONS

On two separate pads (pad 1, syringe material; pad 2, tray material), dispense equal lengths of base and accelerator material side by side on the separate mixing pads, figure 67–1. Care must be taken to prevent the materials from touching, as this starts the chemical reaction.

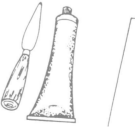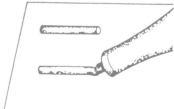

Fig. 67–1. Dispense material onto pad.

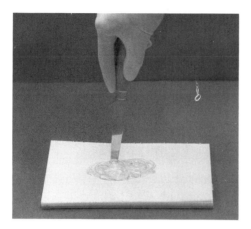

Fig. 67–2. Mix the accelerator into the base paste with tip of spatula.

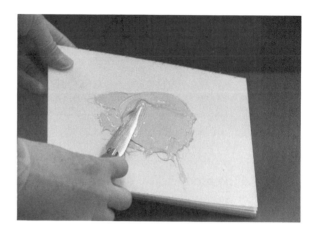

Fig. 67–3. Continue spatulation using flat portion of blade.

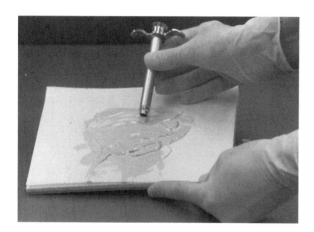

Fig. 67–4. Load syringe from nozzle end of barrel.

Spatulate the Syringe Material

1. Begin by spatulating syringe material.
2. With the tip end of the tapered spatula, incorporate the accelerator into the base paste for five to ten seconds in a circular motion, figure 67–2.
3. Continue spatulation with the flat portion of the blade, using a wide sweeping motion until the mix is free from streaks and is homogeneous in color, figure 67–3.

4. Mix must be completed in sixty seconds or less.
5. Gather syringe material together with spatula, and prepare to load syringe.
6. When using an aluminum syringe, remove plunger and nozzle end.
7. Load the barrel of the syringe by taking the nozzle end of the barrel, and with short, rapid strokes, push the material into the syringe barrel, figure 67–4. If a plastic syringe is used, remove the plunger end only, and load the syringe from the plunger end with the same technique as for an aluminum syringe.
8. Wipe end of barrel with tissue, and replace nozzle tip of syringe.
9. Place plunger in barrel of syringe and expel a small amount of syringe material through the plastic tip to check the flow, figure 67–5.

Spatulate the Tray Material

1. On pad 2, begin to spatulate with second spatula, the tray material in the same manner as for the syringe material. Follow steps 1–4, *Spatulate the Syringe Material.*

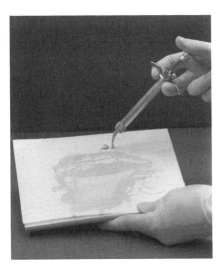

Fig. 67–5. Expel a small amount of syringe material to check the flow.

2. Gather tray material together with spatula, and load prepared tray. Tray material should be evenly distributed over the entire tray.

TAKING AN IMPRESSION

1. Using a typodont, inject the syringe material into each prepared tooth. Start at the most distal cervical step, and fill the cavity from cervical step to occlusal surface, keeping the nozzle tip of the syringe hidden and actually touching the tooth surface being covered. Following this procedure prevents air pockets.
2. Continue expelling the material over the buccal and lingual surfaces. Work as quickly as possible. It is important to finish the syringe application before the impression material becomes too stiff.
3. Push any excess material to form a small ball at the tip of the syringe. Allow the ball to harden (about eight minutes). This

serves as an indicator for timing set material.
4. Position the prepared tray and seat. Place a small portion of this mix against an adjacent tooth outside the operating field to serve as a control sample for determining set.
5. Allow material to set a minimum of eight minutes.
6. Remove from typodont with steady force, and check impression for overall detail. Rinse impression with cold water, dry, and pour in stone. *Note:* Patient impressions must be disinfected prior to being poured (Refer to Chapter 65, page 501).
7. The impression should be poured immediately to prevent dimensional changes caused by continued curing. To avoid having the surface of the cast become porous, the stone should be mixed under vacuum.

CLEANING THE SYRINGE

1. Disassemble syringe.
2. Remove excess material from nozzle tip and barrel of syringe.
3. Remove screw from plunger of aluminum syringe or *O* ring from plastic syringe. Clean excess material from screw or *O* ring. Replace screw; care must be taken not to overtighten screw. With plastic syringe, replace *O* ring.
4. Take brush, wash inside of barrel with water, and dry.
5. Reassemble syringe.

SUGGESTED ACTIVITIES

• Practice spatulating polysulfide impression material, following the step-by-step procedure as outlined in the instructions.
• Take an impression, using a prepared typodont.

Chapter 68: Preparing Silicone Impression Material Using the Putty Tray Technique and a Polyvinylsiloxane Automix Cartridge System

OBJECTIVES:

After studying this chapter, the student will be able to:
- Prepare a custom-made tray using a silicone putty.
- Prepare tray and syringe silicone impression material, and take a quadrant impression of a typodont using the putty custom-made tray.
- Assemble the automix cartridge unit.
- Prepare polyvinylsiloxane impression material using the automix cartridge unit.

INTRODUCTION

Silicone elastomeric impression materials, figure 68–1, are used for taking single-quadrant and full-mouth impressions. The newest silicone impression system in use today uses a moldable puttylike silicone paste material for making a custom-made tray. This material is prepared and placed into a standard stock-tray that retains or holds the puttylike material. The custom-made tray is fashioned before the tooth or teeth being prepared.

The custom-made tray is set aside until the final impression is taken with the low-viscosity syringe impression material. A heavy-body or high-viscosity tray material may be used along with the syringe material. When ready, the syringe and tray materials are spatulated. The syringe material is placed in the syringe and injected onto the prepared tooth or teeth, and the tray material is placed into the putty tray. The custom-made tray is then repositioned over the teeth and allowed to set, between six and eight minutes. This procedure may be referred to as the double- or multiple-mix technique.

MATERIALS NEEDED

- measuring scoop
- 2 mixing pads or measuring cup
- 2 spatulas, stiff
- syringe, aluminum or plastic
- cleansing tissues
- perforated quadrant tray
- plastic separator
- typodont with full crown preparation
- lab knife
- silicone putty paste
- silicone tray material
- silicone syringe material
- catalyst liquid
- paper towels

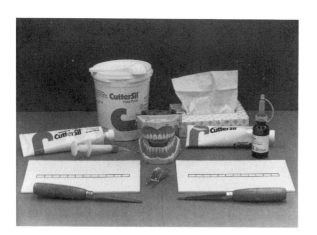

Fig. 68–1. Setup for silicone impression material

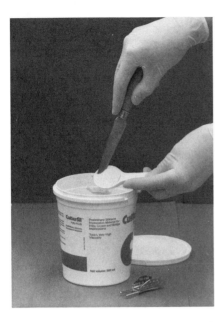

Fig. 68–2. Silicone putty tray material

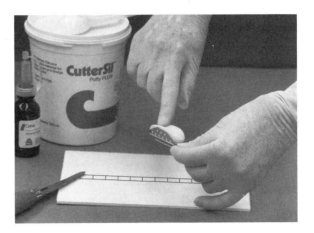

Fig. 68–3. Tray filled with putty material

INSTRUCTIONS

Prepare the Putty Tray

1. Measure one level scoop of silicone putty, and place on mixing pad, figure 68–2.
2. Press putty into the shape of a thin wafer.
3. With spatula, cut shallow grooves (waffle pattern) into putty material.
4. Dispense four drops of catalyst liquid on top of putty material.
5. With spatula, carefully fold and knead liquid into putty for approximately twenty seconds, until the liquid is completely incorporated in the putty and no traces of liquid are visible.
6. Immediately remove putty from mixing pad and vigorously knead with a gloved hand for another twenty-five seconds. *Note:* Should any liquid remain on mixing pad, use putty to blot up remaining liquid from pad.

7. Shape putty into a roll, and place into quadrant tray, figure 68–3.
8. Place plastic separator over top of tray/putty, and position tray over the area of the prepared tooth of the typodont. Apply sufficient pressure to seat tray.
9. Remove putty tray impression from typodont, and set aside to cure, approximately two minutes.
10. Remove plastic separator. Set aside until ready to take final impression, figure 68–4.

Prepare the Syringe and Tray Material

1. On one mixing pad, dispense the required number of graduations of syringe material as directed by manufacturer, figure 68–5.
2. On second mixing pad, dispense the required number of graduations of tray material as directed by manufacturer, figure 68–6.

Spatulate the Syringe and Tray Material

1. On mixing pad with tray material, dispense required amount of catalyst beside, but not touching, tray material.

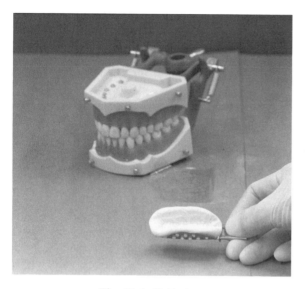

Fig. 68–4. Putty tray

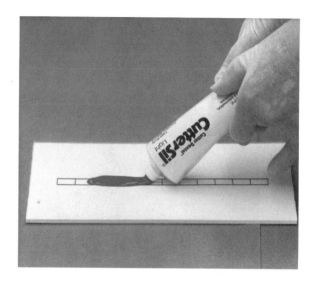

Fig. 68–5. Dispensing syringe material

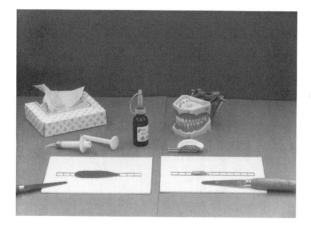

Fig. 68–6. Materials prepared for mixing

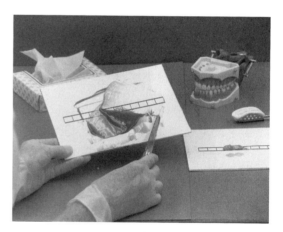

Fig. 68–7. Gathering syringe material for loading

2. On mixing pad with syringe material, dispense required amount of catalyst on top of syringe material.

3. Immediately begin spatulating syringe material to a homogeneous consistency. Spatulation time may vary from thirty seconds to one minute. There should be no trace of catalyst remaining on mixing pad.

4. Gather syringe material with spatula, and prepare to load syringe, figure 68–7. When using an aluminum syringe, remove plunger and nozzle end. Load barrel of syringe by taking nozzle end of barrel, with short rapid strokes, pulling the material into the syringe barrel. If a plastic syringe is used, remove plunger only.

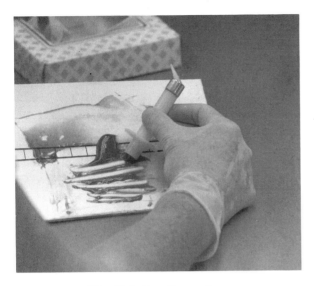

Fig. 68–8. Loading syringe

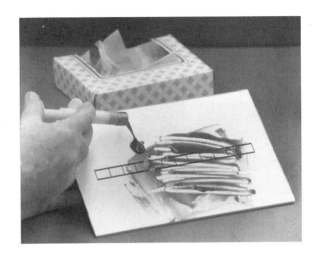

Fig. 68–9. Checking flow of syringe material

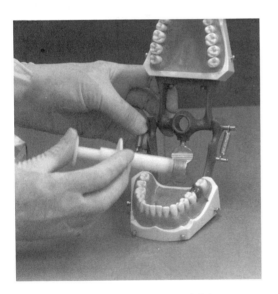

Fig. 68–10. Injecting syringe material into prepared tooth

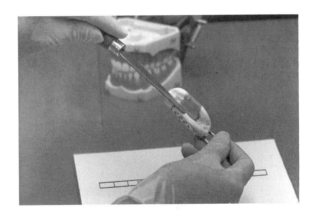

Fig. 68–11. Lining putty custom-made tray

Load syringe from plunger end with the same technique as for the aluminum syringe, figure 68–8.

5. For an aluminum syringe, wipe barrel end with cleansing tissue, replace nozzle tip, and insert plunger into barrel of syringe. With a plastic syringe, wipe plunger end of syringe, and insert plunger. Expel a small amount of syringe material through the plastic tip to check flow, figure 68–9.

6. With syringe, inject material into prepared tooth of typodont. Set aside momentarily, figure 68–10.

7. Immediately spatulate tray material. Gather tray material with spatula, and line putty custom-made tray, figure 68–11.

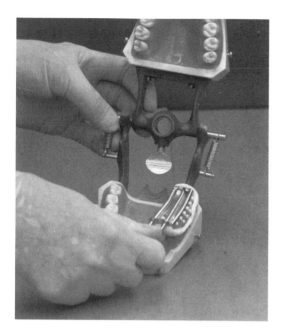

Fig. 68–12. Seating the tray

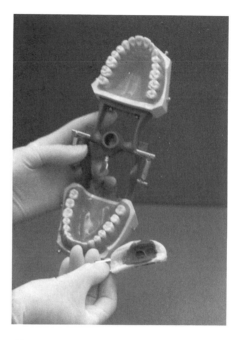

Fig. 68–13. Impression of prepared tooth

8. Seat prepared putty tray over injected syringe material, figure 68–12.
9. Allow material to cure a minimum of six minutes.
10. Remove from typodont with steady force, and check impression for overall detail, figure 68–13. Rinse impression with cold water, dry, and pour in stone. *Note:* Patient impressions must be disinfected prior to being poured in stones (Refer to Chapter 65, page 501).

Clean the Syringe

1. Disassemble the syringe.
2. Remove excess material from nozzle tip and barrel of syringe.
3. Remove screw from plunger of aluminum syringe or *O* ring from plastic syringe. Clean excess material from screw or *O* ring. Replace screw; care must be taken

not to overtighten screw. With plastic syringe replace *O* ring.
4. Take brush, wash inside of barrel with water, and dry.
5. Reassemble syringe.

AUTOMIX CARTRIDGE SYSTEM

Silicone light- and medium-bodied impression materials and polyvinylsiloxane are available in a dual cartridge, or automix system, figure 68–14. With the dual cartridge system, the base paste is in one side of the cartridge, and the catalyst paste in the other. The cartridge is inserted into the automix unit with a trigger-type handle and movable plunger. By pressing the handle, the plunger forces the material through the cartridge. A mixing tip is attached to the cartridge. When the handle is firmly pressed, the plunger will apply pressure to the cartridge forcing the

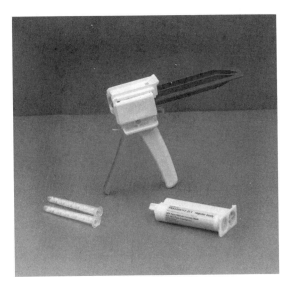

Fig. 68–14. Component parts of automix system

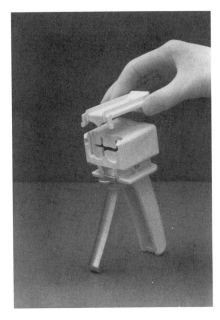

Fig. 68–15. Removing retainer plate

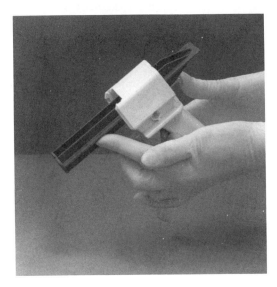

Fig. 68–16. Inserting plunger

material may be expelled directly into the syringe or into the prepared tooth or putty tray.

MATERIALS NEEDED

- automix unit
- dual cartridge, impression material
- mixing tip
- paper towel

INSTRUCTIONS

1. Assemble unit. Remove retainer plate, figure 68–15.
2. Insert plunger by pushing up on the release lever, figure 68–16.
3. Insert dual cartridge into the guide grooves on unit, figure 68–17.
4. Replace retainer plate, figure 68–18. Carefully squeeze handle until plunger makes contact with the cartridge.

material through the mixing tip. As the material is pushed through the mixing tip, the base and catalyst are folded over each other, are mixed together, and a homogeneous mass is expelled from the mixing tip. At this time the impression

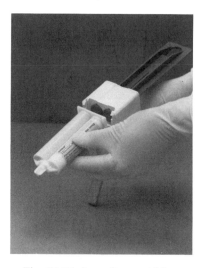

Fig. 68–17. Inserting cartridge

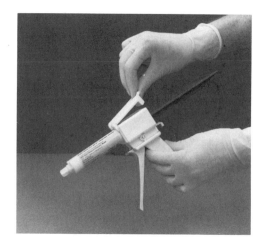

Fig. 68–18. Replacing retainer plate

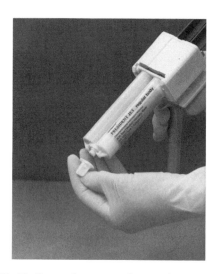

Fig. 68–19. Removing protective cap from cartridge

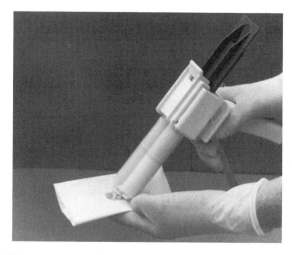

Fig. 68–20. Expelling small amount of base or catalyst

5. Remove protective cap and seal from the cartridge, figure 68–19. Check function of unit by expelling a small amount of material onto a paper towel, figure 68–20.
6. Wipe end of cartridge, and insert mixing tip, figure 68–21. Lock tip into position by giving a one-quarter turn clockwise.

7. Test flow by squeezing handle to expel a small amount of material onto a paper towel, figure 68–22.
8. With firm and continuous pressure, squeeze handle to expel the desired amount of material needed for the procedure, figure 68–23. The flow of material is stopped immediately when pressure on the handle is released.

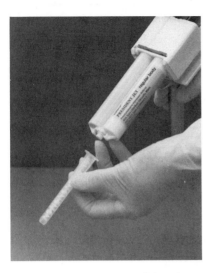

Fig. 68–21. Inserting mixing tip

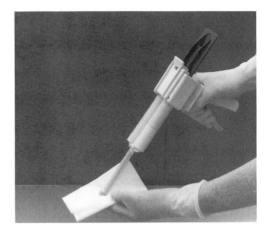

Fig. 68–22. Testing flow of material

9. Load syringe or putty tray directly from the mixing tip. *Note:* Do not remove mixing tip from cartridge. The impression material left in the mixing tip will harden in a few minutes. The tip helps to seal the cartridge opening, preventing the impression material from hardening.

Replacing Used Mixing Tip

1. Remove used mixing tip from cartridge, and throw away.
2. Check for hardened material at the cartridge openings.
3. Expel a small amount of material onto a paper towel.
4. Place new mixing tip on cartridge.

Replacing a Cartridge

1. Press release lever up, and hold in position while removing plunger.
2. Remove retainer plate from unit.
3. Remove cartridge.
4. Insert new cartridge, and throw used cartridge away.

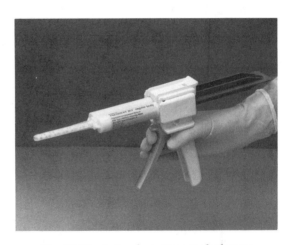

Fig. 68–23. Automix system ready for use

SUGGESTED ACTIVITIES

• Make a custom-made tray with putty silicone paste using a typodont with a full crown preparation.
• Prepare syringe and tray impression material using the double-mix technique.
• Practice assembling and using the automix unit.

OBJECTIVES: After studying this chapter, the student will be able to:
- Review the construction and placement of accurate treatment crowns.
- Develop a well-standardized technique for constructing treatment crowns.

INTRODUCTION

When constructing crowns and bridges, it is necessary to keep the tooth or teeth protected anytime from a few days up to, in some cases, many months. In the latter case, gold castings are often constructed. Placement of accurate treatment crowns and adequate protection and stabilization of the tooth preparation are important for the following reasons:

- To prevent tooth movement and to prevent extrusion of the prepared tooth and/or opposing tooth
- To provide for the patient's comfort
- To sedate the pulp of the tooth
- To protect free gingiva from irritation and resulting recession and to prevent food impaction into the contact areas, resulting in periodontal problems
- To provide for esthetics
- To prevent unnecessary exposure of the tooth to mouth fluids
- To make up for lost function where possible
- To adjust occlusion in many cases

The placement of well-constructed treatment crowns can also have a great effect on the patient's confidence and attitude. If the restorations are uncomfortable or repeatedly come off between appointments, the patient is apt to become irritable and upset.

TYPES OF TEMPORARY COVERAGE

Acrylic Restorations

These are made from acrylic resin as a temporary crown for a tooth until the permanent restoration is placed. They provide a more accurate fit because they are exact replicas of the patient's tooth.

Aluminum and Stainless Steel Crowns

These are manufactured in a series of graduated sizes and in anatomical and nonanatomical forms. They should be used only as an expedient in the rare situation in which, because of time and various other factors, the construction of a plastic temporary is impractical.

Castings

In some cases, particularly for full reconstructions, the temporary castings need to be in place for a prolonged time. If plastic temporaries are used in the posterior teeth and cuspids (canines), it is likely that wear, breakage, tissue reactions, and loosening will occur. In these cases, it is important that the occlusion be maintained in a relatively comfortable and stable state. For these reasons, temporaries are often cast in Type II or III alloys.

Zinc Oxide Eugenol Cements (ZOE)

A ZOE cement can be used alone only in small inlay preparations. However, even in these cases, if time will permit, it is better to place a plastic temporary. ZOE cements are used routinely in a more workable form to cement all of the previously mentioned types of temporaries.

TREATMENT OF THE PREPARED TOOTH STRUCTURE

It is important that the problem of sensitivity (thermal, in the final restoration) be considered as early as when the tooth is prepared. It has been shown that ZOE cements exhibit less leakage than do zinc phosphate cements, and they also have a sedative effect on the pulp. For these reasons and for ease of removal, the temporaries are cemented with ZOE at preparation time. When the restoration is cemented, the tooth is treated with varnish. It is very important that the tooth not be dried so vigorously that the dentin is desiccated (thoroughly dried up). However, in order to place varnish or cement, the tooth must be dry.

MATERIALS NEEDED

- alginate impression material, spatula
- alginate impression tray
- hydrocolloid syringe material
- cotton pellet
- plaster, fast-setting
- self-curing acrylic kit
- dappen dish
- Caps Spatula
- rubber band, heavy
- finishing burs
- pressure pot
- rag wheel and pumice
- plaster bowl
- Carver, Hollenback, or plastic instrument
- scalpel or lab knife
- scissor, curved
- ZOE cement

INSTRUCTIONS

The principle behind constructing a temporary crown is to approximate the original tooth form with certain modifications. In the majority of cases, the original tooth form will be adequate. However, there are cases where the tooth should *not* be duplicated such as the pontic tooth or teeth. In such cases, the original tooth form is modified on a diagnostic cast. That cast is then used in constructing the temporary crown.

1. While waiting for the onset of anesthesia, an *overimpression* is made in alginate. This impression must include, wherever possible, one or more teeth mesially and distally to the tooth to be prepared, figure 69–1.
2. Store this impression in the airtight container. It must be kept moist, as it will not actually be used until after the preparation is completed.
3. The tooth preparation is then accomplished.

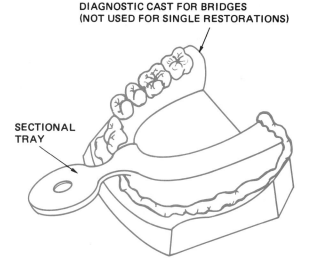

DIAGNOSTIC CAST FOR BRIDGES (NOT USED FOR SINGLE RESTORATIONS)

SECTIONAL TRAY

Fig. 69–1. Taking overimpression

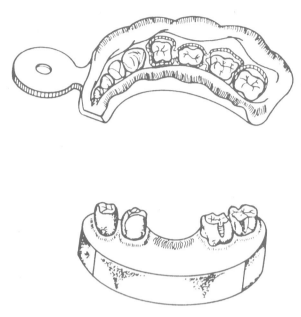

Fig. 69–2. Overimpression and cast of preparation

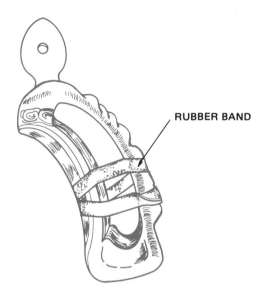

RUBBER BAND

Fig. 69–3. Cast in place in overimpression

4. Make a second alginate impression of the prepared tooth, again taking care to include one or two teeth mesially and distally. Two alternate methods of making this impression follow; either is acceptable.

Method 1
a. Dry the preparation.
b. With finger, wipe some alginate material into the preparation to pick up all details.
c. Place impression tray loaded with alginate material, and hold until set.

Method 2
a. Dry the preparation.
b. Inject hydrocolloid syringe material over entire preparation and margins.
c. Place a small wisp of cotton over the top of the mound of hydrocolloid material.
d. Place impression tray loaded with alginate impression material. The cotton will ensure a good union between the two separate materials. Hold until set.

By the time the alginate has set, the hydrocolloid will be sufficiently cooled.
5. Pour the impression of the preparation in *fast-setting* plaster. Again, be sure to include at least one or two teeth mesially and distally.
6. When this cast has set (two or three minutes), remove from the impression, and trim on model trimmer so that it will fit solidly into the impression taken before the preparation was made, figure 69–2. If the cast does not fit all the way, trim cast with scalpel or lab knife. Check for one or more of the following:
a. Positive blebs (blisters) in the occlusal surfaces of the plaster cast.
b. Insufficient trimming of the plaster cast.
c. Positive blebs on the gingival areas of the plaster cast.
d. Areas of alginate impression that represent deep undercuts in area of attached gingival tissue.
e. Debris in overimpression.

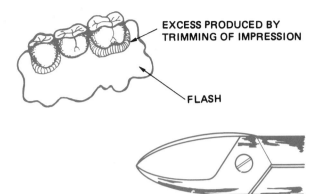

EXCESS PRODUCED BY
TRIMMING OF IMPRESSION

FLASH

Fig. 69–4. Trimming excess acrylic with scissors

7. In dappen dish, mix the resin to a dough stage. Place the bulk of the resin on and around the preparation(s) on the cast that has been trimmed and fitted into the overimpression.

8. Invert the cast into the overimpression, and press firmly to squeeze the excess acrylic around the cast.

9. Use the heavy rubber band to secure the cast and overimpression, figure 69–3.

10. Place in plaster bowl filled with very hot water.

11. Place plaster bowl in pressure pot. Run pressure to 20 pounds, and allow to set for about five minutes.

12. Remove from pressure pot.

13. Separate cast from overimpression.

14. If contour and margins are complete, remove plaster from cast.

15. If not complete, add acrylic to deficient areas by wetting area with monomer, sprinkling area with powder, and placing again in hot water in pressure pot for two to three minutes.

16. Trim gross excess with curved scissors, figure 69–4.

17. Do final trimming with finishing burs.

18. Polish using lathe with pumice and rag wheel.

19. Place acrylic temporary in mouth and adjust occlusion (which will be high in most cases).

20. Cement with ZOE cement. See Chapter 48.

Note: The only significant modification required when constructing temporary bridges is that the pontic (artificial tooth) be waxed up in a soft wax on the study cast and the overimpression made on this cast.

SUGGESTED ACTIVITIES

• Use a typodont with tooth preparations and construct a two- or three-unit temporary restoration.

• Process and finish a temporary restoration, using the detailed information in the chapter.

REVIEW

1. The four types of temporary restorations are constructed of

a. _____

b. _____

c. _____

d. _____

2. The purpose of the treatment restoration is to _____

   _____.

3. The placement of good treatment crowns and the adequate protection and stability of the tooth preparation are important for several reasons. List at least five reasons.

   a. _____

   b. _____

   c. _____

   d. _____

   e. _____

Chapter 70: Single Acrylic Resin Temporary Restorations

OBJECTIVES:

After studying this chapter, the student will be able to:
- Select the necessary materials and proceed to construct an acrylic resin temporary restoration.
- Finish the margins and test the occlusion according to the detailed instructions in the chapter.

INTRODUCTION

The dental assistant should be capable of taking a tray impression of the prepared area and of constructing an acrylic resin temporary restoration. Chapter 69 included the theory and reasons for using such restorations. When a single temporary restoration is desired, the following procedure may be used.

MATERIALS NEEDED

- alginate and tray
- resin powder and liquid
- wax (red)
- dappen dish
- mixing spatula (cement)
- acrylic bur
- bench motor with straight handpiece
- crown and collar scissors
- burlew wheel
- articulating paper
- dental floss
- ZOE cement

INSTRUCTIONS

1. Take an impression of the area to be prepared. (If there are missing teeth or broken cusps that should be included in the temporary, be sure to fill these areas in the mouth with red wax prior to taking the impression.)
2. Store the impression in a moist towel until the temporary is ready to be made.
3. Place several drops of liquid in the dappen dish.
4. Select the proper shade of powder and pour it into the liquid. (The mix should be thick enough to trail 1 to 2 inches from the spatula.)
5. At this point, pour the resin mix into the impression, confining it to the area of the prepared tooth or teeth.
6. When the material reaches the polymerization stage (loses its gloss), place the impression back into the mouth. Hold until the material has set, approximately 2 to 3 minutes. Do not allow the material to become completely hard, only firm.
7. Remove the impression from the mouth, and gradually work the temporary off the prepared tooth. The interproximal excess must be trimmed away to enable the removal of the temporary crown.
8. Continue to work the crown off and on until the temporary acrylic has completely set. At this point, trim the excess away with the crown and collar scissors.
9. Use the acrylic bur to trim the gingival margin making it smooth and flush with the margin of the preparation.
10. Make any necessary corrections by placing the temporary crown on the tooth. Check the occlusion, using the articulating paper, then remove and adjust the occlusion with the acrylic bur. Recheck.
11. Use the burlew wheel to polish the temporary crown. Care must be taken to avoid

removing excess material on the occlusal surface, interproximal areas, or the gingival margin.

12. Because of the accurate fit, a minimum of zinc oxide eugenol should be used for cementation. See Chapter 48.

13. Remove excess cement from the contact area with dental floss.

14. Recheck occlusion with articulating paper. Any marked areas should be removed with the burlew wheel.

SUGGESTED ACTIVITIES

- Use a typodont with prepared teeth. Select a single-tooth preparation; remove one tooth, either mesial or distal, and fill the space with red wax.
- Proceed to construct and finish a temporary acrylic restoration, using the opposing arch typodont to adjust the occlusion.

REVIEW

1. What is the appearance of the acrylic when it reaches the stage of polymerization? _____

Chapter 71: Gypsum

After studying this chapter, the student will be able to:
- Discuss the differences in the structure of dental plaster and dental stone.
- Define the setting time of gypsum (plaster or stone).
- State the difference between wet strength and dry strength of a gypsum product.
- List the factors that influence the strength of plaster or stone.

INTRODUCTION

Gypsum occurs in a massive form as rock-gypsum and is mined in many areas of the United States. This dull-colored rock is a commonly found sulfate mineral. Gypsum ($CaSO_4 \bullet 2H_2O$) is the dihydrate of calcium sulfate ($CaSO_4$). The chemical formula indicates that, in its natural state, calcium sulfate is combined with two molecules of water.

When gypsum is heated, some of the water is driven off and forms plaster or stone. This process is termed *calcination*. The resultant powder can be mixed with water, and gypsum is reformed again.

COMPOSITION

To understand why plaster sets when mixed with water, it is important to know how plaster is made.

Pieces of ground gypsum undergo a chemical change when heated at atmospheric pressure in open kettles. *Calcining* is simply the process of heating the gypsum particles so that some of the water molecules are driven off in the form of steam. As the water molecules are lost, *calcium sulfate hemihydrate* is formed. After calcining, the gypsum powder (plaster) is dry and contains approximately one-half molecule of water. The water leaving the particles as steam produces

pressure that breaks up the particles into finer crystals. They are further dried and ground to provide a variety of particle sizes that provide a plastic (can be poured) mass when mixed with water.

Two basic types of calcium hemihydrate are manufactured. The plaster just described is referred to as the *beta-hemihydrate* form. Gypsum particles heated under steam pressure and in the presence of sodium chloride are designated as *alpha-hemihydrate*, which is the dental stone. This product is used principally for stone dies in the fabrication of metal restorations.

Chemically, plaster and dental stone are identical, but the shapes of the powder particles differ. The powder particles of plaster are generally rough, irregularly shaped, and porous. Similar particles of stone are smooth, regularly shaped, and less porous.

The classification of dental gypsum products used in the American Dental Association (ADA) Specification is presented in the following list:

ADA Specification		Traditional Terminology
Type I	Plaster, impression	Impression plaster
Type II	Plaster, model	Model or lab plaster
Type III	Dental stone	Class I stone or Hydrocal
Type IV	Dental stone	Class II stone, Densite/die stone

527

Impression plaster, Type I, may be used for impressions of the edentulous mouth and for selected prosthetic construction work. Great strength is not desired in impression plaster. For this reason, a higher water to powder ratio is used for mixing impression plaster than is usually employed with other gypsum products. The chief requirement for the mixture is that it be sufficiently thick so that it will not run out of the impression tray as it is inserted into the mouth.

Model plaster, Type II, is generally used for such laboratory work as construction of study models and for articulating stone casts or models.

Dental stone is originally white and cannot be distinguished by appearance from plaster. For this reason, the manufacturer may color the stone buff or one of the pastel shades. The color does not alter the properties of the stone.

There are at least two types of dental stone available. Class I stone is used extensively for the construction of casts. Class II stone is used for dies. A *die* is a reproduction of a single tooth preparation on which a wax pattern is fashioned. The wax pattern is inverted and then cast in metal. A very hard stone cast is required for a die.

Class II stones can be mixed with less water than Class I stones. The surface hardness of a Class II stone is greater than that of a Class I stone.

Because of the uniform shape and size of the powder particles, dental stone can be mixed with less water than plaster. Probably the best way to mix plaster or stone is under vacuum, using a mechanical mixer. In order to get strong and hard plaster, the powder and water must be carefully proportioned. The powder should be weighed on a chemical balance and the water measured in a graduate cylinder.

SETTING REACTION

The setting reaction of plaster and stone is a process of hydration (the addition of water to the powder) and of release of heat, an exothermic reaction.

A few scattered crystals of gypsum are always present in any plaster or stone powder. These crystals (nuclei) act as centers of crystalline growth. The more nuclei present, the more rapid the crystallization.

Water to Powder Ratio

The water to powder ratio determines the physical properties of the final product. Powder particle porosity and size determine the amount of water to use. Because plaster particles are rough, porous, and irregularly shaped, plaster requires more water. This is why set plaster is much weaker than stone. Stone particles are smooth, less porous, and regularly shaped, and therefore require less water.

The overall strength of plaster and stone really depends on the number of nuclei of crystallization present at the time of spatulation. If more water is used than is required, the final strength of the plaster or stone will be weaker, because the nuclei are widely distributed. Therefore, the plaster or stone and water should be accurately measured. When pouring an impression, the consistency of the plaster or stone mix must be thin enough to pour into the impression. Sufficient water must be added so that the powder particles can be stirred or mixed into the water and poured into the impression. This added water is known as "free" or "excess" water. It is driven off as the exothermic reaction occurs.

Setting Time

The setting times of plaster or stone are known as the initial set and the final set. The initial set is the time between the spatulation and the time the mixture loses its gloss and becomes firm or solid enough to handle but is still moist and slightly pliable.

The final set occurs after the plaster or stone has completed its crystallization and all the heat has been driven off. In this stage, the plaster or stone are very hard and fairly dry. As might be expected, the strength of gypsum increases rapidly as the material hardens after the initial setting. Two strengths of the gypsum product are recognized, the wet strength and the dry strength. The wet strength is the strength present when the water is in excess of that required to bring the gypsum back to its natural water content. When the excess water content has been driven off or the model or cast dried, the strength obtained is called the dry strength. The dry strength may be two or more times the wet strength. Factors that influence the setting time of gypsum are:

- refinement
- temperature of water and atmosphere
- time and speed of spatulation
- water-powder ratio
- addition of retarders, accelerators, or other ingredients

SPATULATION

Within limits, the more the water-plaster or stone mixture is spatulated, the quicker it will set. Nuclei and gypsum crystals that start to form will be broken up by spatulation and will result in a greater number of crystals. The amount of spatulation refers to both the time and speed of spatulation.

ACCELERATORS AND RETARDERS

A few accelerators include:

- potassium sulfate 2%
- sodium chloride, very small amounts
- slurry (a watery mixture of insoluble matter)

For example, slurry water is obtained by saving some of the residue from the grinding wheel when plaster models are trimmed.

Retarders, although seldom used, include:

- borax
- hydrocolloid gels
- sodium citrate

REVIEW

1. List the ADA Classification for dental gypsum.

   a. _____

   b. _____

   c. _____

   d. _____

2. What is the process for changing gypsum into dental plaster or stone?

   _____

   _____

3. State the two types of calcium hemihydrate.

_____

_____

4. How do plaster and dental stone differ? _____

_____

_____

5. List five factors that control the setting time of plaster or stone.

a. _____

b. _____

c. _____

d. _____

e. _____

6. Explain how the water-powder ratio can affect the final strength of the gypsum product. _____

_____

_____

7. Define the following:

a. alpha-hemihydrate:_____

b. beta-hemihydrate: _____

c. initial set: _____

_____

d. final set:_____

_____

e. wet strength: _____

_____

f. dry strength:_____

_____

g. free or excess water: _____

_____

Chapter 72: Pouring and Trimming Plaster Models Using an Alginate Impression

OBJECTIVES: After studying this chapter, the student will be able to:
- Use the chemical balance scale for weighing plaster or stone.
- Use a graduate cylinder to measure water.
- Pour impressions in plaster or stone, according to instructions.
- Mark and prepare a maxillary and mandibular plaster model for trimming, using a model trimmer.
- Trim to an acceptable standard a set of plaster models.
- Evaluate trimmed study models.

INTRODUCTION

When mixing any gypsum product with water, one must be careful to avoid incorporating air into the mix. Not only do the air bubbles cause weakness in the model, they also produce surface inaccuracies.

The actual spatulation is done by rapidly stirring the mixture in a rubber plaster bowl with a stiff-bladed metal spatula.

Air is almost certain to be carried into the water if the powder is dumped in or if the water is poured into the powder. For this reason, the powder should be sifted into the water so that air is not introduced at the same time.

In mixing the powder and water together, begin with a circular motion and incorporate all the powder particles. Next, wipe the blade against the side and bottom of the bowl to insure that all the powder is being wetted.

Mixing should be done on a mechanical vibrator, with the bowl placed firmly on the vibrator table. When properly spatulated a plaster or stone mix should be smooth and free from air bubbles.

The amount of time for hand mixing is approximately one to two minutes. Any further mixing is likely to break up the crystals of gypsum that begin to form, which tends to weaken the final product. To obtain the maximum strength, the proportions of water and powder *must be measured.*

When the mixture has been spatulated for approximately one to two minutes, and appears to be smooth and uniform, the plaster/stone can be poured into the impression.

When the models (casts) are thoroughly dried, remove from impression(s), and prepare for trimming with model trimmer.

USING A GRAM CHEMICAL SCALE AND GRADUATE CYLINDER

Materials Needed

- gram chemical scale
- graduate cylinder
- paper cup
- paper towel(s)
- plaster powder
- water, room temperature

Gram Chemical Scale

1. Remove rubber stoppers, and place behind scale.
2. Milligram and gram weights must be at zero, figure 72–1.

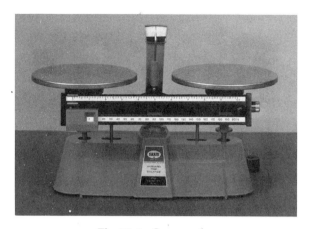

Fig. 72–1. Gram scale

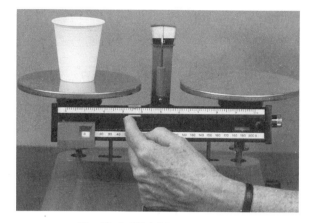

Fig. 72–2. Weighing paper cup

3. Scale must be in balance. If not, add pieces of paper towel to right side of scale until balanced.
    a. Top bar, milligram scale 1/10
    b. Bottom bar, gram scale 10, 20, 30, etc., grams
4. Place paper cup or paper towel on left side of the balance.
5. Balance scale again, using milligram scale. Weigh paper cup or towel, figure 72–2.
6. Set gram scale for given powder ratio, figure 72–3. Add weight of paper cup or paper towel.
7. Measure powder into paper cup or on paper towel until scale is in balance.
8. Remove cup and set aside.
9. Replace milligram and gram weights on zero.
10. Replace rubber stoppers on scale.

Graduate Cylinder

1. Pour room-temperature water into graduate cylinder.
2. Read level of water (meniscus) at prescribed amount, figure 72–4.

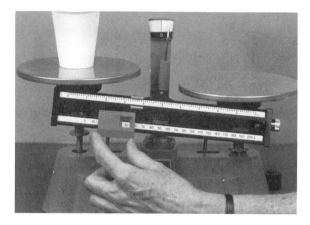

Fig. 72–3. Setting gram scale

POURING THE IMPRESSIONS

Two basic techniques are used for pouring models and establishing a base on them. The *inverted technique* requires a *double pour* with the first mix used for filling the teeth, palate, or tongue areas. The second mix forms the base.

The *boxed technique* employs the use of a wax boxing strip that forms the entire model.

Prior to pouring impressions, use a lab knife to remove excess impression material from the

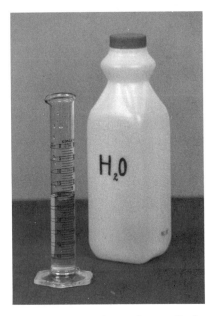

Fig. 72–4. Using the graduate cylinder

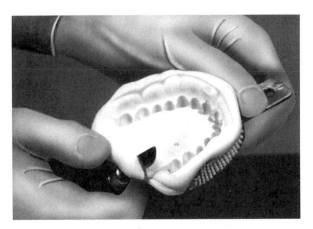

Fig. 72–5. Trimming excess impression material

tuberosity, retromolar pad, and other areas of the impressions. *In doing so, care must he taken to avoid losing any portion of the impression(s).*

Inverted Technique

Materials Needed

- alginate impressions
- plaster bowl
- spatula, plaster
- spatula, small (metal)
- vibrator
- glass slab or tile square
- plaster powder
- water (room temperature)
- lab knife
- gram scale
- graduate cylinder
- Q-tips
- paper cup
- paper towels
- humidor

Ratio

Maxillary teeth/palate	75 gr plaster/37 ml water
Mandibular teeth/ tongue	75 gr plaster/37 ml water
Base for maxillary and mandibular	100 gr plaster/45 ml water

Instructions

1. Weigh plaster in cup or towel.
2. Measure water, and pour into bowl.
3. Rinse impression with cool water.
4. Trim excess impression material from tray. Leave a $1/4''$ (6-mm) margin beyond the impression of the tuberosity or retromolar pad and other areas of the impression, figure 72–5.
5. Remove any visible surface water from alginate impression(s), with Q-tips.
6. Dampen a paper towel, and fold in half diagonally.
7. Place maxillary tray or impression in center of folded towel and approximately 1 to $1^1/2''$ from folded edge. Wrap tray or impression with towel, allowing the three points of the towel to come together at the handle of the tray. The paper towel will

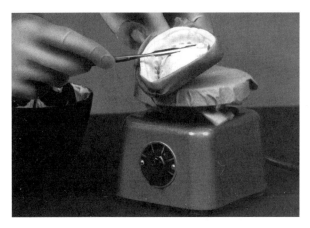

Fig. 72–6. Adding small increments of plaster

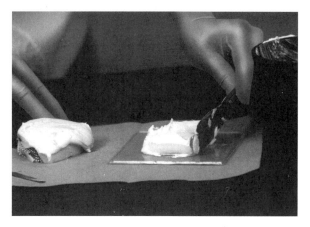

Fig. 72–7. Forming plaster patty

prevent plaster from flowing out of the impression and onto the vibrator. (See figure 72–6.) *Note:* When pouring a mandibular impression, it is suggested that the tongue area be blocked out with a damp paper towel.

8. Sift plaster powder into the water.

9. Allow powder to settle in the water for thirty seconds. This will minimize the incorporation of air into the mix during spatulation.

10. Next, rapidly spatulate plaster for thirty seconds at approximately two revolutions per second.

11. Turn on the vibrator, low speed.

12. Place bowl on vibrator, and thoroughly vibrate plaster for another thirty seconds. Remove bowl from vibrator.

13. Hold prepared tray or impression with paper towel in place, and rest base of tray or impression on vibrator.

14. Use small cement spatula, and begin adding small increments of plaster to the most distal portion of one side of the impression, figure 72–6.

15. Continue to place small increments of plaster in the same area of the impression, allowing each tooth to be filled in succes-

sion. This may necessitate tilting the impression tray until all the teeth are filled. This procedure will prevent the entrapment of air during the process of pouring.

16. Take the plaster spatula, and continue to add small portions of plaster until the impression is filled to its borders.

17. Remove tray or impression from vibrator, and set aside.

18. Remove paper towel from the impression tray.

19. Prepare plaster and water for a second mix.

20. Prepare the second mix of plaster according to previous instructions.

21. Place entire second mix on a glass slab or tile, and form a square, thick patty, figure 72–7.

22. Quickly invert the impression on the patty, which was previously prepared. Seat the patty with sufficient pressure to join the plaster of the patty with the plaster of the impression, figure 72–8. Important: Hold tray handle steady, and hand-vibrate impression, using a fulcrum to support the tray; otherwise, the tray will be buried in plaster, resulting in a shallow base.

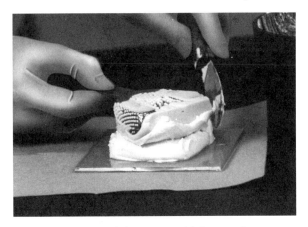

Fig. 72–8. Joining patty with impression

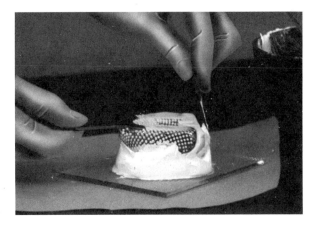

Fig. 72–9. Forming the base

23. Soft plaster can be added along the borders of the base at this time. Likewise, excess plaster may be removed. Keep all walls of the plaster base vertical, figure 72–9. Fill in any voids that may exist. *Do not bury tray into plaster. It will be very difficult to separate model or cast from tray.*

24. Place poured impression(s) in 100% humidity for sixty minutes.

Cleanup

1. Remove excess plaster from bowl and spatulas with paper towel. *Never* wash plaster or stone products down the sink!
2. Wash and dry bowls and spatulas.
3. Clean plaster from vibrator, and return to station.
4. Clean work station.

Boxed Technique

Materials Needed

- alginate impressions
- plaster bowl
- spatula, plaster
- spatula, small (metal)
- vibrator
- plaster powder
- water (room temperature)
- lab knife
- gram scale
- graduate cylinder
- Q-tips
- paper cup(s)
- paper towels
- wax boxing strips
- bowl of hot water
- humidor

Ratio

Maxillary impression	100 gr plaster/49 ml water
Mandibular impression	100 gr plaster/49 ml water
Extra plaster, if needed	50 gr plaster/24 ml water

Instructions

1. Weigh plaster in cup or towel.
2. Measure water, and pour in bowl.
3. Rinse impression with cool water.
4. Trim excess impression material from tray. Leave a 1/4″ (6-mm) margin beyond the tuberosity or retromolar pad and other areas of the impression. See figure 72–5.

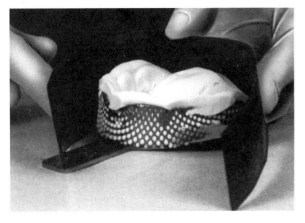

Fig. 72–10. Boxing strip and impression

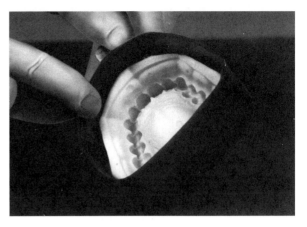

Fig. 72–11. Boxing strip in place

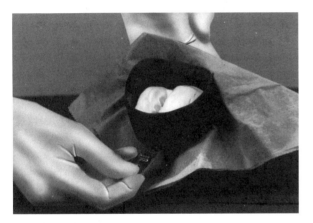

Fig. 72–12. Placement of paper towel

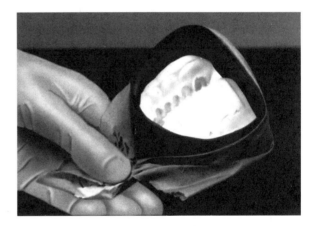

Fig. 72–13. Paper towel in place

5. Remove any visible surface water from alginate impression(s) with Q-tips.
6. Soften boxing strip in bowl of hot water.
7. Place center of boxing strip across posterior part of impression, and bring ends of strip forward, overlapping strip at handle of the tray. Secure overlap by pressing the two ends together, figure 72–10.
8. The boxing strip must be closely adapted to the impression tray with no visible spaces between tray and boxing strip. The walls of the wax boxing strip must be vertical, figure 72–11.
9. Dampen a paper towel, and fold in half diagonally.
10. Place tray or impression in center of folded towel and approximately 1 to $1^1/2''$ from folded edge, figure 72–12. Wrap tray or impression with towel, allowing the three points of the towel to come together at the handle of the tray. The paper towel will prevent the plaster from flowing out of the impression and onto the vibrator, figure 72–13.
11. Sift plaster powder into the water.

12. Allow powder to settle in the water for thirty seconds. This will minimize the incorporation of air into the mix during spatulation.

13. Next, rapidly spatulate plaster for thirty seconds at approximately two revolutions per second.

14. Turn on vibrator, low speed.

15. Place bowl on vibrator, and thoroughly vibrate plaster for another thirty seconds. Remove bowl from vibrator.

16. Hold prepared tray or impression with paper towel in place, and rest base of tray or impression on vibrator.

17. Use small cement spatula, and begin adding small increments of plaster to the most distal portion of one side of the impression.

18. Continue to place small increments of plaster in the same area of the impression, allowing each tooth to be filled in succession. This may necessitate tilting the impression tray until all the teeth are filled. This procedure will prevent the entrapment of air during the process of pouring.

19. Take the plaster spatula, and continue to add small portions of plaster until the impression is filled to top edge of boxing strip.

20. Repeat procedure for mandibular impression, *except to fill in tongue area*, with a rolled, damp paper towel.

21. Place poured impression(s) in 100% humidity for sixty minutes.

22. Remove from humidor, and carefully remove wax boxing strips from impression tray(s). *Boxing strips are reusable.*

23. Separate models from impression. Where necessary, use lab knife to free model from impression. *Caution:* Do not apply force when separating model from impression, as this could cause teeth to be fractured off the model.

Cleanup

1. Remove plaster from boxing strips, and straighten strips by placing in water, then on paper towel to flatten.

2. Following previous instructions, clean equipment and work station.

TRIMMING STUDY MODELS

Materials Needed

- safety glasses
- prepared plaster models
- pencil
- plaster bowl (2)
- plastic apron
- lab brush
- plastic triangle
- lab knife

Instructions

Mark Maxillary Model

1. Using pencil, draw a horizontal line about $1/4''$ distal to the tuberosity or molars, figure 72–14.

2. Mark center tip of maxillary cuspids, and extend line to labial fold, figure 72–15. Mark and draw line division between maxillary central incisors. Extend line on frenum to labial fold, figure 72–16.

3. Mark and draw a straight line from cuspid to midline of maxillary central incisor along the labial fold, right and left sides, figure 72–17.

4. Observe occlusal grooves to determine the angle of the buccal cut.

5. Mark and draw a straight line along the buccal fold from the cuspid to the tuberosity or molar line, right and left sides, figure 72–18.

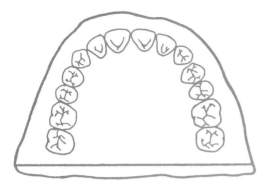

Fig. 72–14. Marking peripheral outline of maxillary tuberosity

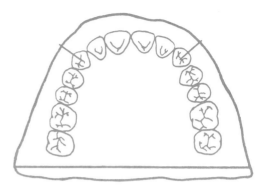

Fig. 72–15. Marking maxillary cuspids

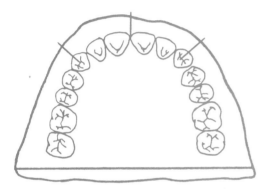

Fig. 72–16. Marking division between maxillary central incisors

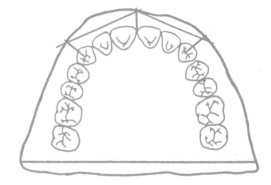

Fig. 72–17. Marking cuspid(s) to midline of maxillary central incisors

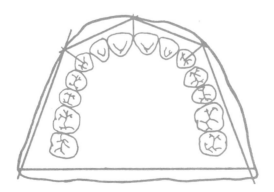

Fig. 72–18. Marking buccal fold from cuspid(s) to molar(s)

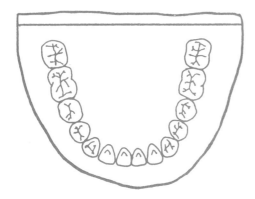

Fig. 72–19. Marking peripheral outline of mandibular retromolar area

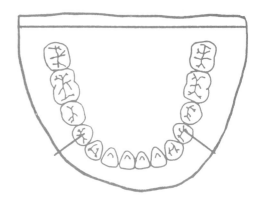

Fig. 72–20. Marking mandibular first premolars

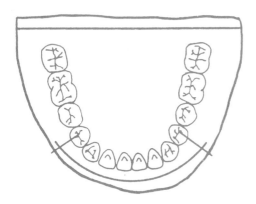

Fig. 72–21. Marking anterior curve from first premolar to first premolar

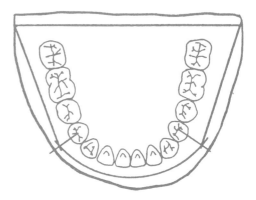

Fig. 72–22. Marking buccal fold from premolar(s) to molar(s)

Mark Mandibular Model

1. Draw a horizontal line ¹/₄″ distal to the retromolar pad or molars, figure 72–19.
2. Mark center tip of first premolar(s), and extend line to buccal fold, figure 72–20.
3. Draw a curved line from first premolar to the opposite premolar and along the labial fold, figure 72–21.
4. Observe occlusal grooves to determine the angle of the buccal cut.
5. Mark and draw a straight line along the buccal fold from the first premolar to the retromolar pad or molar, right and left sides, figure 72–22.

TRIMMING PLASTER MODELS

Note: The student must wear safety glasses and plastic apron!

The Model Trimmer

1. Adjust table to conform to a 90° angle from wheel. Use a plastic triangle (protractor) as a guide.
2. Establish water flow. Turn ON model trimmer switch.

Preparing Models for Trimming

1. Dry models must soak in water for a minimum of five minutes.
2. Using a lab knife, remove excess extension in posterior area(s) that may prevent occlusion of models.

Trimming Procedures

A grinding wheel cuts faster if the operator does not exert tremendous pressure against the wheel. When trimming models, applying light pressure against the wheel is all that is necessary. *Never allow grinding wheel to be used dry.*

1. Invert mandibular model with teeth resting on the countertop. Determine if the base of the model is parallel to the occlusal plane, figure 72–23.
2. Trim base of mandibular model parallel to the occlusal plane. The base should be at least $1/2''$ thick in tongue area, figure 72–24.
3. Trim posterior of mandibular model at right angles to the base, figure 72–25.
4. Occlude maxillary and mandibular models, and trim posterior of maxillary model parallel to the base of the mandibular model, figure 72–26.
5. Occlude models, and trim the base of the maxillary model parallel to the base of the mandibular model, figure 72–27.

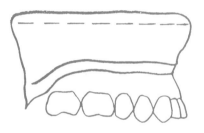

Fig. 72–23. Determining plane of base

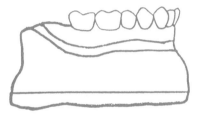

Fig. 72–24. Trimming base parallel with occlusal plane

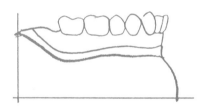

Fig. 72–25. Trimming retromolar area at right angle with base

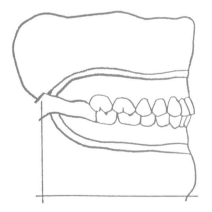

Fig. 72–26. Trimming posterior of maxillary model with models in occlusion

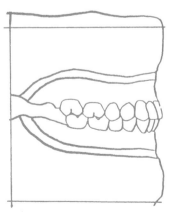

Fig. 72–27. Trimming maxillary base with models in occlusion

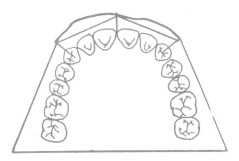

Fig. 72–28. Trimming buccal folds of maxillary model

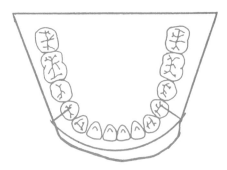

Fig. 72–29. Trimming buccal folds of mandibular model

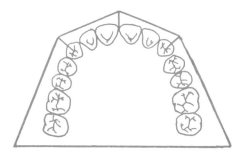

Fig. 72–30. Trimming maxillary angles, cuspid(s) to central incisor(s)

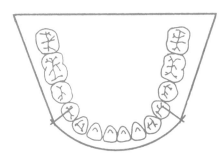

Fig. 72–31. Trimming mandibular anterior curve, on first premolar to first premolar

6. On the maxillary and mandibular models, trim the buccal line parallel to the occlusal grooves and width of the buccal fold, figures 72–28 and 72–29.

7. On the maxillary model, trim from the cuspids to central incisors according to marked lines, left and right side, figure 72–30.

8. On mandibular model, trim from the premolar to opposite first premolar along labial fold and according to marked line, figure 72–31.

9. Occlude both models. With a ruler draw a diagonal line across the maxillary base from the point where the labial and buccal cuts meet (cuspid) to the angle formed where the buccal and tuberosity cuts meet, figure 72–32.

10. Trim occluded models by aligning point of cuspid area in center slot and forward on grinding table. Adjust posterior angle to fall on the center slot and next to grinding wheel. Trim to form a 25° angle, figure 72–33.

EVALUATING TRIMMER STUDY MODELS

1. Models must be trimmed in a symmetrical pattern, figures 72–34 and 72–35.

2. Model must exhibit a 1/2″ base.

3. Trimmed models will sit on end without losing occlusion.

4. All teeth and supporting structures must be present without loss of any anatomy.

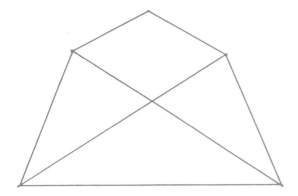

Fig. 72–32. Marking maxillary base for buccal angles

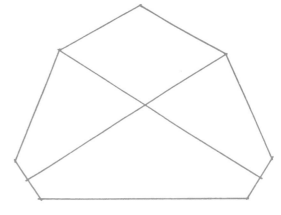

Fig. 72–33. Trimming tuberosity or retromolar angle(s)

Cleanup

1. Clean model trimmer with lab brush. Firmly hold and press lab brush against grinding wheel while using full flow of water.
2. Turn off water. Switch motor to OFF.
3. Remove guide table. Wash, dry, and set aside. Clean out reservoir beneath the motor where plaster accumulates. *Note:* If the reservoir is not kept clean, water backs up, causing the grinding wheel to splash water out.
4. Replace guide table to its correct position on model trimmer.
5. Clean plastic apron with damp towel, fold, and store.
6. Print name on bottom of trimmed models with indelible pen.
7. Trimmed models should be evaluated by both student and instructor.

SUGGESTED ACTIVITIES

- Pour a set of study models from alginate impressions using the inverted technique.
- Pour a set of study models from alginate impressions using the boxed technique.
- Trim each set of study models according to instructions given in this chapter.

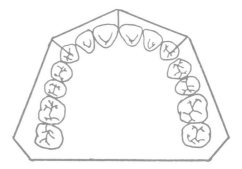

Fig. 72–34. Properly trimmed maxillary model

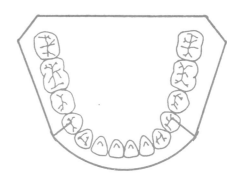

Fig. 72–35. Properly trimmed mandibular model

- Evaluate both sets of study models according to instructions given in this chapter.

OBJECTIVES:

After studying this chapter, the student will be able to:
- Discuss the uses of the articulator.
- Determine the categories of articulators.
- Discuss the variations in technique when using the Stephan articulator as compared to using the Hanau.

INTRODUCTION

The **articulator** is a frame used in prosthetic procedures and other case studies. The frame holds the upper and lower models in correct relationship. The articulator maintains the correct occlusion of the patient's casts or models and represents his or her jaws.

USES OF ARTICULATOR

The articulator is used for (1) carving wax patterns; (2) establishing and studying occlusion in orthodontic cases; (3) studying periodontal malocclusion, inlay techniques, and study model displays; (4) examining typodont models to demonstrate proper occlusion; and (5) examining typodont models with various types of restorations.

Through **articulation**, it is possible to determine the length of the teeth involved when working with a dental prosthesis.

CATEGORIES OF ARTICULATORS

Articulators may vary in construction from a very simple wire construction to a more complex one. However, they are all constructed of metal. The more difficult prosthetics demand the more complicated ball-and-socket types of articulator.

Articulators may be categorized as follows:

- nonanatomical, nonadjustable simple hinge articulator
- semianatomical, semiadjustable articulator
- anatomical, adjustable articulator

Although the word *anatomical* appears in all three categories, none of these devices is truly anatomical. Fortunately, all come close to the reproduction of mandibular movements. Adjustable articulators provide greater adaptability and movement to positional relationships as recorded by the jaws of the patient and provide an opportunity to arrange teeth in harmony with individual jaw movements. This enables the dentist to obtain the best possible esthetic effect.

A function that the clinical dental assistant should perform solo is to mount models or casts in an articulator. Two articulators representative of the categories mentioned will be illustrated, as in all probability the dentist will have both types in the preparation area.

Stephan Articulator

The *Stephan articulator* (Model A) is an example of a nonanatomical device, but it *does* open and close with a spring so that lateral movements can be simulated. The lower bow of the articulator represents the mandible and the vertical support arms from it represent the rami. The technique of mounting a set of models in the Stephan articulator is not difficult; however, the first step is to grind the models so that they will slip easily between its bows, figure 73–1. The hinge represents the temporomandibular joints, and the upper bow represents the maxilla.

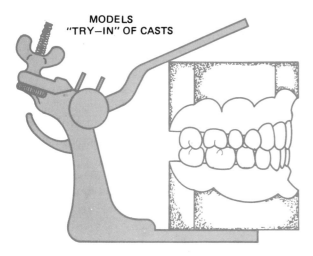

Fig. 73–1. Trying fit of models to articulator

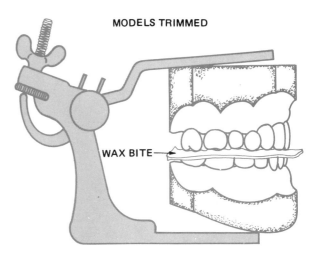

Fig. 73–2. Bows parallel and models trimmed

(For instructions on how to use the Stephan articulator, see Chapter 74.)

The locking nut presets the space between the upper and lower bows. Generally, these bows are set parallel to each another, and the locking nut is tightened in this position. The wax registration is in place during the adaptation. Figure 73–2 shows the parallel position of the bows and the trimmed models with the wax registration in place.

After the models are adapted on the articulator, they are fastened to the bows with plaster, figure 73–3. After the plaster has set, the articulator can be opened and the wax bite removed. This is a routine procedure regardless of the type of articulator used.

Hanau Articulator

The *Hanau* is a semianatomical, semiadjustable articulator. This articulator is used with a face bow for bite registration. The models are mounted between the upper and lower bows in a plane relative to those of the individual patient's mouth. The face bow is in reality a device for taking the bite registration. It consists of a bite fork over which wax is placed prior to having the patient make the registration. The fork is

attached to a bow extending from the opening of the right ear to the left ear. The face bow with the registration and upper model is plastered to the upper bow. The face bow positions the model in the proper anterior-posterior position as well as the proper inferior-superior relationship.

When the case does not call for an exact bite registration, the face bow may not be used, and the Hanau can help achieve the desired results.

Using the Hanau Articulator

1. Make certain the articulator is functioning properly and that all adjustments are free.
2. Check the device to make certain all plaster from the previous use has been removed and the bows are parallel. (The paralleling of the bows in the Hanau is controlled by the incisal guide pin. This pin must be flush with the upper bow, figure 73–4.)
3. Place a rubber band over the articulator. It should rest at three points: the notch in the incisal guide pin, and on the *bar* in the *H* on "Hanau" imprinted on each of the two vertical posts. With the rubber band in place, it will establish the plane of occlusion for the lower model.

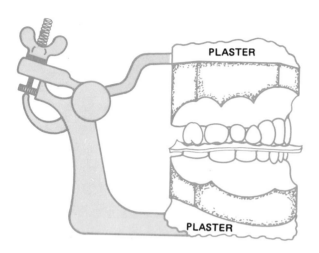

Fig. 73–3. Plastering the bows to the models

4. Place plaster over the ring on the lower bow of the articulator and *force* the lower model down into the plaster until the plane of occlusion of the model is parallel with the plane of occlusion established by the rubber band.

5. Allow the plaster around the lower model to set. Position the upper model, using a wax bite registration.

6. Plaster the upper model to the ring of the upper bow of the articulator, figure 73–5.

7. Remove excesses of plaster to make the mountings as neat as possible. *Note:* When removing the models from an articulator, always clean the parts thoroughly. Coat the articulator with a *thin* film of petrolatum before storing it.

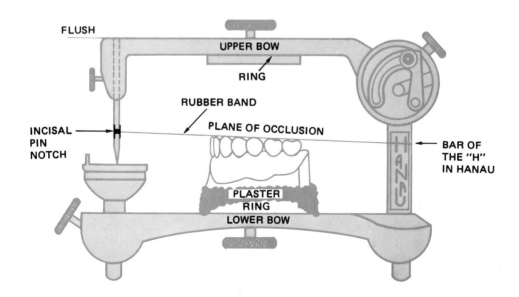

Fig. 73–4. Mounting the lower model in a Hanau articulator

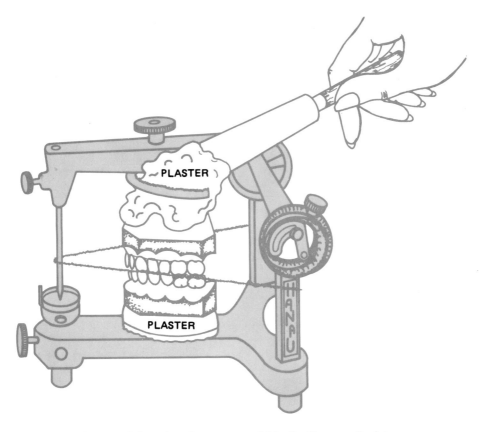

Fig. 73–5. Mounting the upper model in the Hanau articulator

REVIEW

1. What are the three categories of articulators?

    a. _____

    b. _____

    c. _____

2. Give four uses for articulators.

    a. _____

    b. _____

    c. _____

    d. _____

3. Which model is articulated first?_____

_____

_____

4. When is the wax bite registration used in articulating models?_____

_____

_____

Chapter 74: Articulating Dental Models Using a Stephan Articulator _____

OBJECTIVES: After studying this chapter, the student will be able to:
- Review the principles of operating the articulator.
- Select the necessary materials, including the articulator, and proceed to articulate the models.
- Evaluate the articulated models.

INTRODUCTION

After the models have been judged satisfactory, articulation is complete. *Articulating* models is the process of establishing a correct relationship between the upper teeth and the lower teeth. The articulator provides a mechanical means of duplicating the actual movements of the mandible and the maxilla.

MATERIALS NEEDED

- plaster models (trimmed)
- plaster of Paris powder
- water (room temperature)
- spatula, laboratory
- plaster bowl (small)
- glass slab or tile square
- graduated cylinder, in millimeters
- Stephan articulator
- laboratory knife
- scales, gram
- Bunsen burner
- spatula, wax
- base wax

INSTRUCTIONS

1. Place the articulator on the glass slab.
2. Place the trimmed models in occlusion, then in the articulator to determine if the articulator can be used.
3. Warm a square of base wax and obtain a bite relationship, figure 73–2.
4. Mix the plaster of Paris, using 50 gr to 25 cc water.
5. Place a mound of plaster (about five tablespoons) on the lower bow of the articulator.
6. Place the base of the lower model on the articulator and plaster.
7. Smooth sides, but do not allow plaster to work up on the models. Carefully remove the excess. Allow to harden.
8. Lower the top flange of the articulator into place.
9. Mix another plaster of Paris mix.
10. Carefully apply mix on top of model. Be sure to cover articulator completely.
11. Wet your hands, and smooth the plaster mix. Allow it to harden. Do not disturb it until the final set has been completed.
12. Clean up the laboratory.

SUGGESTED ACTIVITIES

- Review Chapter 73, *Principles of Operation of the Articulator*.
- Smooth and finish articulated models. Set them aside for an evaluation of the end product. Use the line graphs of cutting procedures in Chapter 72.
- Warm a square of base wax, and obtain a bite relationship.

Chapter 75: Use of the Boley Gauge

OBJECTIVES:

After studying this chapter, the student will be able to:
- Identify the parts of the Boley gauge.
- Explain when the straight and curved beaks are used on a Boley gauge.
- Give the step-by-step procedure for manipulating the Boley gauge.

INTRODUCTION

The *Boley gauge* shown in figure 75–1 is a *caliper rule* (a tool of measurement with one scale fixed to, or integral with, a graduated straight bar on which the outer scale slides) used to measure the dimensions of teeth.

The metric system is used when reading the Boley gauge. The gauge is graduated in millimeters on the handle, or stationary side, of the beam. The window of the movable arm or beam is fitted with a *vernier* (a small, movable, graduated scale running parallel to the fixed graduated scale). The vernier is used for measuring a fractional part of one of the divisions on the fixed scale. Numbers on the *fixed scale* are written as units; those on the vernier are written decimally,

with the decimal point placed immediately after the unit, e.g., 2.5 mm. Each unit represents 1 mm; each fraction is equal to one-tenth of a millimeter.

There are two sets of markings (numbers) on the fixed scale; both include 0 through 9. Readings can be made from either side of the rule, and, in either case, the space between the numbers is equal to 1 cm. Markings on the vernier equal only nine spaces on the fixed scale.

The *base jaw* is fixed, but the *movable jaw* can be moved in either direction. The *notch* acts as a thumb purchase during adjustment. The *lock* holds the jaws in place after the adjustment so that an exact reading can be made.

The straight (parallel) beaks of the gauge are used for outside diameters and convex curvatures. The *curved beaks* should be used only when measuring concave diameters.

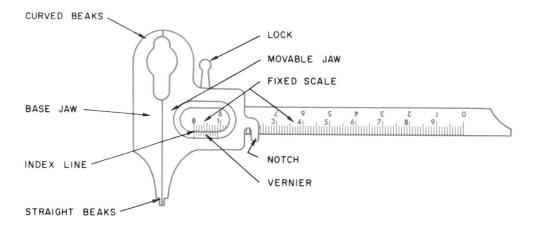

Fig. 75–1. Boley gauge

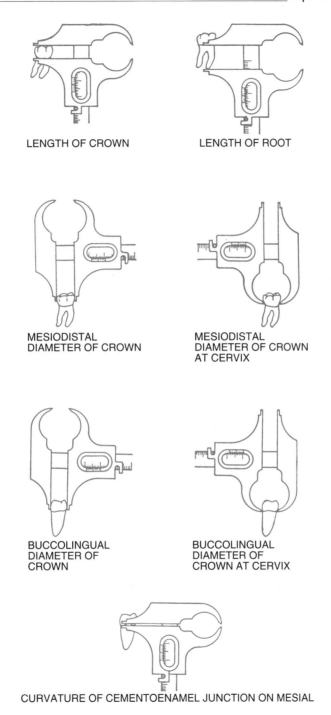

LENGTH OF CROWN

LENGTH OF ROOT

MESIODISTAL
DIAMETER OF CROWN

MESIODISTAL
DIAMETER OF CROWN
AT CERVIX

BUCCOLINGUAL
DIAMETER OF
CROWN

BUCCOLINGUAL
DIAMETER OF
CROWN AT CERVIX

CURVATURE OF CEMENTOENAMEL JUNCTION ON MESIAL

Fig. 75–2. Method of calibrating a posterior tooth (Courtesy Wheeler, R.C., *Tooth Form Drawing and Carving,* **2nd ed., Saunders, Philadelphia, 1986)**

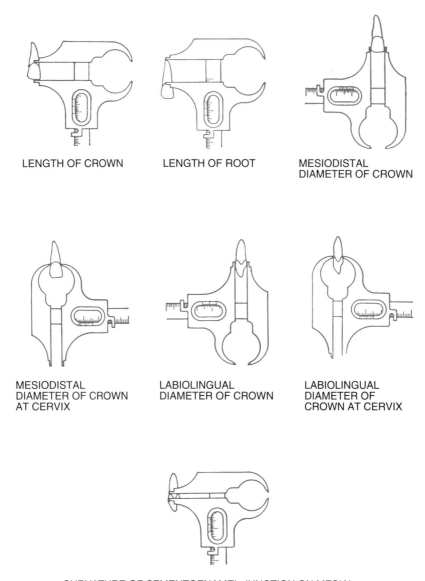

LENGTH OF CROWN

LENGTH OF ROOT

MESIODISTAL
DIAMETER OF CROWN

MESIODISTAL
DIAMETER OF CROWN
AT CERVIX

LABIOLINGUAL
DIAMETER OF CROWN

LABIOLINGUAL
DIAMETER OF
CROWN AT CERVIX

CURVATURE OF CEMENTOENAMEL JUNCTION ON MESIAL

Fig. 75–3. Method of calibrating an anterior tooth (Courtesy Wheeler, R.C., *Tooth Form Drawing and Carving*, **2nd ed., Saunders, Philadelphia, 1986)**

MANIPULATING THE BOLEY GAUGE

Pick up the gauge with the markings facing you. (Tilt the gauge so the light falls on the rule.) Place thumbnail in the notch. Fit the jaws over the object with plenty of room on each side. Hold the base against one side of the object, and push the movable jaw until it touches the opposite side of the object. With the index finger, tighten the lock by pulling it in the direction of the thumb.

Reading the Boley Gauge

Note the 0 on the fixed scale; call that the "zero guide." Now, write down the first number to the left of the *index line*, and nearest the zero guide. This can be done by counting the lines. Put a decimal point to the right of the number. If the index line is to the right of the line on the fixed scale, it indicates a fraction (one-tenth) of a millimeter; if the index line is directly under any line of the fixed scale, that is the measurement in units. Count the divisions to the right of the index line until a line on the vernier exactly coincides with a line on the fixed scale. Place this figure to the right of the decimal point.

SUGGESTED ACTIVITY

- Measure the overall length of an extracted tooth. Measure all the aspects, using the sketches in figures 75–2 and 75–3 as guides. Include the following information: name of tooth; maxillary or mandibular; overall length in millimeters; length of crown; mesiodistal crown; labiolingual or buccolingual crown; mesiodistal neck; labiolingual or buccolingual neck. Turn in the extracted tooth along with your measurements of it to the instructor for evaluation.

Chapter 76: Introduction to the Dental Specialties

After studying this chapter, the student will be able to:
- List and briefly describe the eight dental specialties.
- Describe the role of Dental Public Health as it relates to the entire practice of dental care.
- Discuss the function of official agencies as a part of local, state, and federal dental health programs.
- Describe the role of voluntary agencies in providing dental health care.
- Discuss the most widely accepted theory of the cause of dental caries.
- Discuss the interrelationship of operative dentistry with the dental specialties.
- Discuss complete pediatric dental care and its importance to a lifelong process.
- Determine the various hazards of malocclusion.
- Determine the differences between a removable partial prosthesis and a fixed prosthesis.
- List and describe the types of cast crowns used in fixed prosthodontics.
- Describe the role of the dental laboratory technician in dentistry.
- Determine the difference between radiographs for a periodontal diagnosis and those for other areas of dental care.
- Discuss the various aspects of periodontal care and their impact on total body health.

INTRODUCTION

The purpose of this chapter is to provide the learner with an overview of the field of dentistry. Although some areas have received more emphasis than others, dental practice specialties are greatly interrelated.

Basic educational requirements for the dentist require an undergraduate college degree plus graduation from an approved dental school, accredited by the Commission on Dental Accreditation of the American Dental Association (ADA). The degree usually granted is the DDS (doctor of dental surgery) or DMD (doctor of dental medicine), depending on the granting institution.

Training for specialty practice includes an additional two years of postgraduate and graduate education in the area of specialization. The program must be approved by the Commission on Dental Accreditation of the ADA.

Dentistry is the department of medicine that is concerned with the teeth, oral cavity, and associated parts. Dentistry includes the diagnosis and treatment of defective and missing teeth and oral tissue.

A dental office is a place in which the patient is receives dental service in a dental chair by a dentist or a dental hygienist. The dental office may be located in a hospital, in an industrial plant, in an outpatient clinic, or in a private dental suite.

Research indicates that most of the information that patients retain regarding their teeth is first heard or experienced in a dental office. Dental personnel must, therefore, present the facts and correct any wrong impressions about proper dental care.

THE DENTAL SPECIALTIES

Dental Public Health is involved with the prevention and control of dental diseases, prevention and spread of communicable diseases, and the promotion of dental health through organized and shared community efforts.

Operative dentistry, also called *general dentistry*, is involved with restoring or reforming hard dental tissues.

Pediatric dentistry is involved with preventive and therapeutic care of children from birth through adolescence. Special patients who are afflicted with mental, physical, or emotional problems may also be cared for by the pediatric dentist.

Orthodontics is involved with the supervision, guidance, and correction of malocclusion in the developing and mature dentofacial structures.

Endodontics is involved with the cause, diagnosis, prevention, and treatment of disease or injuries of the dental pulp and associated tissues.

Prosthodontics is involved with the maintenance and reestablishment of oral functions by the restoration of natural teeth or the replacement of missing teeth and related oral and maxillofacial tissues with artificial appliances.

Periodontics is involved with the diagnosis and treatment of disease of the surrounding tissues and supporting structures of the teeth.

Oral and maxillofacial surgery is involved with the diagnosis, surgical, and additional treatment of disease, injury, and defects, including both the functional and esthetic quality of the hard and soft tissues of the oral and maxillofacial areas.

Oral pathology is involved with the study of the cause and nature of the diseases that affect the oral structures and the tissues near them.

PUBLIC HEALTH

In the United States, the responsibility for the health of the people primarily rests in each state. The federal government has definite responsibilities for health and welfare. One of its functions is to provide guidance and assistance to the several states in developing adequate public health services. The Social Security Acts passed by the Seventy-fourth Congress authorized the distribution of funds to improve and enlarge public health services at the national, state, and local levels.

The right of each state to control and safeguard the health of its several communities amounts to police power. It gives to the state government the power to enact laws and to enforce them in order to ensure health, safety, morals, order, comfort, and general welfare.

Health Organizations and Dental Health Education

Dental health education is included in the functions of a number of government agencies. These are called *official agencies* and operate as a part of the local, state, and federal governments.

At the federal level, the U.S. Public Health Service (USPHS), which is an agency within the Department of Health, Education, and Welfare (HEW), assumes a major role in the dental health programs. The USPHS assists the states in planning and promoting dental health programs. This agency helps to formulate policies for dental health programs in industries and provides special studies and surveys for the evaluation of dental health data. Another function of the USPHS is to provide personnel for demonstration programs.

Demonstration programs provided in a number of states by the USPHS show the techniques, the costs, time schedules, and personnel needed for the topical application of stannous fluoride to the teeth of school children. The extensive reports released to the public indicate the value of these caries-prevention methods for areas where other means of providing fluoride are impractical.

The Children's Bureau of the USPHS allocates funds to the states for programs of dental health, specifically for mothers and children. The dental consultant of the Children's Bureau advises state agencies concerning dental programs for handicapped children.

The Department of Education of each state has received from the legislative branch of the state government authority to provide physical examinations of pupils. Where state laws have been enacted in this respect, they frequently employ physicians, dentists, nurses, and other health specialists, including dental hygienists, for the purpose of performing periodic health examinations and inspections. The purpose of these activities is to detect adverse conditions in the school population, to advise concerning the need for care, and to educate parents or guardians and children.

Role of Voluntary Agencies in Dental Health

Voluntary agencies come into existence because of a specific need and are usually organized by groups of people who have either financial resources, professional ability, or just plain community spirit and a willingness to contribute to the same cause. The prime purpose of any voluntary agency is to bring to public attention the need for study, treatment, or prevention of a health hazard within the community. Public interest is stimulated, thus demanding government action.

The professional organizations' role deserves notice, for it is through the contributions of the ADA, the American Dental Hygiene Association (ADHA), the National Education Association (NEA), and a number of others in the field of health and education that authentic dental health information has become available. Through the efforts and controlled research of professional organizations, the aims and purposes for the standards of treatment have been determined.

Four Principles of Establishing a Dental Health Program

Through the ADA Council on Dental Health, four principles were adopted as a basis for dental health programs. Briefly stated, they are:

1. Adequate provisions should be made for research that may lead to the prevention and control of dental diseases.
2. Dental Health education should be included in all education and treatment programs for children and adults.
3. Dental care should be available to all, regardless of income or geographic location. Programs should be based on the prevention and control of dental diseases. Dental caries is the responsibility of the individual, the family, and the community in that order. If the responsibility is not assumed by the community, it should be assumed by the state, and then by the federal government. The community, in all cases, shall determine the methods for providing service in its areas.
4. In all conferences that may lead to the formation of a plan for dental research, dental health education, and dental care, there should be participation by authorized representatives of the ADA.

Dental Disease—A Public Health Problem

Public health authorities recognize a situation to be a public health problem if it is widespread and affects the health and life of a wide portion of the population.

Dental disease is known to be epidemic at all times, occuring early in life for most individuals. Studies indicate that less than 2 percent of the population live the entire life span without some form of dental disease.

According to the ADA, 50 percent of all 2-year-old children have one or more diseased teeth. At 5 years of age, they have three or more cavities in primary teeth. Fourteen percent of them will have cavities in their first permanent molars. The average youth at age 16 will have seven carious (decayed) or restored teeth. Less than 4 percent of high school students are free of decay.

Dental Caries

Of all dental disorders, tooth caries (decay) is unquestionably the most chronic disease affecting the American people. The cause of dental caries has been attributed to a number of factors.

A summary of research conducted by the ADA Advisory Committee on Research in Dental Caries, states the following:

> *Caries* is a bacterial disease of the calcified dental tissues (enamel and dentin), producing a typical and abnormal change in the structure of teeth. The active cause of caries is acid produced on tooth areas, often or long enough to enable the acid there to disintegrate the mineral structure. Many secondary factors determine the growth of the bacteria, affect the concentration and confinement of the acids, and their resistance to attack. Among these factors are (a) diet as it affects oral environment, products of bacterial growth, and tooth structure, and (b) systemic reaction of the individual, including metabolic processes, oral secretions, and tooth construction. Since dental caries is an individual disease,

and *not* communicable, the conditions that allow it to be produced are also individual.

The most widely accepted theory of dental caries, according to the ADA, was expressed as early as 1890 by Dr. W. D. Miller. The theory does not completely satisfy the scientists of research as they continue to strive for a more exact explanation. However, the Miller Theory of Tooth Decay remains a reliable one.

As stated by Miller, the process of dental decay follows several steps:

1. Food debris (carbohydrates and sugars) remain on perfect or imperfect tooth surfaces where the cleaning action of saliva, chewing, or toothbrushing cannot reach or dislodge it.
2. The end-products of bacteria and enzymes of fermentation are in a concentration sufficient to dissolve the mineral content of tooth enamel.
3. Decalcification, once started, progresses until the enamel surface is broken, and the dentin is subjected to the same action.
4. During the process of decalcification, decomposition of the organic structure of the tooth takes place. This process is continuous until the dental pulp is affected.
5. Final putrefaction of the dental pulp occurs. *Putrefaction* means the chemical breakdown of the tissues, causing the formation of a foul smell and destruction of tooth vitality.

The principal acid-producing bacteria in the mouth is *lactobacillus acidophilus*, a lactic-acid–forming bacteria. The chemical action of lactobacillus on a carbohydrate food debris results in fermentation and the creation of lactic acid. Other bacteria found in the mouth may be contributors as well.

Conditions, such as endocrine dysfunction, emotional instability, improper nutrition, and disease provide a systemic environment for the onset of dental caries.

The diagnosis of dental caries, unlike that of many other diseases, is not a difficult matter. Any layman can observe and detect gross tooth decay. However, the problem of diagnosing interproximal caries calls for radiographic interpretation. Refer to Chapter 82 for more information on interproximal radiographic techniques. Unless small cavities are filled as soon as they are found, extensive amounts of tooth structure must be sacrificed in large preparations.

Factors Involved in Dental Decay. It is a common misunderstanding that food debris remaining on the teeth is the only cause of dental decay. There are other factors involved.

Dental plaque. *Dental plaque*, a thin film-like deposit that clings to the teeth, is made up of microorganisms and mucin from the saliva. *Mucin* is a secretion of the mucous membranes. This deposit covers all or part of the crown of the tooth. It must be constantly removed if dental caries is to be controlled.

Dental plaque accumulates on teeth at varying rates. It can be easily removed by thoroughly brushing and flossing, provided it is not permitted to accumulate and become firmly attached to the teeth.

Although the exact nature of dental plaque is not definitely known, there is evidence that it is a protein substance from the saliva in the form of mucin. This substance traps the microorganisms and permits them to grow into a matted mass that adheres to the teeth. The same bacteria, acting on the carbohydrates in the food eaten, makes the plaque acid. Plaque that has reached a pH of 5.0 is known to cause decalcification of tooth enamel.

Dental plaque accumulates even in a clean mouth during hours of rest. Even after teeth have been thoroughly brushed prior to bedtime, plaque tends to cover the teeth, and a person may arise in the morning with a thick film on his or her teeth. In addition to the role plaque plays in initiating dental caries, it is also one of the factors in producing dental calculus (tartar). A rough, spongy surface of calculus acts as a matrix, thus enabling the inorganic salts of the saliva to adhere to the teeth.

Cleanliness of the teeth greatly depends on the stress used by the teeth in the process of cutting and crushing the food. The more vigorous the chewing, the cleaner are the teeth, and the less chance for dental caries. The value of a diet of natural (unrefined), bulky, fibrous foods that are well chewed cannot be overstressed. Of course, such foods do not eliminate the need for a good toothbrushing and flossing.

Materia Alba. *Materia Alba* is a thick cream-colored mass that forms on the teeth when toothbrushing is neglected. This condition occurs when the main food of an individual consists of soft carbohydrates. The food debris adheres to the dental plaque and, by bacterial action, becomes highly acid. This accumulation remains undisturbed around those areas of the teeth that are not cleaned by the action of the tongue and cheeks. The retention of materia alba leads to the decalcification of the enamel and the formation of cavities. These cavities are found around the gingival third of the tooth. Routine brushing after each meal will control the deposits of materia alba.

Congenital Malformations

Congenital malformations, or birth defects, that affect the teeth and facial structure of an individual are cerebral palsy, cleft palate, and cleft lip.

Cerebral Palsy. *Cerebral palsy* is a disturbance of muscular function due to injury of the nervous system during fetal development or during the birth process. The lack of coordination prevents those so affected from receiving dental treatment because of the difficulty in controlling them in the dental chair. Many of these children also have severe orthodontic problems. Because of the unequal tensions exerted by facial muscles, food metabolism may be disturbed, with malformation of teeth as a consequence.

Their problems are definitely within the jurisdiction of those official and voluntary agencies that deal with crippled and handicapped children. Much attention has been focused on this group through efforts of the Association for the Cerebral Palsied. Primarily, this is a fund-raising organization for the relief of afflicted children. Efforts have been made to give special training to dentists and dental hygienists in the treatment of the cerebral palsied child.

Education of parents and guardians in the proper care for the mouths of these children is aimed toward helping the child to care for herself or himself, within her or his own limitations. An important phase of the program for rehabilitation of palsied children is continuous care.

Cleft Palate and Cleft Lip. Cleft palate and cleft lip are two recognized malformations, caused by complete or partial failure of the body parts that form the roof of the mouth to unite during fetal development. The deformity results in the lack of a partition between the nasal cavity and the mouth. Correction is started early in life, as the abnormality makes infant feeding difficult. A series of surgical operations may be necessary to close the cleft(s). Through cooperation of the pediatrician, oral surgeon, dentist, orthodontist, and speech therapist, the cleft palate child can be helped to lead a normal life.

The role of the dental health advisor is to seek out and recommend to parents and guardians of these children the special services available to them. Poverty need not prevent the correction of these conditions, as there are sources and funds from the crippled children's agencies to provide surgical procedures, prosthetic replacements, and corrective speech, to correct such congenital defects.

Periodontal Diseases

The *Journal of the American Dental Association* (*JADA*) offered this contribution:

> The efforts of the dental profession in the field of Public Health Dentistry ought to include a program of preventive periodontia. (*Periodontia* is the science of treating diseases of the supporting tissues of the teeth.) Very often this condition is found to have its inception at an age prior to the teens. If this phase of treatment received emphasis equal to repairing the ravages of dental caries, the interest of our national health economy would be better served.

Because of the involvement of several types of tissues in periodontal disease, no one causative factor can be stated. There appears to be two sets of factors that tend to make an individual susceptible to periodontal disease: (1) deposits of debris on the teeth, such as calculus and food impactions, are classified as *local conditions*; and (2) *systemic conditions* include any irritating force on the tissues, such as dental caries, poor-quality dental restorations, abnormal stress habits (e.g., mouth breathing), tongue thrusts, grinding teeth, and chewing on hard objects (pencils and the like).

Acute Necrotizing Ulcerative Gingivitis. *Acute necrotizing ulcerative gingivitis (ANUG)*, otherwise known as Vincent's infection, is a serious, acute infection of the gingiva that tends to become chronic. Caused by disease-bearing bacteria, it is a disease that attacks the individual with lowered resistance, but it is not considered communicable. The disease responds favorably to thorough removal of calculus and other debris by dental prophylaxis, coupled with a strict program of thorough toothbrushing. Individuals who have the infection should complete a physical checkup to determine the cause of low vitality. Corrections of physical illness and the maintenance of optimal good health are the best preventions.

All cases of the simplest types of gingival inflammation should be regarded as conditions that could lead to more serious periodontal disturbances. For instance, children who have heavy deposits of calculus should be treated as potential cases of periodontal disease in later life. However, ANUG is seldom seen in children.

OPERATIVE DENTISTRY

Operative dentistry, also referred to as *restorative dentistry*, is the branch of oral health service concerned with restoring or reforming hard dental tissues. Operative dentistry is often called *general dentistry*, because it is the branch of dentistry for which a new patient has an initial appointment. Should the services of a specialist be required, the general dentist refers the patient to a specific specialty practice for treatment. The subject of patient referral will be discussed as the various specialties are presented later in this chapter.

The practice of operative dentistry includes the techniques involved in the prevention and restoration of defects, caries, or trauma-related injury in the enamel and dentin of individual teeth. Included in such a practice are amalgam restorations, cast gold inlays, onlays, crowns, direct gold foil restorations, and cosmetic surgery.

Cosmetic dentistry, sometimes termed *esthetic dentistry*, involves the placement of tooth-colored composite resin restorations and veneers that improve the appearance of anterior teeth. Veneers are discussed with crown and bridge replacements.

Composite resins are used to:

- Repair surfaces that are fractured, chipped, or worn.
- Cover badly stained teeth.
- Narrow the diastema (abnormal space between adjacent teeth in the same arch. A wide diastema usually occurs between the maxillary central incisors.

PEDIATRIC DENTISTRY

Pediatric dentistry is the specialty that is limited to dentistry for children. This branch of dental care includes training the child to accept dentistry from birth to the stage of mixed dentition (13 to 14 years). Also included in this dental service:

- Restoring and maintaining the primary, mixed, and permanent dentition.
- Applying preventive measures for dental caries and periodontal disease.
- Preventing, intercepting, and correcting various problems of occlusion.

The pediatric specialist is concerned with the general health of all young patients. The basic needs and special requirements for treatment, along with a preventive plan as the dentition develops, are all of concern to the specialist.

Pediatric dental practice is maintained by referrals from the general dentist, other dental practitioners, and physicians. The general dentist and the specialist must work cooperatively to ensure the ultimate in dental services.

The pediatric specialist follows treatment of the child through the eruption of the second permanent molars. As a general rule, the child is then referred to the generalist at this time.

The Pediatric Dental Office

Preparing a child for dental treatment is an approach very different from that for an adult. Children must be made to feel at home, primarily in a corner of the reception room where furnishings are scaled to a child's size. Small tables, chairs, familiar books, pictures, and toys give the child a sense of belonging. Included could be some dental materials, such as cotton rolls and paper cups. Becoming acquainted with such articles gives the children an introduction to the dental office and helps to hold their interest while waiting.

Controlling Fear

When children are placed in an unfamiliar environment, their first urge is self-preservation. In an unknown situation, the first emotion is fear, accompanied by the reaction to resist. Fear of the unknown, fear of pain, or fear of ridicule cause an urge to flee the situation. The confident parent or guardian can do much to reassure the child that he or she is safe in a new experience. Once a child has a feeling of safety, he or she is more likely to become an interested and cooperative patient. Were the child to discover any doubt in the mind of the parent or guardian, a lack of confidence in the dentist might also occur. In this event, dental treatment would literally become impossible.

Mutual Respect

Most American children have had some introduction to concepts of dental health in the home and possibly at school. The child hears from others their experiences "at the dentist." A youngster knows that teeth need attention. When placed in an adult situation not experienced before, he or she hopes to act like an adult. A child will respect those who respect him and likes to be spoken to as though he understands what is taking place.

The Examination

Unless the first visit is an emergency, the child is thoroughly examined. The child's breath, saliva consistency, gingivae, supporting tissues, and oral mucosa are checked. The examination also includes the tongue, tonsils, and pharynx for normal or abnormal conditions.

The surfaces of the teeth are examined with a mouth mirror and explorer. Carious lesions are charted. The eruption pattern of the teeth is recorded.

Following the examination, when only plaque is found to be present, the crowns of the teeth are polished. If any calculus exists, a prophylaxis is performed by the dentist or dental hygienist.

Medical History. The patient's medical history record is completed by the parent or guardian. The history of the child's infancy will help to provide information on caries prevention, any previous dental experience, allergies, facial habits, and general development of the child. The family's interest in nutrition and preventive dentistry can be determined at the same time.

Preparing the Patient. The assistant approaches the child in a friendly manner, calling the child by name. The patient is invited to go meet the doctor. As the patient is seated, draped, and the chair adjusted, the assistant will explain what is being done. Conversation between the assistant and patient is pleasant and unhurried.

The assistant introduces the dentist to the patient, then gives the dentist a chance to become acquainted with the patient. During this conversation, the dentist will explain, in a positive manner, the use of the equipment in the operatory, the procedure to be followed, and why it is necessary.

To maintain a rapport with the child, the dentist and assistant must function smoothly, quickly, and comfortably for the patient.

The question of rewards for good behavior has been challenged. Some pedodontists feel that the child patient should be given a small gift at the end of each appointment to indicate that the dentist is the child's friend. It is preferable to have the children make their own selection from a chest of small toys. For older children, a word of sincere praise is adequate.

Radiographs. A dental radiographic survey is an important portion of the diagnosis for the pediatric patient. Radiographs will show the condition of the primary teeth and the position and development of the permanent teeth.

Study Models (Casts). Alginate impressions are made for study models that become a part of the diagnosis. Study models in various stages of development provide growth of the dental arches, the supporting structures, and tooth-eruption sequence.

Treatment Plan. The parent or guardian meets in consultation with the dentist and is informed of the treatment required and the fee involved for the treatment plan. The parent or guardian must give signed consent for the treatment.

The responsibility of the administrative secretary includes an accurate file of each referral, and a letter of acknowledgment to the referring practitioner.

Treatment

Acute Infections of the Mucosa. Acute infections of the mucosa are generally of brief duration and may recur from time to time. They are due to specific microorganisms. Some are communicable and, therefore, may become epidemic in schools. These infections involve only the soft tissues of the mouth, lips, nose, and throat.

Herpes Simplex. Herpes simplex is commonly seen in children. The onset of the infection may be severe, with temperature and general weakness. The entire mouth may be highly inflamed and accompanied by vesicles (fluid-filled blisters) on the lips and around the oral cavity. Caused by a virus, herpes simplex may be found in the tissues long after the acute stage is past. It may break out from time to time as the individual's resistance is lowered.

Children suffer considerable discomfort from herpes simplex disease and should be protected from it by providing a healthful school environment, particularly with reference to drinking fountains and other classroom equipment.

Stannous Fluoride. Depending on the tendency toward dental caries, the dentist may prescribe the topical application of stannous fluoride. After the removal of any plaque or calculus, stannous fluoride is applied. These treatments are usually repeated every six months, following the routine prophylaxis. Daily toothbrushing and flossing are a part of ongoing care between prophylaxis appointments.

Pit and Fissure Sealants. If the patient's teeth show a high incidence of caries, *pit and fissure* sealants may be prescribed by the pedodontist. Sealants are used as preventive treatment to seal hard-to-clean, naturally deep and narrow fissures on the occlusal surfaces of primary and newly erupted permanent teeth.

When decalcification has already begun, a composite resin restoration may be placed instead of the sealant. Sealants are not used in teeth that have caries, for which a restoration is indicated.

Restorative Materials. The materials used in pediatric dentistry are the same materials used in the restoration of permanent teeth. Composite resins are used to provide an esthetic quality to anterior teeth and are sometimes placed in primary molars. However, silver amalgam is most frequently preferred for posterior restorations.

Accidental Injury or Traumatized Teeth. Patients who have experienced a fractured or evulsed tooth are always treated as emergency cases. An _evulsed_ tooth is one that has been knocked or torn from its socket.

The person calling in an emergency should be instructed to (1) try to find the tooth, and any fragments, if it is fractured; (2) wrap the tooth in a clean cloth; and (3) immediately bring the patient to the dental office.

The lapse of time from the accident to when the tooth can be repositioned (put back into the socket) should be no more than thirty minutes. If the tooth can be saved, it is positioned in the arch and splinted into place.

Splints are custom appliances whose object is to retain the traumatized tooth (teeth) in approximately the same position in the dental arch as before the injury. The splint may be constructed of cold-cure acrylic and orthodontic wires.

Space Maintainers. Following the premature (early) loss of a primary tooth, a _space maintainer_ is designed to maintain the space until the normal eruption of the permanent tooth.

A space maintainer may be _fixed_ (cemented in place) or _removable_ (can be removed and replaced by the patient). The choice of one type over the other depends on:

- the age of the child
- the number of primary teeth present and of permanent teeth not yet erupted
- the patient's oral hygiene
- the need for a unilateral (one side) or a bilateral (both sides) appliance.

Suggestions Concerning Dental Treatment for Children

Most children will accept dental treatment if:

1. Dental appointments do not interfere with their free time. Release time from school has been sanctioned by school administrators for medical and dental appointments.

2. Make appointments for young children in the early morning, while they are rested and quiet.

3. Schedule older children for early afternoon appointments.

4. Give the apprehensive child longer intervals between appointments to aid in relieving nervous tension.

5. Shorten the dental visit if it is noted that the child has a short interest span. The time may be lengthened as the child matures.

6. Always be truthful about pain with the pediatric patient. Respect the pain tolerance of a child. Avoid hurrying to complete any dental treatment.

7. Use every available means to reduce discomfort for the young dental patient.

Special Problems of the Adolescent

Teenagers are often more difficult to treat than younger children. They may be overtalkative or completely silent. In either case, they are attempting to control fear, but want no one to suspect they are afraid. Both boys and girls are highly emotional during puberty, and their pain tolerance is low. In treating them, as much of the dental equipment (instruments, syringes, and dental handpieces) as possible should be kept out of sight. Teenagers are highly susceptible to impressions. The amount and appearance of dental equipment is frightening even to a well-adjusted adult patient.

Adolescents are seeking careers, and are interested in science. To be allowed to watch what is going on in the dental lab holds their interest. For instance, the pouring of plaster models is an excellent opportunity to stimulate their interest in dental careers.

Subjects that might encourage teenagers to more openly express themselves in a friendly discussion include:

1. Personal cleanliness, good appearance, and social advantage of a fine set of teeth in a healthy mouth.
2. Adequate diet for clear complexions and good teeth. Restriction of sugars, particularly between meals.
3. Stressing the high incidence of dental decay at this age. Regular dental checkups are a must!
4. Stressing safety in relation to teeth. Encourage those involved in competitive (contact) sports to wear mouth guards.
5. Look for nervous habits that may result in future dental deformities.
6. Explain dentistry and dental research as progressive scientific efforts for the teenagers' particular benefit.

Mouth Guards. *Mouth guards* are designed to fit over the full dentition and to protect the teeth from accidental injury. It is constructed of a pliable material and may be custom-molded for a particular patient. Premolded commercial mouth guards (stock guards) can be purchased in assorted mold sizes to approximate the size of the patient's dental arch. These are less accurate in their fit than custom guards but are used by many athletes. They are better than no guard at all.

ORTHODONTICS

Orthodontics is the dental specialty concerned with the study and supervision of the growth and development of dentition and related anatomical structures from birth to maturity. Orthodontics is the science dealing with the prevention and correction of dental and oral anomalies (any deviation from the normal).

Orthodontic patients come to the specialist by referral for both corrective and preventive procedures of evaluation and treatment. Orthodontic treatment may be provided for patients of all ages, including adults. The objective of orthodontics includes the maintenance of the functional relationship of the teeth, dental arches, and supporting structures of the face and skull.

Influence of Function

Function is an important factor in the continued growth and development of the human body. In addition to the influence of function, growth is appreciably affected by, and dependent on, many other factors, namely, heredity, environment, nutrition, and general health.

The orthodontic patient's history is checked for hereditary or physical problems that may affect treatment. The conditions may include heart problems, asthma, diabetes, glandular disturbances, or blood disorders.

Dental health and emotional development are interdependent areas. Maladjustments in emotional development are indicated by habits involving the teeth and structures of the mouth.

Habits Influencing Dentition

Thumb Sucking. *Thumb suckers* are of two types. The first type starts at a very early age and stops when the physiological desire is satisfied. The second type starts again, four or five years later, when the child meets with difficulty. Being unable to progress normally with solutions to problems, the child will regress to an early form of gratification.

From infancy to age 5, defects of the teeth and facial structures are not evident. Beyond age 5, defects of the maxillary arch, the palate, and the anterior teeth will become apparent. Should this occur, the orthodontist may recommend corrective treatment.

Tongue-Thrusting. *Tongue thrusting* places great forward pressure against the maxillary teeth each time the child swallows. The tongue thrust causes the maxillary arch to move forward, with the teeth pushed into a fan-shaped position.

Bruxism. *Bruxism* is the involuntary grinding or clenching of the teeth, other than during normal chewing movements. Bruxism occurs most frequently during sleep, although the grinding sound may also be heard during the waking hours.

Extreme habits of bruxism must be corrected as grinding wears away the enamel and puts pressure on the periodontium. Self-directed suggestions may help patients to overcome their habit. However, a professional psychologist may be called upon, stressing the need to abstain from bruxism.

Mouth Breathing. *Mouth breathing*, referred to as *adenoid breathing*, may or may not be due to an obstruction of the nasal passages of the respiratory system. A physical examination and consultation with the patient's physician may be indicated before plans for orthodontic treatment are determined.

Mouth breathing can cause a pinched face because of the narrowing of the dental arch. Over a period of years, the entire dentofacial structure of the child may be changed because of prolonged mouth breathing.

Malocclusion and Facial Defects

The entire form and function of the face and its structures are directly affected by the manner in which the biting surfaces of the teeth of the maxillary arch meet and close (occlude) with the teeth of the mandibular arch. The exact pattern is called **occlusion**, further defined as the space relation between teeth in the action of closing and chewing.

The establishment of occlusion of the teeth begins at about the sixth month of life and ends with the eruption of the third molars. It may be said that the development of occlusion in an individual is a long and changing process, which begins with inception and continues throughout life.

Malocclusion is any deviation from the normal pattern of occlusion.
Malocclusion tends to:

- Impair mastication.
- Increase the susceptibility to dental caries.
- Encourage periodontal disease.
- Lead to early loss of teeth and abnormal respiratory habits.
- Provoke abnormal mental attitudes in relation to facial esthetics.
- Impair speech.

The Examination

A patient history should be completed during the patient's first visit to the orthodontic office.

The examination includes profile photographs and study models of the patient. If the referring dentist has provided recent radiographs of the patient, these may be used for a comparative diagnosis. However, occlusal, cephalometric, and panoramic radiographs will be necessary for a complete radiographic survey.

Alginate impressions to produce study models and working casts are obtained during the initial visit.

The Case Presentation

The orthodontist will study the diagnostic aids, develop a treatment plan and cost estimate for the patient. These aids will help explain the diagnosis and treatment plan.

The presentation includes the approximate length of treatment and a statement of the responsibility of the patient to ensure the successful completion of the procedure.

Financial Arrangements

The fee for the consultation and case presentation is a separate fee usually paid at the time of the visit. When the patient and person legally responsible for the account agree that treatment should proceed, a contract for services is signed.

If the patient requires restorative dentistry before the teeth are banded, he or she is referred to the general dentist.

When extractions are necessary, they may be performed by the general dentist or an oral surgeon. After the tissues have healed sufficiently to permit banding, an appointment is scheduled.

Oral Hygiene Instructions

Emphasis must be placed on the importance of a clean mouth and teeth during orthodontic treatment.

The teeth and appliances are to be thoroughly brushed after each meal. The orthodontist will recommend a specific type of toothbrush for the patient. Particular attention must be given to the ligature wires, the margins of the bands, and the cervical, lingual, and occlusal surfaces of the teeth.

ENDODONTICS

Endodontics, also referred to as root canal therapy, is the branch of dentistry that specializes in the diagnosis and treatment of the tooth pulp and periapical tissues. This makes it possible to save a tooth that, otherwise, would be lost by extraction.

Although the general dentist may provide endodontic treatment, the option to refer the patient to an endodontist is often chosen.

When endodontic treatment has been successfully completed, the specialist refers the patient to the general dentist. A permanent restoration is then placed.

Some indications for endodontic treatment are:

- The tooth pulp is grossly inflamed or in a necrotic state. *Necrosis* means the death of cells due to the loss of blood supply, bacterial toxins, or physical and chemical damage.
- The tooth can be restored to function after endodontic treatment.

- Endodontia may be chosen in conjunction with periodontal therapy as a means of saving the tooth.
- The natural tooth (teeth) can be maintained in the dental arch following endodontia.

Endodontic treatment is not recommended for teeth that cannot be restored to function or be maintained because of the weakness of the periodontal support. The tooth may become mobile in the socket, because infection or injury has affected the supporting tissues of the periodontium.

Planning for Treatment

The potential endodontic patient may call the dental office complaining of severe pain. Others may complain of intermittent discomfort, with a feeling of tenderness and pressure in a particular area of the dental arch.

The general dentist may see the patient and determine the reasons for the complaints. Usually a dental radiographic of the periapical area is made to determine the degree of disease. If the tooth appears to have involvement of the apex or apices of a multirooted tooth, the patient will be referred to an endodontic specialist for treatment.

Clinical History and Examination

When the patient is referred to the endodontic office, a complete medical and dental history is recorded. Antibiotics may be prescribed before treatment begins. For this reason, any sensitivity to a particular antibiotic must be determined prior to further treatment.

Radiographs. A periapical radiograph is made of the tooth in question. To ensure that no distortion occurs, it may be wise to expose a second film, using a different angulation as a means of comparing the length of the root(s), surrounding alveolus, and periapical tissues.

Palpation and Percussion. Palpation of the tooth and surrounding tissues, and soft tissues of the face and neck is performed by the dentist. *Palpation* means exerting light pressure of the fingers to a body surface.

Percussion involves tapping of a body part to determine the condition of the body parts beneath. In this case, the tooth or teeth in a quadrant are tapped with an object to establish the amount of sensitivity of the tooth in question. Palpation and percussion are used simultaneously.

Thermal Sensitivity. The tooth may be tested for a reaction to hot and cold. A cylinder of ice held in a cotton square is brought into contact with the tooth. The tooth is then touched with heated gutta percha of stick compound.

In a clinical examination, cold will stimulate the sensation of pain. The inflamed pulp violently reacts to the application of heat. Relief from this pain may be controlled by a second application of cold. This condition is termed advanced acute pulpagia. *Pulpagia* means pain in the pulp. The patient is in constant severe pain.

When the tooth lacks sensation to the cold and hot application, an acute apical abscess may be present.

Transillumination. The transillumination test is helpful for teeth in the anterior arch. Because of their position in the arch, a fiber optic light can be placed in the lingual surface. The light will be reflected through the enamel and dentin.

The dentist can compare the translucency of the tooth with that of other teeth in the arch. *Translucency* means that the tooth structure allows the light to pass through, making the inner structures visible.

Electric Pulp Tester. The pulp tester (vitalometer) is used to measure the vitality of a tooth.

It has a control to regulate and limit the voltage during the evaluation.

Because of patient apprehension and fear, the use of the test is explained to the patient before the procedure is begun. The patient is told that a slight tingling sensation may be felt, and as soon as the sensation is registered, the test on that tooth will cease.

A tooth that is hyperreactive will react more readily than a normal tooth. *Hyperreactive* means a greater response to stimuli. A tooth with a hyporeactive (lower response) pulp will react more weakly to the pulp tester stimulus. A tooth with a necrotic pulp will not register at all.

Endodontic Treatment

Vital Pulp Capping. Pulp capping involves traditional methods of therapy to stimulate pulp regeneration. *Indirect pulp capping* is used when there is a danger of exposing the pulp if all carious tissues (enamel and dentin) are removed. *Direct pulp capping* is used to treat a pulp that has been mechanically exposed during an operative procedure of preparing a tooth for a restoration.

Pulpectomy. A pulpectomy involves the surgical removal of the vital pulp of a tooth. The term *pulpectomy* is used as a description of the method used only when removing a vital pulp. Trauma-related injuries of the pulp include cysts, periodontal involvement, and other inflammation.

Pulpotomy. *Pulpotomy* refers to partial removal of a vital pulp that lies within the crown of a tooth, leaving the root portion intact. The object of this procedure is to stimulate the tissue in the root canal(s) to form a bridge of secondary dentin over the pulpal root tissue.

This procedure works well for the young patient when the root portion is not fully developed. Thus, the tooth is retained, allowing full development of the root.

Apicoectomy. An *apicoectomy* is the surgical removal of the apical portion of the tooth. Usually performed along with periapical curettage, it becomes necessary to make a surgical opening in the bone and overlying tissues. *Curettage* is the scraping and cleaning with a dental curette hand instrument.

Postoperative Follow-up

As a general rule, after completion of endodontic treatment, the dentist will request the patient to return at periodic intervals. These intervals may vary from three- to six-month periods up to a period of several years.

A posttreatment radiograph is made to determine the elimination of infections and the extent of regeneration.

PROSTHODONTICS

Prosthodontics is the branch of dentistry that is concerned with the diagnosis, planning, construction, and insertion of artificial devices, or prostheses. A *prosthesis* is the replacement for one or more teeth and associated tissues.

Prosthodontics has three main branches: *removable prosthodontics*, *fixed prosthodontics*, and *dental implants*.

Removable Prosthodontics

The primary objective of *removable prosthodontics* is to replace missing dentition and restore occlusion with an appliance that the patient removes for cleaning and, with little difficulty, repositions.

Two major groups of removable prostheses are *removable partial dentures* and *removable complete dentures*.

A removable partial denture replaces one or more teeth in one arch and is retained and supported by the underlying tissues and some of the remaining teeth.

Removable complete dentures replace all of the teeth in one arch. A full denture is retained and supported by the underlying tissues of the alveolar ridges, hard palate, and oral mucosa.

Removable Partial Dentures. The basic goals of the partial denture are to restore missing teeth and to preserve the remaining hard and soft tissues of the oral cavity. The partial denture is designed to distribute the forces of mastication between the abutments and alveolar mucosa, enabling them to resist the stress of those forces. An *abutment* is a natural tooth that becomes the support for the replacement tooth or teeth.

Advantages of a removable partial include the following:

- Fewer intraoral procedures, chair time, and appointments are necessary.
- Good hygiene of the oral cavity is maintained by the patient, because the prosthesis is removable.
- When several teeth are missing in both quadrants of an arch, a removable partial denture will restore a long span of lost dentition.
- The removable partial denture makes it unnecessary to reduce tooth structure on primary or permanent dentition of children and adolescents. The appliance can also be replaced to compensate for the growth of the child.
- In the case of a cleft palate, the removable appliance may have an added obturator. An *obturator* is that portion of a prosthesis used to close a congenital opening or cleft of the palate.
- The removable prosthesis may be designed to support periodontally involved teeth.

Other Considerations for a Partial Denture

- There must be a number of sufficiently positioned teeth in the arch to support and stabilize a removable prosthesis.

- To retain the appliance, there must be adequate root structure of the remaining teeth.
- The patient must exhibit enthusiasm for maintaining good oral health.

Treatment Planning for a Removable Prosthesis. The treatment plan may involve operative dentistry, periodontic, endodontic, or surgical procedures before the construction of a partial denture. Such treatment must be completed and healing taken place before prosthodontic preparation can begin.

Diagnosis and Treatment Planning. A preliminary appointment is scheduled for examination of the patient. Accurate preliminary impressions for producing study models and working casts are taken. Review Chapters 60 and 61 for more information on taking alginate impressions.

Radiographic films of the partially edentulous mouth are exposed and processed by the assistant. Review Chapter 86 for the technique.

Instant-type (Polaroid) photographs are made of the patient, including full face, frontal view, and profile, with a closeup of the anterior teeth overbite.

Consultation Visit. The dentist explains the diagnosis, the proposed treatment plan, the prognosis, and answers any questions and concerns expressed by the patient.

As with other dental procedures, a cost estimate is prepared and presented to the patient during the consultation visit. The dental laboratory fee for constructing the prosthesis is taken into consideration.

When the patient has accepted the treatment plan, a suitable financial plan is approved, and necessary appointments are made for treatment.

Delivery of the Prosthesis. Usually, a twenty- to thirty-minute appointment is sufficient time to deliver the removable partial denture.

The new prosthesis is disinfected and rinsed before it is placed in the patient's mouth. The

dentist places the appliance in the patient's oral cavity and makes any necessary adjustments.

The patient is then given a short ten- to twenty-minute appointment within a few days after the delivery. At this time, the dentist removes the partial denture, checks the mucosa, and makes any necessary adjustments.

The patient is given a recall appointment, usually several months later. These recall visits are important, and allow the dentist to evaluate the fit and function of the prosthesis. At the same time, the patient's oral hygiene can also be evaluated.

Removable Complete Dentures. *Complete denture prosthesis* is the phase of dental prosthodontics dealing with the restoration of natural teeth and their associated parts in the dental arch with artificial replacements. When one or both dental arches have been rendered edentulous, a full denture is constructed.

Other Considerations for Complete (Full) Dentures

- Extensive bone loss and lack of support for teeth remaining in the arch.
- Remaining anterior teeth that are involved with gross decay, periodontal disease, or abscesses
- Evidence that oral hygiene has been chronically poor
- Totally edentulous patient

The patient's mental and physical capabilities must be such that he or she is able to accept and wear the prosthesis. Impaired health may contribute to a lack of muscle coordination to retain the denture in place.

Diagnosis and Treatment Planning. A preliminary appointment is scheduled for the dentist and the patient to discuss the need for a complete denture. During this visit, the dentist will examine the patient and review the medical history. The dentist will also prescribe radiographs and alginate impressions for study models (casts). Photographs (instant-type) are made of the full face, frontal view, and profile of the patient.

Preparation of the diagnosis, cost estimate, and treatment plans are much the same as for a partial denture prosthesis.

Full Denture Construction. The alginate impressions taken during the preliminary appointment are used to pour stone casts. These may be poured by the assistant or referred to the dental laboratory. Custom denture trays are constructed from the stone casts.

With the custom trays, secondary impressions are taken by using rubber-base, silicone elastomeric impression material, or polysiloxane. These impressions are poured in dense dental stone and create the master casts. Secondary impressions provide the basis for the construction of the prosthesis and, therefore, must be accurate.

The *maxillary impression* must include tuberosities, frenum attachments, and other landmarks of the arch. The *mandibular impression* must include retromolar pads, oblique ridge, mylohyoid ridge, genial tubercles, and the lingual, labial, and buccal frenums.

The dental laboratory will construct a baseplate on the master cast. A *baseplate* is a preformed semirigid acrylic resin material that temporarily represents the base of the denture.

Bite rims, made of several layers of baseplate wax, are built on the baseplates. *Bite rims* register the space provided by the teeth in normal occlusion, or vertical dimension.

The baseplate-bite rim is tried in the patient's mouth, and centric occlusion is established by the dentist. *Centric occlusion* occurs when the jaws are closed in a position that produces maximal contact between the occluding surfaces of the maxillary and mandibular arch.

The final impression involves obtaining the detail of the soft tissues and alveolar ridges.

Zinc oxide eugenol (ZOE) impression paste is flowed into the baseplate.

Artificial teeth are selected according to shade and mold (shape). The tooth-shade selection is made according to the age and skin tone of the patient; natural teeth will darken as a person ages.

The laboratory technician prepares the temporary wax setup of the complete denture(s) on an articulator. This "try-in" consists of the acrylic baseplates, the bite rims, and the artificial teeth set in wax, to resemble gingival tissues. The denture try-in is disinfected before being placed in the patient's mouth.

The try-in assembly is returned to the laboratory technician for processing and completion.

The Immediate Denture. The term *immediate denture* is used to describe a case when the patient's maxillary anterior teeth are the only remaining teeth in the arch. The posterior teeth have been extracted, and the hard and soft tissue areas have completely healed.

After the anterior teeth are surgically extracted, they are replaced by the artificial teeth on the appliance (i.e., the complete denture). Thus, the patient need not be without teeth, and the denture base will act as a splint during the healing process. Normal resorption during healing of the alveolar ridge will cause changes to occur.

Because of the changes, the patient must be advised that an immediate denture will need to be relined or replaced within three to six months of the surgery.

Fixed Prosthodontics

Fixed prosthodontics is the art and science involved with the complete restoration or the replacement of one or more teeth in a dental arch. Fixed prosthodontics is often referred to as *crown and bridge* work.

Fixed prostheses involve the preparation of abutment teeth to support the replacement of teeth with cast metallic restorations. A _pontic_ is the part of the appliance that replaces a missing tooth or teeth. The pontic is fashioned to simulate the incisal edge or occlusal surface of the tooth being replaced. A pontic is the suspended portion of the bridge and has one or more artificial teeth.

The abutment teeth must have vitality and stability to support the pontic of the bridge. These restorations are cemented in place to maintain occlusion in the opposing arch.

Diagnosis and Treatment Planning. The dentist reviews the medical and dental history of the patient. Radiographs and impressions for study models (casts) are made. The patient is scheduled for a second visit.

After reviewing the radiographs and study models, the dentist sees the patient to recommend the type of crown and bridge restoration. The fee is explained for the construction of a custom bridge. Often a sample of a crown and bridge is helpful in the patient's decision to accept the treatment plan. The fee for the construction of a bridge is based on the number of units (abutments and pontics) in the bridge.

Types of Crowns

Full Crowns. A full crown, made of a precious or nonprecious alloy, is precision cast and designed to cover the entire anatomic crown of the tooth. Such a crown is often referred to as a _full-cast crown_.

Veneer Crowns. A veneer crown, also known as a porcelain-fused-to-metal (PFM), is a full crown. For esthetic reasons, much of the surface of the crown is covered with a thin layer (veneer) of tooth-colored material. Because porcelain is frequently used for the veneer, the crown takes its name; however, tooth-colored composite resin materials may be used as well.

Partial Crowns. A partial crown is a cast restoration that covers three or more, but not all,

surfaces of a tooth. A _three-quarter crown_ preparation is made by leaving the facial surface of the tooth intact and by reducing the mesial, distal, and lingual surfaces, with only a slight reduction of the incisal or occlusal surface of a tooth. A _seven-eighths crown_ preparation is made by reducing the entire crown with the exception of the mesio-facial surface near the occlusal.

Impressions for Fixed Prostheses

Polysulfide Impression Materials. Polysulfide impression materials are used for crown and bridge impressions and are especially suitable for details of impression margins. Review Chapter 67 about procedure and Chapter 66 about using a custom acrylic tray.

Silicone-Base Elastomeric Materials. Silicone-base elastomeric materials may also be used for crown and bridge impressions. Silicone material is supplied in two separate forms, syringe-type and tray-type paste. A custom tray is used because of the necessity for coating the tray with adhesive before its use. Review Chapter 68 for the preparation of these materials.

Polysiloxane. Polysiloxane, also called _polyvinylsiloxane_, is supplied in a two-paste system. An extruder gun is used to mix and express the syringe mix into the preparations. The tray is loaded with the putty mix. Review Chapter 68 for complete procedure.

Hydrocolloid Impression Material. To obtain accurate impressions, each step of the manufacturer's instructions must be strictly followed when using reversible hydrocolloid. Correct handling is critical to the success of obtaining the impression. A bite registration is necessary to establish proper occlusal relationship. This is accomplished by using a double-bite hydrocolloid tray. Review Chapters 63 and 64 for hydrocolloid preparation and use.

Role of the Laboratory Technician. The dental laboratory technician performs the procedures in crown and bridge construction, including custom trays, pouring the impressions, preparing single tooth dies, articulating stone casts, producing gold alloy castings, and constructing PFMs. The technician completes the prosthesis the dentist prescribes.

Dental Implants

Dental implants are used as support for replacement teeth, using a device that is placed within the tissues.

Authorities in dentistry highly recommend implants if they are needed. They should be considered only if teeth cannot be saved. An implant should at least have a good prognosis. Determining implant prognosis depends on correct case-treatment planning. In other words, the periodontist or oral surgeon must know the medical and dental history and the quantity and quality of remaining bone structure. If these answers are favorable, then an implant can be done. On the other hand, if a tooth has a poor diagnosis and the gingiva is "seeding" bacteria throughout the mouth, the tooth should be removed. According to Thomas J. Kepic, diplomate, American Board of Periodontology, and practicing periodontist: "Keeping your own teeth is inexpensive relative to implants."

Two most often used dental implants are: *endosseous* (within the bone), and *subperiosteal* (under the periodontium and on the bone).

An alloy of cobalt, chromium, and molybdenum, which are compatible with oral tissue, makes the implant procedure fairly well received by the tissues.

The endosseus implant is set into the bone and protrudes through the oral mucosa. A fixed or removable partial may be attached to the extension(s) of the implant. Endosseus implants may be designed for a single tooth crown or as an abutment for a fixed bridge.

Subperiosteal implants are surgically placed onto the alveolus and under the periosteum. The extensions on this device protrude through the oral mucosa and serve as attachments for a removable partial or full denture.

When a subperiosteal implant is discussed, the patient must be advised that her or his health must be carefully evaluated. This implant procedure involves at least two occurrences of a surgical nature, and the total health of the patient is something to be considered.

The preparation of an arch for a periosteal implant demands an accurate impression of the alveolar bone of the dental arch. To obtain this impression, the tissue must be surgically incised and laid back to expose the alveolar ridge to the impression material.

After the impression has been taken, the surgical wound is cleansed with a natural saline solution, then sutured. A prepared temporary denture is placed over the wound. The objective is to stimulate the tissue and alveolar bone with a protective covering as healing takes place. Approximately four weeks are allowed for healing.

When the appliance is ready for insertion, a second surgical procedure is conducted. The original line of incision is reopened and the tissue retracted once again.

After a thorough cleansing with a saline solution, the sterilized implant is inserted into place over the alveolar ridge. After the implant is seated, the soft tissues are carefully sutured. A temporary denture is worn over, and supported by, the protruding projections of the subperiosteal implant.

Implant procedures may be delivered by a dental team, with an oral surgeon or periodontist performing the replacement portion. An auxiliary member would be the dental laboratory technician.

PERIODONTICS

Periodontics is the branch of dentistry that deals with the cause, prevention, and treatment of periodontal disease. *Periodontia* is a generalized term used to describe the many disorders affecting the surrounding and supporting structures of the teeth.

Periodontal diseases are the most common causes of the loss of teeth in adult life. In most cases, they can be prevented before serious damage occurs. The incidence of periodontal disease is not rare in children, although it is commonly believed to be a degenerative disease with aging adults. It should be noted that cases of periodontal disturbances are being reported in ever-increasing numbers. Review Chapter 19 for a clearer understanding of periodontal support.

The Dental Hygienist in Periodontics

The dental hygienist may very well deliver the initial treatment to the periodontic patient. Licensed and registered, in accordance with the state dental practice act, the hygienist may provide:

- Routine prophylaxis
- Preliminary examination, using a periodontal probe to measure the depth of sulcular pockets and index the areas of gingival resorption
- Alginate impressions for study models (casts)
- Scaling, curettage, and root planing
- Preventive procedures, including application of topical fluorides
- Postoperative care, such as removal of periodontal packs and sutures
- Instruction for the patient in home care, including dietary counseling.

Radiographs

As a diagnostic aid, a special _radiopaque_ grid pattern (uniformly spaced horizontal and perpendicular lines) may be attached to the back of the x-ray film before the film is exposed. When the film is developed, the grid appears around the tooth, thus enabling the periodontist to measure the amount of bone loss. The dentist

will then evaluate the location, amount, contour of the alveolar crest, and continuity of the lamina dura.

Periodontal Examination and Treatment Planning

A normal sulcus is 3 mm deep or less. When the depth is greater than 3 mm, it is termed a _periodontal pocket._

Probing. There are six "readings" that can be made for each tooth in the mouth with a periodontal probe. The _periodontal probe_ is a long, pointed instrument with a scale marked in millimeters. The point of the probe is rounded to avoid patient discomfort or damage to the tissues during probing.

- The periodontal probe is inserted into the depth of the sulcus for three measurements on the facial surface of each tooth in the arch: mesiofacial, facial, and distofacial. This procedure is described as _walking_ the probe around the tooth.
- The probing procedure is repeated for three measurements on the lingual of each tooth: mesiolingual, lingual, and distolingual.
- The entire procedure is repeated for the teeth in the opposing arch. All findings are recorded on the patient's clinical record.

On the conclusion of the examination, the patient may be asked to make another appointment for a diagnosis, prognosis, and to discuss the recommended treatment plan.

If periodontal surgery is a part of the proposed treatment, the patient is made aware of the time that will be necessary for the treatment and subsequent healing.

The patient's commitment to the course of treatment, as well as a vigorous home care program, is essential before treatment can be scheduled.

A cost estimate is developed prior to presenting the treatment plan. Questions and concerns expressed by the patient are patiently heard and answered. Once the patient and periodontist reach an understanding of the financial obligations for the treatment, the appointment schedule is arranged.

Gingivectomy

A *gingivectomy* is the surgical removal of the inflamed and diseased gingivae and of deep suprabony pockets. *Suprabony* means above the bone. A gingivectomy is performed only after a periodontal pocket has failed to respond to scaling and curettage.

A gingivectomy also includes deep scaling and root planing of the root surfaces of a tooth after the diseased tissue has been removed. The purpose of a gingivectomy is the removal of diseased tissue to prevent the spread of disease not only in the oral cavity but also throughout the body.

When a gingivectomy is indicated for both dental arches, each quadrant is treated at a separate appointment on a weekly basis.

Instructions for home care following surgery must be explicit and in written form.

Gingivoplasty

A *gingivoplasty* is the surgical procedure by which gingival deformities are reduced to create normal and functional form.

Gingivoplasty, unlike gingivectomy, is performed in the absence of pockets with the sole purpose of removing excess tissue and recontouring the gingiva. Gingivoplasty may include: (1) tapering the gingival margin; (2) creating a marginal outline; and (3) reshaping the interdental papillae to allow for the passage of food on the free gingiva during mastication.

Osteoplasty

Osteoplasty is the surgical reshaping of the alveolar bone with maintained basic support of the teeth. Osseous (bony) surgery may be either additive or subtractive.

Additive osseous surgery is directed toward restoring the alveolar bone to its original level. This procedure is accomplished by various autoosseous implant bone grafts (auto-; self).

Subtractive osseous surgery procedures are designed to restore the form of the alveolar bone by surgically reducing it. The bony plate is exposed by creating a surgical flap to reveal the bony plate of the alveoli and recontouring the area.

Osseous implants are autogeneous bone grafts that are performed surgically. For instance, the bony implant material may be obtained from the retromolar area of the patient. A mucoperiosteal flap is prepared at the designated site of the implant. Granulated tissue and periodontal fibers are removed with a curette.

The bony tissue is removed from the donor site and placed in the implant area. After the incision is cleansed with a natural saline solution, surgical suturing closes it. A surgical pack is placed over the closed incision. Healing takes place within several days, and the pack and sutures are removed.

Bone allografts are performed surgically by using the demineralized freeze-dried bone of another human (donor). The donor and recipient are sufficiently unlike genetically to interact antigenically.

Preparation of the donor bone tissue involves medical laboratory engineering to remove the mineral salts from the tissue before it is freeze-dried and retained in a bone bank.

During the surgery, the implant tissue will be precisely positioned, and once implanted in the recipient body it will act as an enzyme. When introduced into the body, the implant stimulates the production of antibodies. The antibodies will in turn neutralize toxins, bacteria, or cells and promote healing.

Recent research indicates that the bone allograft procedure lends itself to periodontal surgery and has proven to be highly successful.

Pericoronitis

Pericoronitis is an inflammation or infection of the gingival tissues surrounding the crown of an erupting tooth. The mandibular third molar is frequently involved, with the tendency of food impactions under the loose margins of the gingivae. Cleansing the area is difficult because of the location of the tooth.

Radiographs may determine whether the tooth should be retained or extracted. If the tooth is retained, conservative treatment should be initiated. If the tooth is to be extracted, an antibiotic is normally prescribed prior to surgery.

Acute Necrotizing Ulcerative Gingivitis (ANUG)

Acute necrotizing ulcerative gingivitis (_ANUG_) is a destructive infection of the gingivae. It is characterized by a feeling of illness, bad breath, and appearance of ulcers in the mouth. The thin covering of the ulcer may be easily wiped away, revealing a highly inflamed area that easily bleeds.

The patient is advised to get adequate rest and follow a mild, but nutritionally sound, diet. Smoking, carbonated beverages, and alcohol should be eliminated until the condition improves.

When the acute inflammation has subsided, a complete prophylaxis, scaling, and curettage are in order. Thorough preventive home care, good nutrition, rest, and a periodically scheduled recall visit, as prescribed by the periodontist, can keep the condition under control.

Plaque Control

Dr. Jorgen Slots, newly appointed chairman of the Periodontics Department at the University of Southern California, School of Dentistry, has been conducting microbiologic testing since spring 1992. He can, from a given plaque sample, identify, type, and quantitate up to thirty bacteria known to cause periodontal disease.

Most importantly, he can now also target a specific antibiotic to eradicate those bacteria. It is not a cure, but it does give some important information as to: (1) who is at risk; (2) what is the likelihood of their case worsening; (3) when surgery is necessary if other indicators are unclear; (4) when surgery is not necessary; and (5) when a case is complete. The test, according to Dr. Slots, is easy and relatively inexpensive. The difficulty for some practicing periodontists lies in interpreting the results and putting them in perspective, relative to other tests they conduct. As with all introductions of something new, the learning curve can be very steep.

ORAL AND MAXILLOFACIAL SURGERY

Oral surgery is the science and specialty practice of removing teeth from the oral cavity. _Exodontics_ is the term used to describe the extraction of teeth. Although the general dentist is trained in surgical dental procedures, he or she may choose to refer the more complicated cases to an oral surgeon.

Examination and Treatment Planning

The oral surgeon will examine the surgical patient and confirm findings of the referring dentist.

Radiographs prescribed by the oral surgeon may include periapical, panoramic, temporomandibular (TMJ), extraoral, and occlusal x rays. Radiographs obtained from the referring dentist may be used as a comparison of the patient's condition.

Fees for services must be explained by the specialist and accepted by the patient. In the case of a severe toothache, the patient will require immediate attention.

Fees for elective surgery should be presented prior to any service. In cases requiring hospitalization, the patient's medical and dental insurance must be reviewed.

Pain Control

The level of pain tolerance should be determined early in the treatment plan. Premedication in conjunction with local anesthesia may be prescribed for the apprehensive patient.

For more profound anesthesia, the surgeon may use inhalation of nitrous oxide and select an anesthetic solution of longer duration. Refer to Chapter 42 on local anesthesia.

General anesthesia may be indicated for some oral surgery patients. To ensure the patient's safety, a second professional, such as an anesthesiologist, is present to supervise the administration and monitor the patient's vital signs during surgery.

Special Oral Surgery

Extractions. All extractions are surgical procedures that are rated on a scale from less than difficult to increasingly difficult. Special surgical instruments are used according to the surgical procedure. Review Chapter 36 for information on surgical instruments.

Multiple Extractions. When several teeth are extracted, it may be necessary to reshape the remaining alveolar ridge before placing an immediate denture. This procedure is called an *alveolectomy.*

Impacted Teeth. There are basically two variations of impactions: soft-tissue impactions and bony impactions. A *soft-tissue impaction* may be partially erupted, with a portion of the tooth visible in the mouth. A *bony impaction* is blocked from eruption by both alveolar bone and mucosa. These tissues must be surgically removed before

access to, and removal of, the impaction can be accomplished.

Frenectomy. A *frenectomy* is a surgical procedure to remove a poorly attached facial or lingual frenum. Surgery may involve only a small incision to partially loosen the frenum, complete removal of the frenum, or the frenum may be repositioned. This surgery is generally performed on children to give added mobility to the lip or tongue.

Maxillofacial Surgery

Surgery that deals with the cutting of bone is termed an *osteotomy.* Such dental procedures include the removal of an exostosis.

An *exostosis* is a bony outgrowth that may bilaterally develop in the lingual premolar region of the mandible; this is termed *torus mandibularis.* A torus that develops along the palatine suture is referred to as *torus palatinus.* Surgical removal becomes necessary before a removable partial appliance can be accurately constructed. The tori would interfere with the impression of either arch and subsequent construction of the mandibular lingual bar and saddles and the palatal bar of the maxillary. The need for the same surgery would apply for removable full dentures.

Maxillofacial surgery is performed to modify or correct facial abnormalities, such as a protrusive or retrusive mandible or maxilla. *Protrusive* means projected forward to the position of the opposing arch. In the protrusive position, the mandible would be projected forward in relation to the maxilla. A *retrusive* position of the mandible would be far posterior in relation to the maxilla.

Hospital Dentistry

Hospital dentistry includes both oral surgery and restorative treatment under general anesthesia. Patients unable to receive treatment in the dental office or clinic under local anesthesia are scheduled in a hospital.

In practicing hospital dentistry, the dentist must understand and follow operating room procedures and observe all hospital regulations. Dentist, anesthetist, and hospital staff should consult on the choice of medication, anesthesia, and course of treatment prior to admitting the patient to the operating room. Certain patients, such as small children, the mentally impaired, and the elderly should be thoroughly screened for an existing medical problem they may have prior to hospital treatment.

ORAL PATHOLOGY

Oral pathology is concerned with the etiology and nature of diseases that affect oral structures and regions nearby. *Etiology* is the study and cause of disease.

Oral pathology has been discussed in Chapter 24, *Infectious Disease in the Dental Environment*, and will not be repeated here.

Chapter 77: Principles of Dental Radiography

After studying this chapter, the student will be able to:
- Give a brief history of dental radiography.
- State several characteristic properties of x rays.
- Explain the meaning of ionizing radiation.
- Discuss the three factors that determine the penetrating power of x rays.
- Explain the principles of x-ray generation.
- Describe the basic components of the x-ray machine.
- State the reasons for filtration of the x-ray beam.
- Explain what is meant by *collimation*.
- Discuss the different types of radiation as they relate to dental radiography.

INTRODUCTION

The use of **x rays** in dentistry has gradually increased as a means of studying underlying structures not visible to the eyes. The **radiograph** consists of shadows of a three-dimensional object on film that must be viewed and interpreted by the dental practitioner. The practice of **radiography** requires a basic knowledge of radiation physics and chemistry related to photography plus a high degree of skill and knowledge of **radiation** safety techniques.

When the patient seeks the services of a qualified dentist, a full-mouth radiographic survey is often imperative. At times the patient must be convinced that his or her total health may be in jeopardy because of underlying infections that may not have manifested themselves earlier. The profession of dentistry involves causes, diagnosis, and prognosis of disease; therefore, misconceptions and fears of radiation on the part of the dental patient must be overcome if the diagnostic aid, the dental radiograph, is to be used. **Times of exposure** have been established, and no adverse effect is expected in the person undergoing diagnostic procedures for dentistry if these levels are not exceeded.

BRIEF HISTORY OF ORIGIN OF X RAYS

Wilhelm Conrad Roentgen, a German physicist, discovered x rays in 1895 during his experimentation with a Crookes-type vacuum tube. As he studied the image formed by the rays emanating from the tube, which was covered with black paper, he noticed that when the tube was electrically charged, some unknown rays passing from the tube were affecting a fluorescent tube about two meters away. Unaware of the character of these rays, Roentgen named this radiation "x rays" in order to distinguish them from other types of rays. He read a paper on the subject to the

University of Wurzburg (Germany) Physical Society in 1896. Following the reading of the paper, it was decided by the Society that the rays should be named *Roentgen rays*. Today, the term continues to be used in scientific reference.

Dental radiography is the method of recording images of dental structures on film by the use of *roentgen rays,* or *x rays*. Shortly after the announcement was made that these rays would penetrate substances known to be *impervious* (not permitting passage) to light, the first dental radiographs were produced. The use of radiographs in dentistry today is considered a necessity to a thorough dental examination. *Note:* For all practical purposes, the terms *x ray* and *roentgen ray* may be used interchangeably; both terms have the same meaning. Also, when the operator is speaking with patients, it is good technique to use the term *radiograph* since the operator is not really taking *x rays*.

CHARACTERISTIC PROPERTIES OF X RAYS

X rays are not detected by any of the senses; we cannot see them nor can we taste, feel, hear, or smell them. X rays, like visible light rays, are electromagnetic rays. This means that they have a definite relationship to electric current and a body of matter that possesses the property of attracting other substances, as a piece of iron or steel is attracted by a magnet. These electromagnetic rays differ from the rays emitted (given off) by radioactive particles. Electromagnetic rays consist of pure **energy** rather than separate particles of matter.

The rays are said to radiate, or scatter, in a wheel-shaped path, as waves occur when a pebble is dropped into a pool of water. We refer to the fact that their length varies (from the crest of one wave to that of another) as *wavelength*. The basic difference in the various types of electromagnetic radiation is wavelength. Beginning with the longest wavelengths, the range of electromagnetic radiations includes the following:

- electric waves
- radio, television waves
- microwaves
- radar waves
- infrared rays
- visible light rays
- ultraviolet rays (rays lying beyond the area of vision that must be studied by means of photography, heat effects, etc.)
- photons (x-ray photons are believed to be minute bundles of pure energy that have no mass or electric charge and are produced within the x-ray tube)
- gamma rays (of extremely high penetrating power that move at the approximate speed of light—186,284 miles per second)
- cosmic rays or supervoltage rays

The seven rays appearing at the top of the spectrum are of longer wavelength, lack penetrating power, and are said to produce "**soft**" radiation. The rays with the shorter wavelengths, beginning with ultraviolet rays, are invisible light rays that are able to penetrate solid matter.

X rays and gamma rays are similar and have the same general properties, i.e., they consist of high-energy photons (elemental units of radiant energy), have short wavelengths, and have no mass or electric charge.

Gamma rays, unlike x rays, are produced by the disintegration of certain radioactive elements (radium, uranium, thorium) and are electromagnetic emissions of that particular radioactive substance. Because of their high penetrating power, gamma rays are sometimes used in the medical treatment of deep-seated malignancies.

High-energy photons of x and gamma rays have the ability to pass through gases, liquids, and solids and to ionize the substances they penetrate. Because of their very short wavelength and high penetrating power, x rays and gamma rays are said to produce "**hard**" radiation.

Ionizing Radiation

X rays and other rays of high penetrating power are capable of producing ions, directly or indirectly, in their passage through matter. An **atom** has a nucleus that contains positively charged particles (*protons*); in the orbits around the nucleus are negatively charged particles (*electrons*). **Ionization** occurs when an x-ray **photon** (a high-velocity mass of radiant energy) strikes an atom and causes the negatively charged particles to be ejected from an orbit, figure 77–1. When the balance between the positive and negative particles of the atom is disturbed, the atom becomes unbalanced. This unbalanced atom is called an *ion*. To again achieve a balanced state, it seeks another ion to travel with, thus creating a disturbance or change in the substance. The substance can be organic or inorganic. All forms of radiation are capable of causing ionization of matter.

X rays travel from a common point, as do light waves. They proceed from their source in straight lines and cover an increasingly larger area with lessening intensity. X rays have *frequency*. The shorter the wavelength, the higher the frequency or the greater the number of *oscillations* (waves) emitted per second.

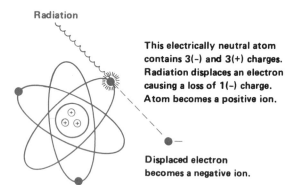

Fig. 77–1. Ionization, showing the removal of an orbital electron by the energy of radiation

The penetrating power of x rays depends on three factors:

1. The wavelength of the rays—the shorter the wavelength, the higher the frequency, the greater the penetrating power.
2. The distance from the source of the x rays to the object—the shorter the distance, the greater the penetrating power.
3. The density of the object penetrated (relative amount of light that the object will allow to pass)—the less the density, the greater the penetrating power of the x rays.

Principles of X-Ray Generation

X rays are produced when any form of matter is struck by electrons traveling at high speed. To accomplish this, it is necessary to have a *source of electrons*, a *high voltage* (electromotive force expressed in units, called **volts**) to accelerate the electrons, and a *target* to stop them.

THE X-RAY MACHINE

Serving as the basis for generating x rays, the x-ray tube within the x-ray head consists of the following components: a **cathode** (negatively charged electrode), containing a filament, which serves as a source of electrons, an **anode** (positively charged electrode, or target), at which the high-speed electrons are directed, figure 77–2. The filament and target are encased within a lead-lined evacuated vacuum tube. Glass used for the vacuum tube is treated with lead, which gives it a bluish-gray appearance, and allows the useful x-ray beam to pass. X rays are produced when the electrons strike the target. In order to function, an electrical current within the tube creates a charge between cathode and anode, propelling the electrons across at very high speeds.

Cathode

The cathode of an x-ray tube is composed of two principal parts: the *filament*, and the *focusing*

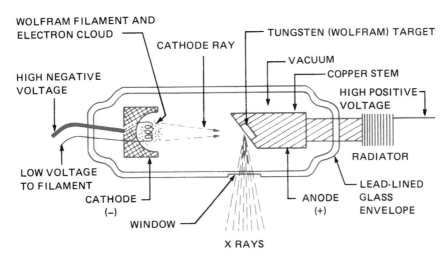

Fig. 77-2. Vacuum tube with components

cup, figure 77-3. The *filament*, the source of electrons within the x-ray tube, is a coil of tungsten (also called wolfram) wire, and is about 0.2 centimeter (cm) in diameter and 1.0 cm in length. It is mounted on two strong, stiff wires that support it and carry the electric current. These two wires lead through the glass tube to serve as connections for the low- and high-voltage source. A **milliampere** (mA) control on a separate side panel provides for fine adjustment of the voltage across the filament, which heats it to a high temperature. Thus, a "cloud" of electrons is produced around the heated coil. The milliampere control regulates the quantity of electrons the filament emits, which in effect regulates the tube current; i.e., the flow of electrons through the tube is measured by the milliammeter.

A filament is located in the focusing cup, figure 77-3, a negatively charged concave reflector cup of molybdenum. The focusing cup electrostatically focuses the electrons emitted by the filament into a narrow beam directed at a small area of the anode called the *focal spot*. The electrons are caused to move in this direction because of the strong electrical force imposed between the cathode and the anode by a high negative charge placed on the cathode and a high positive charge on the anode. The high negative charge of the cathode repels the negatively charged electrons while the positive charge of the anode attracts them.

Anode

The anode is composed of a tungsten target and copper stem. The purpose of the target in an **x-ray tube** is to convert the kinetic (associated with motion) energy of the electrons generated from the filament into x-ray photons. Tungsten is usually selected as target material because of its high atomic number (74)—therefore having many electrons available—high melting point (3370°C), and low vapor pressure, which is important at the high working temperature of an x-ray tube. The tungsten target is embedded in a large mass of copper to help to dissipate (scatter in various directions) the large amount of heat created at the target.

About 1 percent of the energy of the electron beam striking the target is converted into x radiation; approximately 99 percent of the energy becomes heat in the anode structure.

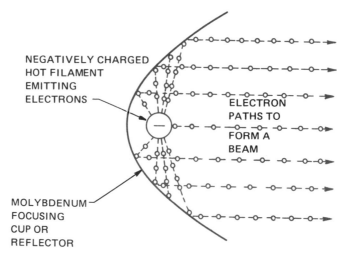

Fig. 77–3. Formation of electron beam by focusing device at the cathode

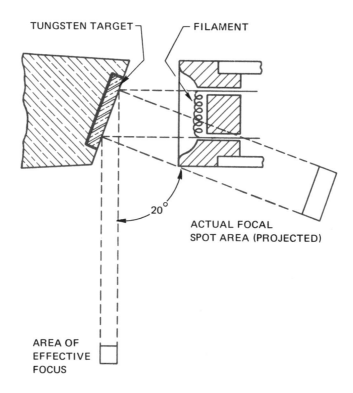

Fig. 77–4. The relationship between the actual focus spot (area of bombardment) and the effective focus as projected from a 20° angle

The angle of the inclination of the target is important, because it partially determines the _focal-spot size_. If the anode is inclined 20 degrees from the vertical and the electrons are projected from the cathode in a rectangular stream, then the projected focal spot can be made square in shape and appreciably smaller than the actual area on the target. Figure 77–4 shows the rectangular stream of electrons bombarding the target, the actual focal spot area projected (area of bombardment), and the area of effective focus.

Power Supply

The primary functions of the power supply are to provide a **current** to heat the x-ray tube filament and to provide a potential difference between the anode and the cathode. These functions are accomplished by the use of a _step-down transformer_ and a _high-voltage transformer_, figure 77–5. These **transformers** and the x-ray tube are contained within an electrically grounded metal housing called the _head_ of the x-ray machine. The transformers are surrounded by an electrical insulating material, usually oil. Depending on the make and size of the **tubehead**, the oil may total as much as five quarts.

The _filament step-down transformer_ reduces the voltage of the incoming current (alternating current) to between 3 and 5 volts. Its operation is regulated by the filament current control (milliamperage switch), which adjusts the current flow through the filament, its heating, and thus the quantity of electrons emitted by the filament.

The output of the _step-up transformer_ is regulated by the **kilovolt** peak (kVp) selector dial. It controls the voltage between the anode and cathode of the x-ray tube. The _high-voltage transformer_ provides the high voltage required by the x-ray tube to accelerate the electrons in order to generate x rays. It accomplishes this by boosting the voltage of the incoming line current to a range of 60 to 90 kilovolts. The 60 to 90 kVp represents the highest, or peak, value of the voltage waves;

i.e., the highest voltage that a given x-ray machine can produce.

The electrons, being negatively charged, will be attracted by a positive charge. The greater the positive charge, the faster the electrons will travel toward it. As the _tube voltage_ is increased, the speed of the electrons toward the cathode correspondingly increases.

The Timer

A timing control device to control the x-ray exposure time is included in the primary circuit of the high-voltage supply. The timer completes the circuit in the high-voltage transformer, and controls the time that the high voltage is applied to the tube and thereby the time during which tube current flows and x rays are produced. To minimize filament use, the timing circuit sends a current through the filament for about half a second to bring it to the proper operating temperature. Once the filament is heated, a time-delay switch applies power to the high-voltage circuit. There is, in many circuit designs, a low-level current passing through the filament that maintains it at a low, safe temperature, so that the delay to preheat the filament before each exposure is shortened.

Some x-ray machine timers are calibrated in fractions of seconds and in whole numbers of seconds. On other timers, the time intervals are expressed as numbers of impulses per exposure. The number of impulses divided by 60 (the frequency of the power source) gives the exposure time in fractions of a second. Thus, thirty impulses is equivalent to a half-second exposure. The x rays are produced only when the operator pushes the button to activate the high electrical input, usually called a _dead-man switch_. On more recently developed timers, this is only a fraction of a second of exposure time. To protect the operator, the switch is usually placed outside the operatory or has a long cord, so that it can be activated while the operator is at least 6 to 8 feet from the tubehead.

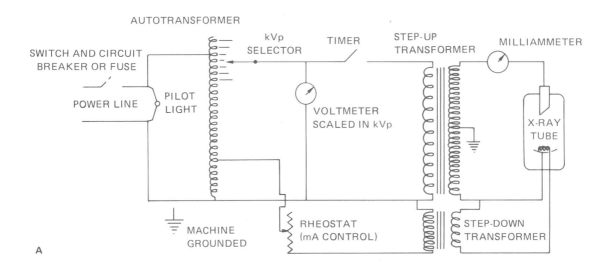

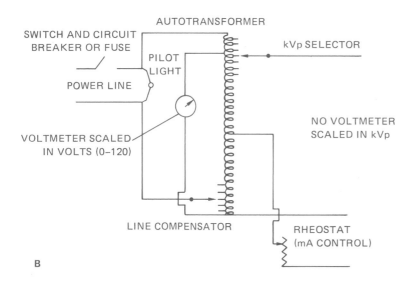

Fig. 77–5. **(A)** A simplified wiring diagram of the basic electrical circuits and parts of an x-ray machine. **(B)** Alternative voltage regulating the system (Courtesy General Electric Company, Medical Systems Division, Milwaukee, WI)

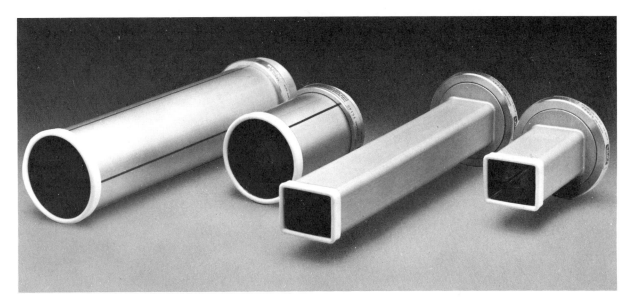

Fig. 77–6. Rinn's lead-lined Position Indicating Devices (PIDs) can greatly reduce the patient's radiation burden and improve radiographic accuracy. Round and rectangular PIDs in 8, 12, and 16" sizes AFD are available for most x-ray machines. (Courtesy Rinn Corporation, Elgin, IL)

Filtration

Although an x-ray beam is composed of x-ray photons (radiant energy) that are arranged according to their wavelength, only those photons with sufficient energy are useful for diagnostic radiographs. Those that are of low penetrating power (long wavelength) contribute to the patient's exposure but not to the information on the film. In the interest of patient safety, a **filter**, an aluminum disk, should be placed over the aperature or window in the head of the x-ray machine to remove the low-energy photons from the beam without affecting those that are able to penetrate the patient and reach the film.

When the amount of filtration for a particular machine is being determined, the operating characteristics of the tube and its housing must be considered. The *inherent filtration* corresponds to the materials that x-ray photons encounter as they travel from the focal on the target to form the useful beam (primary radiation) outside the tube enclosure. These materials include the glass wall of the x-ray tube, the insulating oil that surrounds many of the dental x-ray tubes, and the barrier material used to prevent the oil from escaping through the x-ray window. The tube, surrounded by oil, is encased in a protective metal case called the tubehead, or the tube housing. The window of the tube through which the useful beam passes is chemically treated with lime. Inherent filtration of most x-ray machines ranges from the equivalent of 0.5 to 2 mm of aluminum.

Total filtration is the sum of the inherent filtration plus any added filtration such as aluminum disks. Governmental regulations require that total filtration in a dental x-ray beam be equal to the equivalent of 1.5 mm of aluminum up to 75 kVp, and 2.5 mm of aluminum for all higher voltages.

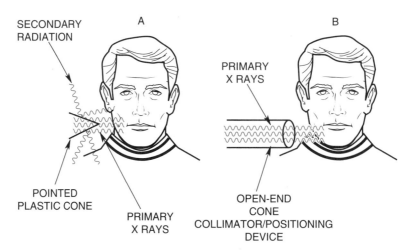

Fig. 77–7. (A) Closed and pointed plastic cone once widely used to collimate the x-ray beam in dental radiography. Originally designed as easy-aiming devices, pointed plastic cones became unpopular when it was discovered that radiation emitted from more than just the tip of the cone; interaction of the primary beam with the plastic cone is a major source of secondary radiation and exposure of the patient's face to long wavelength radiation. The closed and pointed plastic cone has been replaced by the round or rectangular, open-ended, lead-lined or metal collimator positioning device (B) which, because of its shape and composition, eliminates this source of secondary radiation and patient exposure. (Courtesy Edwards, C., M.A. Statkiewicz-Sherer, and E.R. Ritenour, *Radiation Protection for Dental Radiographers*, Mosby, St. Louis, MO, 1984)

Collimation

When an x-ray beam is directed at a patient, some of the x-ray photons are absorbed by tissues, while others pass through to form an image on the film. Many of the absorbed photons generate **scattered radiation**. To minimize the amount of **primary radiation**, collimation reduces the size of the x-ray beam and, thus, the volume of scattered radiation within the patient from which the scattered photons originate.

Cylinder and rectangular **collimators** are used in dental radiography, figure 77–6. These reduce patient exposure and increase film quality.

In many states, radiation protection codes mandate the use of round or rectangular, open-ended, lead-lined cylinders and recommend terminating the use of pointed plastic cones, figure 77–7.

The diaphragm collimator is a thick washer of radiopaque material (usually lead) with an aperature (opening) approximately $2^3/4''$ (7 cm) in diameter. This device is usually placed over the window in the x-ray head through which the x-ray beam emerges. The size and shape of the aperature detemines the size and shape of the useful beam, figure 77–8. The **position indicating device** (PID) also achieves collimation, because it is usually lined with or constructed of radiopaque material and can be cylindrical or rectangular in shape. Rectangular collimators

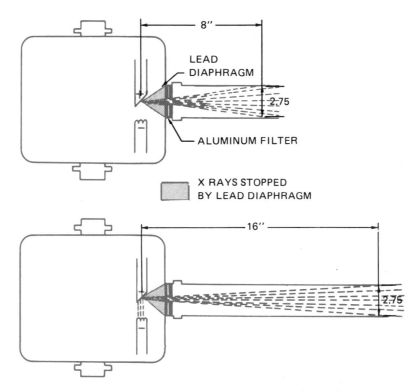

Fig. 77–8. Effects of aperture size on divergence of x-ray beams

limit the beam to a size just larger than the size of an x-ray film. PIDs may vary in length from 8 to 16 inches.

TYPES OF X-RAY RADIATION

There are several types of x-ray radiation, figure 77–9.

1. *Primary radiation* is radiation which emerges from the x-ray tube target (anode), sometimes called direct ray, primary beam, useful beam, or central ray. The **quality** (penetrating power) of this radiation depends upon the correct settings of mA and kVp controls.
2. *Remnant radiation* is all of the x-ray photons that reach their destination (the film) after passing through the object being radiographed and consist of unabsorbed primary and secondary rays generated in the tissue. Remnant rays produce the radiographic image in the form of the **latent image** (not visible until the radiograph is processed).
3. *Secondary radiation* results from interaction between primary radiation and the atoms of an object it contacts. Some of the primary beam will pass through the object with no contact, and some will irradiate atoms of the object. Secondary radiation, therefore, consists of scattered radiation and primary rays, and the amount produced depends on the quality and **quantity** of primary radiation and the atomic

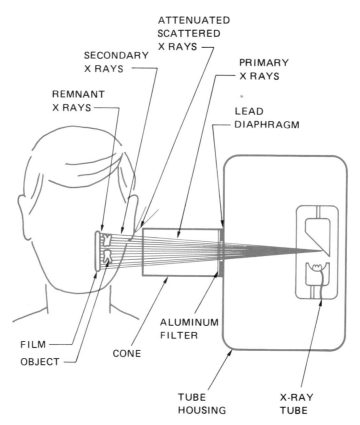

Fig. 77–9. Primary, remnant, secondary, and scattered radiation

number of its tissue source. Elements such as water, body tissue, and wood generate large quantities of secondary radiation. The kVp is the primary factor influencing the production of secondary radiation.

4. *Scattered radiation*, also called secondary scattered rays or secondary scattered radiation, consists of rays from the primary beam that have deflected during their passage through tissues or other substances. These rays may or may not have been attenuated (weakened) by absorption or scattering of the photons. Scatter radiation is all of the radiation that arises from the interaction of the x-ray beam with the atoms of an object in the path of the beam, with associated changes in wavelength.

5. *Stray radiation* consists of all radiation other than the primary or useful beam produced within the x-ray head and is caused by electrons hitting the glass wall and other parts of the x-ray tube rather than the target. Leakage of a faulty tube or tubehead permits stray radiation to escape.

Exposure to any of these types of radiation contributes to the *absorbed dosage*. (This is covered in more detail in Chapter 78.)

REVIEW

1. Who discovered x rays? When and under what circumstances were they discovered? _____

_____

_____

2. Another term for a positively charged electrode is_____.

3. Another term for a negatively charged electrode is _____.

4. What is the function of the step-up transformer? _____

_____

_____

5. What is the function of the step-down transformer?_____

_____

_____

6. The penetrating power of x-radiation is controlled by _____.

7. The amount of current in mA flowing to the x-ray tube is regulated by the

_____.

8. What three factors govern the penetrating power of x rays?

a. _____

b. _____

c. _____

9. X rays are produced when the tungsten target is struck by _____ traveling at high speed.

10. How much of the energy of the electron beam is converted into x rays?

_____

_____

11. Label the following diagram.

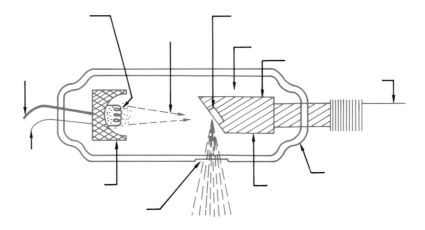

12. The metal case containing the x-ray tube is called the _____.

13. What are the governmental regulations and requirements for total filtration of a dental x-ray beam? _____

_____

_____

14. What is the function of the lead diaphragm in the tubehead? _____

_____

_____

15. Why is the function of an aluminum filter important? _____

_____

_____

16. What are the basic types of x-ray radiation? _____

_____

_____

17. Complete the following diagram by filling in the blank spaces on the arrows.
Use figure 77–9 for any help you may need.

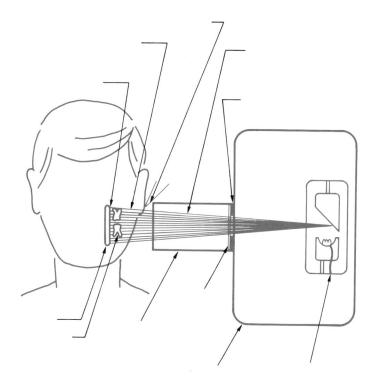

18. What is meant by kilovolts peak? _____

_____

19. The quality of the x-ray beam is controlled by _____

_____.

Chapter 78: Measurement of Ionizing Radiation

INTRODUCTION

Natural (background) radiation or ionizing radiation coming from natural sources has always been a part of human environment. Three *natural* sources include radioactive materials in the earth, cosmic radiation from outer space, and radionuclides (any atomic nucleus specified by its atomic number, atomic mass, and energy state) existing in the human body. A radionuclide is radioactive and disintegrates with emissions of electromagnetic radiations.

The human body contains many radioactive nuclides that exist in small quantities within the tissues. Potassium-40, carbon-14, and strontium-90 are some of the chemical elements. Cosmic radiation (from the sun and stars) varies in intensity at different altitudes of the earth's surface. The higher the altitude, the greater the intensity; the lowest intensity occurs at sea level. Thus far, mankind has been unable to control the quantity of natural radiation.

Manmade, or artificial, radiation includes such sources as dental procedures, medical procedures, nuclear reactors (and the nuclear fuel cycle), and radioactive fallout. Presently, the two largest sources of artificial radiation are medical and dental procedures.

Standards of measurement for ionizing radiation have been developed throughout the world in an attempt to reduce radiation exposure. It is important that the dental radiographer be familiar with these standardized radiation quantities and units.

STANDARDIZATION OF RADIATION MEASUREMENT

In 1921, the medical and dental community formed the British X-ray and Radium Protection Committee to investigate the alarming number of radiation injuries. The unit of measure at that time was the *skin **erythema** dose*, defined as a dose of radiation that caused reddening of the skin following radiation. It is unlikely that it would be necessary to take enough dental films to produce a skin erythema on the patient's face. However, during endodontic treatment, fractures, and other situations when several films are necessary within a short period of time, the limitations of irradiation must be realized.

The International Commission on Radiation (ICRU) was formed in 1925. This commission was charged with the responsibility of defining a unit of exposure in 1928. It was not until 1937 that a report was given to the International Congress of Radiology, defining the **roentgen** (R) as the unit of measurement of exposure to x- and gamma radiation. In 1962, the roentgen was redefined to increase accuracy and acceptability.

Roentgen

A *roentgen unit* (R) can be defined as the amount of x-radiation that will produce one cubic centimeter of air ions (at standard temperature and pressure) carrying one electrostatic (produced by stationary electric charges) unit of either sign (+ or –). The unit of exposure corresponding to ionization in air of one electrostatic unit is 0.001 293 gram of air. Envision a cube of air, 1 centimeter in all dimensions. An x-ray beam passes through it, the x-ray photons strike electrons orbiting around the nuclei of electrically stable air atoms and separate the electrons from their respective nuclei. This action is ionization (ion pair formation); the electron is negatively charged and the remainder of the atom becomes positively charged. When measuring radiation, these charges are collected and counted.

The roentgen (R) has been assigned a quality factor of 1; therefore, 1 R is the traditional unit of x-radiation or gamma radiation, table 78–1.

TABLE 78–1. RADIATION QUALITY FACTORS

Type of Ionizing Radiation	Quality Factor
X-ray photons	1
Beta particles	1
Gamma photons	1
Slow neutrons	3
Fast neutrons	10
Protons	10
Alpha particles	20

Source: Courtesy Edwards, C., M.A. Statkiewicz-Sherer, and E. R. Ritenour, *Radiation Protection for Dental Radiographers*, Mosby, St. Louis, MO, 1984.

Exposure to low levels of radiation may be quantitatively expressed in thousanths of an R, the milli-R or mR. In the near future the roentgen will be replaced by a new unit, the coloumb per kilogram (c/kg); 1 c/kg equals 3.88×10^3R. Refer to table 78–2.

Rad

The **rad** is the unit of absorbed radiation. One unit of rad (*radiation absorbed dose*) is the quantity of energy imparted to a mass of material exposed to any type of ionizing radiation. X- or gamma radiation does not become a *dose* until it is absorbed. A dose may be defined as the total quantity of radiation in roentgens at a given point, measured in air. The dose of ionizing radiation absorbed in human tissue is important in dental radiography, since it is responsible for the biological changes that occur in that tissue and specific area.

Because bone contains calcium and phosphorus it will absorb more ionizing radiation than will soft tissue, which is composed of fat and structures close to that of water. Bone has an effective atomic number (13.8); soft tissue has a lesser atomic number (7.4); the atomic number of water is 7.0. Bone absorbs more ionizing radiation than soft tissue in the diagnostic energy range of 65 to 90 kVp used in dentistry, because the photoelectric process is the dominant mode of energy absorption within this range. (*Photoelectric* pertains to effects produced by increased electrical conduction, as occurs in 65 to 90 kVp.) The higher the atomic number of the material undergoing a photoelectric process, the greater the amount of energy absorbed by that material. With a dental x-ray beam, 1 R will produce an estimated 0.903 rad in soft tissue. In the near future, the rad will be replaced by the gray (Gy); 1 Gy equals 1 joule/kg, which equals 100 rads. Refer to table 78–2.

Quality Factor

The *quality factor* (QF) relates to radiation in terms of biologic effect in body tissue for equal absorbed doses. X rays, beta particles (high-speed electrons) and gamma rays have been assigned a quality factor of 1, and provide the base against which to compare the effectiveness

TABLE 78—2. SUMMARY OF RADIATION QUANTITIES AND UNITS*

Type of Radiation	Quantity	Traditional Unit	SI Unit	Measuring Media	Effect Measured
X or gamma	Exposure	Roentgen (R)	Coulomb per kilogram (C/kg)	Air	Ionization of air
All ionizing radiations	Absorbed dose	Rad	Gray (Gy)	Any object	Amount of energy absorbed by object
All ionizing radiations	Dose equivalent	Rem	Seivert (Sv)	Body tissue	Biological effects

Source: Courtesy Edwards, et al., _Radiation Protection for Dental Radiographers_, Mosby, St. Louis, MO, 1984.

* International System of Units (SI), as developed by the International Committee for Weights and Measures in 1975.

of other types of ionizing radiation in producing biological damage. For example, the specific ionization of fast neutrons is ten times greater than x-radiation in producing a given biological effect and is assigned a quality factor of 10. A neutron is an electrically neutral or uncharged particle of matter existing along with protons in the atoms of all elements (except the mass 1 of hydrogen). Rays of alpha particles, a type of emission produced by a disintegration of radioactive substance (such as uranium and radium) are used only in radiotherapy, table 78–1.

REM

The rem *(roentgen equivalent [in] man)* is the physical and biological effects of the tissues which absorb various degrees of radiation. The rem is the unit of dose equivalent. It is the product of the QF of a particular radiation and the rad dose. In diagnostic radiology, this unit is used to make a comparison between the biological effects of exposure and the various types of radiation. It is generally accepted that 1 R is equal to 1 rad, which equals 1 rem. In the near future the rem will be replaced by the seivert (Sv); 1 Sv equals 100 rem. Refer to table 78–2.

RBE

RBE *(relative biologic effectiveness)* is similar to QF, and is used only in reference to laboratory investigations.

The effects of radiation on living tissue may vary because of the many different physical and biological circumstances. Two generalizations can be made: (1) Ionization is the underlying phenomenon by which changes occur; and (2) all ionizing radiation is hazardous, but the degree of hazard varies.

DOSE-LIMITING RECOMMENDATIONS

Report No. 39 (1971) of the National Committee on Radiation Protection and Measurements (NCRP) establishes certain criteria for the use of radiation on human subjects:

1. Methods providing maximum information with minimum dose should be utilized.
2. Determination should be made as to whether radiation is the preferable agent for performing the survey or study.
3. The possible need for repetition of radiation should be considered in the original plan.

In other words, dental x-radiation should not be used when other media can make the determination.

ALARA

Included in the 1954 report by the NCRP is the stated principle that radiation exposures should be kept "As Low as Reasonably Achievable." The concept of *ALARA* is accepted by all regulatory agencies. The employment of all proper radiation control procedures is the shared responsibility of all persons working in radiology.*

Consumer-Patient Radiation Health and Safety Act of 1981

The Consumer-Patient Radiation Health and Safety Act of 1981 (Appendix B), provides federal legislation requiring the establishment of minimum standards for accreditation of educational programs for persons who administer radiological procedures, and for the certification of such persons. This legislative act was signed by then President of the United States Ronald Reagan in August 1981. The purpose of the act is also to ensure that dental and medical procedures are consistent with strict safety precautions and standards. Legislation governing the practices of radiological technology (radiography, radiation therapy, and nuclear medicine) includes dentists, dental assistants, and dental hygienists.

The secretary for Health and Human Services has the responsibility for establishing minimum standards for certification and accreditation. Individual states are urged to enact similar statutes and to administer appropriate programs for such certification and accreditation.

Maximum Permissible Dose (MPD). The first recommended limits of radiation exposure were developed in 1928 by the NCRP. These limits or guidelines have been revised downward, and the cumulative MPD is now set below levels where any damaging effects have been observed. NCRP Report No. 17 (1954) defined the MPD as "that radiation dose which should not be exceeded without careful consideration of the reasons for doing so." Persons engaged in the operation of x-ray equipment are classified as "occupationally exposed"; however, it is not expected that the absorbed dose that has accumulated over the course of an individual's career (cumulative MPD) will cause any detectable bodily injury to the radiation worker in his or her lifetime.

The NCRP recommends further that the MPD be held to dose limitations. For educational and training purposes it is necessary and desirable that students exposed during educational activities not receive in excess of 0.1 rem per year in the context of their educational activity. This is considered to be a part of the annual dose limit of 0.5 rem for persons under the age of 45, not supplemental to it. Furthermore, operators of x-ray units should be limited to 0.1 R per week.

NCRP Report No. 35 (1970) recommends that the operators in daily contact with roentgen rays receive no more than 0.3 R in any one week; or more than 3 R in a thirteen-week period (calendar quarter); or in excess of 5 R for a year.

The formula for the cumulative MPD is stated in traditional terms as:

$$MPD = 5(N - 18) \text{ rem}$$

This formula was developed by the NCRP and has been used since 1957. The number 5 represents the maximum number of **whole-body** rem that a radiation worker is permitted to receive in any one year. The letter N represents the actual age (in years) of the individual concerned, and the number 18 specifies the legal age at which a person may be employed as a radiation worker.

Problem   Determine the maximum whole-body dose of x-radiation that a 25-year-old radiographer may receive.

* Courtesy of Mosby, St. Louis, MO, by permission.

Solution MPD = 5(N – 18) rem
             = 5(25 – 18) rem
             = 5(7) rem
             = 35 rem

Although the NCRP and similar organizations have no legal status, their suggestions and recommendations are highly regarded. Regulatory bodies have used them to formulate legislation controlling the use of radiation in the dental office.

SUGGESTED ACTIVITY

• Using your own age and the formula for determining cumulative MPD, determine whole-body rem.

REVIEW

1. Two types of ionizing radiation are

   a. _____

   b. _____

2. The first known measurement of a dose of radiation was termed _____

   _____.

3. Presently, the accepted (traditional) unit of exposure is _____.

4. The unit of absorbed radiation is _____.

5. As regards quality factor, which ionizing rays are assigned a value of 1?

   _____

   _____

6. The unit of dose equivalent is _____.

7. State two generalizations that can be made regarding the effects of ionizing radiation on living tissue.

   a. _____

   _____

   b. _____

   _____

8. Who establishes the criteria for use of radiation on human subjects?

_____

_____

9. What are the residual effects of radiation that remain in the body called?

_____

10. List three dose-limiting recommendations established by the NCRP regarding use of radiation.

a. _____

_____

b. _____

_____

c. _____

_____

11. What recently passed legislation provides minimum standards for x-radiation?

_____

_____

12. Define the ALARA concept._____

_____

_____

13. What is the maximum permissible dose (MPD) for a student engaging in radiographic educational activities? _____

_____

_____

Chapter 79: Radiation Protection

INTRODUCTION

The public today is fairly well informed about the hazards of radiation; on the other hand, they are often misinformed. The responsibility for radiation protection of the dental patient lies with the dentist and dental auxiliary personnel. The need for a radiographic examination should be based on obtaining necessary information to enable patient diagnosis by the dental practitioner.

Every exposure of a dental patient to radiation carries with it the dual features of diagnostic benefit and risk of biological harm. Therefore, all exposure to radiation should be kept to the minimum that is necessary to meet specific diagnostic requirements. It should be emphasized that failure to obtain radiographs that are clinically indicated is more likely to harm patients than the slight possibility of suffering radiation injury as a result of exposure. Modern equipment and current safety techniques make the actual hazard from a dental radiograph an improbability.

It should be noted, however, that radiation of any type should be used sparingly and that a record of previous exposures be entered on the patient's chart (Chapters 31 and 32).

BENEFITS OF RADIATION

For a complete dental oral diagnosis, a series of radiographs is extremely important. Many systemic and oral diseases can be detected on radiographs before they are clinically apparent. For example, decay between the teeth can be detected much earlier and more accurately with the aid of radiographs. In addition, abscesses (infection at the root tip), bone diseases, periodontal disease, and the eruption of permanent teeth can be detected with the use of radiographs.

HAZARDS OF RADIATION

All radiation is ionizing radiation and therefore hazardous. However, the *degree* of hazard varies; it depends a great deal on the operator's safety techniques. Ionizing radiation affects living tissue through a process that causes atoms and molecules to become electrically unbalanced. As you remember, (1) all living substances are composed of atoms; and (2) they are arranged in a particular fashion and known as molecules (the smallest particle of a substance that retains the properties of the substance). Atoms prefer to be in balance; in an effort to regain balance after ionization, they may combine with other atoms, creating a new and different substance. This new substance may be harmful to the organ or cell. An example of this is the subtle change from H_2O (water) to H_2O_2 (hydrogen peroxide). The former is essential for a cell, the latter is poisonous.

Effects of Radiation on Cells

A *direct effect* of radiation on a cell occurs when the cell nucleus is hit directly by x rays. The cell either dies immediately or at the time of cell division (**mitosis**).

An *indirect effect* occurs when the hormone balance is altered, or the functions of the cell are changed in a destructive manner. The more cells affected or killed in a body organ, the more rippled that organ becomes. If few alterations occur, the effect may be so slight that the organ functions properly and is unaffected by the radiation.

Some cells are more **radiosensitive** than others. Radiosensitivity is directly proportional to the reproductive cycle of the cell. In other words, the more rapid the mitotic and metabolic activity, the more radiosensitive the cell. Following is a list of cell types ranked from the most radiosensitive to the least radiosensitive. The second list ranks cell types from the least **radioresistant** to the most radioresistant.

Radiosensitive

- germinal cells of the ovary   Most
- seminiferous epithelium of the testes
- blood-forming cells, lymphocytes, and other blood-forming tissues
- intestinal epithelium
- skin   Least

Radioresistant

- glandular tissue (other than genetic) Least
- muscle
- nerve
- bone
- enamel   Most

Radiosensitivity varies among species. Also, there is individual variability depending on the age of the species, the intensity of the x ray, the length of exposure, and the area of exposure.

Somatic Effects

Somatic refers to all body tissue except genetic tissue. Residual effects of radiation that remain in the body are termed **cumulative**. The first signs of radiation illness are blood changes. However, it takes a great deal of *whole-body* exposure to radiation to have this occur. Radiation used in dentistry is termed **specific-area radiation**, as only a small area of the body is exposed. It would take hundreds of times more radiation than a dental x-ray machine is capable of producing to cause even a reddening of the skin.

The lens of the eye is one area of somatic tissue that deserves special consideration. Tissues of the eye are nonrepairable. Even though it would take much more radiation than is used in dentistry to harm the eye, the safest approach is to avoid subjecting the eye to any radiation by asking patients to close their eyes during exposure of the film.

Genetic Effects

All types of radiation, including radiation in the atmosphere, can affect the body. The cumulative effects of radiation on the chromosomes, or genes, is an important consideration, as the possibility of mutations is involved. Mutations may be beneficial or harmful to the species and may not appear for several generations. Because we cannot detect **genetic** effects, it is important that the patient and operator be exposed as little as possible to radiation from medical and dental sources. Proper use of all radiation equipment is imperative.

CONTROL OF PATIENT RISKS

The radiation received by the patient in the usual dental radiographic examination is but a small fraction of the amount that would produce bodily harm. However, the dental auxiliary should make it a habit to ask every patient if he

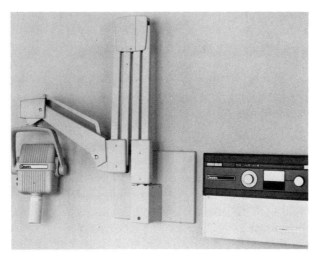

Fig. 79–1. Dental x-ray machine used for intraoral radiographs. GX-1000 with Panelipse II Master Control (GENDEX Corporation, Milwaukee, WI). This control panel permits a choice of milliampe rate and kilovoltage in addition to exposure time and can be used for two different tubeheads.

has been recently exposed to radiation for therapeutic (pertains to the treatment or curing of disease) or diagnostic purposes. *Caution:* If radiation exposure has occurred within the preceding thirty days, the dental auxiliary should consult the dentist before any further exposure occurs.

A policy regarding pregnant patients should be established and strictly observed. Many experts recommend that elective radiographic procedures be postponed until the patient is no longer pregnant.

On a patient's initial visit to the dentist, a thorough clinical examination should be followed by a radiographic survey. The decision to complete a full-mouth survey should depend on the dentist's professional judgment. A complete survey is taken for two reasons: first, to determine the condition of the teeth and underlying bone; second, to establish a basis for future comparison. As a rule, the dentist need not repeat a full-mouth (complete) series for several years unless

the patient has a history of trauma, extensive oral surgery, or orthodontic treatment. Neither the American Academy of Radiology nor the American Dental Association (ADA) is specific about the time interval before repeating a complete oral radiographic survey.

Individual radiographs should be taken whenever necessary for preventive reasons or in cases of a toothache, a loose tooth, pain in the jaw, or to evaluate the progress of dental treatment. Such intraoral radiographs are obtained by use of modern dental x-ray equipment, figure 79–1.

Protective Lead Shields

Occasionally, use of the protective lead apron may cause the patient to question the need for it. Those who question should be reassured by emphasizing the dentist's concern for the welfare of his patients.

Lead aprons are constructed of various light and flexible materials with the thickness of lead

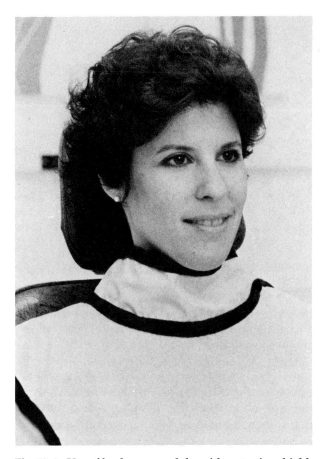

Fig. 79–2. Use of lead apron and thyroid protective shields

varying from 0.25 to 1.25 mm depending on the kVp used; the higher the kVp, the thicker the lead shielding. The apron should be such that it can be draped over the pubis in males and over the lower pelvis in females. Lead aprons should be used to protect *all* patients.

Another shielding device is the lead collar, sometimes called a thyroid protection collar. To achieve more complete patient protection, a thyroid collar should be used in conjunction with an apron, figure 79–2. Both shields should be frequently checked for cracks and defects, since folding the apron or hanging it over a towel rack promotes cracking.

According to the Bureau of Radiologic Health, the use of a leaded thyroid collar is recommended but not required. However, thyroid shields should be used, especially on children, because of the greater sensitivity of the thyroid gland in young people. A study reported in the *Journal of Angle Orthodontists* (47: 17–24, Jan., 1977) indicated that "the use of a thyroid protective collar (shield) is very effective in minimizing radiation exposure to the thyroid during encephalometric examinations. Present scientific evidence does not mandate the use of a thyroid shield but, in time, consumer pressure may force its use". *Note:* A thyroid collar cannot be used effectively with a panoramic x-ray machine because it blocks out parts of the jaws.

RADIATION PROTECTION FOR THE OPERATOR

It is essential to reemphasize that under usual circumstances any patient radiation reduction will have a direct effect on the amount of radiation received by the operator. The term operator includes the dentist and all auxiliaries who expose film. The operator may receive radiation in the form of secondary radiation when the primary beam strikes the patient or objects in the operatory. If the operator foolishly stands in the path of the primary beam, he or she receives radiation exposure. Direct exposure to ionizing radiation is cumulative. In other words, the effects of yesterday's are added to today's and tomorrow's exposures. The resulting accumulation, when great enough, can cause harmful effects. Overexposure may be avoided by observing a few basic rules:

1. Never hold films in the patient's mouth or in any radiographic training mannequin while making an exposure.
2. Never stand in the direct path of the x-ray beam to avoid direct exposure.
3. Always stand behind the tubehead, at least 6 to 8 feet from the patient or behind a lead-lined wall or shield. If a lead-lined booth or barrier is provided, exposures should be made only while the operator is protected by it.
4. Always make certain the x-ray machine meets all standards for operation and safety as regards filtration, shielding, and collimation. Have a periodic check of the x-ray equipment made by a competent radiation-oriented person. Equipment used in measuring the quality and quantity of radiation is expensive, and a thorough knowledge of its use imperative.
5. Wear a personnel monitoring device to detect unwanted exposure.

Film badges are the most widely used type of personnel monitoring device. This inexpensive device records the radiation exposure accumulated over a long period of time. Monitoring companies process the film packet and prepare written reports that state the individual occupational exposure of each person in a particular office or clinic. The film is maintained by the monitoring company and constitutes a permanent legal record of personnel exposure. This service is economical, costing only a few dollars per unit per month. Manufacturers recommend one month as the maximum period of time that a film badge should be worn as an effective monitoring device.

Safety of Shockproof Units

All dental x-ray equipment and tubes are shockproof for the operator and the patient. In self-contained units, the high-voltage elements (x-ray tube and transformer) are immersed in oil in a single, grounded metal container. This oil immersion serves both to insulate the high-voltage circuits and help cool the tube. Insulation of this type eliminates the danger of electric shock if the tubehead is touched during exposure.

SUGGESTIONS FOR THE DENTAL RADIOGRAPHER

Dental radiography is a skill that must be learned and practiced. There are no short cuts to developing a high degree of competence. Effort and self-application are the keys to success. Bear in mind that mistakes will be made. Making these mistakes is a part of the learning process.

The author suggests that DXT TRS* or skulls be used for exposure during the process of learning and prior to patient exposures. This practice

---

* DXT TRS, Rinn Corporation, Elgin, IL.

will help in correcting mistakes in placement of the film, angulation of the cone, and development procedures. An exposure time chart is usually posted near the control panel of the x-ray unit.

INFECTION CONTROL

During the radiographic examination, it will be necessary to work inside the patient's mouth. Infection-control procedures are in order for every patient, to avoid exposure to the operator and cross-infection to other patients. Refer to Chapter 26.

While using properly prepared equipment, infection-control procedures, marked by common sense and good judgment, should be strictly followed.

1. Disinfect all parts of the x-ray unit that will come in contact with the operator's hands during the examination: the control panel, exposure button, the **x-ray cone**, the buttons on the chair, and the door handle to the x-ray cubicle. The barrier technique should be used for any area that has grooves (knobs, buttons, dials). Pieces of clear plastic work well here. Disinfect the flat surfaces where the dental films will be placed.

2. Disinfect, then place clear plastic barriers on the chair; include headrest and armrests.

3. Disinfect, then place clear plastic barriers on the cone and arms of the tubehead of the x-ray unit.

4. Provide a paper cup in which to place exposed film. Place paper cup behind the leaded protective of the x-ray cubicle—not in the operator's pocket!

5. Sterilize instruments used in the patient's mouth after use with each patient.

6. Wear gloves, surgical mask, protective eyewear, and professional gown throughout the procedure to protect yourself.

7. Take all additional precautions with patients identified as high risk to avoid transmitting infection.

Note: Dental personnel should routinely avail themselves of preventive vaccination for hepatitis B and hepatitis D. Presently, there are no vaccinations against tuberculosis, AIDS, or herpes. Refer to Chapter 24.

REVIEW

1. On which basis should radiographs be made? _____

_____

2. Some of the benefits of an oral radiographic series are to detect _____

_____

_____.

3. What is meant by a *direct effect* of radiation? _____

_____.

4. An *indirect effect* of radiation occurs when _____

_____.

5. What is meant by the phrase "radiosensitivity is directly proportional to the reproductive cycle of the cell"? _____

_____

_____

6. Name three body cells that tend to be most radiosensitive.

   a. _____

   b. _____

   c. _____

7. Which three body cells are most radioresistant?

   a. _____

   b. _____

   c. _____

8. What is somatic tissue? _____

_____

9. What is the difference between whole-body and specific-area radiation?

_____

_____

10. Why should the primary beam not be directed toward the eye(s)?_____

_____

11. In establishing limitations of exposure, what procedure should be followed?

_____

_____

_____

_____

_____

_____

12. How can the operator be protected from an unsafe amount of x-radiation?

_____

_____

_____

Chapter 80: Dental X-ray Film

OBJECTIVES:

After studying this chapter, the student will be able to:
- Describe film emulsion and state its purpose.
- Analyze the components of an x-ray film.
- Explain the various film packets.
- Distinguish between different film sizes.
- List the various speeds of film.

FILM COMPOSITION

Dental x-ray film is composed of two principal components: the *base* and the *emulsion*. The base is the supporting material onto which the emulsion is coated. The emulsion is sensitive to x rays and visible light rays and records the radiographic image.

The Base

The base of the x-ray film consists of transparent polyester. Polyester is a compound formed by the reaction between an acid and an alcohol with elimination of water. It is used in making fibers. This transparent base serves to support and retain the emulsion on the film and lends some degree of stiffness throughout the handling of it. Its thickness is approximately 0.2 mm (0.007 inch). A blue tint is added to the polyester during the manufacturing process, which increases the contrast of the exposed and processed film. (This subject will be discussed in Chapter 93.) Added to the film base, on both sides, is a thin adhesive material; this enables the emulsion to adhere to the base material.

The Emulsion

The emulsion of the x-ray film consists of crystals of silver halides suspended in a gelatin matrix (framework). A *halide* is a compound of a halogen (bromine, iodine) with a chemical element (silver, potassium). All halogens are of a closely related chemical family that combine easily with chemical elements. Silver halide is the product of virgin silver dissolved in nitric acid. This silver solution is mixed with potassium bromide to produce silver bromide. To a lesser extent, silver iodide serves as the remainder of the chemical components of the emulsion. Silver iodide adds greatly to the sensitivity of the emulsion, thus reducing the dose of radiation to produce a diagnostic image. The size of the crystals determines the speed with which the emulsion reaction occurs during radiation.

Silver halide crystals (grains) are suspended on both sides of the base, with the gelatin serving to keep the silver grains dispersed. During processing (Chapter 89), the gelatin absorbs the processing solution and thereby allows the chemicals to act on the silver halide grains.

A supercoating on the surface of the film is added to provide a protective barrier during the frequent handling of the film (Chapter 90). This coating is, typically, an additional coating of gelatin. This added coating also helps to protect the film from damage by the rollers of an automatic processor (Chapter 91). The emulsion retains much of its rigidity during normal processing; it has strength when wet but is sensitive to high temperatures.

Intraoral film is supplied by various manufacturers in the United States. Each film is double-coated, i.e., the emulsion is coated on each side of the film base. Double-emulsion "ultraspeed" film is used in modern radiography, because the added thickness of the emulsion allows less radiation to be used when exposing an object.

FILM PACKAGING

The x-ray film is sensitive to such things as light, x rays and gamma rays, various gases and their fumes, and to heat and moisture. Films that are placed within the mouth are termed *intraoral* and, for protection against light and moisture, are individually wrapped in a packet of fairly waterproof material (either white plastic or stippled-surface paper). These materials aid in the retention of the film as it is positioned against the mucosa of the patient. The film is further protected by a black, paper sheath and backed by a thin sheet of lead foil. The *lead-foil backing* prevents much of the secondary radiation, which originates in the tissues of the patient, from **fogging** the film through "backscattering." It also helps to reduce radiation fog during exposure. The metal foil absorbs x rays that have passed through the object and film and helps to reduce exposure of the tissues behind the film. The lead foil is embossed with a pattern that will appear on the film, resulting in a light image of the object if the film is placed with this surface toward the x-ray beam during exposure. To identify the tube side of the film (the surface of the film that is to be placed toward the x-ray source), the manufacturer places a circle or indentation at one corner of the film packet. The side with the depression is placed toward the patient's tongue. After the film is processed, the depression or "dot" is used to identify the patient's right or left side.

Films are packaged as either a single or dual packet, with either a single sheet of film or two sheets of film in each packet. When dual packets are used, the second film becomes a duplicate record.

Dual Film Packets

A dual film packet makes it possible to produce an exact duplicate of a film, thus eliminating the need for additional radiation exposure to the patient.

Original radiographs should *always* be kept in the office with the patient's record. Should the doctor need to refer the patient to another doctor for treatment or verify an insurance claim, dual film packets should be used.

Intraoral films vary only in size and clinical use; the composition of the film is identical.

FILM TYPES

Periapical Film

Current intraoral film sizes are the result of a demonstrated need by the practicing members of the dental profession. The No. 2 (standard size) packet is a *periapical* film that has been traditionally used for adult full-mouth surveys. It is used to record the crowns, roots, and periapical areas of the teeth.

The No. 1, or narrow film, was created as the result of requests from the profession for a film narrow enough to be accepted in the anterior portion of the mouth with less distortion than could be obtained with the use of the standard No. 2 packet.

The No. 0 film packet is half the size of the adult packet and is used for children. This so-called pedo film resulted from the practice of early pedodontists (dentists who specialize in the care of children's teeth) of folding a standard No. 2 size packet in half lengthwise to produce a small packet for small children, figure 80–1.

BiteWing Film

With a wing or tab attached, a No. 2 size periapical film becomes a bitewing. The patient bites on the wing that is placed on the tube surface of the film. This film is used to record interproximal caries and conditions of the alveolar crest. It may be purchased with the wing fixed in position, or a paper loop may be placed over a periapical film. Film holding instruments for

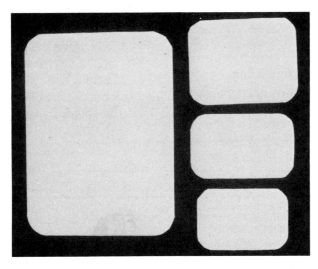

Fig. 80–1. Dental x-ray film is supplied in various sizes. (Left) occlusal film. (Top right) No. 2, Adult posterior. (Middle right) No. 1, Adult anterior. (Bottom right) Child size.

bitewing projections are available (Chapter 82). A child's bitewing consists of a No. 0 or No. 1 size film with a tab attached.

Occlusal Film

An occlusal film is approximately twice the size of a No. 2 film. It is generally used to observe larger areas of the maxilla and mandible than may be seen on a periapical film. The film is held in position by having the patient bite lightly on the film to retain it between the occlusal surfaces of the teeth (Chapter 87).

OTHER INFORMATION

Film Speed

The American National Standards Institute developed a film speed classification that groups x-ray film by speeds ranging from D through F. A represents the slowest speed film (requiring the most exposure); F represents the fastest speed group. Currently, the fastest available film on the market is E speed, as type F has not been released. Of the various types of film, D and E are commercially available. It should be noted that the use of "ultraspeed" film requires precise exposure techniques and darkroom handling (Chapter 90).

Film Storage

Unexposed x-ray film should be stored in a lead-lined container in a location where the atmosphere is cool. X-ray film is inherently sensitive to high temperature, moisture, chemical fumes, and all forms of x-radiation. Since unexposed sensitive materials deteriorate with age, films should be stocked only to the level that they will be used. When the number of unbroken boxes of film is in such excess that they will need storage, they should be placed in the refrigerator and removed at least twelve hours before exposing them. In either case, the time limit indicated by the expiration date printed on the box should be observed and noted.

- Select an outdated film.
- Determine the tube side of the film.
- Carefully break the seal, and open the packet to reveal the components of the packet.

- Observe the transparent film. Is there more than one film present?
- Determine the position of the lead foil backing. Is there more than one sheet of lead backing?
- Observe the black paper. Is there more than one black paper in the packet?

REVIEW

1. What material is used as the base for x-ray films? _____

2. What are the three components of an x-ray film?

   a. _____

   b. _____

   c. _____

3. What is an emulsion? _____

   _____

4. What is the purpose of the lead-foil backing sheet in the film packet? _____

   _____

5. The size of the crystals in the emulsion affects the _____ of the film.

6. Dental films are supplied in the form of _____ that are used for intraoral radiographs.

7. What is the purpose of the supercoating on the film? _____

   _____

8. State the various sizes of intraoral film and the primary use(s) of each.

_____

_____

_____

_____

9. Unexposed dental film should not be used after _____.

Chapter 81: Intraoral Radiographs

INTRODUCTION

A comprehensive understanding of the anatomical arrangement of the internal structure of the mouth with relation to some external **anatomical landmark** aids in positioning the patient in the chair for radiographs. A convenient method is to visualize the part as though it were transparent, so the image of normal structures may be identified in relation to an external landmark.

The relation of the primary beam to the dental area and to the film must be carefully considered. Incorrect placement of the film and inaccurate alignment of the tube are the most common causes of image distortion.

POSITION

Patient Position

The first essential in the standardized procedure is to seat the patient and establish the proper position of the head in relation to the x-ray tube. The chair back and headrest should be adjusted, so the patient's head is properly positioned. If the patient is wearing eyeglasses, they should be removed. Should the patient be wearing a denture, it may remain in place when exposing the periapical of the opposite arch to aid in retention and film holder position. The patient is asked to rinse the mouth with cool water. Should the patient appear nervous or unfamiliar with the routine of radiography, the operator must explain the procedure carefully. This will enable the patient to be more relaxed and cooperative.

Immobilization is imperative, because movements during exposure create a blurred image. Movement of the tubehead and the film packet should be avoided during the exposure. The responsibility for keeping the head and the packet in the established position rests entirely with the operator.

Head Positions for Proper Angulation

For maxillary periapical, interproximal, and maxillary occlusal examinations, the patient's head should be positioned in the headrest, so that the sagittal plane is in a vertical position, figure 81–1. An imaginary line from the **tragus** of the ear (the cartilaginous projection in front of the external auditory meatus) to the **ala** of the nose (the outer side of the nostril) should be horizontal, figure 81–2. The plane of the occlusal surfaces of the maxillary teeth will then be approximately horizontal.

For the mandibular periapical examination, the headrest should be lowered until a line from the tragus to the corner of the mouth is horizontal, figure 81–2. The plane of the occlusal surfaces of the mandibular teeth will then be approximately horizontal when the mouth is open (as required during the exposure). In mandibular occlusal radiography, the head position is altered to suit the desired exposure.

In each instance, the horizontal, or occlusal, plane is considered to be at 0° angulation. Any

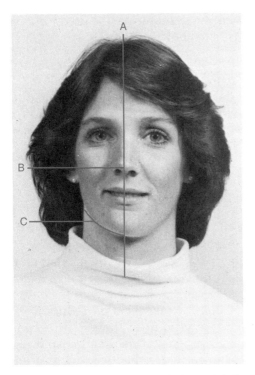

Fig. 81–1. Planes for proper angulation. (A) Sagittal plane. (B) Tip of nose to tragus of ear. (C) One-fourth inch above mandible at apices of mandibular teeth.

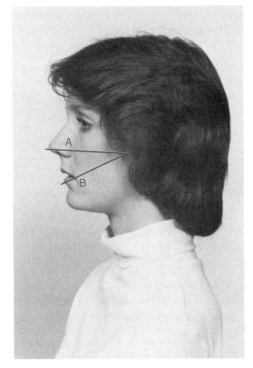

Fig. 81–2. Planes for proper angulation. (A) Ala of nose to tragus of ear. (B) Corner of mouth to tragus of ear.

line or plane intersecting the horizontal plane from above will be at a plus-degree angle to it; any line or plane intersecting it from below will be at a minus-degree angle to it. The angles for the beam of radiation in the procedures are designated as $+°$ or $-°$.

FILM PACKETS

Packet Adaptation

Before intraoral film is exposed, the manner in which the film surface will be presented to the x-ray beam should be carefully considered. An important step to ensure a minimal amount of distortion without discomfort to the patient when the packet is placed in the desired dental area is to preadapt the packet to its exposure position. The packet should never be sharply creased or folded but a corner can be molded over a finger. Adaptation of the packet will do much toward obtaining a satisfactory image. It will minimize the patient's discomfort and shorten the time required for placing the packet.

Placement of Film Packets

Proper placement of the film packet is necessary if excessive bending with resulting distortion of the image and movement during exposure are to be prevented.

When the anterior curvature of the dental arch is sharp, excessive bending of the film may be avoided by inserting a cotton roll between the film and the teeth, thus establishing a rest for the film. Several types of holders for positioning the films are available (Chapters 83, 84, 85).

As all intraoral x-ray film is supplied in packets, it is necessary to place them in the mouth with the correct surface next to the area being exposed. The smooth side of the packet or the so-called *tube side* of the packet is placed toward the teeth (or tube head), and the opposite or opening side of the packet is placed toward the tongue.

In placing the packet in the patient's mouth, some important points should be observed. The packet should never be slid into position because of possible irritation to the oral mucosa. This may cause the patient to gag. Instead, the bitewing packet should be held between the index and middle finger (Chapter 82) of one hand or in a film holder and guided directly to the desired position. *Under no condition should the operator hold the packet in position during an exposure.* Before the exposure is made, the patient should be instructed to relax without changing the position of the packet or the head. In addition, the

following suggestions may be used for a patient who has a tendency to gag:

1. Rinse the mouth with cool water or mouthwash.
2. Ask the patient to breathe deeply and slowly.
3. Ask the patient to hold his or her breath.

Only in rare instances will the dentist prescribe the use of a topical anesthetic.

Exposure Routine

For the patient who has never had a dental x-ray examination, it may be advisable to start a complete periapical survey by making an exposure of a maxillary central incisor region first and then proceeding posteriorly with the balance of the maxillary areas. This procedure is easiest from the standpoint of the patient's comfort. After the maxillary incisor and cuspid regions have been radiographed, the patient will be accustomed to the procedure and will probably find it easier to cooperate when the molar regions are radiographed.

REVIEW

1. The median line of the head should be in the _____ position for routine radiographs.

2. For maxillary exposures, the line from the tragus of the ear to the ala of the nose should be _____.

3. For most mandibular exposures, a line from the tragus of the ear to the _____ is _____.

4. The horizontal or occlusal plane is considered to be at _____ degrees angulation.

5. The angles for the beam of radiation are designated as_____
   and _____.

6. List three suggestions for reducing gagging during radiographic exposure.

   a. _____

   b. _____

   c. _____

After studying this chapter, the student will be able to:
- Prepare a set of four film packets for a bitewing survey.
- Position the cone of the x-ray tubehead for premolar interproximal bitewing exposures.
- Position the cone for molar interproximal exposures.
- Practice placing bitewing films, using a hinged typodont.
- Demonstrate the complete procedure for completing a bitewing survey, using a DXT TRS* mannequin.
- Demonstrate the complete procedure for completing a bitewing survey, using a patient.

INTRODUCTION

Generally, a complete dental radiographic examination, in addition to the periapical films, includes interproximal radiographs of the bicuspids and molars. It is not always necessary or desirable to include interproximal x-ray films of the incisor and cuspid regions.

Certain areas of the teeth cannot be examined except by x-ray films. Cavities may invade the tooth pulp before being discovered by visual examination or periapical film. However, when interproximal film is used, the carious area becomes clearly visible and can be restored before the pulp becomes involved.

PURPOSE

The interproximal (bitewing) examination serves to reveal the presence of interproximal caries, pulp changes (abnormal or otherwise), overhanging restorations, improperly fitted restorative crowns, recurrent caries beneath restorations, and resorption of alveolar bone. It is superior to the periapical examination in certain respects for two reasons:

* Rinn DXT TRS, Rinn Corporation, Elgin, IL.

1. The film surface is placed parallel to the long axes of the crowns of the teeth. The x rays pass through the teeth at nearly a 90° angle, which results in more accurate images of structures, figures 82–1 and 82–2.
2. Images of the coronal and cervical portions of both the maxillary and mandibular teeth, and the alveolar borders of the region are recorded on the same film.

The bitewing film should provide the most accurate representation of the anatomical structure present. There should be no overlapping of the interproximal areas of the teeth. When this occurs, the film should be retaken as it is not useful for diagnosis.

Interproximal film for posterior bitewing exposures is supplied with a tab that extends across the middle of the long aspect of the exposure side of the film packet. Anterior interproximal film has a tab that extends across the short aspect of the exposure side of the film packet.

Periapical film may be used for making interproximal radiographs. When preferred, special tab loops are placed around the film. In the mouth, the tab extends from the film packet between the teeth (the occlusal surfaces of the maxillary and mandibular teeth). The film is held in place by having the patient close his or her teeth firmly on the tab.

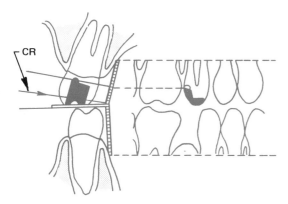

Fig. 82–1. Angle of projection of central ray in bite-wing radiograph that will produce image of caries in a second premolar

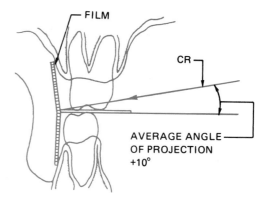

Fig. 82–2. Angle of projection of central ray for bite-wing radiograph—molar

BITEWING TECHNIQUE

Materials Needed

- patient's chart
- basic setup
- film loops
- required number of periapical film
- PID
- paper cup (with patient identification)
- facial tissues
- 2″ × 2″ gauze squares
- cotton rolls
- petroleum jelly
- latex treatment gloves

Preliminary Considerations

It is assumed that the operator has completed disinfection, placed infection-control barriers on the x-ray equipment, and will be using disposable or sterile film-placement accessories.

The operator is attired in a disposable or washable gown, wearing protective eyewear, face mask, and will wear latex treatment gloves.

The patient chart should be available for recording the date, prescription, number of films

exposed, total kVp, and total x-ray exposures (mA). A prescription should always be kept with the patient's records.

Procedural Steps

Prepare the Film

1. Wash and dry your hands.
2. Prepare the film.
   a. Select four No. 2 films.
   b. If you are affixing the tab or loop, assemble all films, making certain the tab is located on the tube side of the film. In placing the loop, allow your index finger to direct the film through the loop. By exerting slight pressure on the film edges, with your thumb and forefinger, the film now has a slight convex shape and will slide easily into the loop, figure 82–3.
   c. Soften the four corners of each film by gently rolling them from the tube side toward the lingual side between the ball of your thumb and forefinger, figure 82–4. *Do not* crease them or use a fingernail to shape them or you will

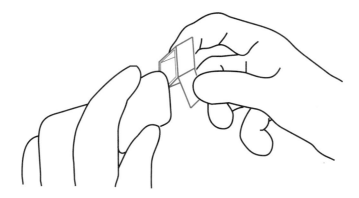

Fig. 82–3. Placing the film loop

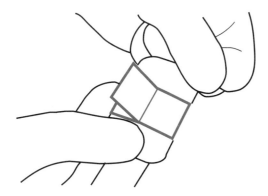

Fig. 82–4. Softening the corners of the film

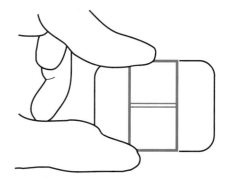

Fig. 82–5. Prepared film

break the emulsion as well as the seal of the packet, resulting in artifacts on the processed film. Place prepared films into a lead-lined storage receptacle.

d. Prepare for placement, figure 82–5. Always position the dot on the film toward the sagittal plane (midline) of the patient. It will appear on the lower corner for the right, figure 82–6, and the upper for the left, figure 82–7.

e. Before positioning film, slide the film back (distally) in the loop for the pre-

molar exposure, figure 82–6. For the molar exposure, slide the film forward (mesially) in the loop, figure 82–7. This will position the tab on the mandibular first molar for either exposure. Figure 82–8 shows four bitewing films with loop and tab in position.

Position the Patient

1. Assemble all necessary equipment: film, paper cup with patient information, and basic setup before the patient is seated.

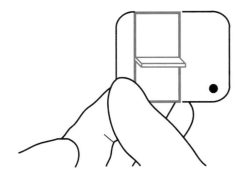

Fig. 82–6. Position of dot, right side

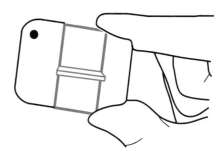

Fig. 82–7. Position of dot, left side

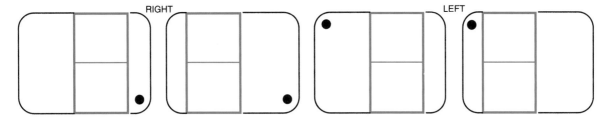

Fig. 82–8. Films with tab / dot in position

   (A) For bicuspid (premolar) film, place so that more of the film is *forward of tab.*
   (B) For molar film, place so that more of the film is *back of tab.*
   (C) Tab will be placed over *mandibular first molar* for both bicuspid (premolar) and molar films.

2. Seat the patient upright in the chair with the head firmly positioned in the headrest.
3. Place the lead apron and protective thyroid collar, figure 79–2.
4. Place the dental napkin, with an additional napkin folded and secured under one clip of the neck chain.
5. Thoroughly wash your hands with germicidal soap and water. Rinse and dry. Don disposable latex treatment gloves.
6. Ask the patient to remove any removable appliance and eyeglasses, if any. Place these items in a safe place, preferably within the patient's view. Direct patient to remove lipstick; offer a tissue. Ask the patient to remove drop earrings if they interfere with the procedure.
7. Lubricate the corners of the mouth, using a small amount of petroleum jelly on the tip of a cotton roll.
8. Using the mouth mirror and a gauze square, examine the mouth. The gauze square will aid in moving and lifting the tongue.
9. Check the x-ray control panel: master switch ON, kVp, mA, and electronic timer.
10. Move the x-ray tubehead to the side (area) of the patient being surveyed.
11. To open the contact areas and interproximals, observe the occlusal surfaces of the

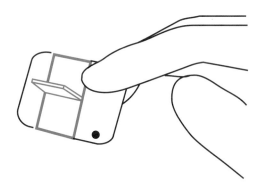

Fig. 82–9. Finger grasp of film

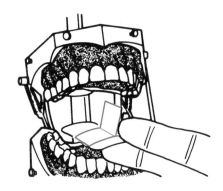

Fig. 82–10. Film in horizontal position using a hinged typodont

teeth. Retract the cheek while standing at the side of the patient, positioning your-self with your eyes on the same plane as the x-ray beam will be directed to. Often, teeth may be rotated or positioned from the normal occlusal pattern.

12. Move the PID into position near the patient's face; adjust the vertical and hori-zontal angulation. Make the exposure.

13. Move the PID away from the patient's face.

14. Remove the film from the patient's mouth, and wipe it free of moisture (saliva), using the folded and secured dental napkin.

15. Drop exposed film into the prepared paper cup; store behind the leaded protective shield until films are processed.

16. Repeat Steps 10 through 15 until all pre-scribed films have been exposed.

Position the Bitewing

1. Select a prepared film from the lead-lined storage box. It is good practice to begin with a premolar exposure, then proceed to the molar area. *Note:* For patient comfort, a moistened 2″ × 2″ gauze square may be placed in the floor of the mouth, at the mesial edge of the film, to cushion the soft tissues.

2. Hold the film with the raised dot toward the apices of the maxillary teeth and with the tab placed distally on the film.

3. With the middle and index finger of one hand, and with the remaining three fingers cupped together, grasp the film between the first joints of the curved fingers and in a diagonal position. This will allow the middle finger to guide the film into posi-tion, as the tip of the index finger rests on the tab, figure 82–9.

4. With the opposite hand, retract the patient's cheek, using the index finger. The pad of the index finger, inserted up to the second joint, should be placed against the mucosa of the cheek. Rotate your wrist and forearm upward, cupping together the remaining four fingers.

5. Carry the film into the mouth in a horizon-tal position, over the tongue, figure 82–10, and gently bring the film into a vertical position as it is placed in the sulcus between the tongue and teeth. With the cheek retracted, bring the tab to rest on the mandibular first molar, figures 82–11 and 82–12.

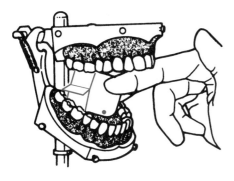

Fig. 82–11. Premolar (bicuspid) placement

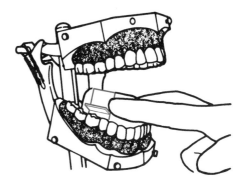

Fig. 82–12. Premolar (bicuspid) placement

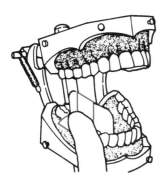

Fig. 82–13. Retention of tab

6. As soon as the packet is in proper position, the operator rotates the index (retraction) finger to stabilize the film by pressing against the tab and the occlusal surface of the mandibular first molar, figure 82–13. (The packet must remain in contact with the lingual mucosa and with the occlusal surface of the molar.)

7. To avoid colliding with the soft tissues in the floor of the mouth, and while continuing to retain the positioned film, gently lift the anterior corner of the packet toward

the median. At no time should the patient be allowed to close on the corner of the film. This causes the film to be driven into the floor of the mouth, resulting in unnecessary pain for the patient, to say nothing of an inferior radiograph.

8. Ask the patient to slowly close on the tab. As the maxillary teeth contact the operator's index finger, the finger is rolled toward the patient's cheek, thus permitting the patient to close on the tab. This places the film half lingually inside the maxillary teeth and half lingually inside the mandibular teeth. The tab should show facially when the cheek is retracted.

9. Fold the extension of the tab on the maxillary facial surface, rather than allowing it to project into the patient's cheek.

10. Position the PID, and adjust vertical and horizontal angulations.

11. Make any final adjustments of the patient's head.

12. Direct the patient to close her or his eyes during each film exposure, to prevent exposure of these sensitive tissues to x-radiation.

13. Direct the patient to temporarily hold her or his breath and not move during the

film exposure, to avoid a blurred image on the radiograph.

14. Step behind the leaded shield. Make the exposure.
15. Remove the film from the patient's mouth and wipe it free of moisture (saliva).
16. Drop exposed film in the prepared paper cup and store behind the leaded shield.

Premolar Bitewing (Right Quadrant)

- Place the film in the film loop, with raised dot toward the apices of the mandibular teeth.
- Follow Procedural Steps, 1 through 16.
- Position the PID, using +5° vertical angulation. Direct the horizontal angulation on the bitewing tab toward the center of the film, between the premolars, and toward the occlusal plane. This angulation will prevent a cone-cut on the processed film, figure 93–4. This projection provides an interproximal image of the distal area of the cuspid, the contacts of the premolars, and the first and second molar on the processed film.

Molar Bitewing (Right Quadrant)

- Place the film mesially in the film loop, with the raised dot toward the apices of the mandibular teeth.
- Follow Procedural Steps 1 through 16.
- Position the PID using a +10° vertical angulation. Direct the horizontal angulation on the bitewing tab toward the center of the film, between the contacts of the first and second molars, and toward the occlusal plane. This projection provides an interproximal image of the distal area of the second premolar, the contacts of the first and second molars and the third molar, plus some of the tuberosity and retromolar area.

Premolar Bitewing (Left Quadrant)

- Place the film distally in the film loop, with the raised dot toward the apices of the maxillary teeth, figure 82–8.

- Angulations and exposures are accomplished in the same manner as for the right premolar quadrant.

Molar Bitewing (Left Quadrant)

- Place the film mesially in the film loop, with the raised dot toward the apices of the maxillary teeth, figure 82–8.
- Angulations and exposures are accomplished in the same manner as for the right molar quadrant.

Finishing Up. When all prescribed film exposures have been completed:

- Return the patient's belongings; dismiss the patient.
- Place films in darkroom for processing.
- Clean and disinfect the x-ray equipment; replace barriers. Sterilize accessories.

SUMMARY

The bitewing examination is considered the least difficult of the intraoral techniques to complete; however, the results of incorrect alignment of the x-ray beam, teeth, and film are often seen on radiographs. Such errors include cone-cutting, overlapped crowns, closed interproximal areas, and improper occlusal planes, Chapter 92.

These errors may be reduced to a minimum by:

1. Determining the correct x-ray beam-teeth-film alignment and the angulation and position of the patient's head.
2. Developing a standardized technique to produce radiographs that are consistently diagnostic.
3. Recording the occlusal plane on a horizontal level.
4. Establishing a positive method to accurately record the interproximal surfaces and contact areas.
5. Eliminating cone-cutting, Chapter 92.

SUGGESTED ACTIVITIES

- Watch a demonstration, then practice placing the film loop on four no. 2 periapical films. Observe the position of the raised dot. Review figure 82–8.
  1. Use a DXT TRS* to position each film. Determine the correct vertical and horizontal angulation of the PID.
  2. Expose the premolar and molar films.
  3. Process the films. Review Chapters 90 and 91. If possible, process half the films manually and half the films in an automatic processor.
  4. Make a list to compare the advantages and disadvantages of each method. *Note:*

* Rinn DXT TRS, Rinn Corporation, Elgin, IL.

It is recommended that the first set of phantom films be self-evaluated and instructor-evaluated, but not graded. This will enable the student to understand how errors can be corrected before attempting a new task.

- Using a fellow student for your patient, seat the person in the dental chair, and make all preparations for a bitewing radiographic survey. Check your procedures under the supervision of the instructor.
  1. Practice placement of the film and angulation of the cone for both the bicuspid (premolar) and molar bitewing films.
  2. Do not turn on the current of the x-ray machine, but perform all the other steps in making a set of bitewing exposures.
  3. Dismiss your patient, and clean up the operatory.

REVIEW

1. List six purposes for an interproximal (bitewing) survey.

   a. _____

   b. _____

   c. _____

   d. _____

   e. _____

   f. _____

2. The images of anatomical structures present on a bitewing film are_____

   _____.

3. How are prepared bitewing films stored prior to placement? _____

   _____

4. How are exposed films stored after exposure and prior to processing? _____

   _____

5. What are the vertical angulations generally recommended in the bitewing technique? _____

   _____

6. The patient's head should be positioned with the occlusal plane _____ and with the sagittal plane _____.

7. Why should a patient close her or his eyes while the film is being exposed?

   _____

   _____

8. The cause of a blurred image on a radiograph is _____

   _____.

9. A cone-cut on a radiograph is due to _____

   _____.

Chapter 83: Bisected-Angle Technique

OBJECTIVES:

After studying this chapter, the student will be able to:
- Describe the basic principle used in the bisected-angle technique.
- Determine the correct angulations for projection of the central ray.
- Demonstrate correct collimator or positioning device and film placement for the maxillary and mandibular arch, using the Rinn Snap-A-Ray holder.

INTRODUCTION

The term *bisected-angle* *technique* describes a method followed for determining the angulation of the x-ray beam. The technique is based on the principle of projecting the x-ray beam at right angles to an imaginary line which bisects (cuts in half) the angle formed by the longitudinal axis of the tooth and the plane of the film packet. This commonly used technique is based on a geometric principle (**Ciezynski's rule of isometry**). Vertical angulation of the central ray is based on this principle, figure 83–1.

The correct angle of projection for the maxillary central area is shown in figure 83–2. If the ray is directed at right angles to the long axis of the teeth, the image in the resultant radiograph will appear elongated, as shown in figure 83–3. If the ray is directed at right angles to the plane of the dental film, the resultant image will appear foreshortened as in figure 83–4. Because it is difficult to determine accurately the position of the bisecting plane, the technique relies heavily on the experience of the operator. To say the least, it is difficult to master the technique. Even the most proficient operator must use approximate

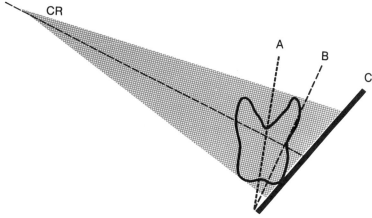

A. longitudinal axis of tooth
B. imaginary bisecting line
C. plane of film
CR central ray

Fig. 83–1. Angulation of the central ray

625

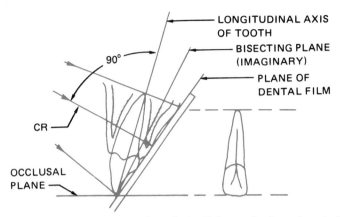

Fig. 83–2. Correct vertical angle (90°) for projection of central ray (CR)

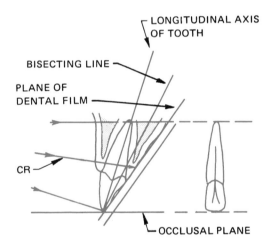

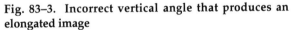

Fig. 83–3. Incorrect vertical angle that produces an elongated image

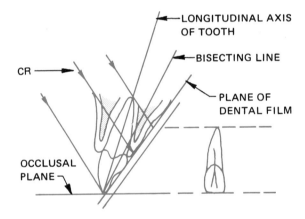

Fig. 83–4. Incorrect vertical angle that produces a foreshortened image

angles based on head position. At best, the bisected-angle angulation technique lacks some accuracy and consistency.

When a high vault of the maxilla causes the packet to assume a more vertical position, the vertical angle should be *decreased* about 5°. When a low vault causes the packet to be less vertical in position, the vertical angle should be *increased* about 5°. In the mandibular region, the

vertical angle is increased 5° when the teeth are inclined or the floor of the mouth is shallow; it is decreased 5° when the teeth are more vertical or the floor of the mouth is deep.

For the *edentulous* (toothless) patient, the film must be placed more nearly horizontal than for the average dentulous mouth. Angulation is increased 5 to 10° more. When surveying the maxillary teeth on children, the angle must be

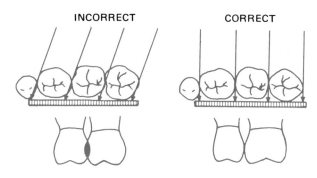

Fig. 83–5. Horizontal angle

increased 5 to 10° because the arch is not fully developed and the film packet is difficult to adapt properly.

PROJECTION OF THE CENTRAL RAY AT A HORIZONTAL ANGLE

The horizontal angulation is determined by directing the central ray through the interproximal spaces (between the teeth) without overlapping adjacent teeth. Examples of correct and incorrect horizontal projections are illustrated in figure 83–5.

Both the vertical and horizontal angulations are dependent on specific head positioning of the patient and correct film placement for success with the bisected-angle technique. Dimensional distortion is an inherent characteristic of this technique.

SIZE AND NUMBER OF FILMS

As the form of the dental arch is studied, it becomes obvious that variation of width and depth can be noted. Using a nineteen- or twenty-film full-mouth survey is now becoming a more common practice. This particular arrangement produces better end results, although it uses a greater number of films. The film placement shown in figure 83–6 will be doubled, producing eight maxillary periapical films, and either seven

or eight mandibular periapical films plus four bitewing radiographs to complete the survey. Depending on the width of the mandibular central to cuspid region, two central-lateral films may be taken or one film with the centrals centered on the film and one on which the laterals will appear. This type of survey uses two sizes of film; the No. 2 (standard) size is used in the posterior regions and for bitewings; and the No. 1 (narrow) for the anterior survey.

The No. 1 (narrow) size film used for the anterior exposures permits a greater degree of patient comfort and lesser tendency for the film to bend and produce distortion. Since each No. 1 film will cover two teeth and their related interproximals, the placement of the cone for the anterior radiograph becomes less complicated than with the use of three No. 2 films for anterior projections.

RINN SNAP-A-RAY FILM HOLDER

Use of a film holder will help to place and stabilize the dental film as it is placed in the mouth. The Rinn Snap-A-Ray can be used, if you prefer to do your own angle bisecting. It is often used for selected single exposures.

The horizontal angulation is determined by directing the central ray at right angles to the tooth and film. The x-ray beam must be aimed through the interproximal spaces to avoid overlapping of tooth structures.

Both angulations depend on specific head positioning of the patient and correct film placement for successful performance of this technique. The Rinn Snap-A-Ray is rather versatile as long as the limitations of the procedure are understood.

Parts of the Holder

The Rinn Snap-A-Ray holder has a pronged end, which is used for anterior maxillary and mandibular projections, figure 83–7. On the

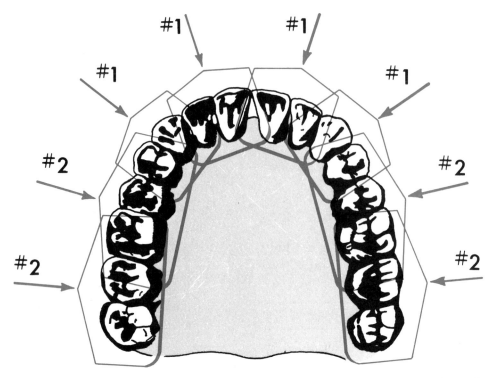

Fig. 83–6. Maxillary arch showing correct film position and projection of the x-ray beam for each periapical radiograph of the teeth

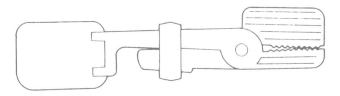

Fig. 83–7. Film in position in holder for anterior areas (Courtesy Rinn Corporation, Elgin, IL)

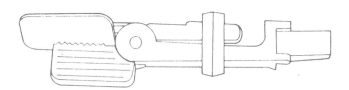

Fig. 83–8. Film in position in holder for most posterior areas (Courtesy Rinn Corporation, Elgin, IL)

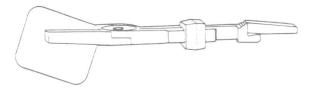

Fig. 83–9. Film in position in holder for mandibular third molar area. The tilt of the film has been exaggerated to conform to the contour of the mandible. (Courtesy Rinn Corporation, Elgin, IL)

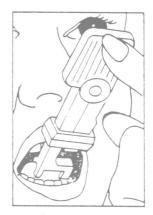

Fig. 83–10. Film placed in holder for mandibular central/lateral incisors

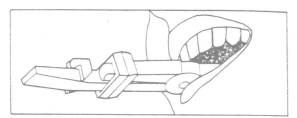

Fig. 83–11. Film placed in holder for maxillary posteriors

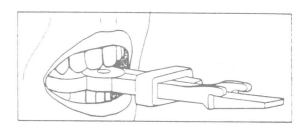

Fig. 83–12. Film placed in holder for mandibular posteriors

opposite end is a biting surface with a narrow and a wide jaw and a sliding friction ring that serves to lock the film in position. These biting surfaces are used for maxillary and mandibular posterior projections. The narrow jaw is most generally used for mandibular posteriors, figure 83–8. The wide jaw is generally used with maxillary posteriors.

Preliminary Considerations

It is advisable to start with the maxillary incisor area, then proceed to the posteriors. Always adjust the tubehead or Position Indicating Device for vertical and horizontal angulation, keeping the end of the collimator or PID and tubehead parallel with the film. Place the PID close to, but not touching, the patient's face; this will ensure proper density and contrast for each film, refer to Chapter 94.

Head positions for the maxillary periapical examination, and for the mandibular periapical projections are covered in Chapter 81 and in figures 81–1 and 81–2.

Film Placement

1. Position film for anterior exposures.
   a. Use No. 1 or No. 2 film; place vertically in mouth.
   b. Soften the corners of the film between thumb and forefinger. Place film in the pronged end of the holder, with dot in the slot. *Do not* crease the film.
   c. Carry the film into place. *Do not* slide into position.
   d. Instruct patient to close firmly but gently to maintain the position of the film by resting teeth in grooves on opposite side of holder. Have patient retain the film

MAXILLARY ARCH

AREA	CONE PLACEMENT-VERTICAL AND HORIZONTAL "RAY"	AVERAGE VERTICAL ANGULATION
Central/Laterals	Center incisors on film. Central ray directed between central/laterals. Horizontal ray side of nose on ala/tragus line.	+40°
Cuspids	Center cuspid on film. Central ray directed at distal of cuspid. Horizontal ray on ala/tragus line.	+45°
Bicuspids (premolars)	Film placed to cover distal of maxillary cuspid. Central ray directed below pupil of eye. Horizontal ray on ala/tragus line.	+30°
Molars	Film placed to cover distal of maxillary second bicuspid. Central ray directed in a line with the outer canthus of eye. Horizontal ray on ala/tragus line.	+20°

MANDIBULAR ARCH

Central/Laterals	Center incisors on film. Central ray directed between central/laterals. Horizontal ray just above lower border of mandible.	−15°
Cuspids	Center cuspid on film. Central ray directed at distal of cuspid. Horizontal ray along lower border of mandible.	−20°
Bicuspids (premolars)	Film placed to cover distal of mandibular cuspid Central ray directed approximately at mesial of mandibular first molar. Horizontal ray just above lower border of mandible.	−10°
Molars	Film placed to cover distal of mandibular second bicuspid. Central ray directed distal of second molar, approximately in a line with the outer canthus of eye. *Note:* For third molars, film may have to be placed further back in mouth in order to have full view of roots—PID will then have to be moved back also.	−5°

Fig. 83–13. PID placement and angulation, Rinn Snap-A-Ray Holder

holder with tips of fingers, and at the same time, push downward on the opposite end of the holder; the mandibular teeth will act as a fulcrum for the maxillary placement. The opposite retention would be used for the mandibular projections, figure 83–9.

e. Use the PID Placement and Angulation Chart (refer ahead to figure 83–13) for centrals or laterals and cuspids, figure 83–10.

2. Position film for posterior exposures, figures 83–11 and 83–12.

a. Use No. 2 film; place horizontally in mouth.

b. Soften the corners of the film between thumb and forefinger. Place it in the jaw (biting surface) of the holder with the dot in the slot, figure 83–8. *Do not crease the film.* Slide friction ring into position, with just enough pressure to hold the film securely.

c. When using the wide biting surface of the holder for maxillary areas, you can position the film farther away from the lingual surface of the teeth by having the patient bite close to the outer edge. By so doing, the maxillary edge can be brought to the roof of the mouth and the lower edge away from the crowns of the teeth as far as the width of the Snap-A-Ray jaw will permit. This will position the film almost, if not parallel to most maxillary posterior teeth, figure 83–11. The mandibular posterior technique is the reverse of the maxillary area, figure 83–12.

d. Use the Cone Placement and Angulation Chart, figure 83–13, for premolars and molars.

SUMMARY

Placement and retention of the packets are the primary responsibility of the operator. Digital retention (the patient holds the film packet in place, using his fingers and light pressure to prevent movement) should be avoided if possible. The operator should *never* hold the film. Disposable styrofoam blocks and plastic film holders are used as a matter of preference in most offices.

Supplementary views of teeth are often necessary to reveal some aspect of dental structure that may be hidden when a standard placement and projection are used. In such instances, the horizontal angle, the vertical angle, and the method of placement may vary. In all cases, the important thing to remember is to *avoid shaping the film to the arch*—a flat film surface must be ensured regardless of the procedure used.

SUGGESTED ACTIVITIES

• Practice exposing periapical films, using a dental x-ray training (DXT TRS*) mannequin or skull, and the Snap-A-Ray.
• Process and evaluate films for their diagnostic quality.

* Rinn DXT TRS, Rinn Corporation, Elgin, IL.

REVIEW

1. In the bisected-angle technique, state the principle that must be considered to produce an accurate image on the film. _____

   _____

   _____

2. If the central ray is directed at right angles to the long axis of the teeth, _____ of the image will result; if the ray is directed at right angles to the plane of the dental film, the image will appear _____.

3. For a high vault of the maxilla, the vertical angulation should be _____
   _____; for a low vault, the vertical angulation
          (increased, decreased)
   should be _____.
                    (increased, decreased)

4. Overlapping images of properly aligned teeth on dental films generally
   indicates incorrect _____ projection.

5. Three methods used to retain film during exposure are:

   a. _____

   b. _____

   c. _____

Chapter 84: Rinn Bisected-Angle Technique

OBJECTIVES:

After studying this chapter, the student will be able to:
- Assemble the Rinn bisecting-angle components for anterior film placement.
- Assemble the BAI instruments for the posterior left maxillary and right mandibular film placement.
- Assemble the BAI for the posterior right maxillary and left mandibular film placement.
- Place the correct film in each BAI.
- Demonstrate correct film and collimator or position indicating device (PID) placement for each region of the oral cavity, using a 12-inch PID.

INTRODUCTION

The Rinn bisecting-angle instruments (BAI) are designed to reduce to a minimum some of the variables of angulation, specific head positioning, and dimensional distortion. These inherent characteristics of the bisected-angle technique may be reduced by:

1. Automatically indicating the correct horizontal and vertical angulation, thus eliminating the need for numerically setting the angulation and for placing the patient's head in a predetermined position.
2. Simplifying the technique, making it easy to master and teach.
3. Standardizing the technique, making accurate duplication of postoperative radiographs the same as the preoperatives.
4. Minimizing curved film plane distortion, (Chapter 92).
5. Eliminating cone-cutting, (Chapter 92).

RINN BAI INSTRUMENTS COMPONENTS

1. **Bite blocks**—designed to hold all sizes and brands of periapical x-ray film. BAI bite blocks differ for anterior and posterior, figure 84-1.
2. Aiming rings—plastic rings used to bring the film "on target." Aiming rings for anterior and posterior films differ, figure 84-2.
3. Indicator rods (arms)—two-pronged rod used by inserting into openings (holes) on the bite block. Anterior and posterior aiming rods differ, figure 84-3.

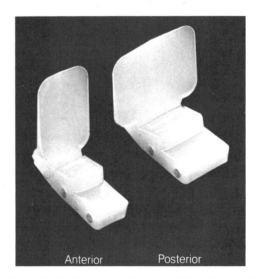

Anterior   Posterior

Fig. 84-1. BAI bite blocks (Courtesy Rinn Corporation, Elgin, IL)

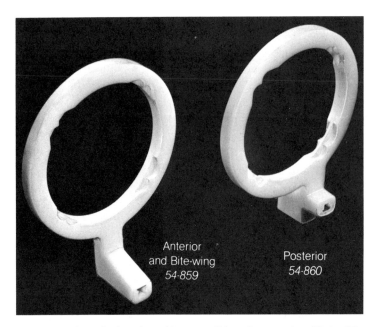

Fig. 84–2. Rinn aiming rings (Courtesy Rinn Corporation, Elgin, IL)

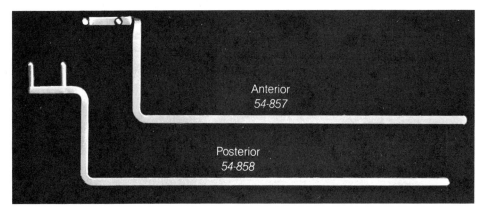

Fig. 84–3. Rinn indicator rods (arms) (Courtesy Rinn Corporation, Elgin, IL)

Assembly Instructions

The same procedure for assembly of the BAI components is followed for all instrumentation, figure 84–4. However, prongs of the posterior rod should be positioned in the openings on the left side of the bite block for left maxillary and right mandibular placement. This is accomplished by inverting the assembled components. Position the prongs in the right side of the bite block for right maxillary and left mandibular projections. Assembled components must be inverted.

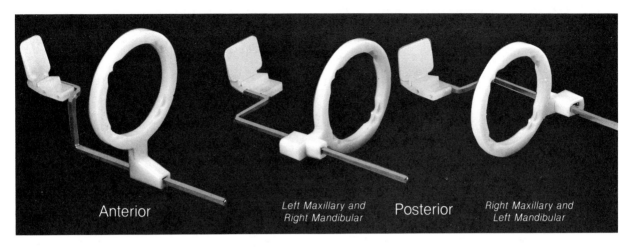

Fig. 84–4. Rinn BAI components properly assembled (Courtesy Rinn Corporation, Elgin, IL)

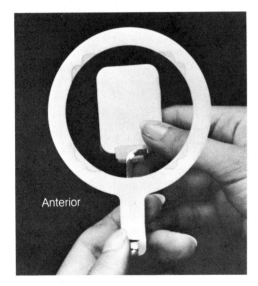

Fig. 84–5. Anterior instrument is correctly assembled with film "on target."

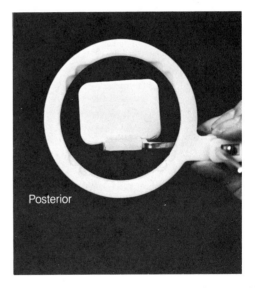

Fig. 84–6. Posterior instrument is correctly assembled with film "on target."

The angled portion of the indicator rod must be positioned away from the biting surfaces of the bite block.

1. Insert the two prongs of the indicator rod into holes in the bite block.
2. Insert indicator rod into aiming ring slot.

3. Flex backing plate of bite block to open film slot for easy insertion of film packet. Make sure the film packet is inserted completely into the slot, with the dot in the slot.
4. Instrument is correctly assembled when film can be seen through aiming ring "on target," figures 84–5 and 84–6.

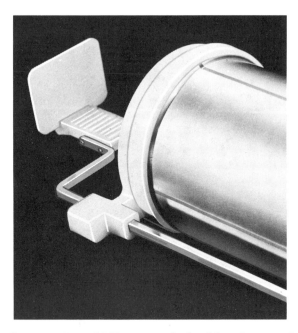

Fig. 84–7. Round PIDs are set flush with and centered on the aiming ring. Shown with XCP bite block. (Courtesy Rinn Corporation, Elgin, IL)

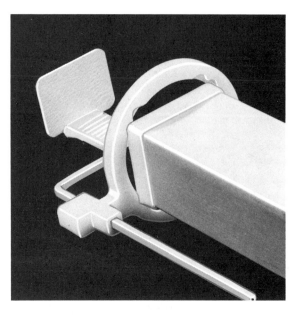

Fig. 84–8. Rectangular PIDs fit into indented alignment guides on the anterior and posterior aiming rings. Shown with XCP bite block. (Courtesy Rinn Corporation, Elgin, IL)

5. Place the Position Indicating Device (PID). When using the round PID, set it flush and centered on the aiming ring. The arm of the indicator rod should run parallel with the PID, figure 84–7. The rectangular PID fits into indented guides on the aiming ring for anterior and posterior films. These guides are provided for vertical and horizontal placement, figure 84–8.

MAXILLARY INCISOR REGION

1. Assemble anterior instrument, figures 84–4 and 84–5, and insert film packet vertically into anterior bite block, pushing film packet all the way into slot. Plain side of film packet should be positioned away from backing plate toward the aiming ring. Narrow #1 film may be used.

This requires an individual exposure for lateral incisors.

2. Center film packet on central incisors. Entire horizontal length of bite block should be utilized to position film as posterior as possible.

3. With bite block placed on incisal edges of teeth to be radiographed, instruct patient to close slowly, but firmly, to retain position of film packet. A cotton roll may be placed between mandibular teeth and block for patient comfort.

4. Slide aiming ring down the indicator rod to skin surface, and align the PID of the x-ray unit in close approximation to aiming ring and centered, figure 84–9.

5. Press x-ray machine activating button, and make exposure.

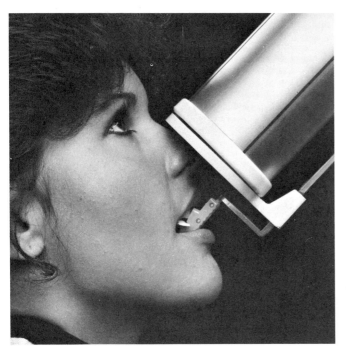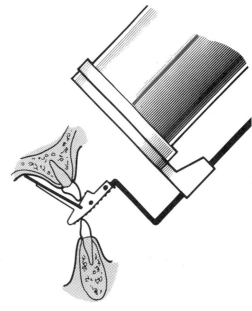

Fig. 84–9. Maxillary incisor region (Courtesy Rinn Corporation, Elgin, IL)

MAXILLARY LATERAL INCISOR REGION

1. Assemble anterior instrument, figures 84–4 and 84–5, and insert film packet vertically into anterior bite block, pushing film packet all the way into slot. Plain side of film packet should be positioned away from backing plate toward the aiming ring. Narrow #1 film is required.
2. Center film packet on lateral incisor, positioning film as close as possible to lingual surface of teeth.
3. After the bite block is positioned on incisal edges of maxillary teeth to be radiographed, instruct the patient to protrude lower jaw and close slowly, but firmly, to retain position of film packet. A cotton roll may be placed between mandibular teeth and block for patient comfort.

4. Slide aiming ring down the indicator rod to skin surface, and align the PID of the x-ray unit in close approximation to aiming ring and centered, figure 84–10.
5. Press x-ray machine activating button, and make exposure.

MAXILLARY CUSPID REGION

1. Assemble anterior instrument, figures 84–4 and 84–5, and insert film packet vertically into anterior bite block, pushing film packet all the way into slot. Plain side of film packet should be positioned away from backing plate toward the aiming ring. Narrow #1 film is recommended. When using #2 films, slightly roll upper anterior corner of film packet to facilitate positioning.
2. Position film packet with cuspid and first bicuspid (premolar) centered on film.

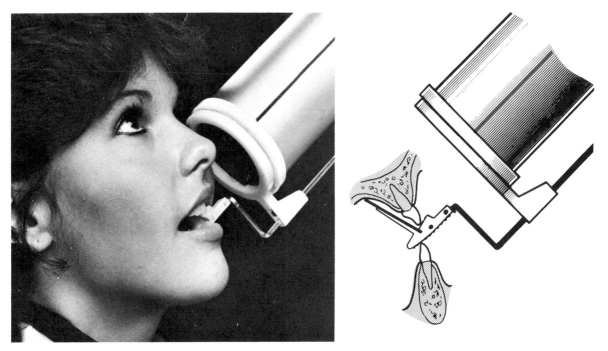

Fig. 84–10. Maxillary lateral incisor region (Courtesy Rinn Corporation, Elgin, IL)

Place film as close as possible to lingual surface of teeth.

3. With bite block positioned on maxillary teeth to be radiographed, instruct patient to close slowly, but firmly, to retain position of film packet. A cotton roll may be placed between mandibular teeth and block for patient comfort.

4. Slide aiming ring down the indicator rod to skin surface, and align the PID of the x-ray unit in close approximation to aiming ring and centered, figure 84–11.

5. Press x-ray machine activating button, and make exposure.

MAXILLARY BICUSPID (PREMOLAR) REGION

1. Assemble posterior instrument, figures 84–4, 84–6, and insert film packet horizontally into posterior bite block, pushing film packet all the way into slot. Plain side of film packet would be positioned away from backing plate toward the aiming ring. Slightly roll upper anterior corner of film packet to facilitate positioning.

2. Center film packet on the second bicuspid (premolar), positioning as close as possible to lingual surfaces of teeth.

3. With bite block positioned on the occlusal surfaces of the maxillary teeth to be radiographed, instruct patient to close slowly, but firmly, to retain position of film packet. A cotton roll may be placed between mandibular teeth and block for patient comfort.

4. Slide aiming ring down the indicator rod to skin surface, and align the PID of the x-ray unit in close approximation to aiming ring and centered, figure 84–12.

5. Press x-ray machine activating button, and make exposure.

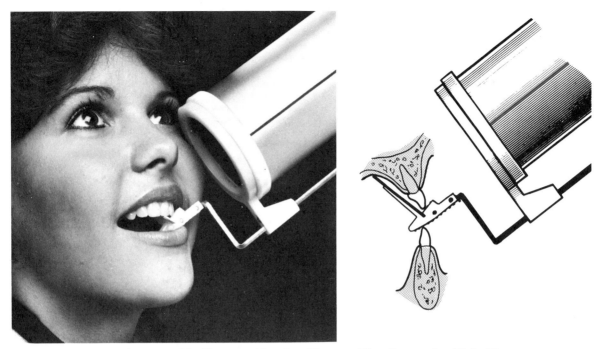

Fig. 84–11. Maxillary cuspid region (Courtesy Rinn Corporation, Elgin, IL)

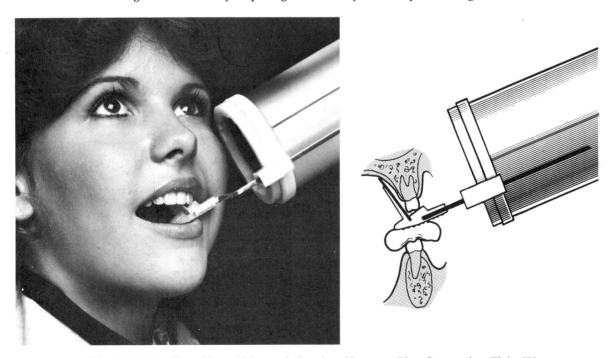

Fig. 84–12. Maxillary bicuspid (premolar) region (Courtesy Rinn Corporation, Elgin, IL)

MAXILLARY MOLAR REGION

1. Assemble posterior instrument, figures 84–4 and 84–6, and insert film packet horizontally into posterior bite block, pushing film packet all the way into slot. Plain side of film packet should be positioned away from backing plate toward the aiming ring. Slightly roll upper posterior corner of film packet to facilitate positioning.
2. Center film packet on second molar, positioning as close as possible to lingual surfaces of teeth.
3. With bite block positioned on occlusal surfaces of the maxillary teeth to be radiographed, instruct patient to close slowly, but firmly, to retain position of film packet. A cotton roll may be placed between mandibular teeth and block for patient comfort.

4. Slide aiming ring down the indicator rod to skin surface and align the PID of the x-ray unit in close approximation to aiming ring and centered, figure 84–16.
5. Press x-ray machine activating button, and make exposure.

MANDIBULAR INCISOR REGION

1. Assemble anterior instrument, figures 84–4 and 84–5, and insert film packet vertically into anterior bite block, pushing film packet all the way into slot. Plain side of film packet should be positioned away from backing plate toward the aiming ring. Narrow #1 film may be used.
2. Center film packet on central incisors, positioning as close as possible to lingual surfaces of teeth to be radiographed.
3. With bite block placed on edges of mandibular incisors, instruct patient to

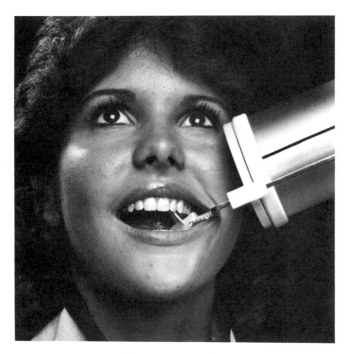
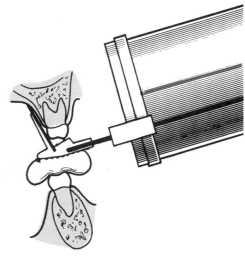

Fig. 84–13. Maxillary molar region (Courtesy Rinn Corporation, Elgin, IL)

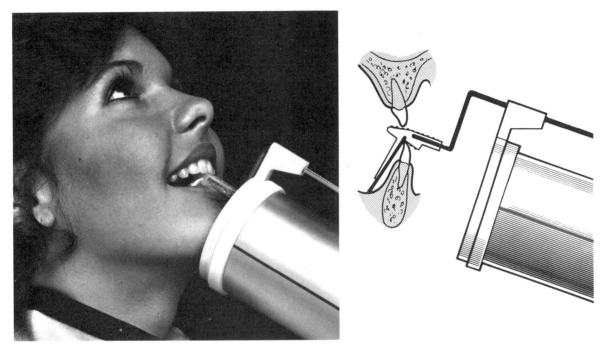

Fig. 84–14. Mandibular incisor region (Courtesy Rinn Corporation, Elgin, IL)

close slowly, but firmly, to retain position of film. A cotton roll may be placed between maxillary teeth and block for patient comfort.

4. Slide aiming ring down the indicator rod to skin surface, and align the PID of the x-ray unit in close approximation to aiming ring and centered, figure 84–14.

5. Press x-ray machine activating button, and make exposure.

MANDIBULAR CUSPID REGION

1. Assemble anterior instrument, figures 84–4 and 84–5, and insert film packet vertically into anterior bite block, pushing film packet all the way down into slot. Plain side of film packet should be positioned away from backing plate toward the aiming ring. Narrow #1 film may be used. When using #2 film, roll lower anterior corner of film packet slightly to facilitate positioning.

2. Center film packet on cuspid and first bicuspid (premolar), positioning as close as possible to lingual surfaces of teeth to be radiographed.

3. With bite block placed on edges of mandibular teeth to be radiographed, instruct patient to close slowly, but firmly, to retain position of film. A cotton roll may be placed between maxillary teeth and block for patient comfort.

4. Slide aiming ring down the indicator rod to skin surface, and align the PID of the x-ray unit in close approximation to aiming ring and centered, figure 84–15.

5. Press x-ray machine activating button, and make exposure.

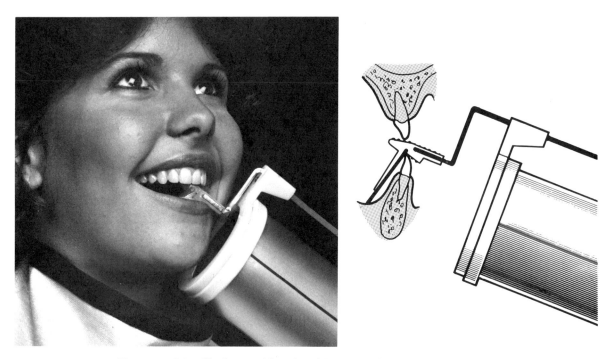

Fig. 84–15. Mandibular cuspid region (Courtesy Rinn Corporation, Elgin, IL)

MANDIBULAR BICUSPID (PREMOLAR) REGION

1. Assemble posterior instrument, figures 84–4 and 84–6, and insert film packet horizontally into posterior bite block, pushing film packet all the way into slot. Plain side of film packet should be positioned away from backing plate toward the aiming ring. Roll lower anterior corner of film packet slightly to facilitate positioning.

2. Center film packet on second bicuspid (premolar), positioning as close as possible to lingual surfaces of teeth to be radiographed.

3. With bite block placed on occlusal surfaces of mandibular teeth to be radiographed, instruct patient to close slowly, but firmly, to retain position of film. A cotton roll may be placed between maxillary teeth and block for patient comfort.

4. Slide aiming ring down the indicator rod to skin surface, and align the PID of the x-ray unit in close approximation to aiming ring and centered, figure 84–16.

5. Press x-ray machine activating button, and make exposure.

MANDIBULAR MOLAR REGION

1. Assemble posterior instrument, figures 84–4 and 84–6, and insert film packet horizontally into posterior bite block, pushing film packet all the way into slot. Plain side of film packet should be away from backing plate and toward the aiming ring. Roll lower posterior corner of film packet slightly to facilitate positioning.

2. Center film packet on second molar, positioning as close as possible to lingual surfaces of teeth to be radiographed. Anterior

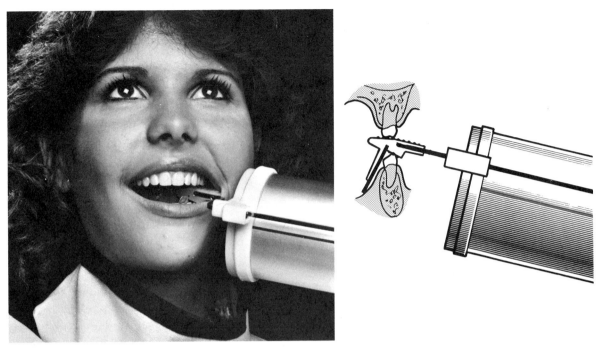

Fig. 84–16. Mandibular bicuspid (premolar) region (Courtesy Rinn Corporation, Elgin, IL)

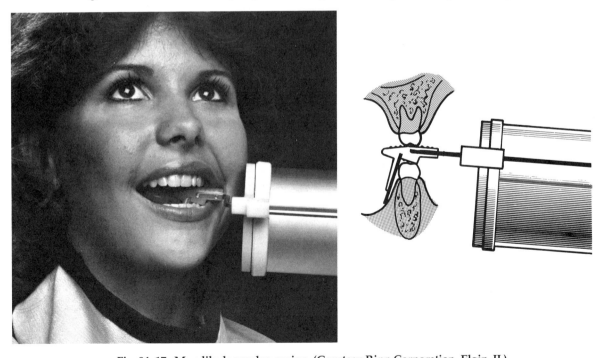

Fig. 84–17. Mandibular molar region (Courtesy Rinn Corporation, Elgin, IL)

border of film packet should align with distal portion of second bicuspid (premolar).

3. With bite block placed on occlusal surfaces of mandibular teeth to be radiographed, instruct patient to close slowly, but firmly, to retain position of film packet. A cotton roll may be placed between maxillary teeth and block for patient comfort.

4. Slide aiming ring down the indicator rod to skin surface, and align the PID of the x-ray unit in close approximation to aiming ring and centered, figure 84–17.

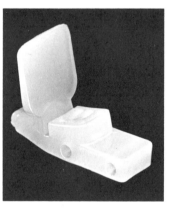

Fig. 84–18. BAI anterior bite block (child) (Courtesy Rinn Corporation, Elgin, IL)

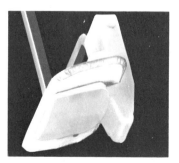

Fig. 84–19. Posterior bite block (child) (Courtesy Rinn Corporation, Elgin, IL)

5. Press x-ray machine activating button, and make exposure.

RADIOGRAPHIC TECHNIQUE FOR THE CHILD PATIENT (BAI)

The full-mouth survey for children is possible with a maximum of six to eight films. As with the adult patient, exposure should be kept to a minimum, under strict adherence to the ALARA concept (Chapter 78).

A No. 0 film is placed in the child's mouth with a plastic holder. The anterior bite block is reduced in size from that used for adults, to accommodate a vertically positioned film. The backing plate is cut down to a level slightly lower than the height of the film. The length of the bite block biting surface remains the same as that used in the conventional technique, as do the aiming rings and indicator rods (arms).

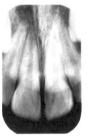 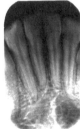

Fig. 84–20. Incisor films (child) (Courtesy Rinn Corporation, Elgin, IL)

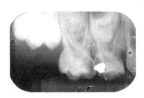 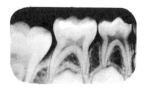

Fig. 84–21. Posterior films (child) (Courtesy Rinn Corporation, Elgin, IL)

Anterior Region

1. Assemble the anterior instrument, figures 84–4 and 84–5, and insert a No. 0 film packet vertically into anterior bite block, figure 84–18.
2. Follow Steps 1 through 4—incisor region and conventional BAI technique.
3. Check the exposure chart before activating the exposure button. A child's tissue is less dense, thus the exposure time will be less than for an adult.

Posterior Region

1. Assemble the posterior instrument, figures 84–4 and 84–6, and insert a No. 0 film horizontally into posterior bite block, figure 84–19.
2. Follow Steps 1 through 4—posterior region and BAI technique.
3. Check exposure time. Press activating button and make exposure.

Note: Typical exposures for children are shown in figures 84–20 and 84–21.

SUGGESTED ACTIVITIES

- Under the supervision of the instructor, prepare and place film in a DXTRR phantom or skull. Use the Rinn BAI and an 8-inch PID.
- Expose and process the film for diagnostic quality.

REVIEW

1. In what ways does use of the Rinn BAI instruments reduce the inherent characteristics of the bisected-angle technique? _____

_____

_____

2. What is the purpose of a cotton roll when placing the block with the film?

_____

_____

_____

3. Narrow films are recommended for which areas? _____

_____

_____

4. No. 0 films are recommended for which patients? Areas? _____

_____

_____

Chapter 85: Paralleling Technique

OBJECTIVES:

After studying this chapter, the student will be able to:
- Compare the bisecting-angle technique with the paralleling technique.
- State the principles for the projection of the central ray with the paralleling technique.
- Differentiate between disadvantages and advantages of the paralleling technique.
- Determine the proper film placement and angulation of the central ray for various areas of the oral cavity, using the paralleling technique.

INTRODUCTION

The paralleling technique has proven to be a practical one for periapical radiography in the dental practice. The value of the dental x-ray examination depends on the quality of processed films and their interpretation. A good-quality radiograph should show dental structures clearly and accurately.

It has been established that the bisected-angle technique (Chapter 83), produces certain undesirable radiographic results. The most objectionable is dimensional distortion.

PARALLELING TECHNIQUE

Along with the advantages of the paralleling technique, there are disadvantages. First, there is the problem of attaining parallel film placement in all areas of the oral cavity. Parallelism is rather easily established in the mandibular molar region, where the lingual alveolar process is relatively thin; therefore, the film can be placed closer to the teeth. In the maxillary molar and premolar (bicuspid) region, it is necessary to position the film at the midline of the palate and some distance from the teeth. In the maxillary anterior region, narrow films must be used, and as a result, often no more than one tooth is satisfactorily shown. The same problem holds for the mandibular anterior teeth.

The previous problems can be somewhat minimized by utilizing a styrofoam bite block or plastic film holder. Both permit the film to be brought to the center of the vault, nearly parallel with the teeth, without discomfort to the patient. Of the several types of accessory devices for holding the film in position, experience has shown that they should be **radiolucent** (permitting the passage of x rays), economical, easy to use, and capable of withstanding sterilization, or disposable.

The paralleling technique for periapical radiography will minimize dimensional distortion and result in a more true anatomical relationship and size. It involves placing the plane of the film parallel with the long axes of the teeth. Basic to any technique is the principle that image sharpness is primarily affected by increased anode-film distance (AFD), the size of the focal spot of the central ray, and motion, figure 85–1. The paralleling technique favorably meets this criteria.

When a longer position indicating device (PID) is used (and the anode-film distance increased), the x rays reaching the film tend to be more nearly parallel, and magnification of the image is decreased. Because magnification is less, it is possible to position the film farther away from the teeth in a plane parallel to the long axes. As with any technique, every effort must be made to eliminate motion of the patient

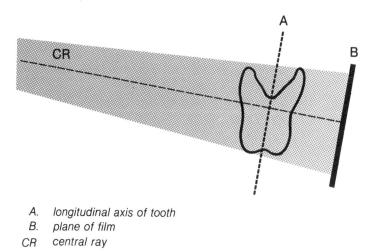

A.   longitudinal axis of tooth
B.   plane of film
CR   central ray

Fig. 85–1. Angulation of the central ray (Courtesy Rinn Corporation, Elgin, IL)

or vibration of the tubehead during the exposure. Such motion increases the focal-spot size and results in a hazy or blurred image.

When done properly, the paralleling technique will produce diagnostic intraoral radiographs with less distortion of the images (teeth and surrounding structures) than those produced with the bisected-angle technique. (Refer ahead to figures 85–2 and 85–3).

Certain essentials must be maintained for successful completion of this technique.

1. Keep the film flat; use an accessory device.
2. Position the film, except in the mandibular molar area, lingually as far as possible to cover the apices of the teeth.
3. Position the film parallel with the long axes of the teeth.
4. Increase the AFD to minimize dimensional distortion.
5. Keep the face of the open PID parallel with the plane of the film and thus ensure that all of the film is covered by the x-ray beam.

For anterior maxillary and mandibular film exposures, use No. 1 film, placed in a vertical position. For posterior maxillary and mandibular projections, use No. 2 film placed in a horizontal position.

Film Placement

It is important to remember that the position of the film must be more lingually placed for mandibular exposures, and near center of the vault for the maxillary.

1. Center the film in the holder by sliding it along the backing support of the holder, with the dot in the slot. Make certain the film is secured with the edge completely in the slot and with the plain side of the film away from the backing plate toward the aiming ring.
2. Soften the lingual (palatal) corners of the film between the thumb and forefinger.
3. Introduce the film and backing support in a slanted position, with the film parallel to the long axes of the teeth. Seat the biting

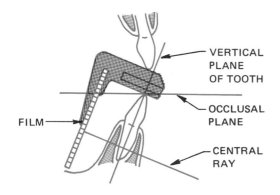

Fig. 85–2. Film placed in disposable holder for mandibular central or lateral exposure

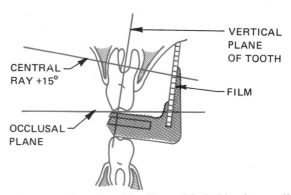

Fig. 85–3. Film placed in disposable holder for maxillary molar exposure

surface of the holder on the biting edges of the teeth under survey.

4. Ask the patient to close the opposing teeth on the block to retain the film. *Note:* When using a disposable film holder or an XCP holder with an aiming ring, the biting portion that extends facially beyond the incisal or occlusal surfaces of the teeth will indicate the horizontal center of the film, figures 85–2 and 85–3.
5. Position the face of the open cone parallel to the plane of the film, which should then direct the central ray toward the center of the film and perpendicular to the film and object.

SUMMARY

With the central ray directed perpendicularly to the two planes (the film and the teeth), a truer profile and relative registration of the shadow images are the result on the radiograph. This technique also employs a slightly increased object-film distance and an increased AFD. Some advantages of this technique include:

1. Sharpness of details.
2. Minimal enlargement and control of malar bone shadow.
3. Images of teeth nearly anatomically accurate from right-angle exposures and flat surfaces of film.
4. Alveolar crest in true relationship to the teeth.
5. Increased film clarity and contrast.

SUGGESTED ACTIVITY

• Demonstrate (to the class) the paralleling technique, indicating the x-ray tube and central ray, the film and the object. Under supervision of the instructor, practice preparation and placement of the film, using a DXT TRS* phantom or skull. Position the cone. Expose and process the films for diagnostic quality.

* Rinn DXT TRS, Rinn Corporation, Elgin, IL.

REVIEW

1. What are some of the advantages of the paralleling technique? _____

_____

_____

_____

2. What are the disadvantages of the paralleling technique? _____

_____

_____

_____

3. What are the requisites of any accessory device used for positioning? _____

_____

_____

_____

Chapter 86: Rinn Extension Cone Paralleling Technique (XCP)

OBJECTIVES:

After studying this chapter, the student will be able to:
- State the principles used as a basis for the Rinn Extension Cone Paralleling Technique (XCP), using a 12- or 16-inch PID.
- Discuss four advantages of the XCP Technique.
- Assemble the components of the Rinn XCP instruments.
- Determine the proper position of the film, cone, and paralleling instruments for the anterior film exposures.
- Determine the proper position of the film, cone, and paralleling instruments for each posterior quadrant of the oral cavity.

INTRODUCTION

Paralleling techniques require the use of a film-holding device. One of the most commonly used is the Rinn XCP instrument* (extension cone paralleling).

Extension cone paralleling (XCP) is a practical technique for periapical radiography that minimizes dimensional distortion and presents the objects being radiographed in their true anatomical relationship and size. A film-holding device, very similar to that used for the bisected-angle technique, will direct the position of the film and position indicating device (PID) to meet the principles of the paralleling technique. This systematic procedure is based on the following principles:

1. Paralleling the film with the longitudinal axes of the teeth to diminish dimensional distortion.
2. Increasing the anode-film (source) distance (AFD) to avoid image enlargement and *adumbration*; i.e., the images of the teeth are overshadowed by an object, as occurs with the superimposition of the malar bone over the apices of the teeth on a maxillary posterior film.

* Rinn XCP instrument, Rinn Corporation, Elgin, IL.

3. Directing alignment of the x-ray beam to assure correct vertical and horizontal angulation.

Advantages of the XCP technique include:

1. Simplicity—eliminates the need for predetermined angulation and positioning of the patient's head.
2. Adaptability—can be used in most offices regardless of space limitations by rotating the chair or the patient's head.
3. Reliability—anatomical accuracy of tooth size and length and size of canals is assured.
4. Results—radiographs that reproduce anatomical structures in their normal size and relationship, free of distortion with minimal superimposition of the zygomatic shadow and exhibiting maximum detail and definition.

RINN EXTENSION CONE PARALLELING (XCP) INSTRUMENT COMPONENTS

Bite Blocks

Designed to achieve true parallelism of the longitudinal axes of the teeth and the plane of the film, XCP bite blocks have greater length to the grooved biting surface than those used for the bisected-angle technique. The backing plate for the anterior instrument is positioned at right angles to the biting surface. Anterior and posterior XCP bite blocks differ, figure 86–1.

Aiming Rings

Plastic rings used to bring the film "on target." The same rings are used for both bisecting-angle

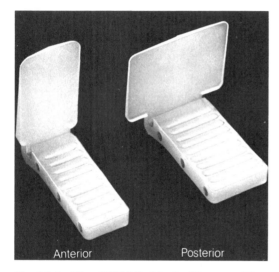

Fig. 86–1. Rinn XCP bite blocks (Courtesy Rinn Corporation, Elgin, IL)

instruments (BAI) and XCP. Aiming rings for anterior and posterior films differ.

Indicator Rods (Arms)

The same rods are used for both BAI and XCP. Anterior and posterior rods (arms) differ.

ASSEMBLY INSTRUCTIONS

Figure 86–2 shows the properly assembled XCP instrument components. The angled portion of the indicator rod must be positioned away from the biting surfaces of the bite block.

1. Insert the two prongs of the indicator rod into the holes of the bite block. On anterior three-hole blocks, use the two forward holes (away from the backing plate). The third opening is for use when the bite block needs to be shortened for an extremely narrow arch, figure 86–3.
2. Insert indicator rod into aiming slot, figure 86–4.
3. Flex backing plate of bite block to open film slot, for easy insertion of film packet. Make sure the film packet is inserted completely into the slot, with the dot in the slot, figure 86–5.

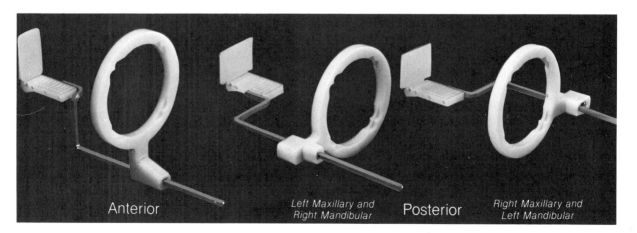

Fig. 86–2. Rinn XCP instrument components properly assembled (Courtesy Rinn Corporation, Elgin, IL)

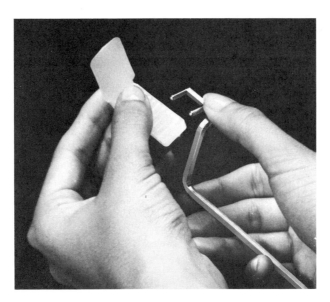

Fig. 86–3. Insert the two prongs of the indicator rod into openings in the bite block as shown. On three-hole blocks, use the two forward holes (away from the backing plate). The third opening is for use when the bite block is shortened for pedo technique.

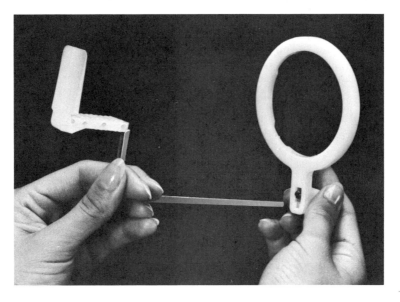

Fig. 86–4. Insert indicator rod into the aiming ring slot.

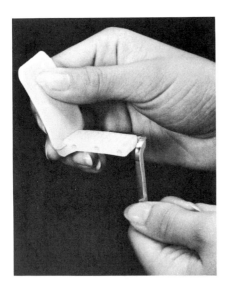

Fig. 86–5. Flex backing plate of bite block to open film slot.

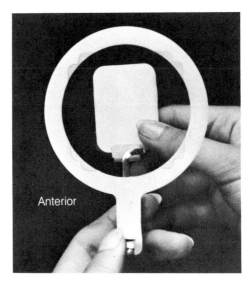

Fig. 86–6. Anterior instrument is correctly assembled with film "on target."

4. When assembling an anterior instrument, make sure that the film is "on target," figure 86–6.

PLACING THE FILM INSIDE THE MOUTH

Hold the instrument by the paralleling rod and ring. For maxillary films, tilt the top portion of the film toward the center of the mouth, making a *V* shape with the bite block, figure 86–7. Keeping this angle, guide the bite block up to contact the tooth of interest. This will avoid scraping the film across the intraoral tissues.

For mandibular films, lift the tongue with your index finger, and allow the lower border of the film packet to slide into place between the tongue and lingual side of the teeth. Keep the film approximately 1/4 inch away from the lingual side of the teeth. Do not place the film in direct contact with the lingual surface of the teeth.

When instructing the patient to bring the teeth together on the bite block, use the phrase, "Slowly, close, please." This will allow you to keep the film where it was placed and to remove your finger before the teeth close on it.

MAINTAINING PATIENT COOPERATION

Place and expose the film as quickly as possible. Remove the film as soon as it has been exposed. At best, this procedure is not a comfortable one for many patients. Keeping the film in the patient's mouth for as short a time as possible, tends to increase patient cooperation.

Begin with the easiest films, probably the maxillary anterior. With these successfully accomplished, the patient is likely to cooperate for t' ε remaining exposures.

Be as quick and gentle as possible. Be sure of yourself. Learn as much of the procedure as you can by practicing and learning it as much as you can before actually exposing a full-mouth series of radiographs on a patient.

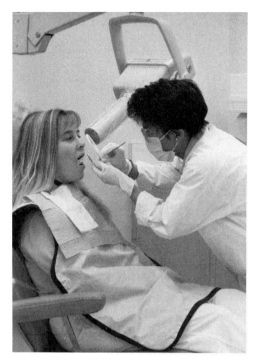

Fig. 86–7. Placing the film in the mouth, making a *V* shape with the bite block (Courtesy Registered Dental Hygiene Program, Pasadena City College, Pasadena, CA)

MAXILLARY INCISOR REGION

1. Assemble anterior instrument, and insert film packet vertically into anterior bite block, pushing film packet all the way into slot. Plain side of film packet should be positioned away from backing plate. Narrow #1 film may be used. This requires an individual exposure for lateral incisors.
2. Center film packet on central incisors while viewing through the aiming ring. Entire horizontal length of bite block should be used to position film as posterior as possible.

3. With the front edge of bite block placed on incisal edges of teeth to be radiographed, instruct patient to close slowly, but firmly, to retain position of film packet. A cotton roll may be placed between mandibular teeth and block for patient comfort.
4. Slide aiming ring down the indicator rod to skin surface, and align the PID of the x-ray unit in close approximation to aiming ring, centered and parallel to rod, figure 86-8.
5. Press x-ray machine activating button, and make exposure.

MAXILLARY LATERAL INCISOR REGION

1. Assemble anterior instrument, and insert film packet vertically into anterior bite block, pushing film packet all the way into slot. Plain side of film packet should be positioned away from backing plate. Narrow #1 film is required.
2. Center film packet on lateral incisor while viewing through the aiming ring. Entire horizontal length of bite block should be used to position film as posterior as possible.
3. With front edge of bite block on incisal edge of tooth to be radiographed, instruct patient to close slowly, but firmly, to retain position of film packet. A cotton roll may be placed between mandibular teeth and block for patient comfort.
4. Slide aiming ring down the indicator rod to skin surface, and align the PID of the x-ray unit in close approximation to aiming ring, centered and parallel to rod, figure 86-9.
5. Press x-ray machine activating button, and make exposure.

MAXILLARY CUSPID REGION

1. Assemble anterior instrument, and insert film packet vertically into anterior bite

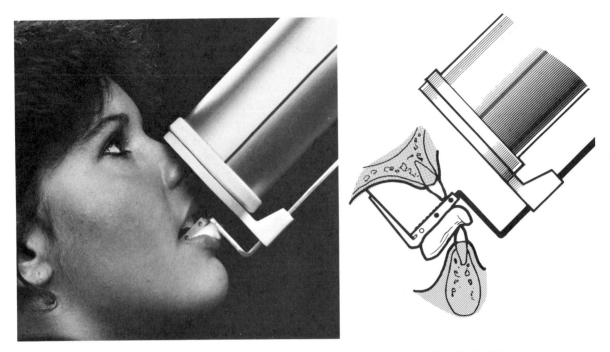

Fig. 86–8. Maxillary incisor region (Courtesy Rinn Corporation, Elgin, IL)

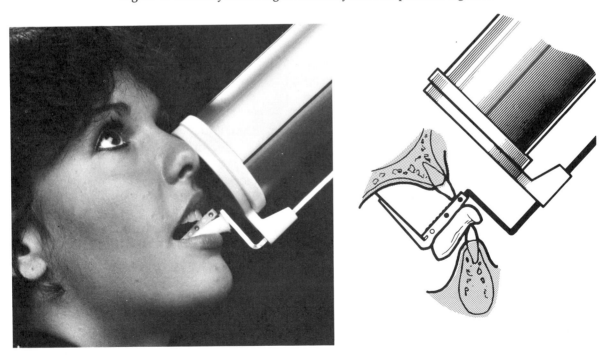

Fig. 86–9. Maxillary lateral incisor region (Courtesy Rinn Corporation, Elgin, IL)

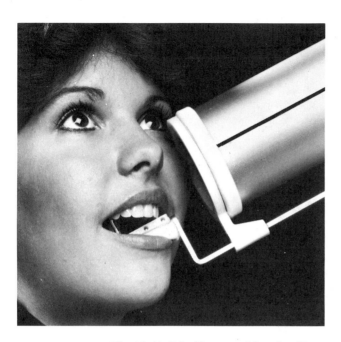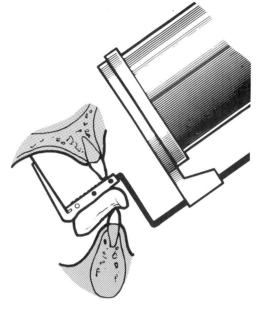

Fig. 86–10. Maxillary cuspid region (Courtesy Rinn Corporation, Elgin, IL)

block, pushing film packet all the way into slot. Plain side of film packet should be away from backing plate. Narrow #1 film may be used. When using #2 film, slightly roll upper anterior corner of film packet to facilitate positioning.

2. Position film packet with cuspid and first bicuspid (premolar) centered on film while viewing through the aiming ring. Entire horizontal length of bite block should be used to position film as posterior as possible.

3. With bite block placed on maxillary teeth to be radiographed, instruct patient to close slowly, but firmly, to retain position of film packet. A cotton roll may be placed between mandibular teeth and block for patient comfort.

4. Slide aiming ring down the indicator rod to skin surface, and align the PID of the

x-ray unit in close approximation to aiming ring, centered and parallel to rod, figure 86–10.

5. Press x-ray machine activating button, and make exposure.

MAXILLARY BICUSPID (PREMOLAR) REGION

1. Assemble posterior instrument, and insert film packet horizontally into posterior bite block, pushing film packet all the way into slot. Plain side of film packet should be positioned away from backing plate. Slightly roll upper anterior corner of film packet to facilitate positioning.

2. Center film packet on second bicuspid (premolar) while viewing through the aiming ring. Entire horizontal length of bite block should be utilized to position film in mid-palatal area.

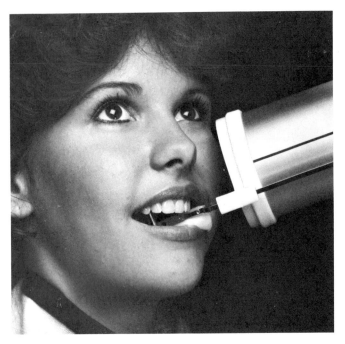
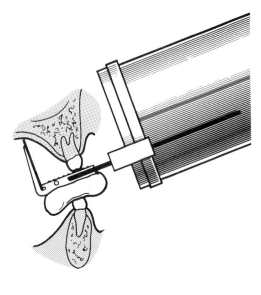

Fig. 86–11. Maxillary bicuspid (premolar) region (Courtesy Rinn Corporation, Elgin, IL)

3. With bite block placed on occlusal surfaces of teeth to be radiographed, instruct patient to close slowly, but firmly, to retain position of film packet. A cotton roll may be placed between mandibular teeth and block for patient comfort.

4. Slide aiming ring down the indicator rod to skin surface, and align the PID of the x-ray unit in close approximation to aiming ring, centered and parallel to rod, figure 86-11.

5. Press x-ray machine activating button, and make exposure.

MAXILLARY MOLAR REGION

1. Assemble posterior instrument, and insert film packet horizontally into posterior bite block, pushing film packet all the way into slot. Plain side of film packet should be positioned away from backing plate. Slightly roll upper posterior corner of film packet to facilitate positioning.

2. Center film packet on second molar while viewing through the aiming ring. Entire horizontal length of bite block should be utilized to position film in mid-palatal area.

3. With bite block placed on occlusal surfaces of teeth to be radiographed, instruct patient to close slowly, but firmly, to retain position of film packet. A cotton roll may be placed between mandibular teeth and block for patient comfort.

4. Slide aiming ring down the indicator rod to skin surface, and align the PID of the x-ray unit in close approximation to aiming ring, centered and parallel to rod, figure 86-12.

5. Press x-ray machine activating button, and make exposure.

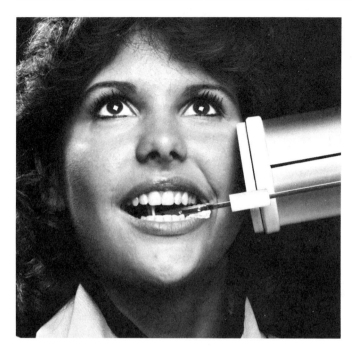

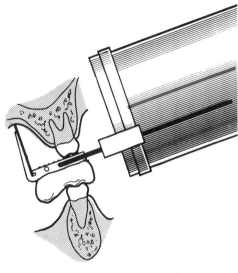

Fig. 86–12. Maxillary molar region (Courtesy Rinn Corporation, Elgin, IL)

MANDIBULAR INCISOR REGION

1. Assemble anterior instrument, and insert film packet vertically into anterior bite block, pushing film packet all the way into slot. Plain side of film packet should be positioned away from backing plate. Narrow #1 film may be used.
2. Center film packet on central incisors while viewing through the aiming ring. Lingual placement of film packet should be as posterior as anatomy will allow.
3. With bite block placed on incisal edges of teeth to be radiographed, instruct patient to close slowly, but firmly, to retain position of film packet.* A cotton roll may be placed between maxillary incisors and block for patient comfort.

4. Slide aiming ring down the indicator rod to skin surface, and align the PID of the x-ray unit in close approximation to aiming ring, centered and parallel to rod, figure 86–13.
5. Press x-ray machine activating button, and make exposure.

MANDIBULAR CUSPID REGION

1. Assemble posterior instrument, and insert film packet vertically into anterior bite block, pushing film packet all the way into slot. Plain side of film packet should be positioned away from backing plate. Narrow #1 film may be used. When using #2 film, roll lower anterior corner slightly to facilitate positioning.
2. Position film packet with cuspid and first bicuspid (premolar) centered on film

* film should be straightened as patient closes and floor of the mouth relaxes.

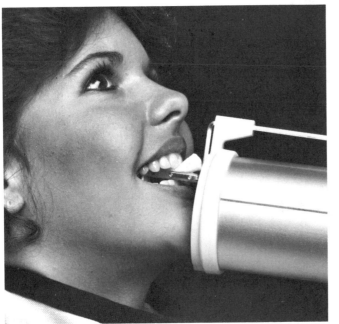

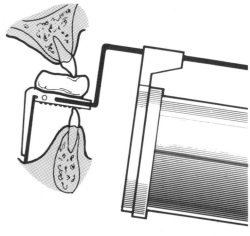

Film should be straightened as patient closes and floor of the mouth relaxes.

Fig. 86–13. Mandibular incisor region (Courtesy Rinn Corporation, Elgin, IL)

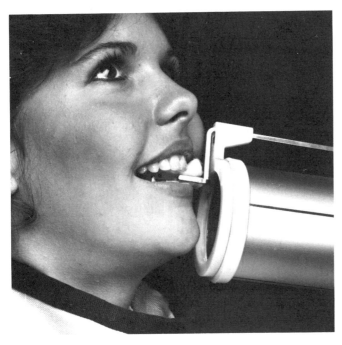

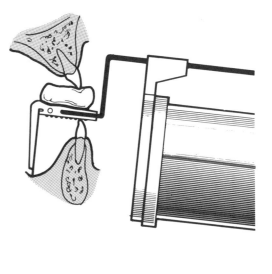

Fig. 86–14. Mandibular cuspid region (Courtesy Rinn Corporation, Elgin, IL)

while viewing through the aiming ring. Lingual placement of the film should be as posterior as anatomy will allow.

3. With bite block placed on mandibular teeth to be radiographed, instruct patient to close slowly, but firmly, to retain position of film packet. A cotton roll may be placed between maxillary teeth and block for patient comfort.

4. Slide aiming ring down the indicator rod to skin surface, and align the PID of the x-ray unit in close approximation to aiming ring, centered and parallel to rod, figure 86–14.

5. Press x-ray machine activating button, and make exposure.

MANDIBULAR BICUSPID [PREMOLAR] REGION

1. Assemble posterior instrument, and insert film packet horizontally into posterior bite block, pushing film packet all the way into slot. Plain side of film packet should be positioned away from backing plate. Roll lower anterior corner of film packet slightly to facilitate positioning.

2. Position film packet with second bicuspid (premolar), centered on film while viewing through the aiming ring. Lingual position of film packet should be as medial as anatomy will allow.

3. With bite block placed on occlusal surfaces of mandibular teeth to be radiographed, instruct patient to close slowly, but firmly, to retain position of film packet. A cotton roll may be placed between maxillary teeth and block for patient comfort.

4. Slide aiming ring down the indicator rod to skin surface, and align the PID of the x-ray unit in close approximation to aiming ring, centered, and parallel to rod, figure 86–15.

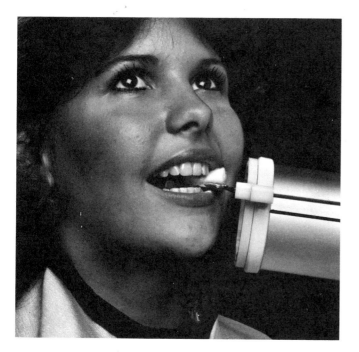
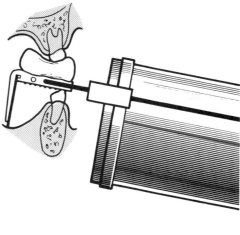

Fig. 86–15. **Mandibular bicuspid (premolar) region (Courtesy Rinn Corporation, Elgin, IL)**

5. Press x-ray machine activating button, and make exposure.

MANDIBULAR MOLAR REGION

1. Assemble posterior instrument, and insert film packet horizontally into posterior bite block, pushing film packet all the way into slot. Plain side of film packet should be away from backing plate. Roll lower posterior corner of film packet slightly to facilitate positioning.
2. Position film packet with second molar centered on film while viewing through the aiming ring. Lingual position of film should be as medial as tongue attachment will allow. Anterior border of film will align with distal portion of second bicuspid (premolar).
3. With bite block placed on occlusal surfaces of mandibular teeth to be radiographed, instruct patient to close slowly, but firmly, to retain position of film. A cotton roll may be placed between maxillary teeth and block for patient comfort.
4. Slide aiming ring down the indicator rod to skin surface, and align the PID of the x-ray unit in close approximation to aiming ring, centered, and parallel to rod, figure 86–16.
5. Press x-ray machine activating button, and make exposure.

VARIATIONS OF THE CONVENTIONAL XCP PROCEDURE

There are cases when the conventional XCP technique must be varied to achieve the desired results. Selected variations are added to this chapter, as XCP is the only such technique shown in the book.

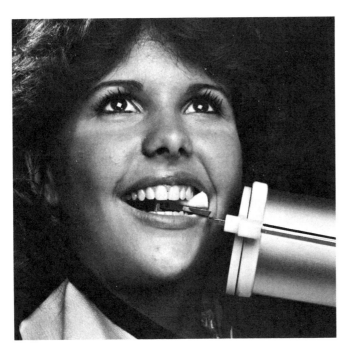
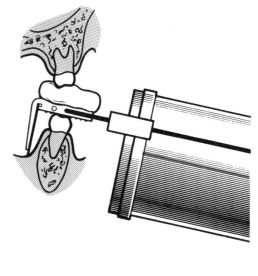

Fig. 86–16. Mandibular molar region (Courtesy Rinn Corporation, Elgin, IL)

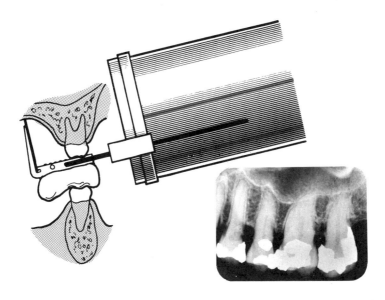

Fig. 86–17. Variation problem—low palate (Courtesy Rinn Corporation, Elgin, IL)

Maxillary Posterior Region

Low Palates. Parallelism between the film and long axes of the teeth is difficult to accomplish in patients with low palatal vaults. If the discrepancy from parallelism does not exceed 15°, the resultant radiograph is usually acceptable, figure 86–17.

By using a two-cotton roll technique (one on each side of block), the film can be paralleled with the long axes, but the area of periapical coverage will be reduced, figure 86–18. This may prove adequate in many instances, particularly if the teeth have short roots.

Increasing Periapical Coverage. Greater periapical coverage than can be obtained with the conventional technique may be desired in certain instances.

This can be accomplished by increasing the vertical angulation 5 to 15° more than the instrument indicates, figure 86–19.

Increasing Periapical Coverage. By altering the relationship of the film to the teeth on a horizontal plane, various aspects of multirooted teeth can be projected on the radiograph, figures 86–19, 86–20.

Mandibular Bicuspid (Premolar) Region

Overcoming Inadequate Periapical Coverage. With an excessive mandibular occlusal curve or in patients with long bicuspids, the conventional technique may result in inadequate coverage. Two methods are suggested to overcome this problem.

1. Projection of the bicuspid images higher on a conventionally positioned film can be accomplished by increasing the vertical angle negatively 5 to 15° more than the XCP instrument indicates, figure 86–21.
2. By placing the film vertically rather than horizontally in the posterior instrument and using a two-cotton roll technique (one on each side of the block), complete

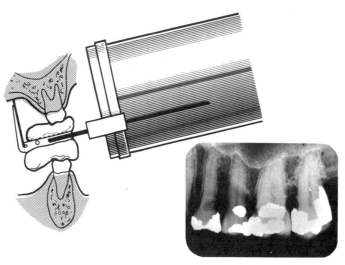

Fig. 86–18. Low palate solution (Courtesy Rinn Corporation, Elgin, IL)

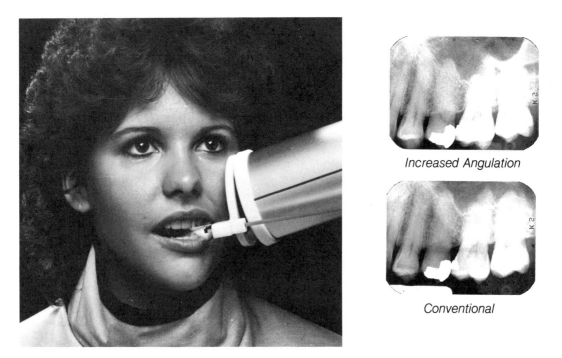

Increased Angulation

Conventional

Fig. 86–19. Variation problem—increasing periapical coverage (Courtesy Rinn Corporation, Elgin, IL)

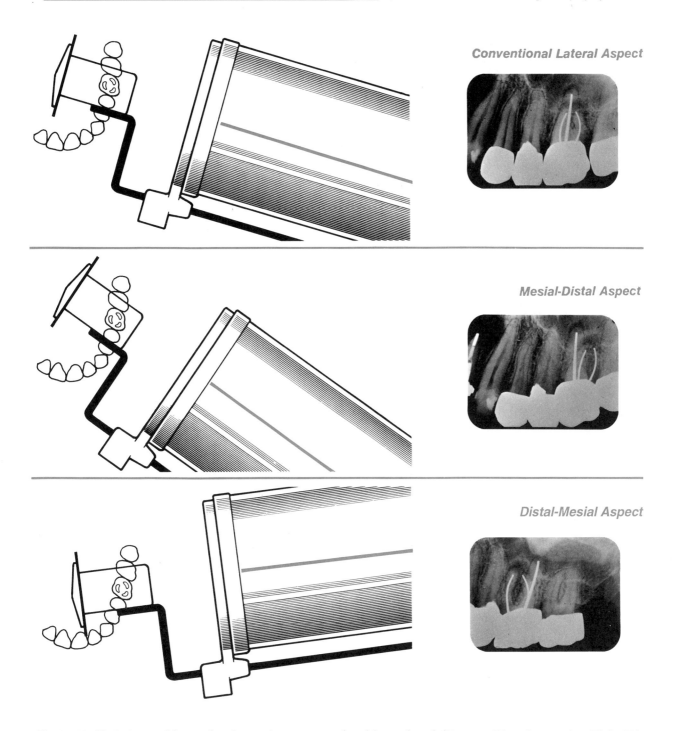

Fig. 86–20. Variation problem—showing various aspects of multirooted teeth (Courtesy Rinn Corporation, Elgin, IL)

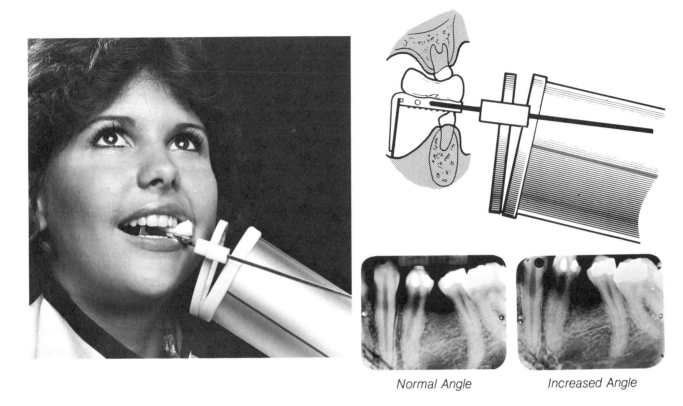

Normal Angle   Increased Angle

Fig. 86–21. Inadequate periapical coverage—Method #1 (Courtesy Rinn Corporation, Elgin, IL)

visualization of the bicuspid region will be accomplished. The purpose of the second cotton roll between the block and the mandibular bicuspids is to prevent unnecessary impingement of the film on the floor of the mouth, figure 86–22.

Partially Edentulous Technique

The XCP instruments can be used in radiography of partially edentulous mouths by substituting a cotton roll or block of styrofoam (or a similar radiolucent material) for the space normally occupied by the crowns of the missing teeth and then following standard procedure, figure 86–23. Care must be taken to angle the film at approximate parallelism to missing teeth.

Completely Edentulous Technique

When all the teeth are missing, cotton rolls, blocks of styrofoam or a combination of both can be used with the XCP instruments, as illustrated. The thickness of the cotton rolls or styrofoam will determine the amount of film coverage of the edentulous ridges. The instrument is positioned in the mouth with the film parallel to the ridge area being examined. The patient closes, holding the film in position, and the standard procedure is followed, figure 86–24.

Technique for Limited Operatory Space [XCP Only]

It is well-known that some x-ray procedures cannot be used in some offices because of limited space. Space is not a limiting factor with the

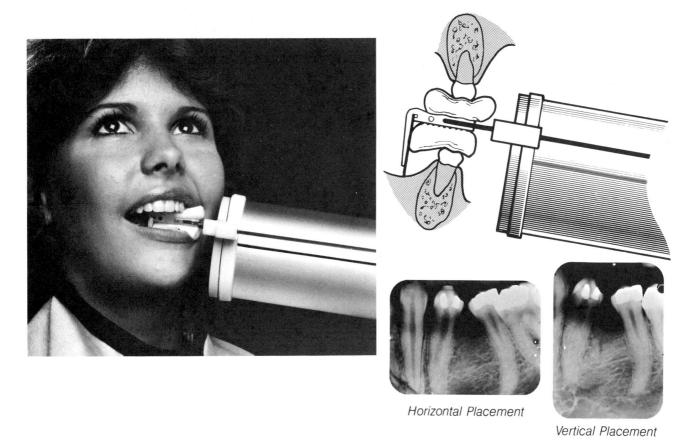

Horizontal Placement

Vertical Placement

Fig. 86–22. Inadequate periapical coverage—Method #2 (Courtesy Rinn Corporation, Elgin, IL)

XCP technique, because the patient no longer needs to be maintained in the standard dental radiographic posture. By rotating or tipping the patient's head or by adjusting the dental chair to a convenient position, it is always possible to align the extension tube (PID) with the XCP instrument regardless of space limitations or restricted mobility of the x-ray unit, figure 86–25.

SUGGESTED ACTIVITIES

- Under the supervision of the instructor, assemble the XCP instruments.

- Using a DXT TRS mannequin, place the film. Have the film placement checked by the instructor. Expose and develop the films. It is recommended that the first set of radiographs be carefully evaluated but not graded. This should eliminate some student stress when trying an unfamiliar procedure.
- Using a fellow student, practice placing film and instruments without exposure. Fellow students are most willing to give feedback on the comfort or discomfort of film placement.

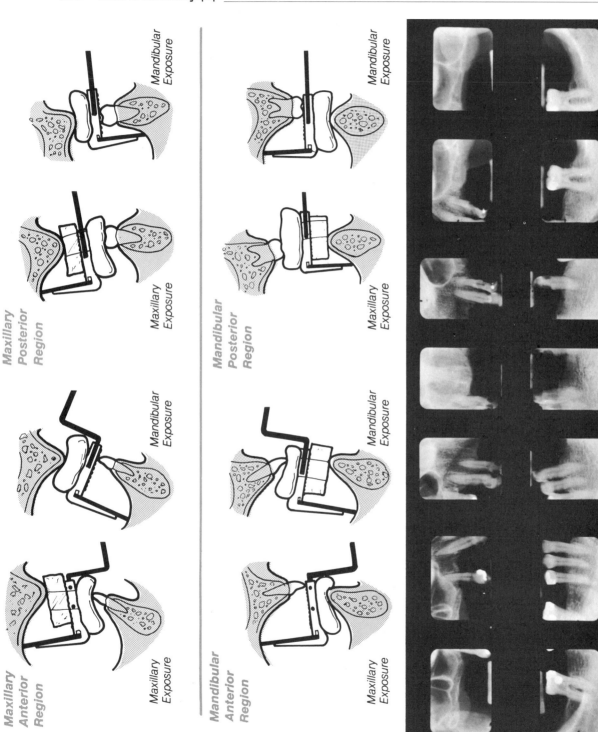

Maxillary Anterior Region

Maxillary Exposure

Mandibular Exposure

Maxillary Posterior Region

Maxillary Exposure

Mandibular Exposure

Mandibular Anterior Region

Maxillary Exposure

Mandibular Exposure

Mandibular Posterior Region

Maxillary Exposure

Mandibular Exposure

Fig. 86–23. Partially edentulous technique. *Note:* Exposure times should be reduced 25 percent from that of a standard technique (Courtesy Rinn Corporation, Elgin, IL)

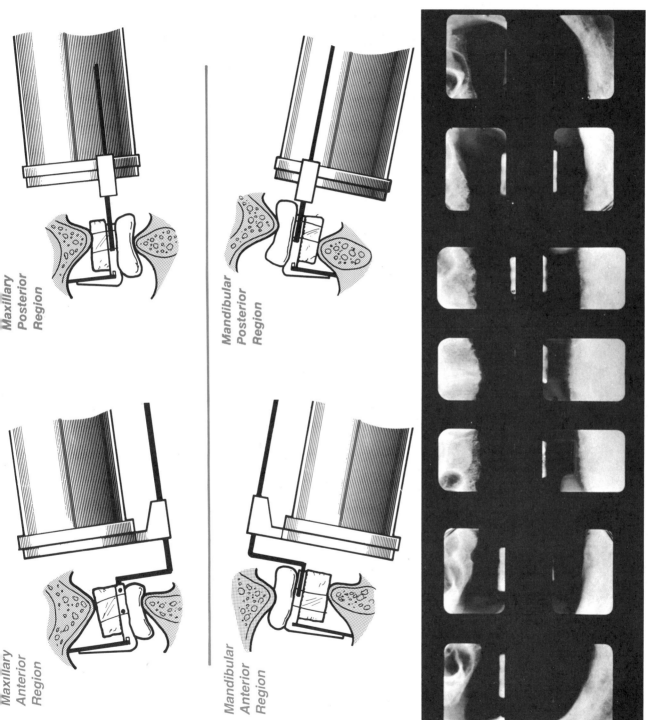

Maxillary Posterior Region

Mandibular Posterior Region

Maxillary Anterior Region

Mandibular Anterior Region

Fig. 86–24. Completely edentulous technique. *Note:* Exposure times should be reduced 25 percent from that of a standard technique (Courtesy Rinn Corporation, Elgin, IL)

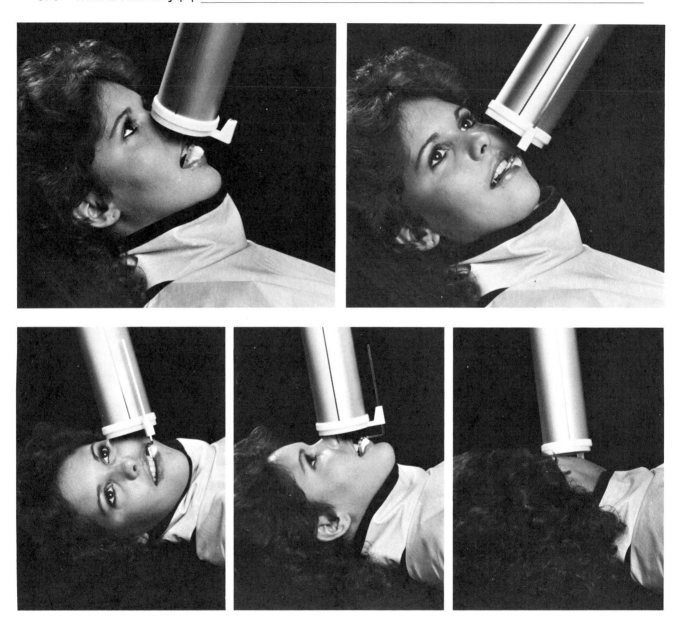

Fig. 86–25. Top: Patient and chair may be inclined to any position, because the XCP instrument aligns the x-ray tubehead in the correct angulation to the teeth regardless of patient position. These photos show the patient at approximately a 45° angle. Note that, by turning the patient's head, the posterior as well as anterior radiograph may be obtained easily.

Bottom: Alignment of the PID with the XCP instrument can also be accomplished with the patient in a supine position. This requires minimal maneuvering of the x-ray unit with the final alignment being made by adjusting the patient's head. Placement of the film is simplified and well tolerated by the patient in this position. (Courtesy Rinn Corporation, Elgin, IL)

REVIEW

1. State the principles used for the XCP technique. _____

   _____

   _____

2. List four advantages of using the XCP technique.

   a. _____

   b. _____

   c. _____

   d. _____

Chapter 87: Occlusal Film Examination

OBJECTIVES:

After studying this chapter, the student will be able to:
- Define an occlusal film examination.
- List six conditions that can be detected by an occlusal film examination.
- Determine the angle of projection of the central ray for occlusal radiographs.
- Practice placing and exposing periapical x-ray films.

INTRODUCTION

The occlusal film examination is so-called because the film packet is placed in the occlusal plane for exposure. Such exposures show sectional views of large dental areas on one film. In cases where periapical packets cannot be used, the occlusal packet is the logical substitute. The image on the occlusal film discloses conditions that cannot be recorded conveniently on any other film.

Industrial and automobile accidents have greatly increased the incidence of jaw fractures. In an examination of such conditions, the dentist cannot always be satisfied with the information provided by extraoral radiographs. If the maxillae are involved, a few additional exposures may be necessary to detect obscure (not easily seen) and hairline fractures that would have an important influence on occlusion and the maxillary sinuses. Often, these added exposures must be made from several different angles.

ADVANTAGES

The occlusal film is particularly useful in revealing fractures of the palate and alveolar processes of the maxilla, as well as various portions of the mandible. Therefore, if the patient can open his or her mouth wide enough to insert the occlusal packet, valuable x-ray information may be secured. In cases where the patient suffers from trismus (lockjaw) or any severe form of mental affliction or disease that prevent the use of periapical or interproximal examination, occlusal packets can be slid between the teeth and radiographs made.

In addition, occlusal film has distinct applications in making rapid surveys of the teeth and jaws. It is of value in locating impacted teeth, foreign bodies, and calculi in the salivary ducts; in determining the extent of lesions, such as cysts, osteomyelitis, and some forms of malignancies; in recording changes in the size and shape of the dental arches; in showing the presence or absence of supernumerary teeth (particularly in the cuspid region); in observing the condition of the upper jaw following operations for closure of cleft palate; in revealing odontomata (an anomaly in tooth development, particularly of the hard tissues) that has blocked the eruption of teeth; in examining edentulous areas at the site of root fragments, cystic growths, necrotic areas, etc.; and in locating areas of destruction in malignancies of the palate.

ANGULATION

The position of the patient and the tubehead, the correct angle for projection, and the normal occlusal radiographs for the anterior and posterior areas of the maxilla and anterior areas of the mandible are illustrated in figures 87–1 through 87–5.

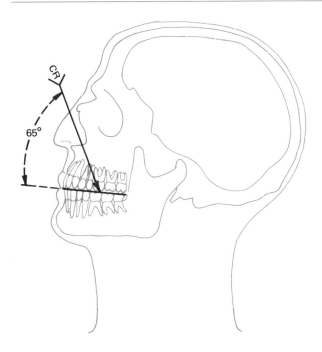

Fig. 87–1. Angle for projection of central ray for maxillary occlusal radiograph—anterior

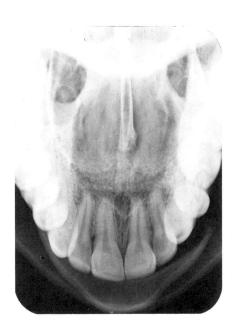

Fig. 87–2. Maxillary occlusal radiograph—anterior

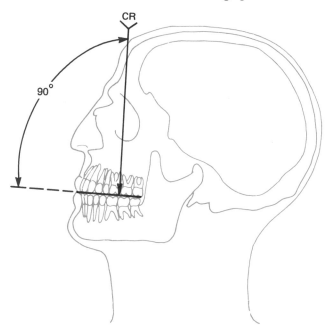

Fig. 87–3. Angle for projection of central ray for maxillary occlusal radiograph—posterior

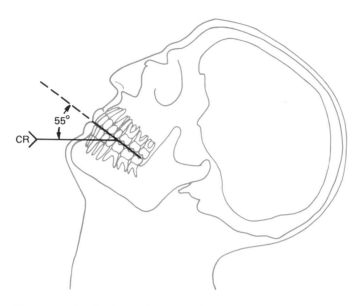

Fig. 87–4. Angle for projection of central ray for mandibular occlusal radiograph—anterior

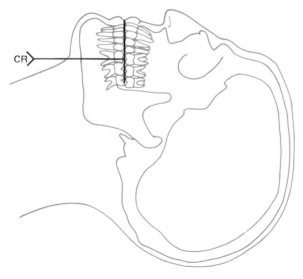

Fig. 87–5. Angle for projection of central ray for mandibular occlusal radiograph—anterior

FILM PLACEMENT [MAXILLARY]

1. Seat the patient in an upright position in the dental chair. The maxillary occlusal plane must be parallel with the floor.
2. Place the smooth side of the film packet toward the maxillary teeth. Instruct the patient to close the teeth firmly on the packet to stabilize the film's position.
3. Check the film that extends beyond the biting surfaces to make certain it remains parallel with the floor.
4. Instruct the patient to maintain this position and to close her or his eyes during the exposure of the film.
5. Using an 8-inch position indicating device (PID) and +65° to +90° angulation, bisect the angle of the curvature of the palatal vault and the plane of the film, figures 87–1 and 87–3.

FILM PLACEMENT [MANDIBULAR]

1. Position the patient in the dental chair, with the head as far back as possible. This will place the inferior border of the mandible at a right angle to the floor.
2. Bring the 8-inch PID in close proximity to the chin, before placing the film.
3. Place the smooth side of the film toward the mandibular teeth. Instruct the patient to close the teeth firmly on the film packet to stabilize its position.
4. Check to determine the plane of the film.
5. Using an 8-inch PID, and 55° to 90° vertical angulation, proceed to expose the film, figures 87–4 and 87–5.

SUGGESTED ACTIVITY

- Practice the placement of occlusal x-ray films, using the 12-inch bisected-angle technique and the Dental X-ray Training (DXTRR) phantom. You may expose the film and process it. *Be sure to check all procedures with your instructor.*
1. Angulation of the cone should be practiced before you turn on the current.
2. Position the patient (a fellow student) for all four occlusal radiographic exposures. Place the film and practice angulation of the cone. *Do not expose the film.*
3. Position four occlusal films in the DXTRR phantom. Make four exposures. Process.

REVIEW

1. Define an occlusal film examination. How is it placed and what does it show?

_____

_____

_____

2. Name six advantages of using occlusal films for radiographic examination.

a. _____

b. _____

c. _____

d. _____

e. _____

f. _____

3. Describe the angle of projection of the central ray for

a. maxillary anterior occlusal radiograph _____

_____

b. maxillary posterior occlusal radiograph _____

_____

4. Describe the angle of projection of the central ray for

a. mandibular anterior radiograph_____

_____

b. mandibular posterior radiograph_____

_____

Chapter 88: Extraoral Radiography

OBJECTIVES:

After studying this chapter, the student will be able to:

- Demonstrate the procedure for lateral jaw radiographs.
- Define panoramic radiography.
- Differentiate between the advantages and the limitations of panoramic radiography.
- Demonstrate loading cassette films and seating patients for the films.

INTRODUCTION

Extraoral x-ray films are exposed with the film outside the mouth. They are valuable for examining the body and ramus of the mandible, the temporomandibular joint, the maxilla, and other areas of the face.

As previously mentioned, cartons of extraoral film must be opened and the film holder or **cassette** loaded in the darkroom. The methods of making some of the more frequently used extraoral radiographs of the head and its parts are shown in figures 88–1 and 88–2. In both cases, the ray is directed at an angle of approximately +25°.

Dental x-ray units are *not* designed for making radiographs of the torso or other extremities. When dental x-ray units are used for this purpose, the patient is subjected to a greater radiation than he or she would be if proper equipment were used. Dental x-ray equipment should be used for this purpose *only in an emergency.*

BODY OF THE MANDIBLE (Lateral Jaw)

The patient's head is positioned with the maxillary occlusal plane horizontal. The cassette or cardboard film holder is placed at the desired side of the head, between the headrest pad and

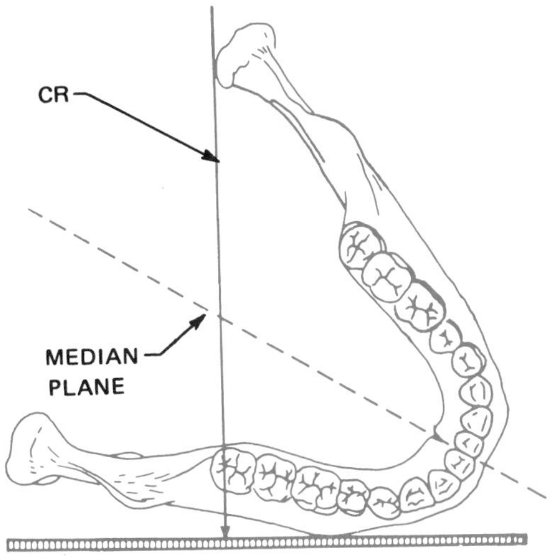

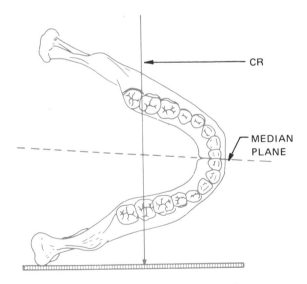

Fig. 88–1. Angle for projection of central ray for mandibular lateral jaw radiograph

Fig. 88–2. Angle for projection of central ray for extraoral radiograph of ramus of mandible

the patient's head, with the front edge of the film held in the patient's hand. *The longer dimension of the film is positioned horizontally*, and the plane of the film is approximately vertical. The patient's head is rotated until the nose is 1/4 inch from the surface of the film holder. The chin is elevated moderately and the teeth held in normal occlusion. The sagittal plane of the patient's head remains vertical at all times. The vertical angulation is 17° upward. The point of entry for the central ray is 1/2 inch below and behind the angle of the undesired side of the jaw. The horizontal angulation is chosen so that the face or axis of the x-ray head parallels the top edge of the film holder. *A paper clip fastened at the center of the lower edge of the tube side of the cardboard film holder is useful to identify the film that is used on the patient's right side.* Refer to the manufacturer's instructions for time of exposure.

CONDYLE (Lateral Jaw)

The patient's head is positioned with the maxillary occlusal plane horizontal. The cassette or film holder is placed on the side of the head with its longer dimension vertical and centered over the desired condyle. It is held in this position by pressure exerted upon the back of the film by the palm of the patient's hand. *The position indicating device (PID) is removed* from the x-ray machine. The vertical angulation setting is 5° upward. The point of entry for the central ray is at the *mandibular foramen* (not the mental foramen) on the undesired side of the jaw. The x-ray machine is placed in contact with the patient's cheek and the horizontal angulation determined so that the face or axis of the x-ray machine parallels the medial sagittal plane of the patient. Before the film is exposed, the patient is instructed to open his or her mouth to its fullest extent. Refer to manufacturer's instructions for time of exposure.

PANORAMIC RADIOGRAPHY

Panoramic radiography is another type of extraoral radiography. This technique records all the dental arches on one film, figure 88–3. It uses

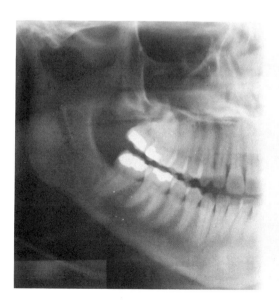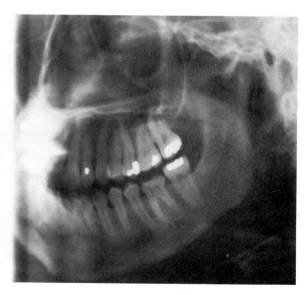

Fig. 88–3. Panoramic survey

a principle called **tomography** wherein the x-ray tube and film are rotated about a pivot point that is located at the level of the selected plane of tissue to be exposed. The recording of the dental arches and their adjacent structures is achieved by moving the cone and the film through the x-ray beam with an equal linear velocity.

Making a panoramic radiograph is similar to taking several photographs of a scenic valley in which the camera is moved to the right or left for each photograph. When all the pictures are developed, they can be pieced together and placed into one panoramic picture of the valley. Panoramic radiographs make it possible to take several pictures of the dental alveolar structures and have them laid out side by side automatically on one film.

In figure 88–4, the film unit is in the same horizontal plane as the tubehead, with the position for the patient's chin in a fixed, preset position. The control panel on most units allows for variation in patient size. The operator's manual provided with the panoramic unit gives further information and technique for use of that

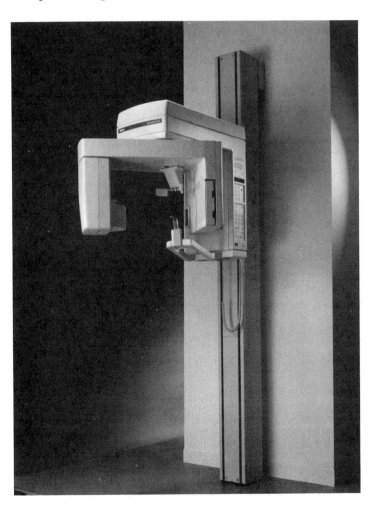

Fig. 88–4. Orthoralix SD (Courtesy GENDEX Corp.)

particular machine. Some of the advantages of using a panoramic radiograph are that

- a wider scope of examination is provided
- the machines are preset and simple to operate
- screening technique for large numbers of people is made available
- it is easy to use for difficult patients
- radiation exposure to the patient is low

Some of the limitations of the panoramic technique are that

- it produces slight magnification and overlapping of images
- image definition and detail are not as precise as with the conventional intraoral radiograph
- the initial cost and space required for the unit may be prohibitive

The addition of panoramic radiography to the dental field has been but one example of the continuing research done to improve the quality of dental health.

SUGGESTED ACTIVITIES

- Load a cassette or cardboard film holder under the supervision of the instructor.
- Seat a fellow student, and follow the step-by-step procedure for making a lateral jaw radiograph. Do not expose the film. Check your procedure with the instructor.
- Visit a dental clinic or office that uses a panoramic radiograpic unit. Ask to see the operator's manual for the unit. Discuss the advantages and limitations of the unit with the personnel who use it.

REVIEW

1. What are the two major areas that require a lateral jaw radiograph?

    a. _____

    b. _____

2. List three advantages of using panoramic radiography.

    a. _____

    b. _____

    c. _____

3. Cite three limitations of panoramic radiography.

    a. _____

    b. _____

    c. _____

INTRODUCTION

When a photographic emulsion, once exposed to x-radiation, is placed in a chemical solution (the developer) and the bromine is taken away from the silver, the black metallic silver remaining behind forms the image. The removal of the bromide from the metallic silver is chemically known as **reduction**.

Chemical reducers have an affinity for oxygen that must be kept within narrow bounds. The reducer must liberate the metal from its salt while in the developing solution. Such reducing agents must be able to reduce the exposed silver halide *without* affecting unexposed silver halide. *Note:* This chemical reduction is *not* to be confused with the operation known as *reducing* of a detail film, which is the weakening of an overdense image; the term refers simply to the removal of silver to produce a less dense image and is not used in the chemical sense.

CHEMISTRY OF DEVELOPMENT

Developer is the solution that reduces the exposed area of the emulsion so that it will be visible to the human eye. It is generally composed of hydroquinone, elon, sodium sulfate, and other chemicals in solution. The function of the developer is to bring out the latent image of the object exposed and one which is contained in the silver halide granules of the film emulsion. Two chemicals used in the developing solution that are reducing agents and have a definite action on the photographic emulsion are:

1. *Hydroquinone*—chemically derived from benzine (a coal-tar distillate). Images developed with hydroquinone come up slowly and gain **density** steadily; it must be used together with other agents to attain successful results.

2. *Elon*—monomethyl paramidophenol sulfate (a by-product of the manufacture of dyes, treated with alcohol). Elon, when used alone in the developer, brings the image up quickly all over the film and gains density slowly.

Hydroquinone is affected readily by the slightest change in temperature, but elon is not affected to any great degree by a slight change of temperature. These differences in the developing agents depend on the chemical nature of the chemicals themselves and constitute what is referred to as the *reduction potential* of the developer. A developer of high reduction potential enables the solution to develop at a more even rate under adverse conditions such as low temperature (near 60°F, 15.6°C) or the presence of halide.

Hydroquinone has a low potential. Slower reaction brings up the highlights of the image first, with shadows not appearing until after the highlights are somewhat developed. Hydroquinone gives **contrast** to the image. Elon has a high potential and starts development quickly

681

producing **detail.** Thus, if both detail and contrast are desired, chemical agents of both high and low potential must be used.

These agents cannot develop at all unless they are used in an alkali medium. The energy of the medium depends on the amount of alkali present. Too little alkali will slow the action of the developer; too much alkali will tend to result in chemical fog. As alkalis soften the gelatin of the emulsion, too much alkali in the solution will produce overswelling, causing frilling or blisters on the film. In developing, the alkalis generally used are the carbonates; sodium carbonate is one. It is used in a form that contains 98% carbonate and a small amount of residual water.

Because developers have great affinity for oxygen and because of the oxygen in the air, solutions containing only the developing agents and alkali will spoil rapidly by the process of oxidation. By adding sulfite of soda, the developer is protected from oxygen, and its life is prolonged.

The developing process will probably be too rapid if a developing solution with a reducer, a preservative, and an alkali is used. Therefore, it is necessary to have potassium bromide in the developer, which acts as a restrainer; it prevents too rapid developing and fogging of the transparent areas of the film.

Distilled water should be the vehicle for all developing solutions. Water containing chemicals may combine with the chemicals of the developing solution and have a damaging effect on the silver halide salts of the emulsion.

CHEMISTRY OF FIXATION

After development of the film, the undeveloped silver halide salts are removed by immersion of the film in what is called the *fixer.* A universally used substance that will dissolve silver bromide is *sodium thiosulfate,* known as hyposulfite of soda, or *hypo.*

Fixing is accomplished by means of the hypo only, but chemicals remove a good deal of the alkaline chemicals carried over from the developer into the fixing bath. To avoid neutrality of the fixer, a large amount of a weak acid is added; the best for the purpose is *acetic acid.* Acetic acid in its diluted form is a vinegar resulting from the fermentation of alcohol.

It is important not to overwork the fixer bath, because it will become saturated with silver and the film will carry this silver into the water bath. Therefore, the film should be properly washed between the developer bath and the fixer; otherwise, the silver salt will adhere to the processed film and, in time, will decompose into silver sulfide, causing a yellowish-green stain on the film. The temperature of the fixing bath solution should be 68–70°F (20–21°C); the time is usually twenty to thirty minutes.

The most common hardening agent in the fixer is *potash alum.* Alums have the property of shrinking and hardening gelatin.

PROCEDURE OF WASHING

The actual time of washing may best be understood by remembering that, as the washing proceeds, the amount of hypo remaining in the gelatin emulsion is continually halved in the same period of time. An average film will give up one-half of its hypo in two minutes, so that at the end of two minutes one-half the hypo will be remaining in it; after four minutes, one-quarter; after six minutes, one-eighth, and so on. In a short time, the amount of hypo remaining on the emulsion will be minimal. However, this assumes that the film is continually exposed to circulating water. During processing, films should always be washed between solutions. After fixing, they should remain in running water for at least 30 minutes before drying.

The temperature of the water in which the films are washed is of great importance. If the temperature is too high, the films will become pitted or **reticulated**. This is caused by the softening of the emulsion. Keeping the water bath under 70°F (21°C) is recommended. Reticulation can also be caused by sudden temperature changes between the solution and the water bath.

REVIEW

1. Explain the chemical composition of the developer. _____

_____

_____

2. What is the function of the developer? _____

_____

3. What is the chemical composition of the fixer? What is the action of each chemical used? _____

_____

_____

4. What is the function of the fixer? _____

_____

5. After fixing, how long should the film be washed and at what water temperature? _____

6. If the film is placed in a 60°F solution (fixer or rinse water) after being developed in a 70°F solution, what will be the result? _____

_____

7. What should be the temperature of the water bath? _____

OBJECTIVES:

After studying this chapter, the student will be able to:
- List the three basic principles for effective darkroom procedure.
- List and explain the twelve steps in proper darkroom procedure.
- Remove films and attach them to a holder.
- State the importance of using care when processing film.

INTRODUCTION

There are three basic principles for effective darkroom procedure. They are:

1. Absolute cleanliness.
2. Absolute light-tight security.
3. Proper use of time and temperature techniques.

Within the framework of these fundamentals lies a step-by-step procedure that will ensure consistency, accuracy, and error-free processing. Explanations and reasons for these steps follow.

MATERIALS NEEDED

- tank with developing solutions
- tank with fixing solution
- tank with water bath
- water thermometer
- stirring rods
- interval timer clock
- x-ray hangers
- safety light
- disposable treatment gloves or plastic examination gloves
- processing chart
- fan

INSTRUCTIONS

Preparing

1. Enter darkroom, figure 90–1. Wipe all work surfaces.
2. Check temperature of solutions. Thoroughly stir solutions.
3. Set interval timer according to manufacturer's directions.
4. Label hanger with name, date, and number of films.
5. Turn off utility light.
6. Turn on safety light.
7. Don gloves.
8. Remove film carefully from film packet, being mindful of finger marks and scratches that damage the film.
9. Clip films on hanger.
10. Recheck films for security of attachment.

Developing

1. Immerse hanger with films attached into the developing tank; agitate hanger up and down five times.
2. Place hanger on side of tank, making certain that all the films are below the level of the solution and do not touch the wall of the tank or one another.
3. Set timer. Lower lever on timer.

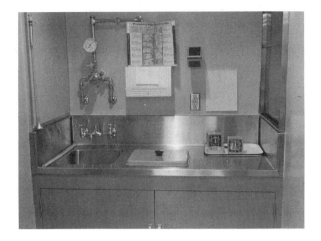

Fig. 90–1. A clean and well-equipped darkroom

Rinsing

1. When timer rings, lift and drain excess developer from hanger.
2. Agitate up and down gently in water bath ten times to rinse as much of the developing solution from the films and film hanger as possible.
3. Drain excess water from hanger.

Fixing

1. Place films and hanger in fixing bath; agitate to remove any air bubbles from the films.
2. Set timer for at least twice the time of the developing or approximately ten minutes. A "wet reading" may be made after three minutes. Return the films to the fixing bath to complete the recommended period.
3. When timer rings, lift hanger and drain excess fixer.

Washing

1. Agitate hanger in water bath ten times.
2. Hang rack on side of tank, making certain that the water level is sufficient to cover

the films. Wash in running water for a *minimum of twenty minutes* (more time is preferred).

Drying

1. Remove films from the water bath, and hold under the cold water tap. Allow the water to run over films and clips.
2. Test the surface of the films by gently rubbing them *with water running* between the thumb and forefinger. They should be free of any residual solution and feel clean to the touch.
3. Hang films up to dry, making certain the air is circulating and the fan is on.
4. Do not attempt to remove films from the hanger until they are *completely dry.*
5. Clean working surfaces and film hangers to remove solutions.

RATIONALE

Wiping Working Surfaces

The first step to undertake when entering the darkroom is to wipe off all work surfaces. Frequently, someone may have inadvertently sprinkled some developer or fixer on the work surfaces; these droplets subsequently evaporate and leave a highly concentrated crystalline residue of processing chemicals. If film is dropped or placed in contact with this chemical combination, it will become spotted, often in such a manner as to indicate possible pathology on the processed film.

Stirring Solutions

Both developer and fixer should be stirred with separate stirring rods. These rods should be washed in water between each stirring operation. The reason is relatively simple; the chemicals of both developer and fixer are heavier than water and tend to settle to the bottom of the tank inserts. Processing without stirring produces a developing "tree" whose films are quite dark at the bottom of the rack, possibly reasonably accurate in the middle, and very frequently quite light at the top. Therefore, for overall consistency of radiographic result, thorough stirring is essential.

Determining Temperature

As mentioned, an effective temperature range is generally between 68 and 70°F (20–21°C). When developers are used at temperatures below 65°F, they may not be effective. Chemicals used at temperatures above 75°F present two problems: (1) reticulation, a condition in which the emulsion softens and tends to slide off the film base; and (2) demands on accuracy, in terms of processing time, that are unjustified. This situation implies the availability of both hot and cold water inflow to the tank.

Referring to the Time-Temperature Chart

The following chart contains recommended time for a given temperature to achieve complete development of the film.

Temperature of Developer	Time
60–62°F	9 minutes
64–66°F	7 minutes
68–70°F (optimum temperatures)	5 minutes
72–76°F	4 minutes
78–80°F	3 minutes

Fixing time: 10 minutes
Washing time: 20 minutes

Setting the Timer

The time should correspond to the recommended time for the temperature available in accordance with the charts published by each manufacturer for each solution.

Opening the Film

The white work light should be turned off before the film packet is opened, and the red safety light should be turned on. Care must be taken when opening dental film and extracting the film from the covering in order to avoid injury of the emulsion through crimping, scratching, or finger marking. Fingernail markings appear as moon-shaped images on the developed film. This damage usually occurs at the time the film is softened before it is placed in the mouth or at the time the bitewing tab or strip is placed on the film. Crimping of the emulsion may occur as the film is placed in the film holder prior to exposure or as the film packet is opened. If the film is grasped by the fingers, marks may occur on the emulsion as the packet is opened and placed on the hanger. These fingerprints will remain on the film. The packet should be grasped between the thumb and the second finger by its long axis, using the index finger as a pressure fulcrum causing the film to bend only enough to permit the opposing hand to grasp the tab, figure 90–2. The film should be opened halfway and the protective papers pulled back to expose one-half of the film. This permits the film to be grasped on one edge as the opposite edge is introduced into the hanger without the necessity of removing the film from the packet manually, figure 90–3.

Securing the Film

All too frequently, films are lost from the processing hanger in the tank because of improper fastening of the film. This problem can be eliminated by introducing the film to a clip hanger in the following manner:

1. Grasp hanger with clips in an "up" position, figure 90–3.
2. Depress selected clip key.
3. Place film on the edge nearest the embossed dot, and introduce the upper edge of the clip at a 45° angle. While holding the film at this angle, release the clip key. This will permit the film to be grasped

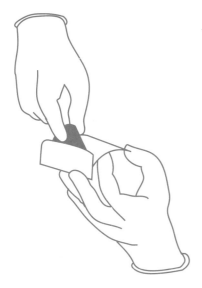

Fig. 90–2. Opening the film packet

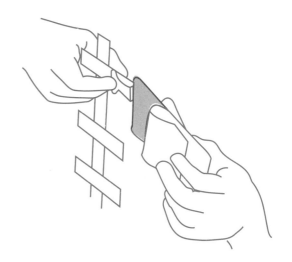

Fig. 90–3. Placing clip on the film

by the *three* securing prongs rather than the *one* central prong frequently employed.

4. Test the security of each film on the hanger by *gently* tapping each with the superior surface of your index fingertip; if the film is not secure, it will fall off before you immerse the hanger in the developer.

Immersing the Film and Starting the Timer

In as simple an action as the immersion of the hanger, specific procedural steps must be followed. The hanger and its films should be immersed in the stirred developer, then lifted out completely from the developer, and then reimmersed in the developer. Set the timer according to the manufacturer's direction. The reason for this is relatively simple to explain once the problem is understood. There are small globules of air suspended in the solutions. Because the film surface is dry as it enters the solution, these air bubbles are frequently attracted to the surface of the film where surface tension will cause them to cling to the emulsion.

This, in turn, prevents the developer from reaching the emulsion, causing one or more white spots to appear on the radiograph. To prove this point, slowly immerse your hand or arm in a tub of freshly drawn water. You will notice how small bubbles form on the surface of your hand or arm. Lifting this part of your arm out of the water and reimmersing it now prevent the formation of air bubbles. Thus, surface tension is destroyed when the surface is fluidized.

Removing and Washing the Film

When the assigned time for development expires and the timer rings, it is necessary to remove the hanger from the developing compartment. Tilt the hanger over the developer to drop any excess developing solution into the compartment. Wash thoroughly in the clean, running water of the water bath compartment for at least thirty seconds. This implies, of course, that there is flowing water in the wash compartment.

Large quantities of valuable chemicals are lost in hanger movement from one compartment to another, because the clips of the hanger tend to retain a substantial amount of fluid. The hanger should be given a quick vertical shake over the appropriate compartment, then turned diagonally and again shaken over the same compartment. This action will reduce the loss of developing fluids.

Fixing the Film

There is a simple formula for proper fixation; it is 3 + 7 = 10. At the end of *three minutes*, the film may be removed from the fixing solution and quickly washed by dipping the water bath, for study or "wet reading." If, however, the film is to remain in a permanent record, *it must be returned to the fixing solution for a period of no less than seven minutes*, for a total of *ten minutes*. In the event the film has been allowed to remain out of the fixer sufficiently long to dry, wash it in the circulating water bath before placing it in the fixer, and allow a full ten minutes for fixing.

Note: If the proper exposure is observed and the temperature of the solution does not exceed 70°F (21°C), it is reasonably impossible to "overdevelop" and becomes impossible to "overfix."

Washing and Wiping the Film

Following fixation of the film, a second wash period removes all chemical residue from the hanger and films. This wash period should be approximately thirty minutes in the flowing water bath. Again, within the limitations of cleanliness and temperature, one cannot reasonably "overwash."

Remove films from the water bath, and hold under the *cold water* tap. Allow the water to run over the hanger, clips, and film. Test the surface of the films for any residual chemicals with the water still running over them. The films will have a slick surface if they are not completely washed; this residue will gather at the lower surface of the films as they dry. *Gently, and with the tap still running, rub the films* between the ball of the thumb and fingers until they feel clean to the touch. Shake the excess water from the hanger and films; then, using a strip of *clean, natural sponge*, gently wipe the excess water from the films or tap hanger on finger over water bath or sink to shake off excess water. Agitate films in Photo Flo preparation for five to ten seconds.

Drying the Films

Hang the films in the drying area until they are crispy and crackling dry. Any residual moisture in the emulsion offers the serious risk of a scarred film surface. Do not attempt to remove and mount films until they are completely dry.

Note: Clean the surfaces of the working area of the darkroom and film hangers. Such a simple safeguard can eliminate many future problems.

SUGGESTED ACTIVITIES

- Practice removing film from the film packets; use outdated film for this purpose.
- Practice clipping the films in the film clips on the hanger, taking care to follow the steps of the procedure outlined in this chapter.

REVIEW

1. State the three basic principles for effective darkroom procedure.

    a. _____

    b. _____

    c. _____

2. If you see a moon-shaped object or image on the film after it has been developed, what would this indicate? When is this condition most likely to occur?

    _____

    _____

3. Where should the clip be placed on a film? _____

    _____

4. List the twelve steps for proper darkroom procedure.

    a. _____

    b. _____

    c. _____

    d. _____

    e. _____

    f. _____

    g. _____

    h. _____

    i. _____

    j. _____

    k. _____

    l. _____

5. To decide the time needed for a particular temperature of solutions, what should the operator do? _____

   _____

   _____

6. Why are films frequently lost from the processing hanger and into the tank?__

   _____

   _____

7. Why should the solutions be stirred before submerging the films?_____

   _____

   _____

8. What is the simple formula for proper fixation?_____

   _____

9. Why is it necessary to return the film to the fixing bath after wet reading? Why are care and precision important when processing film?_____

   _____

   _____

10. What materials are needed in film processing by the time-temperature method?_____

    _____

    _____

11. How long must the films hang in the fixing bath before a wet reading can be obtained?_____

12. Why is it necessary to return the film to the fixing bath after a wet reading?

    _____

Chapter 91: Automatic Processing

OBJECTIVES:

After studying this chapter, the student will be able to:
- Describe the procedure for developing film, using an automatic processor.
- Compare hand-processing with automatic processing of radiographic films.
- Develop a technique for processing radiographs while observing basic principles of automatic processing.

INTRODUCTION

Automatic film processing is a technique that depends on the interrelation of mechanics, chemicals, and film. Automatic processors use a roller transport system to move the film through the developer, fixer, and wash and dry cycles. Special chemicals have been developed to meet the needs of this processing device, figure 91–1.

In addition to very quickly developing and fixing the image on the film, the processing chemicals must prevent excessive swelling, a slippery or gummy emulsion, and must allow the film to be rapidly washed and dried. Equally important is the use of a replenisher solution for chemicals.

Automatic processors may be loaded in a conventional darkroom with a safelight or can be loaded in daylight, should there be a daylight loader unit mounted on the processor. Some makes require plumbing. An automatic processor *does* require an electrical source for the rollers and heater bar.

Manufacturers will recommend chemical solutions that are compatible with a particular model and brand name. The developer and fixer tanks have a capacity of 1 quart each, and the slightly larger wash tank contains $1^1/_2$ quarts.

BASIC PRINCIPLES OF OPERATION

Depending on the brand name and model, instructions for use may slightly vary; however, there are basic principles that apply to automatic processors, figure 91–2.

1. Set the base of the unit on a level surface. Be sure the surface is stable, so chemicals do not splash or spill.
2. Remove the cover, and note the three tanks.
3. Fill tank to the recess level with room-temperature distilled water.
4. Remove the developer tank to prevent any contamination of the developer solution.
5. Fill the fixer tank with 1 quart of solution. Pour carefully to avoid splashing.
6. Reinsert developer tank and empty 1 quart of developer into it. Pour carefully to avoid splashing.

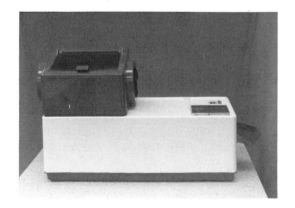

Fig. 91–1. Automatic film processor

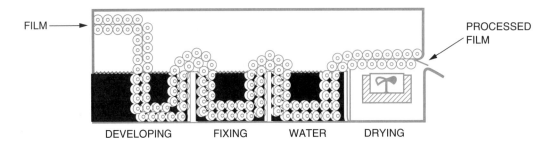

FILM → PROCESSED FILM

DEVELOPING   FIXING   WATER   DRYING

Fig. 91–2. Schematic drawing of a typical automatic film processor

7. Insert the transport (roller) system. Carefully lower into place. Be sure the transport sits squarely.
8. Place the cover and film receptacle.
9. Plug the line cord into a 115 V socket. You are now ready to process films.
10. Refer to the manufacturer's guideline for exposure to obtain best-quality radiographs.
11. Follow the instruction manual for processing films.

HELPFUL HINTS FOR USING AN AUTOMATIC PROCESSOR

1. To minimize the possibility of deposits of chemical particles that may float in the wash tank, *change the water every day.*
2. Check daily the chemical levels in the developer and fixer tanks. If necessary, replenish processing solutions.
3. Maintain a log of the number of films processed as an accurate record. Change chemicals every 300–350 films or every two weeks, whichever is sooner. Place the calendar date of the most recent change in a conspicuous location. Update the entry when you change the chemicals.
4. Strictly adhere to the manufacturer's instructions for care and maintenance of an automatic processing device.

* Rinn DXT TRS, Rinn Corporation, Elgin, IL.

SUGGESTED ACTIVITIES

- Make certain the three tanks are filled before the electrical source is plugged in. Some models of automatic processors have a temperature control; temperatures should range between 70 and 82°F.
- Make certain the unit is operational.
- Check the quality and consistency in processing film. Make sure you include the following points:
  1. Process an unexposed film; the unexposed film should be perfectly clear.
  2. Momentarily expose a film to room light, then process; the light-exposed film should be completely black.
  3. Process a double-film packet that has been exposed using a DXT TRS* mannequin or skull.
     a. Mount one of these radiographs in the corner of a view box, and retain it as a standard reference radiograph.
     b. Periodically, place another radiograph next to the standard reference radiograph.
     c. Compare the density and contrast of the two radiographs.
  Note: Be sure both radiographs used for comparison were exposed using the identical technique factors.

REVIEW

1. Automatic processing is based on three interrelated factors. What are they?

    a. _____

    b. _____

    c. _____

2. How is the film moved through the automatic processor? _____

    _____

    _____

3. State three advantages for use of an automatic processor:

    a. _____

    b. _____

    c. _____

4. What methods may be used to check the quality and consistency in processing a film?

    a. _____

    b. _____

    c. _____

    d. _____

OBJECTIVES:	After studying this chapter, the student will be able to: • List five factors to consider when reviewing radiographs. • Explain the difference between *radiopaque* and *radiolucent*. • Describe the appearance of various tooth structures on a radiograph. • Identify the anatomical landmarks of the maxilla and mandible on x-ray films.

INTRODUCTION

A thorough knowledge of radiographic anatomy is a prerequisite in evaluating normal radiographic images. The operator must have a thorough knowledge of the anatomy of the head and all the landmarks of the skull. *Note:* Refer frequently to figure 92–1 as the structure of the head is discussed.

The many variables to be considered in interpretation of radiographs include: (1) relationship of adjacent teeth; (2) length of the cusp; (3) degree of the axial inclination of the mandibular and maxillary teeth; (4) pathological processes; and (5) physiological stress.

Radiopaque and **radiolucent** are terms used to describe the darkness or lightness of **images** in radiographs. Radiopaque refers to anatomical areas that appear lighter in radiographs. This results from more x rays being absorbed by the object. Radiolucent areas are those that appear darker, such as the periodontal ligament. This results from more x rays passing through the area to expose the film.

DENSITY OF TOOTH STRUCTURES

Enamel, Dentin, and Cementum

Because tooth substance is the densest component of the human body, it absorbs more x rays than any other tissue of comparable size and thickness. The normal tooth has an outer covering called enamel, a middle layer called dentin, and cementum that covers the root. Dentin and cementum have nearly the same capacity to absorb x rays; therefore, radiographic evidence does not differentiate between the two. Both present a uniform gray or white radiographic shadow with no evidence of particular structure or shape.

The coronal portion of the tooth covered by a thin layer of enamel is revealed in radiographs as a homogeneous cap that has greater whiteness than that of the dentin. The line of demarcation between enamel and dentin is sharp and clearly defined. In normal teeth the enamel is of uniform density except in depressions, which are situated chiefly on the mesial and distal aspects of the crown. Because the enamel is thinner, less radiation is absorbed and the darkness of that particular portion of the radiograph increases. Some of the small areas that are difficult to interpret may simulate dental caries and present difficulties in radiographic interpretation of the separate parts. The teeth most likely to reveal these normal anatomical differences are the lower cuspids and bicuspids, followed in frequency by the corresponding teeth in the maxilla.

The Pulp Chamber and Root Canals

The pulp chamber and root canals are continuous cavities within the teeth. They contain soft tissue that absorbs fewer x rays than the surrounding dentin does; therefore, a dark shadow is produced within the shadow of the tooth itself.

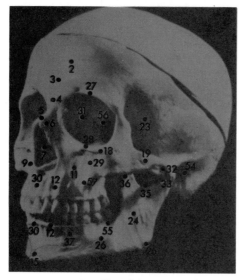

A.   Facial Bones

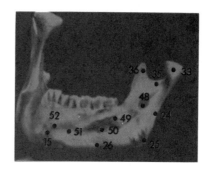

B.   Medial Aspect of Mandible

LEGEND

1 Forehead	29 Zygomatic process
2 Frontal bone	of maxilla
3 Glabella	30 Alveolar process
4 Frontonasal suture (nasion)	31 Orbit
5 Bridge of nose	32 Articular eminence
6 Nasal bone	33 Mandibular condyle
7 Nasal cavity	34 Glenoid fossa
8 Nostrils	35 Mandibular notch
9 Anterior nasal spine	36 Coronoid process
10 Ala of nose	37 Mental foramen
11 Canine fossa	38 Median palatine suture
12 Alveolar ridges	39 Palatine bone
13 Labial commissure	40 Transverse palatine suture
14 Chin	41 Greater palatine foramen
15 Symphysis menti	42 Incisive foramen
16 Inner canthus of eye	43 Nasal septum
17 Outer canthus of eye	44 Posterior nasal spine
18 Cheekbone	45 Vomer
(zygomatic bone)	46 Lateral pterygoid plate
19 Zygomatic arch	47 Medial pterygoid plate
20 Temporomandibular	48 Mandibular foramen and
articulation	lingula
21 Tragus	49 Mylohyoid ridge
22 Auricle	50 Submaxillary depression
23 A. Temple	51 Sublingual depression
B. Temporal fossa	52 Genial tubercles
24 Ramus of mandible	53 Styloid process
25 Angle of mandible	54 External auditory meatus
26 Body of mandible	55 External oblique ridge
27 Supraorbital ridge	56 Optic foramen
28 Infraorbital ridge	57 Maxilla

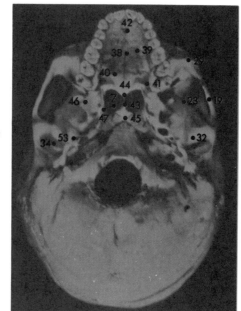

C.   Hard Palate and Adjoining Structures.

Fig. 92–1. Anatomical landmarks of the skull showing (A) facial bones, (B) medial aspect of mandible, and (C) hard palate and adjoining structures

The shape of the pulp chamber is, on the whole, fairly constant, and there is a general pattern for each of the various types of teeth. It is common for some teeth to show an elongation or an increase in the size of one or more of the *cornua* (projections). This may be of great importance in the preparation for restorations. In children of normal health and development, the size of the pulp chamber is rather large. As they grow older, most persons reveal considerable reduction in the size of the pulp chamber. This narrowing of the pulp chamber, regarded as a part of the aging process, is due to the deposition of dentin on the walls of the pulp chamber. The change may be seen in both the coronal portion and the root canals.

The lumen of the roots usually tapers gradually toward the apex. Some roots show slight local alterations and constrictions in the width of the canal. Although teeth may complete their growth and the root canals converge toward the apex, one must remember that there are considerable variations in the appearances of different teeth. The root canal in a developing tooth differs from that of a fully developed tooth. The canal in children is wider and, more importantly, the lumen diverges toward the apical end, which causes this portion of the canal to be funnel-shaped. The dental papilla lies in the wide apex.

The most recently developed portion of dentin is very thin, so that the walls of the root canal are chisel-shaped at the apex. It is important to note, however, that the lamina dura extends to the very tip of the dentin where it continues over the free margin of the dental papilla. This observation is very significant when infection at the apex of an incompletely developed root is considered. As the person gets older and the root formation nears completion, the walls of the canal become parallel and converge. The divergent walls of the root canal permit the differentiation of an incompletely formed root from one that has developed and later undergone external resorption. In the latter case, the root may be short but the canal walls, although they may fail to meet, converge toward the apex.

The Alveolar Process

As a structural material, *cancellous bone* is homogeneous, although it differs mechanically from compact bone in that it possesses less strength. Cancellous bone is usually found where the chief function of the bony structure is to transmit tensile and compressive strains.

The maxilla and mandible are made up of outer and inner alveolar plates of bone, termed *cortical plates*, which serve as cortices of the alveolar process. The tooth socket is lined by a thin layer of dense cortical bone called the *lamina dura*. Beyond the lamina dura, the spongy cancellous bone serves to support the teeth and to anchor them to the mandible or maxilla. On the lingual and labial surfaces of the spongy bone are covering plates of dense bone named *alveolar plates*. The alveolar plates, spongy bone, and the lamina dura

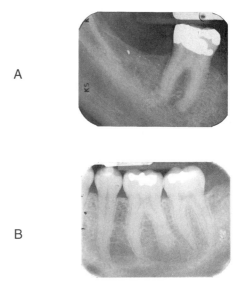

Fig. 92–2. The alveolar process with (A) the mandibular canal visible, (B) the periodontal ligament and lamina dura

are termed the *alveolar process*, figure 92–2. The radiolucent parts of spongy bone when viewed on a radiograph are called *medullary* spaces; the thin radiopaque lines separating them are called *trabeculae*.

Adjacent to the lamina dura lies the *periodontal ligament*. This is delicate, thin, vascular tissue of a density insufficient to absorb any appreciable amount of x rays. On the other side of the ligament lies the lamina dura, which does cast a shadow. With a dense structure on either side of the ligament, the space that the ligament occupies appears as a thin dark line.

The bone adjacent to the periodontal ligament lines the tooth socket. In common with cortical bone, it is denser than the adjacent cancellous bone. Because of its density, this layer of bone (the lamina dura) is revealed in radiographs as a thin white line. This line is of utmost importance in radiographic interpretation. If one bears in mind the great variety of shapes of the roots of teeth and the physical factors that enter into the production of the shadow of the lamina dura, it is easy to understand why there must be great radiographic differences in the lamina dura. Differences in thickness, density, shape, and the number of shadows would be expected merely from the study of cross sections of sockets as seen in dried skulls. All these differences in the radiographic appearance of lamina dura have no clinical significance as long as the lamina dura is continuous around the root.

The essential factor in the radiographic interpretation is that the shadow of the lamina dura must be continuous throughout its extent. Any deviation from this, any slight deficiency or discontinuity is highly suggestive and probably indicative of an abnormal condition.

The Maxilla and Mandible

It is important to note that no radiographic differentiation is possible between the cancellous bone of the alveolar process and the cortical plates that cover the lingual and buccal aspects of those processes. In the maxilla, the whole of the supporting bone, extending from the alveolar crest to the floor of the antrum and the nasal fossa, commonly presents a uniform appearance. The mandible, however, usually does not present a uniform pattern. The maxilla has a finer network pattern that is seen in the mandible of the same person.

LANDMARKS OF THE MAXILLA

There are two maxillary processes that, together, form the upper jaw. Each bone, consisting of four processes, also contains a large air-filled cavity within it called the *maxillary sinus*.

The Malar Bone

The prominence of the cheek is produced by the *malar bone* and *zygomatic process*. Only the inferior portion of the zygomatic process appears in intraoral radiographs. A gray or white shadow, depending on the thickness of the bone and the proportion of dense bone, is seen. The extent of the inferior border varies, beginning over the second bicuspid or first molar area and extending backward, usually beyond the limits of the film. The lowest part of the bone may be situated above the first molar or, less often, the second molar from which it passes backward and upward with varying degrees of sharpness. Depending on anatomical and technical factors, the relation of the shadow of the malar bone to the shadow of the roots of the teeth is variable.

Intraoral radiographs of the malar bone gives this relationship a *U* appearance that overlies the larger shadow of the antrum as a whole. Since the limbs of the *U* are made up of dense cortical bone, they present a white shadow that is accentuated by the dark background of the antrum or sinus.

The Nasal Septum

The nasal fossae often appear in the radiograph as dark shadows, at least in some part, because they contain air. Since the lower portions of the inferior turbinate (osseus) bone occupy some part of the nasal fossae, the dark area is not of uniform density. The nasal septum, which presents a gray or white dividing shadow of variable width, separates the fossae.

The nasal fossae are roughly pear shaped when seen in the large extraoral radiographs made in the posterior and anterior projection. In the intraoral radiographs, only portions of the fossa are seen. These shadows, resembling the letter *W*, have rounded inferior margins, with the nasal septum forming the central portion of the letter.

The nasal septum commonly presents a wide radiopaque shadow as it usually deviates slightly from the midline. A hazy gray shadow may be seen arising from the lateral wall of both fossae, which may extend to the septum or may fall short by a considerable distance. This shadow represents the anterior portions of the inferior turbinate bones. In the midline, at the inferior aspect of the nasal fossa, there usually is a small white inverted *V* that represents the anterior nasal spine. This shadow often is projected over that of the incisive foramen, giving the latter a heart-shaped appearance.

The relationship between apices of the upper incisors and the nasal fossae, which varies considerably, depends on the length of the roots of the teeth and the depth of the subnasal bone. In making radiographs of the upper incisor region, the angle of the central ray is directed downward in such a way that the true relationship of the incisors to the fossa is distorted; therefore, care must be exercised in interpreting the relationship of the two.

Alveolar Process

The alveolar process is a part of the maxilla (and mandible) and forms the investing and supporting tissues for the teeth.

Palatine Process

The superior surface of the palatine process forms a part of the floor of the nasal cavity; the inferior surface of the palatine process forms the roof of the mouth, figure 92–1C (#39). The following structures which are located in the palatine process may be seen on an intraoral radiograph.

Incisive Foramen

In the palate, at the junction of the apex of the premaxilla and the maxillary process, is the incisive foramen, figure 92–3A. It varies widely in shape from a mere slit to a round, oval, heart-, diamond-, or pear-shaped structure. This foramen transmits the nasal palatine nerves and vessels. The radiographic interpretation of this structure is important, because it is often mistaken for a pathological process and is sometimes the site of a cyst.

In radiographs made using the correct technique for the central incisor, the shadow of the incisive foramen almost always occupies a position in the midline of the maxilla. If the central rays are directed from the region of the lateral incisor, the shadow of the foramen may be projected toward the opposite side of the midline. This often leads to erroneous interpretation. Radiography deals with shadows, and in many cases anatomical relationships are grossly distorted.

Although there are great variations in the size, shape, and position of the normal incisive foramen, there is one invariable finding: When the foramen and apex of the normal incisor are superimposed by radiographic projection, the lamina dura and the apex of that tooth are intact.

Median Palatine Suture

In radiographs of the maxillary central incisor region, a radiolucent line extends from the alveolar crest to the posterior aspect of the palate. Sometimes, a short funnel-shaped widening

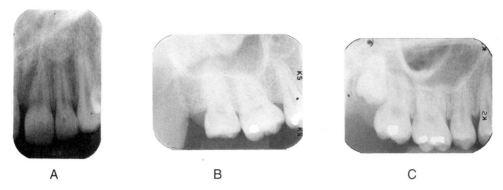

A   B   C

Fig. 92–3. Radiographs showing (A) anterior periapical, incisive foramen, (B) maxillary periapical, maxillary tuberosity and coronoid process, and (C) zygomatic or malar bone and maxillary sinus

appears in the anterior, which may be mistaken for an abnormality. The margins of the suture are lined by cortical bone; therefore, there is a radiopaque border along the edge of each maxilla.

The Coronoid Process

Numerous anatomical structures appear in radiographs of the maxillary third molars. One of these structures is the coronoid process, which may be mistaken for a retained root or an unerupted tooth.

The coronoid process usually appears as a cone-shaped shadow with the apex, which may be blunt or relatively pointed, directed upward and forward, figure 92–3B. The density of the shadow varies considerably from a faint haziness to a well-defined radiopaque shadow. This latter appearance is likely to be mistaken for that of a tooth. The true nature of the shadow may be demonstrated simply by making radiographs with the mouth wide open, in which case the shadow will disappear or the position will be altered sufficiently to make it obvious that it could not have represented a tooth.

Maxillary Sinus

The maxillary sinus, a cavity and bone which contains air, is revealed in radiographs as a dark shadow, figure 92–3C. As in all normal cavities and bone, the margins of the cavity consist of a thin layer of dense bone, the cortex, which appears as a thin white line in radiographs. Because there are differences in the thickness of the walls and the width of the sinus, the dark shadow of the antrum is not uniformly dense throughout.

The maxillary sinus is the largest of the paranasal sinuses. It is subject to both structural and pathological variations, and special problems may arise by reason of its relationship to the teeth.

The maxillary sinus is present at birth. Usually by age 6, it begins to enlarge, having descended to the level of the middle meatus. At puberty, the sinus has expanded, so that the floor is level with the base of the nose. Continued expansion occurs, and by adulthood the floor of the sinus has extended to the level of the alveolar process. This expansion may continue, so that it involves the palate and the tuberosity distal to the third molar. Because the sinus may become exposed during extraction of maxillary bicuspids, these extensions of the sinus are clinically important.

The relationship of the sinus to the teeth is not a constant one. The width of bone between the roots of the teeth and the floor of the sinus varies in thickness. The bone is thin; the roots of the

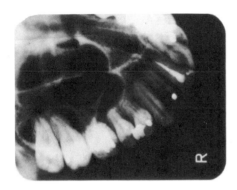

Fig. 92–4. Maxillary cuspid—molar region

teeth may form elevations on the floor of the sinus, and these elevations form recesses. Septa may also divide the sinus into two or more cavities.

The maxillary sinus is revealed as a dark shadow with a thin white cortical border. The radiographic characteristics of this cortical line are important because they often serve to differentiate a normal antrum from a pathological lesion closely resembling the antral shadow. Although the cortex of the sinus is always continuous, there are appearances that suggest small interruptions in the line; these are only a simulation of interruptions.

In intraoral radiographs, the sinus cavity is usually seen to extend from the bicuspid area to the tuberosity, figure 92–4. The anterior aspect of the sinus may be bluntly pointed, rounded, or even flat. Where the anterior wall of the sinus meets the floor of the nasal fossa, an inverted Y-shaped shadow appears, the diverging limbs of which represent the sinus wall in the cortex of the nasal fossa that curves anteriorly. The leg of the letter, or the long line, represents the lateral cortex of the nasal fossa passing backward to the pharyngeal end. This Y-shaped shadow is of value in differentiating some cysts in this region, for it tends to be obliterated in such conditions.

In some cases of doubt, the persistence of the shadow may be evidence against the presence of a lesion.

LANDMARKS OF THE MANDIBLE

At birth, the mandible is in two pieces, joined at the midline by soft tissue only. Within a year after birth, the suture is usually closed.

Mental Process or Ridge

The anterior and inferior aspect of the chin is usually thickened by the presence of a triangle of smooth and shiny denser bone, which stands out above the surface of the adjacent bone. This dense ridge of bone extends from the symphysis of the mandible to the region of the bicuspid. It is called a mental process or mental ridge and varies in different persons. It is more visibly pronounced on a person with heavy bones than one with light bones, thus showing corresponding differences on radiographs. In conventional intraoral radiographs the apex of the triangle may or may not be apparent, depending on the actual depth of the mandible at this side. When the apex is present, it appears to be formed by two dense lines that converge toward the midline. On some occasions, the density of the whole triangle is so great that it interferes with the clear view of the apices of the incisors, figure 92–5C.

Genial Tubercle

In the midline of the lingual surface of the mandible, there frequently may be seen an elevation situated well below the roots of the incisors representing the genial tubercles, figure 92–5A. In periapical radiographs, they appear as a localized area of increased density with a small dark spot, the lingual foramen, in the center. In occlusal radiographs showing the floor of the mouth, this tubercle protrudes, sometimes

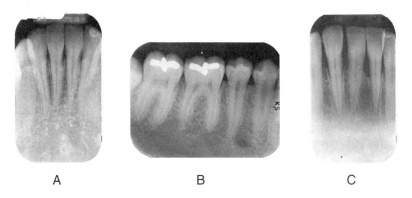

A   B   C

Fig. 92–5. Radiographs showing (A) genial tubercules and lingual foramen, (B) mental foramen (mandibular periapical), (C) mental process or ridge (mandibular periapical)

quite extensively, from the surface of the bone, suggesting to the inexperienced observer that an abnormality is present.

The Mental Foramen

The position of the mental foramen is variable, common sites being at or just below the apex of the second bicuspid or a little medial to and below the apex, figure 92–5B. The mental foramen appears on the radiograph as an area of radiolucency. The shadow may be oval, round, oblong, or any regular shape, or there may be no shadow at all. When present, it varies in size from a few millimeters to a centimeter or more.

Poor angulation sometimes results in a radiolucent area, the mental foramen appearing at the apex of a mandibular bicuspid. In this position, it may be mistaken for a pathological condition; therefore, it is very important to observe that the superimposition of the shadows of the root and foramen are not associated with any discontinuity of the lamina dura. Many teeth are needlessly removed because the superimposition of the mental foramen and root is misinterpreted as disease. It is an axiom that periapical disease should not be diagnosed from radiographs in the absence of discontinuity of the lamina dura.

A

B

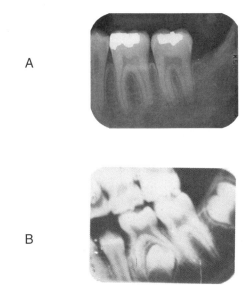

Fig. 92–6. Mandibular molar film showing (A) external and internal oblique ridges, and (B) mixed dentition (mandibular canal not obvious)

The Mandibular Canal

The mandibular canal commences at the mandibular foramen in the ascending ramus. It passes downward until it arrives at the body of the mandible where it turns forward to pass into the anterior portion of the bone. The mandibular

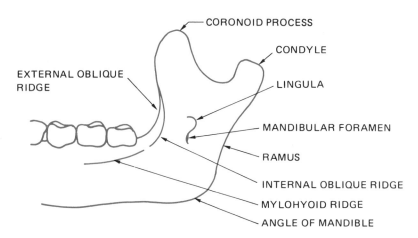

Fig. 92–7. Lingual aspect of the mandible

foramen varies greatly in its radiographic manifestations. Usually it appears as a funnel-shaped area of increased radiolucency with wide variation in the width, length, and depth of the funnel.

The mandibular canal, being a space in bone, appears as a dark shadow in radiographs. Because it is a normal anatomical space, it is lined by a cortical layer of bone. Although such shadows are observed, there is no one typical radiographic image because of the wide variations in the appearance of the canal, figure 92–6B. In most people, the canal appears as a dark, narrow ribbon between two white lines. However, in others, it is not even apparent but is seen as two faint, more or less parallel, white lines without any intermediate alteration in bone density.

Most commonly, the canal lies immediately below the roots of the molars and a little distance below the roots of the bicuspids. It often seems that the apices of the teeth in the mandibular canal coincide, ordinarily with a separation between them. One cannot assume that, because the apices appear to project into the canal, they actually do so. Rarely do the apices enter the canal, and even when they do, there may be no reliable evidence of this fact.

Nutrient Canals

Blood vessels lying in channels or grooves traverse the maxilla and mandible to supply the teeth and gingival tissues. Except for the mandibular canal, these vascular channels usually do not appear on radiographs. However, occasionally it is possible to see them. Radiographs may reveal vascular markings on the walls of the maxillary sinus; or they may be seen in the mandible, most frequently in the incisor region. These channels appear as dark linear shadows situated between the roots of adjacent teeth and more or less parallel with them. The canals fall short of the gingival crest and disappear at various distances below the level of the root apices.

External Oblique Ridge

On the external surface of the mandible is a ridge that descends along the ramus of the mandible and passes downward and outward to become the external oblique ridge, figures 92–6A and 92–7.

If this ridge continues past the third molar, it proceeds downward and forward on the outer part of the body of the mandible, terminating at or above the lower border. This structure may appear on the radiograph as a radiopaque line traversing the mandibular third molar region.

Internal Oblique Ridge and Mylohyoid Ridge

On the internal aspect of the ramus of the mandible is a prominent ridge that passes downward and forward from the ramus to the third molar. This is called the internal oblique ridge. On a radiograph it may show as a thin white line and is usually inferior to the external oblique ridge. The mylohyoid line, or ridge, is a ridge formed from the attachment of the mylohyoid muscle. It may appear to be in the same alignment as the internal oblique as if it were a continuation of that ridge. However, the mylohyoid is more horizontal along the inside of the mandible and below the posterior or molar region.

Coronoid Process

The coronoid process of the ascending ramus varies markedly in different persons. The process is usually cone shaped. The appearance of the coronoid process was covered in Radiographic Landmarks of the Maxilla.

SUGGESTED ACTIVITIES

- Study figure 92–1. Cover the legend, and identify as many of the numbered areas as possible. Repeat the activity.
- Using a full-mouth series of x-ray films, locate as many of the landmarks of the maxilla as you can. List each one and indicate which of the films showed those with normal radiographic appearance. List those with variations within the normal, and indicate which film you viewed to detect it.
- Locate as many landmarks as you can while viewing films of the mandible.
- On a sheet of paper list all the radiographic landmarks on one side and all the radiolucent on the other. Place "max" for maxillary or "mand" for mandibular after each one.
- Locate landmarks that you may expect to find in a panoramic radiograph.

REVIEW

1. List five factors to consider when reviewing radiographs.

   a. _____

   b. _____

   c. _____

   d. _____

   e. _____

2. What normal radiolucent landmark on the mandible could be misinterpreted as an abscess? _____

3. What causes an area to appear radiolucent? _____

_____

4. The thin radiopaque lines separating the medullary spaces are called _____

_____.

5. List as many maxillary landmarks as you would be able to see in a radio-graph. Write the appropriate word, radiopaque or radiolucent, after each.

_____

_____

_____

6. List as many mandibular landmarks as possible noting which are radiopaque and which are radiolucent._____

_____

_____

_____

Chapter 93: Quality Analysis of Radiographs

INTRODUCTION

As dental radiographs are now accepted as routine in dental practice and are generally accepted by the public, the operator of the dental x-ray equipment must not fail to exhibit "reasonable and ordinary skill" in this area of dental care. Radiographs must be on file with the patient's record for future use. They must be factual and provide evidence of the need for operative dental procedures and, on occasion, in court.

One must remember that, in a court of law, the best evidence is factual. However, mere introduction of radiographs in court is not assurance of their value if the films are inadequate because of poor placement, exposure, or processing.

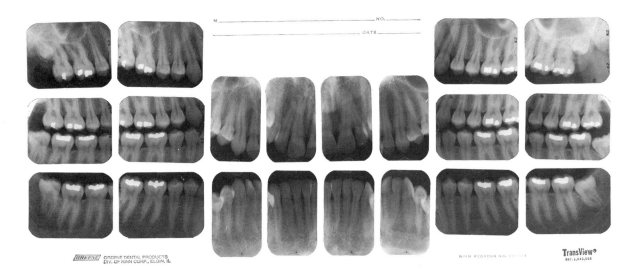

Fig. 93–1. Complete radiographic series (Courtesy Rinn Corporation, Elgin, IL)

COMPLETED RADIOGRAPHS

Images

Two terms which may be used to describe the darkness or lightness of images in the completed radiograph are *radiopaque* and *radiolucent*. Radiopaque objects are those that create a whiter shadow on the film by blocking x rays affecting the film emulsion, (i.e., enamel, bone). Radiolucent images occur when x rays are allowed to pass through the object and still expose the film, creating darker shadows, (i.e., soft tissue, sinuses). The following radiographs show a basic selection of landmarks that may be visible on radiographs placed in the proper area for a complete periapical series, or a bitewing series. Figure 93–1 shows an actual example of a complete radiographic survey, i.e., a "full-mouth" series, including bitewings.

PERIAPICALS

Maxillary Central Incisor

- both centrals
- mesial of adjacent laterals
- median palatine suture
- incisive foramen
- nasal fossa
- crowns, roots, and alveolar crest

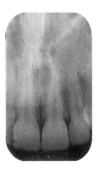

Maxillary Central and Lateral Incisor

- central and lateral
- half of adjacent central
- median palatine suture
- incisive foramen
- crowns, roots, and alveolar crest

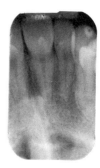

Maxillary Cuspid

- cuspid crown and apex
- oblique view of first bicuspid (premolar)
- bifurcation of first bicuspid (premolar)
- alveolar crest

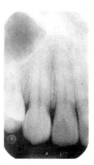

Maxillary Bicuspids (Premolars) and First Molar

- distal of lateral cuspids, bicuspids (premolars), and first molar apices
- maxillary sinus

- zygomatic process (malar bone)
- oblique view of crowns and roots

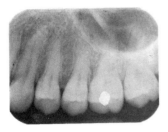

Maxillary Molar

- second bicuspid (premolar) and molar apices
- maxillary sinus
- maxillary tuberosity
- crowns, roots, and alveolar crest
- zygomatic process

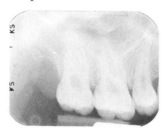

Maxillary Impacted Third Molar

- distal of second bicuspid (premolar)
- all molars
- maxillary tuberosity
- zygomatic process

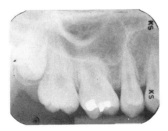

Mandibular Central-Lateral Incisor

- central and lateral incisors
- half of adjacent central
- lingual foramen
- genial tubercules
- crowns, roots, and alveolar crest

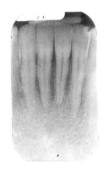

Mandibular Cuspid

- cuspid and first bicuspid (premolar)
- half of lateral incisor
- oblique view of second bicuspid (premolar)
- crowns, roots, and alveolar crest

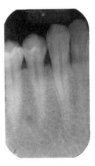

Mandibular Bicuspids (Premolars), First, and Second Molar

- distal of cuspid
- first and second bicuspids (premolars)
- first and second molars
- crowns, roots, and alveolar crest
- mental foramen

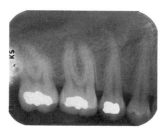

Mandibular Impacted Third Molar

- distal half of first molar
- molar contacts opened
- mandibular canal
- oblique ridges
- crowns, roots, and alveolar crest

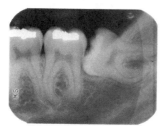

BITEWINGS

Bicuspid (Premolar) Bitewing

- distal of upper and lower cuspids
- upper bicuspid (premolar) contacts
- lower bicuspid (premolar) contacts

- accurate pulp chambers
- crowns and alveolar crest

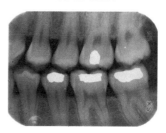

Molar Bitewing

- distal second bicuspid (premolar)
- all molars, impacted third molars
- area of third molar, if none present

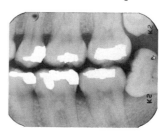

THE RADIOGRAPHIC IMAGE

The radiographic image is a graphic representation of the internal structures of an object placed in the path of the x-ray beam. The primary objective is to obtain maximum differentiation of tissues on the film. This differentiation is realized only when the film has four visual qualities: radiographic **detail**, radiographic **density**, radiographic **contrast**, and radiographic **distortion** (or lack of it). Although the quality of the x-ray beam depends on certain factors concerned with the production of the beam, the visual (diagnostic) quality of the radiograph depends on:

- *Radiographic detail:* The sharpness of the image, or the clean-cut outlines or borders of the images on the radiograph. (The greatest single cause of loss of detail, or lack of sharpness, is motion of the patient, the tubehead, or the film.)

- *Radiographic density:* The overall degree of darkening of the exposed film and the amount of light transmitted through the film. Overall density depends on the number of photons absorbed by the film emulsion and is controlled by varying the milliamperage and exposure time.
- *Radiographic contrast:* The difference in densities (black, white, and various shades of gray) on adjacent areas of the film. Contrast is generally controlled by using a fixed exposure time and milliamperage but varying the kilovoltage.
- *Radiographic distortion:* Factors that tend to increase or decrease the size of the object and to change the shape of the object. Both detail

and contrast are reduced by *fog.* Fog is produced by secondary radiation, faulty darkroom technique, use of an unsafe safelight, darkroom leakage, or by using outdated x-ray film.

EXPOSURE FACTORS

Exposure Time (Seconds)

If two radiographs are taken of the same area using a fixed milliamperage and kilovoltage BUT VARYING THE EXPOSURE TIME, the one taken at the longer exposure time will display a greater overall density; see art.

Milliamperage (mA)

If radiographs are taken of the same area using a fixed exposure time and kilovoltage BUT

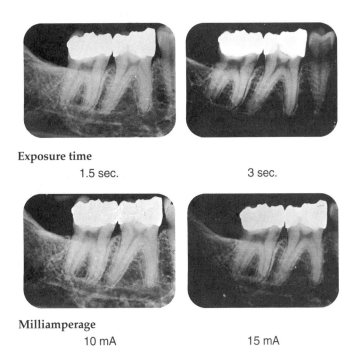

Exposure time

1.5 sec.   3 sec.

Milliamperage

10 mA   15 mA

Fig. 93–2. Exposure time and milliamperage

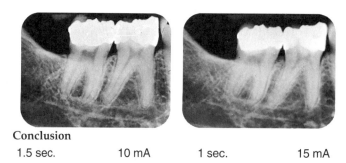

Conclusion

1.5 sec.   10 mA   1 sec.   15 mA

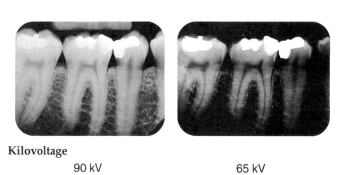

Kilovoltage

90 kV   65 kV

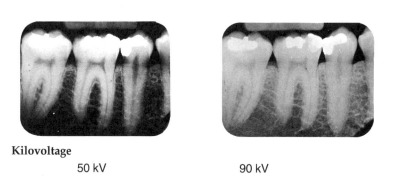

Kilovoltage

50 kV   90 kV

Fig. 93–3. Kilovoltage and contrast

VARYING THE MILLIAMPERAGE, the overall density will be increased as the milliamperage is raised (see art, page 709).

Conclusion

Because both exposure time and milliamperage control the density of a radiograph, they can be combined as a single factor known as milliampere-seconds (mAs); see art, page 710.

Example:
$$\left.\begin{array}{rclcl} 5\,mA & \times & 3 & sec. & = & 15\,mAs \\ 10\,mA & \times & 1.5 & sec. & = & 15\,mAs \\ 15\,mA & \times & 1 & sec. & = & 15\,mAs \end{array}\right\} = \text{Constant Density}$$

Note: It is recommended that maximum milliamperage be used to permit the shortest exposure time.

Kilovoltage

If two radiographs are taken of the same area using a fixed exposure time and milliamperage BUT VARYING THE KILOVOLTAGE, the one taken with the greater kilovoltage will display a greater density and a diminished contrast; see art, page 710.

A radiograph taken with LOW KILOVOLTAGE will display HIGH CONTRAST, because the number of densities that comprise the image are relatively few because of the limited penetrating power of the x-ray beam. This is known as *short-scale* contrast: densities are limited and change abruptly from black to white.

A radiograph taken with HIGH KILOVOLTAGE will display LOW CONTRAST, because the

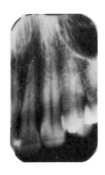

Fig. 93–4. Elongation

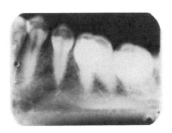

Fig. 93–5. Foreshortening

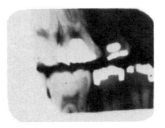

Fig. 93–7. Cone-cut

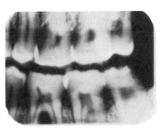

Fig. 93–8. Overlapping

Inadequacy	Causative Factor	Inadequacy	Causative Factor
Elongation (Figure 93–4)	Insufficient vertical angulation	Density Too Light	Insufficient exposure Insufficient development
Foreshortening (Figure 93–5)	Excessive vertical angulation		Excessive fixation
Partial Image (Figure 93–7)	Cone-cut (either incorrect direction of central ray or incorrect film placement)		Solutions too cold Use of aged, contaminated, or poorly mixed solutions Outdated films
	Incompletely immersed in processing solutions		Wrong side of film placed toward tube (leaded side of packet toward teeth)
	Film touched other film or side of tank during processing	Too Dark	Excessive exposure Excessive development Too warm temperature of developer Unsafe safelight Exposure to overhead light (may be black after processing)
Overlapping (Figure 93–8)	Incorrect horizontal angulation (central ray not directed through inter-proximal)	Artifacts Pattern (Figure 93–12)	Foil side of film placed next to teeth
No Image	Machine not functioning properly	Dark Lines (Figure 93–13)	Moon-shaped mark left by fingernail
	Machine not turned on during exposure		Film bent or creased
	Film placed in fixer before developer		Wrapper sticking to film when opened due to excess saliva of patient (not drying film surface after exposure)
Blurred Image (Figure 93–9)	Movement of film, patient or tube during exposure		
	Film exposed a second time		Static electricity (film removed with force before processing)
Stretched Appearance of Teeth or Supporting Tissues (Figure 93–10)	Film plane was bent, not flat, overcontoured	Stains and Spots	Finger marks Unclean hanger and/or clips Developer, fixer, water, or dust splatter
Fog Chemical Fog	Deterioration of processing solutions		Splattering dry films with solutions or water
	Imbalance of chemicals in solutions		Air bells adhering to film surface (insufficient agitation of films)
Radiation Fog (Figure 93–11)	Improper storage of film (both unused and exposed prior to processing)	(Figure 93–14)	Insufficient rinsing after developing before fixing
Light Fog	Exposure to light (either before or during processing)		Overlapping of films in tanks or on drying racks
(Figure 93–16)	Unsafe safelight Darkroom leak		Paper wrapper stuck to film during processing
Reticulation	Sudden temperature changes between processing solutions and wash water	Latent Film Figure 93–15)	Incomplete processing and/or rinsing
		Discoloration	Too warm a storage place Stored too close to chemicals

Fig. 93–6. Radiographic inadequacies and causative factors

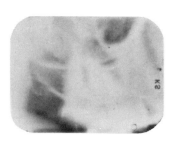

Fig. 93–9. Blurred image

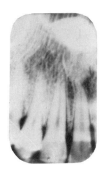

Fig. 93–10. Results of film bending

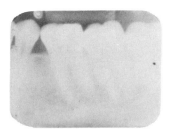

Fig. 93–11. Film fog

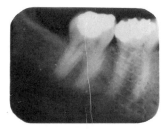

Fig. 93–12. Embossed pattern

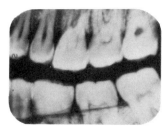

Fig. 93–13. Dark line

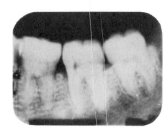

Fig. 93–14. Incomplete film washing during processing

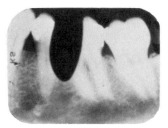

Fig. 93–15. Incomplete fixing process. Two films were probably touching each other.

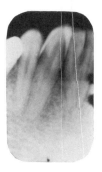

Fig. 93–16. Light leak

number of densities in the image are increased because of the greater penetrating power of the x-ray beam. This is known as *long-scale* contrast, because additional densities are recorded on the film and the result is a more gradual change from black to white. These added densities may detract from the esthetic quality of the image, *but* they also may reveal information that is obscured on the more esthetic, high-contrast radiograph; see art, page 710.

Film Inadequacies

Several factors contribute to inadequate radiographic images and render them useless for proper diagnosis, as seen in figures 93–4 and 93–5. Figure 93–6 lists some common inadequacies and their causative factors (illustrated in figures 93–7 to 93–16). Care must be taken to avoid such results when making and handling radiographs.

RESULTS

By developing a systematic procedure for the bitewing survey, diagnostic films will be accomplished, figures 93–17 to 93–19.

SUGGESTED ACTIVITY

- Select a mounted periapical radiographic survey. Identify as many landmarks as possible. List them according to individual radiograph, using the completed radiographs presented in this chapter as an aid.

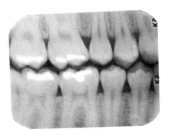

Fig. 93–17. Bicuspid (premolar) film

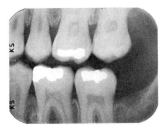

Fig. 93–18. Molar film

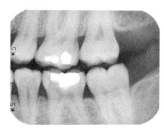

Fig. 93–19. Molar film (third molars are missing)

REVIEW

1. What are the four visual qualities a diagnostic radiograph should possess? Briefly explain each.

   a. _____

   _____

   _____

   b. _____

   _____

   _____

   c. _____

   _____

   _____

   d. _____

   _____

   _____

2. What is the greatest single cause of loss of detail or sharpness of a radiographic image? _____

3. How does fogging of film occur? _____

   _____

4. Using a fixed mA and kVp, how does increased exposure time affect a radiograph? _____

   _____

   _____

5. Using a fixed exposure time and kVp, how does increased mA affect a radiograph? _____

_____

_____

6. Using a fixed exposure time and mA, how does increased kVp affect a radiograph? _____

_____

_____

7. What is meant by "short-scale" contrast? _____

_____

8. What is meant by "long-scale" contrast? _____

_____

9. Low kilovoltage will result in _____ contrast; high kilovoltage will result in _____ contrast.

10. Name the three stages during which inadequacies may occur.

a. _____

b. _____

c. _____

11. Elongation and foreshortening of the image are due to improper _____.

12. What would be the reason for reticulation of the image? _____

_____

_____

Chapter 94: A Program of Quality Assurance for Dental Radiography

OBJECTIVES:

After studying this chapter, the student will be able to:
- Define the term *quality assurance* as it relates to dental radiography.
- Identify the components of a quality assurance program.
- Explain the function of a reference film.
- Explain the rationale for using a film monitoring device.

INTRODUCTION

The term *quality assurance* in dental radiography describes a systematic approach to control and ensures that all components in a radiographic system are functioning at an acceptable level of proficiency.

An established *quality assurance program* should maintain a standard of operation that will produce quality dental radiographs while reducing the level of ionizing radiation to both patient and operator.

The first step in a quality assurance program is to establish a reference of baseline value by which the x-ray equipment and film processing system can be monitored before a problem occurs that could adversely affect the diagnostic quality of the radiographs. A program of this type has been shown to lower the level of radiation exposure to patients through the decrease in the number of retakes.

X-RAY UNIT

Monitoring of generators (transformers) and other electronic components (kVp, mA, and timer) of the unit should be tested by a qualified physicist or x-ray engineer at least once a year.

ASSESSMENT PROGRAM FOR DARKROOM

Test Safelight or Other Light Leakage

1. Take an exposed film to darkroom.
2. Close darkroom door and turn on safelight.

3. Remove film from packet, and place on clean, dry countertop.
4. Place a coin in the center of unwrapped film.
5. Allow the coin to remain on film for five minutes.
6. After five minutes remove coin, and process film.
7. If processed film shows an outline of the coin, the film is being fogged by faulty safelight or other darkroom leakage.
8. Should #7 occur, replace safelight, or take steps to eliminate the cause.

Daily Evaluation of Processing Solutions

1. Check solution levels to be certain that the developer and fixer will cover the films on the top clips of hanger(s).
2. Fresh developer or replenisher should be added to maintain a proper level in developer tank. The level of the fixer may be restored with fresh fixer.
3. Change solutions at regular, prescribed intervals.

Evaluation of X-Ray Machine and Processing Chemicals, Using a Step Wedge

1. Place metal-alloy step wedge on top of an unexposed intraoral film packet, figure 94–1.
2. Position cylinder or positioning indicating device (PID) over step wedge, allowing $1/4$ inch distance between the end of cylinder or PID and the top step of the wedge.

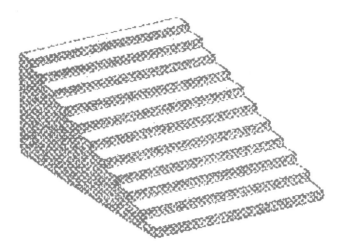

Fig. 94–1. Step wedge

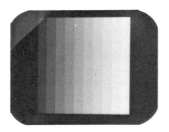

Fig. 94–2. Radiograph of step wedge

3. Expose the film, using the recommended exposure factors.
4. Process in fresh chemicals. It is important to use fresh chemicals for the first test, because subsequent tests will be based on this initial test film.
5. The processed radiograph should reveal ten distinct steps of the wedge (normal contrast), figure 94–2. If the steps are lost on the lighter end of the scale, radiographs may be underexposed, requiring either an increase in exposure time or milliamperage (mA).

* Rinn DXT TRS, Rinn Corporation, Elgin, IL.

Should some of the steps be lost on the darker end of the scale, the radiograph is overexposed and will require a decrease in exposure time or mA.

Note: An increase in kilovolt peak (kVp) will increase density but will decrease contrast (Chapter 93).

6. The developing solution can be checked daily, using the step wedge, following Steps 1–4. The solution is still functioning properly if all ten steps continue to appear. When the chemicals becomes exhausted, steps on the lighter end of the scale will begin to fade. This is the time to change the developer and fixer solutions.

Reference Film

The use of a reference film is another method to monitor film quality. Be sure to include these steps:

1. Expose periapical film, using DXT TRS* or skull.
2. Process film in fresh solutions using the time-temperature method.

3. When dry, tape radiograph to a corner of a viewbox.
4. Compare all subsequent radiographs to the reference film to determine film density and contrast.

   Note: If overall film quality is reduced and all factors of exposure have been correct, it is apparent that the chemicals are depleted. Change processing solutions.

Monitoring of Other Equipment

The viewbox should be checked periodically. Fluorescent tubes that show blackening at the ends should be replaced.

Retakes

Retake films may be made only when proper diagnosis cannot otherwise be accomplished, and by prescription of the dentist.

RADIATION SAFETY ASSURANCE—PATIENT AND OPERATOR

Patient

1. X-ray exposure to the patient must be based on diagnostic need.

2. Use a lead apron and thyroid shield or collar.
3. Use D or E speed film.
4. Use high kVp technique.
5. Use open-ended, lead-lined cylinder or PID. The rectangular PID is considered ideal, Chapter 77.
6. Use appropriate techniques in exposing and processing radiographs.

Operator

1. Monitoring devices or "film badges" are recommended to provide a useful record of occupational exposure.
2. Use of an accepted radiographic technique observing all safety practices

SUGGESTED ACTIVITIES

- The student should test the darkroom for safelight or other light leakage.
- Using the step wedge, the student should expose, process and evaluate a radiograph.

REVIEW

1. What is a reference film?_____

   _____

2. Give the step-by-step procedure for checking safelight and other darkroom light leakage.

   a. _____

   _____

   b. _____

   _____

c. _____

_____

d. _____

_____

e. _____

_____

f. _____

_____

g. _____

_____

h. _____

_____

3. What is the main reason for establishing a quality assurance program?

_____

4. What should a properly exposed and processed step wedge radiograph reveal?

_____

5. If the steps are lost on the lighter end of the scale in a step wedge radiograph, this indicates _____.

6. Name the six steps that can reduce patient radiation.

a. _____

b. _____

c. _____

d. _____

e. _____

f. _____

Chapter 95: Mounting Dental Radiographs

INTRODUCTION

Dental mounts should be stiff and have a sufficiently glazed surface to promote permanent filing of radiographs. Their construction should ensure that the films remain rigid and securely in place.

Mounts come in various sizes and with 1, 2, 4, 7, 14, 16, 18, 20, and 28 windows. Bitewing mounts have either 2 or 4 windows. The most commonly used periapical mounts have 16 and 18 windows.

TYPES OF MOUNTS

Clear Plastic Mounts

Advantages
- Reasonable price
- Little storage problem
- Water repellent
- Reusable
- Easy to handle

Disadvantages
- Subject to scratches
- Crack, split (cannot be reused)
- Glare of surrounding films inhibits diagnosis

Plastic Mounts

Advantages
- Same as for clear plastic
- Frosted quality cuts out light glare

Disadvantages
- Same as for clear plastic

Cardboard Mounts

Advantages
- Block out view of any object detracting from film
- Cheaper than plastic

Disadvantages
- Soil easily
- Absorb water
- Film is not held tightly
- Bend and break easily
- Difficult to mount films
- Seldom reusable

When bitewing films are mounted, the operator must keep in mind that the center of the mount is the median line and that the distal portion of the area appears along the right margin of the film and is, therefore, the left-hand side of the dental arch. If it appears along the left margin, the right side is indicated. This view of the films when mounted represents the facial aspect to the operator.

MATERIALS NEEDED

- 2- or 4-window mount for bitewing and 16- or 18-window mounts for periapical

- Developed films
- Rubber finger cot or white cotton gloves

INSTRUCTIONS

1. Cover the index finger with the rubber finger cot. Hold the film edgewise with the thumb and forefinger to avoid leaving finger marks on the film.
2. If using gloves, make certain they are clean and as free of lint as possible.
3. Determine the right side of the film
   a. Convex dot toward the operator
   b. Second molar appears along distal margin of the film; bicuspid area along the mesial margin of the film
   c. Occlusal line curves slightly upward from mesial to distal
   d. Place film in horizontal position in the right of the median line for the left side; to the left for the right side
4. Mount the anterior (premolar area) films toward the center of the mount; mount the molar areas toward the outer margins.
5. Hold film with the convex side of the dot TOWARD the operator.
6. Hold mount in one hand and place film in mount with the other hand.

SUGGESTED ACTIVITIES

- Practice mounting bitewing films and peri-apical films through the use of films that are kept on file.
- When you have mounted one set and viewed it for accuracy, select another set and repeat the procedure.
- Practice this procedure until you can do it rapidly and without error.

REVIEW

1. Give two desirable qualities for dental film mounts.

   a. _____

   b. _____

2. What are three advantages of clear plastic mounts?

   a. _____

   b. _____

   c. _____

3. How many windows are on a mount for bitewing films?_____

4. How many windows are on a mount for a full set of periapical radiographs?

_____

5. If the bitewing films are mounted properly, which way does the occlusal plane curve? _____

6. Describe how the operator can tell which is the patient's right side on a full-mouth set of radiographs. _____

_____

Chapter 96: Labeling and Filing Dental Radiographs

OBJECTIVES:	After studying this chapter, the student will be able to: • Name three reasons for keeping dental radiographs. • Determine proper storage. • State the proper labeling and filing procedure for dental radiographs.

INTRODUCTION

All x-ray films of a patient should be kept in the same envelope and filed alphabetically in a steel cabinet. Drawers should accommodate envelopes without crowding or without excess space. Because dental films are the property of the dentist, it is essential that they be kept in a cool, dry place that is as nearly fireproof as possible. Films may become crimped or soiled because of moisture. Care should be taken that the films are not bent, scratched, or otherwise damaged—this impairs their diagnostic value.

All files should be kept for at least a period of five years as a means of comparing progress of dental treatment; as a legal protection in case of malpractice suits; to indicate the necessity of operation and the results obtained; and for identification of deceased persons after ordinary characteristics of identification no longer exist.

MATERIALS NEEDED

- steel cabinet
- manila envelope (size needed for film mount)
- mounted films

INSTRUCTIONS

Film Mount

1. Write patient's name in full on top line, indicated by:
   M _____
   (Example: Mrs. Janet W. Smith)

2. Write date radiographs were taken on second line, indicated by:
   DATE_____
3. Fill in the number according to the patient file system on line indicated by:
   NO. _____
   NUMBER OF FILMS: _____
4. Fill in the dentist's name and who referred the patient on lines indicated by:
   DR._____
   REFERRED BY_____

Film Envelopes

1. Write patient's full name in the upper left corner of envelope:
   - Last name, title, first name, and middle initial
   - **Example:** Smith, Mr. James Lowell
     Smith, Ms. Martha Louise
     Smith, Mrs. Mary T. (Russell J.)
     Smith, Mrs. Jane L.
2. Place envelope in the indexed section of file indicated by the first letter of the last name.
   - Alphabetize according to first three letters of last name and initials of first name.
   - **Example:** James, Mrs. Susan R.
     Jamison, Mr. Robert T.
     Jorgensen, Miss Sarah L.
     Jorgensen, Mr. Thomas D.
     Juergens, Mrs. Lillian M.
3. *Never seal envelopes.*

REVIEW

1. Give three reasons for keeping radiographs for at least five years.

   a. _____

   b. _____

   c. _____

2. Describe proper storage for mounted radiographs. _____

   _____

   _____

3. List the four items necessary on the label for the x-ray mount.

   a. _____

   b. _____

   c. _____

   d. _____

4. How should the film envelope be filed? _____

   _____

Appendix A: A Guide to Daily Food Choices

Food Guide Pyramid

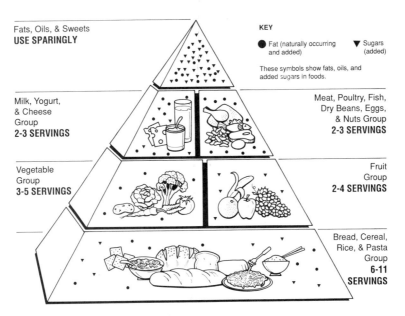

Fats, Oils, & Sweets
USE SPARINGLY

KEY
● Fat (naturally occurring and added)   ▼ Sugars (added)

These symbols show fats, oils, and added sugars in foods.

Milk, Yogurt, & Cheese Group
2-3 SERVINGS

Meat, Poultry, Fish, Dry Beans, Eggs, & Nuts Group
2-3 SERVINGS

Vegetable Group
3-5 SERVINGS

Fruit Group
2-4 SERVINGS

Bread, Cereal, Rice, & Pasta Group
6-11 SERVINGS

Source: U.S. Department of Agriculture, Washington, DC.

726

A Sample Label: Macaroni and Cheese

Nutrition Facts

Standardized — Serving Size: 1/2 cup
Servings Per Container: 4

Amount Per Serving

Calories 260   Calories from Fat 120 — *New*

% Daily Value* — *New*

Total fat 13g	20%
Saturated Fat 5g	25%
Cholesterol 30mg	10%
Sodium 660mg	28%
Total carbohydrate 31g	11%
Dietary Fiber 0g	0%
Sugars 5g	
Protein 5g	

New

Vitamin A 4% • Vitamin C 2% • Calcium 15% • Iron 4%

* Percents (%) of a Daily Value are based on a
2,000 calorie diet. Your Daily Values may vary
higher or lower depending on your calorie needs.

Nutrient		2,000 Calories	2,500 Calories
Total fat	Less than	65g	80g
Sat. fat	Less than	20g	25g
Cholesterol	Less than	300mg	300mg
Sodium	Less than	2,400mg	2,400mg
Total carbohydrate		300g	375g
Fiber		25g	30g

— *New*

1g Fat = 9 calories
New — 1g Carbohydrate = 4 calories
1g Protein = 4 calories

Source: *Wellness Letter*, March 1993, by permission.

Appendix B: Consumer-Patient Radiation Health and Safety Act of 1981

Subtitle I—Consumer-Patient Radiation Health and Safety Act of 1981

SHORT TITLE

[42 USC 10001] note.

Sec. 975. This subtitle may be cited as the "Consumer-Patient Radiation Health and Safety Act of 1981."

STATEMENT OF FINDINGS

[42 USC 10001.]

Sec. 976. The Congress finds that—
(1) it is in the interest of public health and safety to minimize unnecessary exposure to potentially **hazardous radiation due to medical and dental radiologic procedures;**
(2) it is in the interest of public health and safety to have a continuing supply of adequately educated persons and appropriate accreditation and certification programs administered by State governments;
(3) **the protection of the public health and safety from unnecessary exposure to potentially hazardous radiation due to medical and dental radiologic procedures and the assurance of efficacious procedures are the responsibility of State and Federal governments;**
(4) persons who administer radiologic procedures, including procedures at Federal facilities, should be required to demonstrate competence by reason of education, training, and experience; and
(5) the administration of radiologic procedures and the effect on individuals of such procedures have a substantial and direct effect upon United States interstate commerce.

STATEMENT OF PURPOSE

[42 USC 10002.]

Sec. 977. It is the purpose of this subtitle to—
(1) provide for the establishment of minimum standards by the Federal Government for the accreditation of education programs for persons who administer radiologic procedures and for the certification of such persons; and
(2) **insure that medical and dental radiologic procedures are consistent with rigorous safety precautions and standards.**
[bold type added]

DEFINITIONS

[42 USC 10003.]

Sec. 978. Unless otherwise expressly provided, for purposes of this subtitle, the term—
(1) "radiation" means ionizing and nonionizing radiation in amounts beyond normal background levels from sources such as medical and **dental radiologic procedures;**
(2) "radiologic procedure" means any procedure or article intended for use in—
   (A) The diagnosis of disease or other medical or **dental conditions** in humans (including diagnostic X-rays or nuclear medicine procedures); or
   (B) the cure, mitigation, treatment, or prevention of disease in humans;
that achieves its intended purpose through the emission of radiation;
(3) "radiologic equipment" means any radiation electronic product which emits or detects radiation and which is used or intended for use to—
   (A) diagnose disease or other medical or **dental conditions** (including diagnostic X-ray equipment); or

(B) cure, mitigate, treat, or prevent disease in humans; that achieves its intended purpose through the emission or detection of radiation;

(4) "practitioner" means any licensed doctor of medicine, osteopathy, **dentistry**, podiatry, or chiropractic, who prescribes radiologic procedures for other persons;

(5) "persons who administer radiologic procedures" means any person, other than a practitioner, who intentionally administers radiation to other persons for medical purposes, and includes medical radiologic technologists (**including dental hygienists and assistants**), radiation therapy technologists, and nuclear medicine technologists;

(6) "Secretary" means the Secretary of Health and Human Services; and

(7) "State" means the several States, the District of Columbia, the Commonwealth of Puerto Rico, the Commonwealth of the Northern Mariana Islands, the Virgin Islands, Guam, American Samoa, and the Trust Territory of the Pacific Islands.

PROMULGATION OF STANDARDS

[Regulation. 42 USC 10004.]

Sec. 979. (a) Within twelve months after the date of enactment of this Act, the Secretary, in consultation with the Radiation Policy Council, the Administrator of Veterans' Affairs, the Administrator of the Environmental Protection Agency, appropriate agencies of the States, and appropriate professional organizations, shall by regulation promulgate minimum standards for the accreditation of educational programs to train individuals to perform radiologic procedures. Such standards shall distinguish between programs for the education of (1) medical radiologic technologists (including radiographers), (2) **dental auxiliaries (including dental hygienists**

and assistants**),** (3) radiation therapy technologists, (4) nuclear medicine technologists, and (5) such other kinds of health auxiliaries who administer radiologic procedures as the Secretary determines appropriate. Such standards shall not be applicable to educational programs for practitioners.

[Regulation.]

(b) Within twelve months after the date of enactment of this Act, the Secretary, in consultation with the Radiation Policy Council, the Administrator of Veterans' Affairs, the Administrator of the Environmental Protection Agency, interested agencies of the States, and appropriate professional organizations, shall by regulation promulgate minimum standards for the certification of persons who administer radiologic procedures. Such standards shall distinguish between certification of (1) medical radiologic technologists (including radiographers), (2) **dental auxiliaries (including dental hygienists and assistants),** (3) radiation therapy technologists, (4) nuclear medicine technologists, and (5) such other kinds of health auxiliaries who administer radiologic procedures as the Secretary determines appropriate. Such standards shall include minimum certification criteria for individuals with regard to accredited education, practical experience, successful passage of required examinations, and such other criteria as the Secretary shall deem necessary for the adequate qualification of individuals to administer radiologic procedures. Such standards shall not apply to practitioners.

MODEL STATUTE

[42 USC 10005.]

Sec. 980. In order to encourage the administration of accreditation and certification programs by the States, the Secretary shall prepare and transmit to the States a model statute for radiologic procedure safety. Such model statute shall provide that—

(1) it shall be unlawful in a State for individuals to perform radiologic procedures unless such individuals are certified by the State to perform such procedures; and

(2) any educational requirements for certification of individuals to perform radiologic procedures shall be limited to educational programs accredited by the State.

COMPLIANCE

[42 USC 10006.]

Sec. 981. (a) The Secretary shall take all actions consistent with law to effectuate the purposes of this subtitle.

(b) A state may utilize an accreditation or certification program administered by a private entity if—

(1) such State delegates the administration of the State accreditation or certification program to such private entity;

(2) such program is approved by the State; and

(3) such program is consistent with the minimum Federal standards promulgated under this subtitle for such program.

(c) Absent compliance by the States with the provisions of this subtitle within three years after the date of enactment of this Act, the Secretary shall report to the Congress recommendations for legislative changes considered necessary to assure the States' compliance with this subtitle.

[Report to Congress.]

(d) The Secretary shall be responsible for continued monitoring of compliance by the States

with the applicable provisions of this subtitle and shall report to the Senate and the House of Representatives by January 1, 1982, and January 1 of each succeeding year the status of the States' compliance with the purposes of this subtitle.

(e) Notwithstanding any other provision of this section, in the case of a State which has, prior to the effective date of standards and guidelines promulgated pursuant to this subtitle, established standards for the accreditation of educational programs and certification of radiologic technologists, such State shall be deemed to be in compliance with the conditions of this section unless the Secretary determines, after notice and hearing, that such State standards do not meet the minimum standards prescribed by the Secretary or are inconsistent with the purposes of this subtitle.

FEDERAL RADIATION GUIDELINES

[42 USC 10007.]

Sec. 982. The Secretary shall, in conjunction with the Radiation Policy Council, the Administrator of Veterans' Affairs, the Administrator of the Environmental Protection Agency, appropriate agencies of the States, and appropriate professional organizations, promulgate Federal radiation guidelines with respect to radiologic procedures. Such guidelines shall—

(1) determine the level of radiation exposure due to radiologic procedures which is unnecessary and specify the techniques, procedures, and methods to minimize such unnecessary exposure;

(2) provide for the elimination of the need for retakes of diagnostic radiologic procedures;

(3) provide for the elimination of unproductive screening programs;

(4) provide for the optimum diagnostic information with minimum radiologic exposure; and

(5) include the therapeutic application of radiation to individuals in the treatment of disease, including nuclear medicine applications.

APPLICABILITY TO FEDERAL AGENCIES

[42 USC 10008.]

Sec. 983. (a) Except as provided in subsection (b), each department, agency, and instrumentality of the executive branch of the Federal Government shall comply with standards promulgated pursuant to this subtitle.

[Regulations.]

[38 USC 101 et seq.]

(b)(1) The Administrator of Veterans' Affairs, through the Chief Medical Director of the Veterans' Administration, shall, to the maximum extent feasible consistent with the responsibilities of such Administrator and Chief Medical Director under subtitle 38, United States Code, prescribe regulations making the standards promulgated pursuant to this subtitle applicable to the provision of radiologic procedures in facilities over which the Administrator has jurisdiction. In prescribing and implementing regulations pursuant to this subsection, the Administrator shall consult with the Secretary in order to achieve the maximum possible coordination of the regulations, standards, and guidelines, and the implementation thereof, which the Secretary and the Administrator prescribe under this subtitle.

[Report to congressional committees.]

(2) Not later than 180 days after standards are promulgated by the Secretary pursuant to this subtitle, the Administrator of Veterans' Affairs shall submit to the appropriate committees of Congress a full report with respect to the regulations (including guidelines, policies, and procedures thereunder) prescribed pursuant to paragraph (1) of this subsection. Such report shall include—

(A) an explanation of any inconsistency between standards made applicable by such regulations and the standards promulgated by the Secretary pursuant to this subtitle;

(B) an account of the extent, substance, and results of consultations with the Secretary respecting the prescription and implementation of regulations by the Administrator; and

(C) such recommendations for legislation and administrative action as the Administrator determines are necessary and desirable.

[Publication in Federal Register.]

(3) The Administrator of Veterans' Affairs shall publish the report required by paragraph (2) in the Federal Register.

(NOTE: Bold print has been added.)

Glossary of General Terms

Abrasion Wearing, grinding, or rubbing away by friction. Pathological wearing away of dental hard tissue by friction.

Abscess A localized collection of pus in a limited area.

Abscess, periapical A localized area of pus formed in the alveolus, at the apex of the root tip.

Abscess, periodontal A localized area of acute or chronic inflammation, containing pus, found in the periodontal tissues.

Absorption The taking up of a material, usually of a liquid or a gas by a solid.

Abutment A tooth, root, or implant used for the support or retention of a fixed or removable prosthesis.

Accelerator A chemical that increases the rate of a chemical reaction.

Acrylic An organic resin from which various types of dental appliances, retainers, and devices are constructed.

Activator A chemical or form of energy that excites another chemical to accelerate a reaction.

Acute Having a short and relatively severe course, as opposed to chronic.

Addiction Drug-oriented behavior that includes the compulsive abuse of the drug, an obsession to secure its supply, and great difficulty to discontinue its use.

Adhesion The force that causes unlike molecules to attach to each other. The state in which two surfaces are secured together by chemical forces, mechanical interlocking forces, or both.

Adrenalin Epinephrine. A vasoconstrictor.

Aerobes A variety of bacteria that must have oxygen in order to grow.

Agar-agar A polysaccharide extracted from seaweed and used as the active ingredient in a reversible or irreversible impression material.

AIDS Acquired immunodeficiency syndrome.

Alginate See *Hydrocolloid, irreversible*.

Allergen An antigenic substance that can trigger the allergic state.

Allergy An immunological response to an antigen that results in impaired function.

Alloy The combination of two or more metals, excluding mercury.

Alveolar bone That part of the alveolar process that lines the sockets into which the roots of the teeth are affixed.

Alveolar mucosa The mucous membrane covering the basal part of the alveolar process and continuing to form the lining of the cheeks and the floor of the mouth.

Alveolar process The extension of the maxilla and mandible that surrounds and supports the teeth and forms the dental arches.

Alveoli The cavity within the alveolar process in which the root of the tooth is held in position.

Amalgam The combination of a dental alloy with mercury.

Amalgam carrier An instrument for carrying small masses of triturated amalgam to a prepared cavity.

Amalgam carver An instrument used to carve the anatomy of a freshly condensed amalgam restoration.

Amalgam condenser An instrument used for condensing or packing amalgam into the cavity preparation.

Amalgamation The reaction that occurs between mercury and a dental alloy.

Amalgam well A metal cup that holds the triturated amalgam.

Anabolism The process of converting nutrients to build body cells and substances.

Anaerobes A variety of bacteria that grow in the absence of oxygen and are destroyed by the presence of oxygen.

Anaphylaxis An allergic reaction that may be immediate, severe, and fatal.

Anatomy The study of the structure of the body and its parts.

Anemia A deficiency in the quality of hemoglobin of the blood and a diminished red blood cell count.

Anesthesia The loss of feeling or sensation.

Anesthetic A drug that produces the loss of feeling or sensation.

Angle former A dental hand instrument used to refine line and point angles in the internal outline and retention form of a cavity preparation.

Angle, line The junction of two walls (tooth surfaces) of a cavity preparation.

Angle, point The junction of three walls (tooth surfaces) of a cavity preparation.

Anode The electrically positive terminal in an x-ray tube.

Anodontia A lack of initiation stage that results in a congenital absence of the teeth.

Antagonists Teeth in opposing arches that contact each other.

Anterior Toward the front.

Anterior teeth The maxillary and mandibular incisors and cuspids.

Antibiotic A chemical substance that is able to inhibit the growth of, or to destroy, bacteria and other microorganisms.

Antibody A protein produced by the body in response to a foreign substance that reacts specifically with that substance.

Antigen A substance that can incite the production of specific antibodies and can combine with those antibodies.

Antihistamine Drugs that counteract the release of histamine in allergic reactions.

Antiseptic A substance that inhibits or kills microbes.

Apex The anatomical area at the end of the tooth root.

Aphthous ulcer A viral infection that causes recurring outbreaks of blisterlike sores inside the mouth and on the lips.

Apical Pertaining to the apex.

Appliance A device used to provide function to therapeutic effect.

Apposition The body's process of laying down new bone. Also the deposition of the matrix for the hard dental structures.

Arch See _Mandibular arch_ and _Maxillary arch_.

Articular disc A cushion of tough specialized connective tissue within the temporomandibular joint. Also known as the meniscus.

Articulator A mechanical device that represents the temporomandibular joints to which upper and lower casts of the dental arches may be attached to simulate mouth functions.

Articulation The contact relationship of upper and lower teeth as they move against each other.

Asepsis Absence of pathological microorganisms.

Astringent An agent that is applied topically to control moderate bleeding by causing capillaries to contract.

Attrition Loss of tooth structure due to wear.

Autoclave A sterilizing device employing steam under pressure.

Axial An imaginary plane that runs parallel to the long axis of a tooth.

Back order Notification from a supplier that an item is out of stock.

Bacteria One-celled microorganisms with certain characteristics. Some, but not all, are pathogens.

Base The layer of cement that acts as an insulator and protective barrier under a restoration.

Benign Doing little or no harm. Not malignant.

Bevel A slanting of the enamel margins of a tooth preparation. A cut with an angle of more than 90° with a cavity wall.

Bevel, full A bevel involving the entire wall of a cavity preparation.

Bevel, long A bevel involving more than the external one-third of a cavity wall but no more than the external two-thirds.

Bicuspid See _Premolar_.

Bifurcation The anterior area where roots divide in a two-rooted tooth.

Bilateral Pertaining to both sides.

Bile A secretion of the liver that is stored in the gallbladder.

Bin-angle An instrument having two off-setting angles in its shank.

BIS-GMA A polymer that is formed by the reaction of bisphenol A and glycidyl methacrylate and that, when reacted with diacrytes, forms the polymer used in pit and fissure sealants and in composite restorative materials.

Bite An occlusal record of the relationship between the upper and lower teeth.

Blade The sharpened working end of a dental hand instrument.

Bleaching The use of chemical oxidizing agents to lighten discolored teeth.

Bonding The force by which a substance is secured in intimate contact with another substance. Bonding may be mechanical, chemical, or physical.

Bridge A prosthetic device consisting of artificial teeth (points) that is supported by cementing it to abutment teeth.

Broach An instrument with barbs protruding from a metal shaft. Used in endodontic treatment.

Buccal Pertaining to or adjacent to the cheek.

Buffer A substance in solution capable of neutralizing both acids and bases.

Bur A rotary cutting instrument made of steel or tungsten carbide manufactured with cutting heads of various shapes and sizes.

Bur, friction-grip A bur with a smooth shank that is held in place in the plastic or metal chuck of a handpiece.

Bur, latch-type A bur with a notched hand that fits into a latch-type contra-angle handpiece.

Burnish The process of smoothing a metal surface by rubbing.

Burnisher A dental hand instrument used to smooth the edges at the margin of a metal restoration and the tooth surface.

Calcification The process by which organic tissue becomes hardened by the deposit of calcium and other mineral salts.

Calculus A hard mineralized deposit attached to the teeth.

Canal The pulp chamber of a root.

Canine See *Cuspid*.

Canker sore See *Aphthous ulcer*.

Capsule A metal, plastic, or premeasured cap that contains the dental alloy and mercury that are triturated to form the dental amalgam.

Carcinoma A malignant epithelial neoplasm that tends to invade surrounding tissue and to metastasize to distant regions of the body.

Caries Dental decay. An infectious disease that progressively destroys tooth substance.

Caries, recurrent Decay occurring beneath the margin of an existing dental restoration.

Carotid Either one of the two main arteries of the neck.

Carrier An individual who harbors disease organisms without being ill with the disease. The party to a dental contract that may collect premiums, assume financial risk, pay claims, and/or provide administrative services. Also known as third party.

Cartilage A flexible, white tissue around the ends of bones and joints.

Carver An instrument used to shape a plastic material such as amalgam or wax.

Cast Replica of the teeth or dental arch that is used as a working model.

Catabolism The process of breaking down foodstuffs to produce energy.

Catalyst A material that initiates a chemical reaction.

Cavity A lesion or hole in a tooth.

Cavosurface The junction of the cavity and the exterior tooth surface.

Cavosurface, angle An angle in a cavity preparation formed by the junction of the wall of the cavity with the exterior tooth surface.

Cavosurface, bevel A bevel found at the cavosurface angle of the cavity preparation.

CDA Certified dental assistant; one who has passed a national examination in chairside assisting.

Cellulitis An inflammation that spreads through the substance of the tissue or organ.

Cementoclast A specialized cell that causes resorption of the roots of primary teeth during exfoliation.

Cementoenamel junction The junction of the enamel of the crown and the cementum of the root.

Cementum The substance covering the root surface of the tooth.

Centric occlusion When the jaws are closed in a position that produces maximal stable contact between the occluding surfaces of the maxillary and mandibular teeth.

Ceramics The art of making dental restorations from fused porcelain.

Cerebellum A major division of the brain.

Cerebrum The largest portion of the brain.

Chisel An instrument for cutting or cleaving tooth structure in the preparation of cavities.

Cingulum A bulge or prominence of enamel found on the cervical third of the lingual surface of an anterior tooth.

Clasps The attachments of a partial denture that grasp the natural teeth.

Cleft A vertical fissure.

Cleoid A carving instrument with a blade shaped like a pointed spade. Claw-like.

Coagulant An agent that promotes the clotting of blood.

Collimation The elimination of peripheral radiation.

Colloid A suspension of particles in a dispersion medium such as water. Its two phases are *sol* (liquid) and *gel* (solid).

Composite Formulations of resins used for restorative purposes.

Compressive stress The stress that occurs when an applied force pushes against a material.

Concave Inward curvature.

Condense To insert and compress a dental material into a prepared cavity.

Condenser A dental hand instrument used to pack plastic-type restorative material into a cavity preparation.

Consultation The joint deliberation, usually for diagnostic purposes, between two or more practitioners or between patient and practitioner.

Contour The shape, form, or surface configuration of an object.

Contra-angle An instrument having two or more off-setting angles. See also *Handpiece*.

Convex Outward curvature.

Corrosion A chemical reaction of a nonmetallic substance with a metal.

Cotton pliers Pliers designed with plain or serrated point that are used as part of the basic dental setup. Also known as college pliers.

Cross-linked polymers Polymers that are three-dimensional network molecules.

Crown, anatomic The portion of the tooth that is covered with enamel.

Crown, cast A cast restoration that covers the entire portion of a tooth that is normally covered with enamel.

Crown, clinical That portion of the tooth that is visible in the mouth.

Curette A hand instrument with sharpened curved blade that is used with a scraping motion.

Curettage Scraping or cleaning with a curette.

Curing The act of polymerization.

Curve of Spee The slightly curved plane of the occlusal surfaces of the posterior teeth.

Cusp A pointed or rounded eminence on the surface of a tooth.

Cusp of Carabelli The "fifth" cusp located on the lingual surface of many maxillary first molars.

Cuspid An anterior tooth with long thick root.

Cyanosis A lack of oxygen that causes a bluish tinge to the skin.

Cyst An abnormal space developed by a membrane and filled with fluid or semifluid material.

Dappen dish A small clear glass mixing vessel.

Decalcification The loss of calcium salts from the enamel. The first step in the decay process.

Decay See *caries*.

Deglutition The act of swallowing.

Dental hygienist A licensed preventive oral health professional who provides educational, clinical, and therapeutic services.

Dentin The material forming the main inner portion of the tooth structure.

Dentinocemental junction The line of union of the cementum and dentin of the tooth.

Dentinoclast A specialized cell that causes the resorption of the roots of deciduous teeth during exfoliation.

Dentition Natural teeth in the dental arch.

Denture A substitute for missing teeth. May be complete (full) or partial.

Denture, duplicate A second denture intended to be a copy of the original.

Dependents Generally the spouse and children of a covered individual, as defined in a contract.

Dew point The temperature at which condensation occurs.

Diagnosis Recognizing a departure from normal and distinguishing one disease or condition from another.

Die A replica of a single tooth or several teeth on which a restoration is fabricated.

Diplococci Pair-forming cocci.

Disaccharide A sugar consisting of two monosaccharides joined together.

Disc Rotary instruments made of various abrasive materials, commonly using a metal or paper backing.

Disclosing solution A dye applied to the teeth to stain plaque.

Discoid A spoon-shaped instrument with a cutting edge around the total periphery.

Disinfectant An agent used to kill pathogenic microorganisms without necessarily sterilizing the material.

Disinfection The process of killing pathogenic agents by chemical or physical means. It does not include the destruction of spores and resistant viruses.

Disposable Supply items that are used once and then discarded.

Distal Away from the midline.

Dorsum The upper surface of the tongue.

Droplet infection See *Infection, droplet*.

Ductility The ability of a material to withstand permanent deformation under tensile stress without fracture.

Ectoderm The outer embryonic tissue layer.

Edema Excessive accumulation of fluid in the tissue spaces.

Edentulous Without teeth. Usually meaning having lost all natural teeth.

EFDA Extended function dental auxiliary. Also known as an expanded function dental auxiliary.

Elastic limit The maximum stress that a structure or material can withstand without being permanently deformed.

Elasticity Pertains to the ability of a body that has been changed or deformed under stress to again assume its original shape when the stress is removed.

Elastomer A generic term for all substances having the physical properties of rubber.

Embrasure A V-shaped space in a gingival direction between the proximal surfaces to two adjoining teeth in contact.

Embryology The study of development during the first eight weeks of pregnancy.

Emulsifier A material used to help mix an oily substance with water.

Enamel The hard tissue that covers the anatomic crown of the tooth.

Endoderm The inner embryonic tissue layer.

Epinephrine See *Adrenalin*.

Epithelium The covering of the internal and external surfaces of the body.

Epithelium, oral The tissue serving as the lining of the mouth tissue surfaces.

Equilibration The act of putting the mandible in a state of balance with the maxilla.

Erosion The superficial wearing away of tooth substance not involving bacteria.

Erythrocytes Red blood cells.

Eruption The migration of a tooth into functional position in the oral cavity.

Etch Treating enamel with phosphoric acid to provide retention for resin sealants, restorative materials, or orthodontic brackets.

Etching, acid A procedure in which an acid solution or gel is used to etch tooth enamel.

Ethics That part of philosophy that deals with moral conduct, duty, and judgment.

Etiology The causes of disease.

Eugenol A pale colored liquid obtained from clove oil and other natural sources.

Eustachian tube The narrow tube leading from the middle ear and opening into the nasopharynx.

Excavator, spoon A dental hand instrument with a sharp, bowl-shaped edge that is used to remove carious dentin.

Excision Cutting away or taking out.

Exfoliation The normal process by which primary teeth are shed.

Exodontics The science and practice of removing teeth.

Exothermic The heat given off during a chemical reaction.

Expendables Supply items that are relatively small in cost and that are used up in a short period of time, i.e., mouth mirrors.

Explorer A dental hand instrument with a fine tip that is used to detect caries and rough areas on the tooth surface.

Exposure Uncovering, as in exposing a pulp via the opening in the wall of the pulp chamber. Also when producing a radiograph, exposing the dental film and tissues to ionizing radiation.

Extrude The migration of a tooth out of its normal occlusal position due to absence of opposing occlusal force, as when the contacting tooth in the opposite arch has been lost. Also to force out, that is, dispense, impression material from an extruder gum.

Fabrication Constructing or making a restoration.

Facial Refers collectively to both the labial and buccal surfaces.

Fetus The developing child from the third through the tenth lunar month.

File A metal instrument with ridges or teeth on its cutting surfaces.

Finish line The point at which the cavity preparation meets the external surface of the tooth.

Fissure A deep groove or cleft, commonly the result of the imperfect fusion of the enamel.

Fistula An abnormal tract connecting two body surfaces or organs or leading from an internal cavity, or tooth root, to the body surface.

Flow Continued change in shape under a static load. Also known as creep or slump.

Fluorosis Mottled enamel caused by excessive fluoride intake.

Foramen A natural opening in bone or other structure.

Force Any push or pull energy exerted on matter.

Forceps An instrument used for grasping or applying force to teeth, tissues, or other instruments.

Form, outline The curved shape and border of the restoration and of the tooth.

Form, retention The shape given to the tooth surfaces (cavity walls) to prevent the dislodgement of the restoration.

Fossa A hollow, grooved, or depressed area in a bone or tooth.

Fracture To break apart or rupture.

Framework The metal skeleton that provides a basic support for the saddle and the connectors of the removable partial denture.

Frenum A fold of mucous membrane attaching the cheeks and lips to the upper and lower arches, in some instances limiting the motions of the lips and cheeks.

Fulcrum The point or support on which a level turns.

Furcation The anatomical area of multi-rooted tooth where the roots divide.

Gag reflex Protective mechanism located in the posterior of the mouth. Contact with this area causes gagging, retching, or vomiting.

Gagging The retching action caused by touching the posterior area (soft palate) of the mouth.

Gauges Instruments used to measure dimensions.

Gel The solid phase of a colloid.

Gelation Process by which a colloid changes from the sol to the gel state.

Gelation temperature The temperature at which the colloid changes from the sol (liquid) to the gel (solid) state.

General Anesthesia A state of unconsciousness produced by chemical induction.

Generic Applies to drug (product) names that any business form may use.

Germicide A solution capable of killing all microorganisms except spores.

Gingiva The fibrous tissue covered by epithelium that immediately surrounds a tooth and is continuous with its periodontal ligament and with the mucosal tissues of the mouth (plural, gingivae).

Gingiva, attached The portion of the gingiva extending from the gingival margin to the alveolar mucosa.

Gingiva, free That part of the gingivae that surrounds the tooth and is not directly attached to the tooth surface.

Gingival curettage The removal of soft tissue comprising of pocket wall (sulcular or crevicular epithelium) by scraping with periodontal instruments.

Gingival margin The most coronal portion of the gingiva surrounding the tooth.

Gingival margin trimmer A dental hand instrument designed to bevel the cervical cavosurface walls of the cavity preparation.

Gingival sulcus The shallow furrow formed where the gingival tip meets the tooth enamel.

Gingivectomy The excision of the soft tissue wall of the periodontal pocket when the pocket is not complicated by extension into the underlying bone.

Gingivitis Inflammation of the gingiva characterized clinically by changes in color, gingival form, position, surface appearance, and the presence of bleeding and/or exudate. Also known as Type I periodontal disease.

Gingivitis, HIV Inflammation of the gingiva characterized by a bright red linear border along the free gingival margin. Also known as atypical gingivitis.

Glossitis Inflammation of the tongue.

Glucose Form of sugar found in the blood as well as in some foods.

Glutaraldehyde A high-level disinfectant.

Glycogen A polysaccharide composed of glucose molecules.

Gram-negative bacteria Bacteria that are not stained by Gram stain.

Gram-positive bacteria Bacteria that are stained by Gram stain.

Granulation tissue New tissue formed in the healing process.

Groove A shallow line on the surface of a tooth.

Hand instruments Instruments used under hand direction as opposed to motor-driven instruments.

Handpiece An instrument to hold rotary tools in a dental engine and connect them with the power source.

Handpiece, air driven An air-driven turbine handpiece that may reach speeds from 300,000 to 800,000 rpm.

Handpiece, contra-angle An extension attached to a straight handpiece to form an offset angle.

Handpiece, high speed A dental handpiece that rotates at between 100,000 and 800,000 rpm.

Handpiece, low speed A dental handpiece that rotates at between 6,000 and 10,000 rpm.

Handpiece, right-angle An extension attached to a straight handpiece to form a right angle.

Handpiece, straight A low-speed handpiece that may be used to hold rotary instruments. Also used to hold contra-angle and right-angle handpieces.

Hardness The ability of a material to resist permanent indentation or scratching.

Hatchet An angled hand-cutting instrument used to develop internal cavity form.

Hemorrhage An abnormal loss of large quantities of blood.

Hemostat A scissorlike surgical instrument with a static-type lock used to help hold an object or tissue.

Hepatitis A An inflammation of the liver transmitted through contact with contaminated food or water. Also known as infectious hepatitis.

Hepatitis B A viral infection of the liver. Also known as serum hepatitis.

Herpes simplex A viral infection that causes recurrent sores.

Histamine A natural substance released when the body comes into contact with certain substances to which it is sensitive.

Histodifferentiation The developmental stage where cells differentiate and become specialized.

Histology The study of the composition and function of tissues.

HIV Human Immunodeficiency Virus is a disease that invades the body and generally develops into AIDS (Acquired Immunodeficiency Syndrome).

Hoe A dental hand instrument, used with a pull motion, that has the working blade at a right angle to the long axis of the handle.

Homogeneous A mix with a uniform quality throughout.

Hormones Substances produced in one part of the body that specifically influence cellular activities in another part.

HVE High-volume evacuator. Used to remove excess fluids and debris from the oral cavity.

Hydrocolloid A colloid solution in which water is used as the dispersing medium. Also a type of impression material.

Hydrocolloid, irreversible A hydrocolloid that once a solid will not return to the liquid phase. Alginate impression materials.

Hydrocolloid, reversible A hydrocolloid that may repeatedly be taken from sol to liquid phase. Agar impression materials.

Hygroscopic Tending to absorb water for the air.

Hypercementosis Abnormal thickening of the cementum.

Hyperplasia An abnormal increase in the number of normal cells in the normal arrangement of tissue.

Hyperreactive A greater than normal response to stimuli.

Imbibition To take on water.

Immunity The ability of the body to resist a specific infection.

Immunity, acquired Immunity acquired either by having a disease or through vaccination.

Immunity, natural Immunity with which the individual was born.

Immunoglobulin Antibodies or antibodylike protein molecules, usually part of the gamma globulin portion of the blood.

Impaction Any tooth that remains unerupted in the jaws beyond the time at which it should normally be erupted.

Impaction, bony A tooth that is blocked by both bone (alveolus) and tissue (mucosa).

Impaction, soft tissue A tooth that is blocked from eruption only by gingival tissue.

Impression compound Thermoplastic impression material that is rigid at mouth temperature.

Incisal Biting edge of an anterior tooth.

Incise To cut or tear.

Incisor Anterior teeth with thin and sharp cutting edge.

Incubation period The time between the infection of the individual by a microorganism and the first manifestation of the disease.

Infection, droplet The type of infection transmitted by the droplets of water such as from sneezing or from handpiece spray.

Infection, self Infective microorganisms present in the patient's mouth cause infection when they get into the bloodstream during dental surgery. The patient infects himself.

Infectious hepatitis See *Hepatitis A.*

Infiltration Technique of applying anesthetic solution in the area immediately surrounding the tooth or teeth.

Inflammation The sum of the reactions of the body to injury.

Initiation The beginning development of a tooth.

Initiator Reactive material that starts a chemical reaction.

Inlay A cast restoration prepared outside the mouth and cemented in a cavity preparation that is designed to restore one, two, or three surfaces of the tooth. The remaining tooth margins are intact.

Interdental See *Interproximal.*

Interproximal Between the proximal surfaces of adjacent teeth.

Invaginate To fold inward.

Iodophors Disinfectants that are used in differing strengths as a surgical scrub and as a surface disinfectant.

Ion An atom or group of atoms that carry a positive or negative electrical charge.

Ionomers Powders in a variety of shades with water-soluble polymers and copolymers of acrylic acid as the liquids.

Irreversible Incapable of returning to the original state.

Junction Coming together.

Junction, cementoenamel See *Cementoenamel junction.*

Junction, dentinocemental See *Dentinocemental junction.*

Kaposi's sarcoma A form of cancer that usually begins with skin lesions.

Kilovolt Unit of electrical potential equal to 1,000 volts.

Labial Of, or pertaining to, the lip.

Lactose A disaccharide consisting of one molecule of glucose and one of galactose.

Lamina dura Thin, compact bone lining the alveolar socket.

Lateral Toward the side.

Leakage Penetration of fluids between a dental restoration and the surrounding tooth.

Lesion A broad term describing tissue damage caused by either injury or disease.

Leukocytes White blood cells.

Leukoplakia White patches that occur in the mouth.

Ligament A band of tough tissue that helps keep an organ in place or connects the ends of bones where they form joints.

Ligature Cord, thread, or stainless steel wire used to bind teeth together or to hold structures in place.

Liner, cavity A dental material that seals the dentinal tubules and insulates the pulp against thermal changes.

Lingual Of, or pertaining to, the tongue.

Lobe A developmental segment of a tooth.

Local anesthesia Deadening of sensation of a specific area through the administration of a drug that blocks nerve condition.

Lumen The space within a tube, such as a blood vessel or needle.

Luting Bonding or cementing two unlike substances together.

Macrodontia Abnormally large teeth.

Macrophage A large mononuclear phagocyte.

Malignant Tending to become progressively worse and to result in death.

Malleability The ability of a material to withstand permanent deformation under compressive stress without rupture.

Malocclusion When the teeth in the upper and lower jaws do not come together correctly.

Malpractice Professional negligence.

Mamelon A rounded eminence on the incisal edge of a newly erupted incisor.

Mandibular arch The teeth in position in the alveolar process of the mandible. Also known as the lower jaw.

Mandrel A mounting device with a screw and a threaded end or a snap-on attachment to hold the disc in a dental handpiece.

Margin In cavity preparations, the outside limit of the preparation.

Materia alba White curds of matter composed of dead cells, food, and other components of the dental plaque.

Matrix band A short strip of thin steel or plastic used to form the missing wall(s) of a cavity preparation and support restorative material.

Maxillary arch The teeth in position in the alveolar process of the maxilla. Also known as the upper jaw.

Meatus An external opening of a canal.

Meniscus The bottom of the elliptical curve where the water touches the dry side of the container. See also *Articular disc.*

Mercury (Hg) A heavy metal that is fluid at room temperature and has a silvery appearance.

Mesenchyme The meshwork of embryonic connective tissue in the mesoderm from which are formed the connective tissues of the body, and also the blood and lymphatic vessels.

Mesial Toward the midline.

Mesoderm The middle embryonic tissue layer.

Metal A chemical element, which is crystalline in structure and has a melting and setting (freezing temperature) point.

Metabolism The process involved in the body's use of nutrients.

Metastasis The distant spread of the tumor cells from the site of origin.

Microdontia Abnormally small teeth.

Microorganism A living organism so small that it is only visible with a microscope.

Mobility Movement of the tooth within its socket.

Model Replica typically made of a gypsum product (a cast).

Modulus of elasticity A measure of the rigidity or stiffness of a material at stresses below its elastic limit.

Molar A posterior tooth with a broad occlusal surface for chewing.

Molecule The smallest part of a compound that retains all the properties of the compound.

Monangle An instrument having one off-setting angle in its shank.

Monococcus A single coccus.

Monomer Molecule with a single mer, or unit.

Morphodifferentiation The stage of development at which the basic form and relative size of the tooth are determined.

Mucosa A mucous membrane consisting of an outer epithelial layer and a connective tissue layer.

Mucus Secretions of the mucous membranes.

Mulling Continuation of the amalgamation process in which the pestle is removed from the capsule and the mixing of the dental amalgam is continued for two or three seconds to collect the mass.

Mutation Abnormal development caused by genetic changes.

Nasmyth's membrane The enamel cuticle partially remaining on a tooth surface after tooth eruption.

Natal Related to birth.

Natal teeth Erupted teeth present at birth.

Necrotic Dead cells or tissues that are in contact with living cells.

Negligence The failure to use due care or the lack of due care.

Neoplasm A tumor that may be benign or malignant.

Nib   The working end or face of a dental hand instrument with a smooth or serrated surface.

Nutrients   Substances used by the body in growth and maintenance.

Occlusal   The chewing surfaces of the posterior teeth.

Occlusion   The contact between the maxillary and mandibular teeth in all mandibular positions and movements.

Odontology   A study of the external form and relationship of the teeth.

Onlay   A cast restoration designed to restore the occlusal surface, the mesial-distal or lingual-facial margins, and frequently two or more cusps of the occlusal surface of a posterior tooth.

Opaque   The ability to block light.

Opportunistic disease   A disease that normally would be controlled by the immune system but cannot be controlled because that system is not functioning properly.

Osteoblasts   The cells responsible for bone formation.

Osteoclasts   The cells responsible for bone restoration.

Overhang   Excess restorative material projecting over the cavity margin.

Palatal   Area involving the palate, or roof, of the mouth.

Palate, hard   The bony anterior of the roof of the mouth.

Palate, soft   The posterior tissue portion of the roof of the mouth.

Palpation   An examination technique of the soft tissues with the examiner's hand or finger tip.

Papilla   Gingiva filling the interproximal spaces between adjacent teeth. Projection located on the dorsum of the tongue that contain receptors for the sense of taste (plural, papillae).

Papilla, incisive   A rounded projection at the anterior end of the palatine raphe.

Palpitation   Unusually rapid heart beat.

Partial denture   Prosthetic device containing artificial teeth supported on a framework and attached to natural teeth by means of clasps.

Pathogen   A microorganism capable of causing disease.

Pathology   The study of disease.

Pellagra   A disease caused by a niacin deficiency.

Percussion   An examination technique that uses sharp, short blows to the involved tooth with a finger or instrument.

Periodontal scaling and root planing   The procedure designed to remove the microbial flora and bacterial toxins on the root surface or in the pocket, calculus, and diseased cementum and dentin.

Periodontal ligament   The tissues that support and anchor the tooth in its socket.

Periodontitis   Inflammatory and destructive disease involving the soft tissue and bony support of the teeth.

Periodontitis, HIV   Periodontal lesions associated with AIDS. Also known as *AIDS virus—associated periodontitis.*

Peristalsis   The wavelike muscle action that moves food through the digestive system.

pH   A scale of 0 to 14 that expresses the acidity or alkalinity of a solution, with a pH 7 being considered neutral.

Pharmacology   The study of drugs, especially as they relate to medical uses.

Physiology   The study of the functions of the body systems.

Pit   A pinpoint depression on the surface of a tooth.

Pit and fissure   Faults that are the result of non-coalescence of enamel during tooth formation.

Plaque   A soft deposit on the teeth consisting of bacteria and bacteria products.

Plaques   Clearly circumscribed lesions larger than 1 cm.

Pneumocystis carinii pneumonia (PCP)   A particular type of lung disease associated with AIDS.

Polymer Molecules made up of many mers, or units.

Porcelain Ceramic containing minerals held together by glass.

Porosity Voids in a material that reduce the apparent density.

Portepolisher A cleansing and polishing hand instrument constructed to hold a wooden point.

Posterior Toward the back.

Posterior teeth The maxillary and mandibular premolars and molars.

Predetermination An administrative procedure whereby a dentist submits the treatment plan to the third party before treatment is initiated. Also known as pretreatment estimate.

Premolar A posterior tooth with points and cusps for grasping, tearing, and chewing.

Process A prominence or projection of a bone.

Proliferation To grow and increase in number.

Prophy angle See _Handpiece, right-angle._

Prophylaxis, oral A scaling and polishing procedure performed to remove coronal plaque, calculus, and stains to prevent caries and periodontal disease.

Prosthesis A replacement for a missing body part.

Proximal Nearest or adjacent to.

Proximal walls The tooth surface, mesial or distal, that is nearest to the adjacent tooth.

Pulp The vital tissues of the tooth consisting of nerves, blood vessels, and connective tissue.

Pulp capping Application of a material to a cavity preparation that has exposed or nearly exposed the dental pulp.

Pulpectomy The surgical removal of a vital pulp from a tooth.

Pulpal floor The floor of the cavity preparation, horizontal to the pulpal area of the tooth.

Pulpitis Inflammation of the dental pulp.

Pulpotomy The partial excision of the dental pulp.

Pumice Ground volcanic ash that is used for polishing.

Purchase order A form authorizing the purchase of specific supplies from a specific supplier.

Pus Thick, opaque, often yellowish fluid that forms at the site of an infected wound.

Putrefaction The decomposition of proteins with the production of foul-smelling products.

Q.I.D. Latin term used in prescription, meaning four times per day.

Quadrant One of the four sections, or quarters, of the mouth.

RDH Registered dental hygienist. See _Dental hygienist._

Reamer An instrument with a tapered metal shaft, more loosely spiraled than a file, used to clean and enlarge a root canal.

Recession Loss of part or all of the gingiva over the root of a tooth.

Regeneration The process by which lost tissue is replaced by a tissue similar in type.

Requisition A formal request for supplies.

Resorption The body's process of removing existing bone.

Retainer matrix A mechanical device designed to engage the ends of the matrix band and tighten the matrix around the tooth.

Retarder A chemical that decreases the rate of a chemical reaction to allow a longer working time.

Retention The result of adhesion, mechanical locking, or both.

Rickets A disease caused by a vitamin D deficiency.

Ridge A linear elevation on the surface of a tooth. Also the remaining bone of the alveolar process in an edentulous arch.

Ruga A fold in the mucosal tissue found on the roof of the mouth and in the stomach (plural, rugae).

Saddle The portion of the removable appliance that rests on the oral mucosa covering the alveolar ridge. It also retains the artificial teeth.

Sarcoma A malignant neoplasm of the soft tissues arising from supportive and connective tissue such as bone.

Scaling A treatment procedure necessary to remove hard and soft deposits from the tooth's surface.

Schedule of benefits A list of covered services that assigns each service a sum that represents the total obligation of the plan with respect to payment for such service. Also known as table of allowances.

Scurvy A disease caused by a vitamin C deficiency.

Sealant Polymeric material that is used to penetrate pits and fissures to protect against caries.

Sedatives Drugs that reduce excitability, create calmness, and allow sleep to occur as a secondary effect.

Sepsis The presence of disease-producing microorganisms.

Serum hepatitis See *Hepatitis B.*

Shaft The elongated stem of an instrument that is designed for grip and to give leverage.

Shank The tapered position of the dental hand instrument between the handle and the blade. The portion of a bur that fits into the dental handpiece.

Shear strength Stress required to rupture a material in which one portion is forced to slide over another position.

Sign Objective evidence of disease that can be observed by someone other than the patient.

Sinus An air-filled cavity within a bone.

Sol Colloidal system (liquid) in which the dispersed phase is solid and the continuous phase is liquid.

Spirochetes Unicellular bacteria that have flexible cell walls, are capable of movement, and have a wavelike or spiral shape.

Spores Protective form taken by some bacteria in order to withstand adverse conditions.

Staphylococci Cocci that form irregular groups or clusters.

State Dental Practice Act The law that contains the legal restrictions and controls on the dentist, dental auxiliaries, and the practice of dentistry within each state.

State Board of Dental Examiners The administrative board assigned to interpret the implement regulations under the state dental practice act. It also supervises and regulates the practice of dentistry within the state.

Sterilization The process by which all forms of life are completely destroyed within a circumscribed area.

Stones Mounted rotary instruments used for polishing and refining restorations.

Strain The distortion of change produced in a body as the result of stress.

Streptococci Chain-forming cocci.

Stress The internal reaction, or resistance, within a body to an externally applied force.

Subcutaneous Below the skin.

Succedaneous That which follows.

Sucrose Table sugar.

Sulcus A groove or depression. See also *Gingival sulcus* (plural, sulci).

Supernumerary Any tooth in excess of the thirty-two normal permanent teeth.

Supine Positioned lying on the back with the face up.

Symptom Subjective evidence of a disease that is observed by the patient.

Syncope A temporary loss of consciousness caused by an insufficient blood supply to the brain. Also known as fainting.

Syndrome A particular group of signs and symptoms that occur together.

Syneresis To lose water by evaporation due to exposure to air.

Synthetic phenols Compounds with broad-spectrum disinfecting action.

Syphilis A sexually transmitted disease caused by *Treponema palladium.*

Tarnish Simple surface discoloration of a silver alloy.

Temporary filling Material used to fill a tooth until cavity preparation or placement of a final restoration.

Temporomandibular joint The articulation of the mandible with the temporal bone.

Tensile strength Stress required to rupture a material when it is pulled apart

Tetanus An infection producing neurotropic poison that causes muscle spasms and rigidity. Also known as lockjaw.

Thermal expansion The increase in volume of a material that is caused by a temperature increase.

Thermoplastic The property of becoming softer on heating and harder on cooling, the process being reversible.

Thrombosis A blood clot that blocks the artery where it forms.

Thrush Candidiasis of the oral mucosa.

Tofflemire A matrix retainer and band system used to replace the missing wall of a tooth while the restoration is being placed.

Torque A rotational force.

Trabecular bone Bone spicules in cancellous bone that form a network of intercommunicating spaces that are filled with bone marrow.

Tragus The cartilaginous projection anterior to the external opening of the ear.

Transaction Any charge, payment, or adjustment that is made to a patient account.

Translucency The relative amount of light transmitted through an object.

Trauma Wound or injury.

Trifurcation Division into three.

Trismus Partial contraction of the muscles of mastication causing difficulty in opening the mouth.

Triturate To combine a dental alloy with mercury mechanically.

Tuberculosis A disease caused by the tubercle bacillus.

Tumors Solid lesions larger than 1 cm.

Ulcer Craterlike break in continuity of the mucosa.

Ultimate strength Maximum stress a material sustains before it fractures.

Ultrasonic scaling The use of an ultrasonic scaler to remove mineralized deposits from the tooth surface.

Ultraviolet light Light that is just beyond violet in the spectrum and that serves to begin a polymerization reaction in certain sealant and composite resin materials.

Undercut The portion of a tooth that lies between the height of contour and the gingivae.

Universal System Identification of the teeth by numbering the permanent teeth from 1 to 32. Primary teeth are lettered from A to T.

Varnish Resin surface coating formed by evaporation of a solvent.

Vasoconstrictor Agent that shrinks blood vessels.

Veneer A layer of tooth-colored material (composite or porcelain) that is bonded or cemented to the prepared tooth surface.

Ventral Refers to the front or belly side of the body.

Vermilion border The exposed red portion of the upper and lower lip.

Virulence The relative capacity of a pathogen to overcome body defenses.

Virus Submicroscopic infectious agents.

Viscosity The property of liquid that causes it not to flow.

Wall, axial A portion of the prepared tooth near the pulpal area and parallel with the long axis of the tooth.

Wedelstaedt chisel A dental chisel with a modified curved shank.

Young's frame A U-shaped metal or plastic frame used to hold rubber dams in place.

Glossary of Radiographic Terms

Ala (of the nose) The outer side of the nostril.

Ampere Unit of quantity of electrical current; the amount of flow of electrons through a circuit.

Anatomical landmark An anatomical structure that serves to orient and identify other structures in the region.

Anode A positive electrode that attracts negative ions. In the dental x-ray tube, it incorporates the tungsten target.

Atom The smallest particle of an element that is capable of entering into a chemical reaction.

Attenuation The process of absorption of the x-ray beam as it passes through matter and thus becomes weaker.

Autotransformer A device that compensates the incoming, or line voltage, as it comes into the dental x-ray machine.

Bite block A device used to hold the mouth open during operative and oral surgery procedures.

Bisected-angle A technique for taking radiographs based on the principle of directing the central rays perpendicularly to an imaginary line that bisects the angle formed by the long axis of the teeth and the plane of the film.

Cassette A lightproof container with intensifying screens in which external x-ray films are placed for exposure to x-ray radiation.

Cathode A negative electrode that attracts positive ions. In the dental x-ray tube, it incorporates the tungsten filament.

Cathode ray The ray of electrons leaving the cathode to bombard the target of the anode; travels at about $1/3$ the speed of light.

Ciezynski's rule of isometry "The normal ray is directed perpendicularly to a plane which lies midway between the plane of the teeth desired and the plane of the film." Ciezynski, 1907.

Circuit A flow of electrons from one point to another, beginning to end of the current.

Collimation Reduces the size of the x-ray beam and the volume of scattered radiation.

Collimator The diaphragm placed at the base of the cone (usually of lead, to restrict the size of the beam).

Cone The device projecting from the tubehead that indicates and directs the primary beam of x ray.

Current A flow of electrons passing a given point.

Energy The capacity to do work. Kinetic energy is active or expended energy, and potential is inactive energy.

Erythema A temporary redness of the skin caused by exposure to radiation in excessive amounts.

Film A thin piece of transparent polyester coated with gelatin of emulsion in which radiation of light-sensitive crystals are suspended.

  contrast Referring to film contrast, it is the difference between the black, white, and various shades of gray on adjacent areas of the film.

  density (1) As applied to radiographs, the term refers to the degree of blackening of the film and the amount of light transmitted through the film. (2) Object density refers to the object's resistance of x ray passing through it.

  dental radiography The method of recording images of dental structures by the use of roentgen rays or x rays.

  detail As applied to radiographs, the term refers to the sharpness of the image.

  distortion On an x-ray film, that which tends to increase the size of the object and the shape of the object.

extraoral Radiographic film used outside the mouth (panoramic, lateral jaw, etc.).

intraoral Radiographic films used inside the mouth (bitewings, periapicals, etc.).

screened Radiographic film that is exposed by the blue light being emitted from screens that are placed adjacent to the film. These screens are affected by the x rays, creating a blue light. The process is usually used in extraoral radiography and uses cassette holders.

Filter The material (usually aluminum) placed at the base of the cone to absorb the weak, unuseful x rays.

Fogging As related to radiographic film, the darkening of all or parts of the film by other means than the primary beam (chemical, light, etc.).

Frequency The number of cycles, wavelengths, or revolutions completed in a unit of time.

Genetic Those body tissues related to chromosomal or genetic reproduction of the species.

Image Pertaining to the radiographic representation of dental structures as they are presented on an exposed, processed film.

radiolucent Those images on the film that appear darker; the darkness is related to the lack of density of the object which allows more x ray to go through it and expose the film. Restorative materials, certain diseases and soft tissues will appear radiolucent on a radiograph.

radiopaque Those images on the film that appear whiter or lighter; the lightness is related to the density of the object being exposed (bone, enamel, dentin). Certain restorative materials of dense metallic structure will also appear radiopaque on a radiograph.

Ion An atomic particle or atom carrying an electrical charge, either positive or negative.

Ionization The process by which a balanced atom becomes an unbalanced atom, or particle, with an electrical charge of positive or negative.

Kilovolt A unit of energy equal to 1000 volts (electromotive force) (kVp abbrev.).

Latent image The radiographic representation of dental structures on an exposed but not completely processed film (it is invisible).

Milliamperes A unit of energy equal to 1/1000 of an ampere (mA abbrev.).

Mitosis The point of cell division that involves the chromosomes of the nucleus.

Ohm A unit of electrical resistance.

Oscillations Fluctuations, variations, complete cycles of waves.

Osteology The science of the structure and function of bones.

Panoramic radiography A type of extraoral radiography whereby both dental arches are exposed and presented on the dental film.

Photon A high-velocity mass of x-ray energy.

Position indicating device (PID) A device used to direct and restrict the central beam in dental radiographic technique.

Quality As applied to ionizing radiation, the term refers to the penetrating power of the rays. When applied to radiographic films, the term describes the visual or diagnostic characteristics of the film produced.

Quantity As applied to ionizing radiation, the term refers to the amount of x rays produced and flowing through the x-ray beam.

Radiation Radiant energy, a form of kinetic or active energy that has no mass and propagates through space or matter in waves of electromagnetic force.

cumulative A descriptive term for the effects of radiation in biological tissues.

hard A term used to describe shorter, high-frequency wavelengths of radiation.

heterogeneous X-radiation of mixed wavelengths produced in the vacuum tube.

homogeneous X-radiation of similar wavelengths produced in the vacuum tube.

leakage   Rays that leave the x-ray machine any place other than the cone.

primary   Useful rays projected from the target and leaving the cone.

remnant   Radiation that has passed through the object to expose the film and produce an image. It is the image-forming radiation.

scattered   Radiation that may be deflected from matter and travel in directions not planned by the procedure.

secondary   Rays that have passed through matter, or the primary radiation that has interacted with matter.

soft   A term used to describe longer, lower frequency wavelengths of radiation.

stray   Rays that flow from parts of the tube other than the target.

Radiation absorbed dose (rad)   One unit of radiation absorbed by matter. Equivalent to 1 roentgen.

Radiation equivalent man (REM)   The unit of radiation for an absorbed dose of radiation by man. Equivalent to 1 RBE.

latent period   The period between the exposure to radiation and the time when the effects become visible.

median lethal dose   The amount of radiation that will kill half of the population of a certain species.

specific-area   Radiation exposure in a very specific area at one time of exposure.

threshold dose   The dose of radiation below which there is no clinical effects of ionizing radiation.

whole-body   Radiation exposure over the entire body at the same exposure time.

Relative biological effectiveness   The unit of radiation absorbed by biological tissue (RBE). Equivalent to 1 rad.

Radiation therapy   The use of radiation to eliminate irregularly developing cells that are detrimental to the surrounding tissues (i.e., cancer cells). Usually very high dosages of radiation are required for this medical technique.

Rem (roentgen equivalent [in] man)   Unit of dose equivalent, or the absorbed dose of any type of ionizing radiation that produces the same biological effect as 1 rad; equivalent to 10 milliseivert.

Radiograph   Consists of shadows of a three-dimensional object on film that can be viewed and interpreted.

Radiography   (1) The art or science of making radiographs, (2) the act of making a radiograph.

Radioresistent   In relation to cellular tissue, those cells that are not particularly sensitive to ionizing radiation.

Radiosensitive   In relation to cellular tissue, those cells that are particularly sensitive to ionizing radiation.

Reduction   The removal of the bromide from the metallic silver when the film emulsion is being affected by the developer. (There is another definition involving "reducing" or lightening a dark image on a film with a special chemical.)

Reticulated   As related to film emulsion, fine pitting or wrinkling of the emulsion resulting from great temperature differences between the developer and fixer.

Roentgen   (abbrev. R) An international unit based on the ability of radiation to ionize air. The unit of exposure corresponding to ionization in air of one electrostatic unit in 0.001293 gram of dry air.

Roentgenology   That part of radiology pertaining to roentgen rays (mechanically produced or generated x rays).

Somatic   All body tissues but genetic tissues.

Time of exposure   The factor of time, usually a fraction of a second, to allow the x ray to be produced and leave the cone to go through the object and expose the film.

Tomography   A general term describing radiographic techniques that section certain body planes and "lay them out flat" on the film.

Tragus (of the ear)   The cartilaginous projection in front of the external auditory meatus.

Transformer   Steps up or steps down the voltage to necessary levels needed to produce high kVps or low Mas in the dental x-ray unit.

Tubehead or **tube housing**   Part of dental radiography that incorporates the Coolidge vacuum tube, the filters, the collimator, and the cone.

Volt   The unit of electrical pressure necessary to produce a current of 1 ampere through a resistance of 1 ohm.

Voltage   The potential or electromotive force of an electric charge, expressed in volts.

Wavelength   The distance between the crest of one wave and the crest of the next one, as related to electromagnetic radiation.

X rays   A type of electromagnetic radiation with wavelengths between 1000 angstrom units and 10–4, approximately. They are invisible, odorless, travel at the same speed as light, and were discovered by Wilhelm Conrad Roentgen in 1895.

X-ray tube   An enclosed, glass vacuum tube in which x rays can be generated.

References

Accepted Dental Therapeutics, 40th ed. Chicago: American Dental Association, 1984.

ADA Council on Dental Materials, Instruments, and Equipment. Recommendations in radiographic practices: An update. *JADA* 119: 115–117, 1989.

ADAA Principles of Ethics and Code of Professional Conduct. Chicago: American Dental Assistants Association, 1980.

AIDS fuels global rise in TB cases. *The Atlanta Journal*, June 15, 1990.

The AIDS Epidemic: Turning a Corner. Condensed form Network News. National AIDS Network, 1990.

AIDS program, centers for infectious diseases. *AIDS Weekly Surveillance Report.* Atlanta: Centers for Disease Control, May 16, 1988.

AIDS: The disease and its implications for dentistry. *JADA* 15: 395–403, 1987.

Air-water spray caution urged. *CDA Journal* 18(13): 6, 1991.

American Dental Association principles of ethics and code of professional conduct. *JADA* 117: 657–661, 1988.

The American Dental Association Regulatory Compliance Manual. Chicago: American Dental Association, 1990.

Are we closer to a cure for AIDS? *Women's World* XII(3): 30, 1991.

Baker, R. Are We Closer to a Cure for AIDS? San Francisco: AIDS Foundation (SFAF), 1991.

Barnard, C., and J. Illman. *The Body Machine.* New York: Multi-Media Publications, 1981.

Barton, R.E., S.R. Matteson, and R.E. Richardson. *The Dental Assistant*, 6th ed. Malvern, PA: Lea and Febiger, 1988.

Bhaskar, S.N. *Synopsis of Oral Pathology*, 7th ed. St. Louis, MO: Mosby, 1986.

Biological indicators for verifying sterilization. *JADA* 117: 653, 1988.

Boyd, W. *An Introduction to the Study of Disease*, 10th ed. Malvern, PA: Lea and Febiger, 1988.

Caldwell, E., and B. Hegner. *Health Assistant.* Albany, NY: Delmar, 1980.

Carlson, A.J., and V. Johnson. *The Machinery of the Body*, 5th ed. Chicago: The University of Chicago Press, 1961. [Currently out of print.]

Chambers, D.W., and R. Abrams. *Dental Communication.* Norwalk, CT: Appleton-Crofts, 1986.

The changing epidemiology of hepatitis B in the United States. *JADA* 263(9), 1990.

Chasteen, J.E. *Essentials of Clinical Dental Assisting*, 4th ed. St. Louis, MO: Mosby, 1989.

Chernega, J. *Emergency Guide for Dental Auxiliaries*, 2nd ed. Albany, NY: Delmar, 1994.

Christensen, G.J. Glass ionomers as a luting material. *JADA* 120(1): 59–62, 1990.

Connors, K., and Y. Lomeli. The use and abuse of gloves in dentistry. *California DAA Journal* 2(2): 17, 1988.

C.O.N.T.R.O.L.: The Infection Control Newsletter 6(9). Fruit Heights, UT: I.C. Publications, 1991.

Controlling anxiety in the dental office. *JADA* 113: 728–735, 1986.

Cottone, J.A. Recent developments in hepatitis: New virus, vaccine, and dosage recommendations. *JADA* 120(5): 501–508, 1990.

Cousins, N. Head First: the Biology of Hope. New York: Dutton, 1989.

Davis, W.L. *Oral Histology: Cell Structure and Function.* Philadelphia: Saunders, 1986.

Dental Assisting National Board. 1991–1992 Certification for Dental Assistants—Dental Assisting National Board Examinations. Chicago: Dental Assisting National Board, 1991.

Dental Consultants, Inc. (DCI). *The Dental Advisor: The Quarterly for the Dental Profession* 4(2), June 1987; 6(2), June 1989. Ann Arbor, MI: DCI.

Dentist's Desk Reference: Materials, Instruments and Equipment, 2nd ed. Chicago: American Dental Association, 1983.

Dietz, E.R. The dental assistant's role in preparing the anesthetic syringe. *JADAA* 56: 26–27, 1987.

Dietz, E.R. Pit and fissure sealants. *JADAA* 57: 11–17, 1988.

Dietz, E.R. Update: Dental office waste management. *Dental Economics* 80(90): 62–67, 1990.

Disinfecting impressions. *Dental Product Report* 26(7), 1988. Skokie, IL: MEDEC Dental Communications.

Dorland's Illustrated Dictionary, 27th ed. Philadelphia: Saunders, 1988.

Edwards, C., M.A. Statkiewicz-Sherer, and E.R. Ritenour. *Radiation Protection for Dental Radiographers.* St. Louis, MO: Mosby, 1988.

Eggleston, D. Gloves—EDA and OSHA Approval. Newport Beach, CA: Gloves Clubs, 1992.

Employee Right to Know: Compliance Programs for Dentists. Academic Products, 1988.

Enter Hepatitis C. *Consumer Reports* 55(6), 1990.

Erlich, A. *Business Administration for the Dental Assistant*, 3rd ed. Champagne, IL: Colwell Systems, 1988.

Ehrlich, A. *Nutrition and Dental Health*, 2nd ed. Albany, NY: Delmar, 1994.

Erlich, A. Update 1990: diseases of major concern to dental health personnel. *JADAA* 59(6): 16–18, 1990.

Facts about AIDS—for the Dental Health Team. Chicago: American Dental Association, 1988.

Farman, A.G. Concepts of radiation safety and protection. *JADAA* 60(1): 11–14, 1991.

Farman, A.G. Radiographs, Pitfalls and Errors. Chicago: American Dental Assistants Association, 1990.

Farman, A.G., and A.E. Curran. Biologic effects of radiation and radiation safety and protection. *JADAA* 60(1): 11–14, 1991.

Farman, A.G., and A.E. Curran. Film, Darkroom and Processing. Chicago: American Dental Assistants Association, 1990.

Federal Register 52(163): 31852–31886, August 24, 1987.

Finkbeiner, B.L., and J.C. Patt. Office Procedures for the Dental Team, 2nd ed. St. Louis, MO: Mosby, 1985.

Garcia, N. Hazard communication. *CDAA Journal* 4(1): 10, 1990.

The glass ionomer cement. *JADA* 120(1): 1929, 1990.

Gray, H. *Gray's Anatomy.* New York: Bounty Books, 1977.

Greenfield, J. *A Workable Solution to Disease Transmission Control in the Dental Practice.* Sacramento: The Institute of Dental Environment, J. Productions, 1987.

Guidelines for Compliance with OSHA: Hazardous Communication, Release, Response, and Infection Control Plans. Region IX Manual. Sacramento, California Dental Association, 1989.

Handle with Care: A Hazards Communication Program for Dentistry. Reprint from *ADA News*, Apr. 25 and Sept. 19, 1988. In compliance with Occupational Safety and Health Administration (OSHA) regulations.

Handpiece sterilization procedures. *Dental Product Report* 21: 47–51, 1987.

Handwashing. *Dental Product Report* 25(2): 85–89, 1991.

Harrah, J. *Dental Charting.* Cupertino, CA: Professional Publishers, 1992.

Harris, N.O., and L.S. Scheirton. Pit and Fissure Sealants: A Self-Study Course. Chicago, IL: American Dental Hygienists Association, 1985.

Hazard Communication: A Compliance Kit, J–7. Washington, DC: U.S. Department of Labor, OSHA, 1988.

Hazardous Materials, Confusion, Frustration and Anxiety. Reprint from *CDA Journal* 17(12): 32–34, 1989.

Healthcare Leaders National Forum on AIDS and Hepatitis B. *Dental Products Report* 24 1–2, 1990.

Infection control in the dental office. *ADA News* 22(22): 1–10, 1991.

Infection Control in the Dental Office. Dental Radiography Series, Health Sciences Publication N-415. Rochester, NY: Eastman Kodak Co., 1990.

Infection control practices for dentistry. Occupational Safety and Health Administration (OSHA). *Federal Register* 56(41): 375–382, 1991.

Infection Control '91 Report. Perio Support Products. Irvine, CA: 1991.

Infection control procedures and products. *JADA* 117: 293–301, 1988.

Introduction to Glass Ionomers, pp. 26–28. Norristown, PA: Premier Sales Corp., 1990.

Koester, K. Your right to know. *Dental Assisting Journal* 2(4): 29–31, 1988.

Leimone, C.A., and E.M. Earl. *Dental Assisting Basic and Dental Sciences.* St. Louis, MO: Mosby, 1988.

Logan, M.K. The legal importance of patient records. *Dental Teamwork* 1: 226–228, 1988.

McCarthy, F.M. *Medical Emergencies in Dentistry*, 3rd ed. Philadelphia: Saunders, 1982.

Macdonald, G. Chemical hazards: Regulations, identification and resources. *CDA Journal* 17(12): 32–34, 1989.

Malamed, S.F. *Handbook of Medical Emergencies in the Dental Office*, 3rd ed. St. Louis, MO: Mosby, 1987.

Manson-Hing, L.R. *Fundamentals of Dental Radiography.* Malvern, PA: Lea and Febiger, 1985.

Massler, M., and I. Schour. *Atlas of the Mouth, in Health and Disease*, 2nd ed. Chicago: American Dental Association, 1982.

Miles, D.A., M. VanDis, C. Jensen, and A. Feretti. *Radiographic Imaging for Dental Auxiliaries.* Philadelphia: Saunders, 1989.

Miller, B.F., and C. Keane. *Encyclopedia and Dictionary of Medicine, Nursing and Allied Health*, 2nd ed. Philadelphia: Saunders, 1978.

Miller, B.F., and C. Keane. *Encyclopedia and Dictionary of Medicine, Nursing and Allied Health*, 5th ed. Philadelphia, Saunders, 1992.

Miller, C.H. Implementing and office infection control program. *JADAA* 59(6): 11–15, 1990.

Miller, C.H. Instrument sterilization. *JADAA* 59(2): 4–5, 1990.

Milliken, M.E. *Understanding Human Behavior*, 4th ed. Albany, NY: Delmar, 1987.

National Council on Radiation Protection No. 35. Bethesda, MD: Health and Human Services Publications, Federal Drug Administration 84-8225, 1984.

National Research Council. *Health Effects of Exposure to Low Levels of Ionizing Radiation.* Washington, DC: National Academy Press, 1990.

OSHA moves to hasten compliance with infection control guidelines. *Dental Product Report* 22: 59–67, 1988.

Pampalone, B. Meeting OSHA requirements: Document your procedures. *JADAA* 61(1): 9, 1992.

Phillips, R.W. *Elements of Dental Materials for Dental Hygienists and Assistants*, 4th ed. Philadelphia: Saunders, 1984.

Phillips, R.W. *Skinner's Science of Dental Materials*, 8th ed. Philadelphia: Saunders, 1982.

Recommended infection control practices for dentistry. *Morbidity and Mortality Weekly Report* 40(22): 224–235, 1991.

Risk Management Series, a Manual, pp. 1–23. Chicago: American Dental Association, 1987.

Runnells, R.R. *Infection Control and Hazards Management*. Fruit Heights, UT: I.C. Publications, 1989.

Schaefer, M.E. Infection control, OSHA, and a hazards communication program. *CDA Journal* 18(8): 53–58, 1990.

Silverman, S. Oral findings in people with or at risk for AIDS: A study of 375 homosexual males. *JADA* 112(2): 187–192, 1986.

Sterilizers and Sterilization Devices. In: *Dentist's Desk Reference: Materials, Instruments and Equipment*, 2nd ed. pp. 390–401. Chicago: American Dental Association, 1983.

Torres, H.O., and A. Erlich. *Modern Dental Assisting*, 4th ed. Philadelphia: Saunders, 1990.

U.S. Department of Health and Human Services, Public Health Service. Preventing the Transmission of Hepatitis B, AIDS, and Herpes in Dentistry. Atlanta: Centers for Disease Control, 1987.

Waste handling and processing standards developing for dentistry. *Dental Products Report* 23: 46–63, 1989.

Wilkens, E.M. *Clinical Practice of the Dental Hygienist*, 6th ed. Malvern, PA: Lea and Febiger, 1989.

Index